Essential Echocardiography

Timothy M. Maus
Christopher R. Tainter
Editors

Essential Echocardiography

A Review of Basic Perioperative TEE and Critical Care Echocardiography

Second Edition

Springer

Editors
Timothy M. Maus
Department of Anesthesiology
University of California
San Diego Health
La Jolla, CA
USA

Christopher R. Tainter
Department of Anesthesiology
University of California
San Diego Health
La Jolla, CA
USA

ISBN 978-3-030-84348-9 ISBN 978-3-030-84349-6 (eBook)
https://doi.org/10.1007/978-3-030-84349-6

This Springer imprint is published by the registered company Springer Nature Switzerland AG
The registered company address is: Gewerbestrasse 11, 6330 Cham, Switzerland

To Molly, for your unwavering love; to my Dad, for your caring love and support throughout my life; and to William, Owen, Winston, and Porter, for the overwhelming joy you bring to our lives.

– Timothy M. Maus

To my loving wife, who tolerated countless hours of writing and editing, to my supportive family who created and developed me, and to all of the patient people who have learned from or taught me anything.

– Christopher R. Tainter

Preface

Echocardiography and point-of-care ultrasound play an invaluable role in the management of hemodynamically unstable patients. Transesophageal echocardiography (TEE) has a well-established history of utility in cardiac operating rooms, and the advances and increased availability of TEE, along with the portability of transthoracic echocardiography (TTE), have propelled both modalities outside of the cardiac operating room realm. Whether in the emergency department, intensive care unit, inpatient unit, or operating room with high-risk surgical patients, echocardiography's ability to monitor cardiac function, assess response to interventions, and quickly diagnose causes of hemodynamic instability have made it a necessary skill for practitioners in this era of medicine.

Utilizing both two-dimensional echocardiography and Doppler imaging, numerous causes of hemodynamic compromise can be identified that may warrant immediate intervention. Recognizing myocardial ischemia, pericardial tamponade, left ventricular outflow tract obstruction, severe valvular abnormalities, hypovolemia, venous air embolism, and pulmonary emboli can directly affect patient management and outcomes. In addition, important extra-cardiac causes of instability can be identified with ultrasound as well, including pneumothorax and other lung pathology, aortic aneurysm or dissection, intraperitoneal or intrathoracic hemorrhage, and deep vein thromboses.

The editors of this textbook hope to encourage and educate interested practitioners regarding the utility of basic echocardiography in everyday practice. The intention is to create an easily approachable and well-illustrated text as a resource to learn the principles of perioperative and critical care echocardiography and integrate its use into clinical practice. While numerous comprehensive echocardiography textbooks exist, this text differs by offering a unique perspective for emergency and critical care providers as well as noncardiac anesthesiologists. Therefore, advanced topics such as determinations for valvular repair versus replacement are omitted. Instead, there is a distinct emphasis on identifying normal versus abnormal anatomic and physiologic states, commonly encountered pathologies, and emergent causes of hemodynamic instability.

Essential Echocardiography, 2nd Edition: A Review of Basic Perioperative TEE and Critical Care Echocardiography contains several key additions while staying true to the intention of the first edition serving as a guide and providing a framework for the readers as they are introduced to the application of critical care and basic perioperative echocardiography. The addition and integration of transthoracic echocardiography within the core echocardiography topics allows a unified approach to both image interpretation and identification of pathology regardless of the modality. The textbook concludes with a section on critical care ultrasonography including lung, abdominal, and vascular imaging as well as assessments of volume status and detection of hemodynamic shock. Understandably, it is often intimidating to learn a new skill such as echocardiography. The gentle approach of the authors helps to allay those fears and minimize the frustration that often comes with learning a new skillset. Material is presented in an understandable fashion, building upon basic physiologic principles. It is also important to remember that a multimodal approach to learning echocardiography is key, including echocardiography simulation and repetitive hands-on application during patient care. Often valuable insight can be gained by performing even a portion of an exam, and the learner doesn't have to be an expert to acquire relevant information.

In addition to helping the practitioner who is seeking to implement the use of TTE and TEE into their clinical practice, this text is intended as an aid for those who are seeking certification in echocardiography, including passing the Basic PTEeXAM® and the CCEeXAM®. Each chapter in this book is designed to address the core competencies that are tested in these exams and prepare the practitioner for either or both certifications. Each chapter now concludes with board review style questions to further cement core concepts and aid in retention. In addition to being a valuable and practical guide to obtaining certification, we hope that this textbook becomes a practical resource for the application of echocardiography into your clinical practice.

La Jolla, CA, USA — Timothy M. Maus
La Jolla, CA, USA — Christopher R. Tainter

Contents

Contributors

Dalia Banks Department of Anesthesiology, University of California San Diego Health, La Jolla, CA, USA

Michael Benggon Department of Anesthesiology, Loma Linda University, Loma Linda, CA, USA

Kenneth Chen Department of Medicine, Division of Pulmonary, Critical Care, and Sleep Medicine, University of California San Diego Health, La Jolla, CA, USA

Christine Choi Department of Anesthesiology, University of California San Diego Health, La Jolla, CA, USA

Brett Cronin Department of Anesthesiology, University of California San Diego Health, La Jolla, CA, USA

Michele Curtis Department of Anesthesiology, University of Utah School of Medicine, Salt Lake City, UT, USA

Byron Fergerson Department of Anesthesiology, University of California San Diego Health, La Jolla, CA, USA

Kirill Gelfenbeyn Department of Anesthesiology, University of California San Diego Health, La Jolla, CA, USA

Neal Gerstein Department of Anesthesiology and Critical Care Medicine, University of New Mexico School of Medicine, Albuquerque, NM, USA

Andrew Goodrich Department of Anesthesiology, University of California San Diego Health, La Jolla, CA, USA

Patricia Guan Department of Anesthesiology, University of California San Diego Health, La Jolla, CA, USA

Seth T. Herway Department of Anesthesiology, University of California San Diego Health, La Jolla, CA, USA

Diana Hylton Department of Anesthesiology, University of California San Diego Health, La Jolla, CA, USA

Ian Joel Department of Medicine, Los Robles Regional Medical Center, Thousand Oaks, CA, USA

Swapnil Khoche Department of Anesthesiology, University of California San Diego Health, La Jolla, CA, USA

Perin Kothari Division of Cardiothoracic Anesthesiology, Department of Anesthesiology, Perioperative, and Pain Medicine Stanford University School of Medicine, Stanford, CA, USA

Gerard Manecke Department of Anesthesiology, University of California San Diego Health, La Jolla, CA, USA

Timothy M. Maus Department of Anesthesiology, University of California San Diego Health, La Jolla, CA, USA

Tariq Naseem Department of Anesthesiology, Cedars-Sinai Medical Center, Los Angeles, CA, USA

Liem Nguyen Department of Anesthesiology, University of California San Diego Health, La Jolla, CA, USA

Quoc-Sy Nguyen Department of Anesthesiology, University of California San Diego Health, La Jolla, CA, USA

Sonia Nhieu Department of Anesthesiology, Kaiser Permanente Santa Clara Medical Center, Santa Clara, CA, USA

E. Orestes O'Brien Department of Anesthesiology, University of California San Diego Health, La Jolla, CA, USA

Sophia P. Poorsattar Department of Anesthesiology and Perioperative Medicine, University of California, Los Angeles Medical Center, Los Angeles, CA, USA

Ramon Sanchez Department of Anesthesiology, University of California San Diego Health, La Jolla, CA, USA

Christopher R. Tainter Department of Anesthesiology, University of California San Diego Health, La Jolla, CA, USA

Suraj Trivedi Department of Anesthesiology, University of California San Diego Health, La Jolla, CA, USA

Eric Tzeng Department of Anesthesiology, University of California San Diego Health, La Jolla, CA, USA

Gabriel Wardi Department of Emergency Medicine and Department of Medicine, Division of Pulmonary, Critical Care, and Sleep Medicine, University of California San Diego Health, La Jolla, CA, USA

Joshua Zimmerman Department of Anesthesiology, University of Utah, Salt Lake City, UT, USA

Department of Anesthesiology, University of Utah School of Medicine, Salt Lake City, UT, USA

Part I

Basic Perioperative and Critical Care Echocardiography

1 Introduction to Basic Perioperative and Critical Care Echocardiography: Examination, Certification, Indications, and Contraindications

Timothy M. Maus, Christopher R. Tainter, and Seth T. Herway

Abbreviations

TEE	Transesophageal echocardiography
TTE	Transthoracic echocardiography
NBE	National Board of Echocardiography
CME	Continuing medical education
ASA	American Society of Anesthesiology
SCA	Society of Cardiovascular Anesthesiologists
ASE	American Society of Echocardiography
FAST	Focused assessment with sonography for trauma
DICOM	Digital Imaging and Communications in Medicine

Introduction

While echocardiography originated in the realm of cardiologists and the birth of transesophageal echocardiography occurred in the perioperative setting by cardiac anesthesiologists, its evolution continues to broaden well past these two arenas. The use of transesophageal echocardiography in noncardiac surgery and intensive care settings has become well-established, including a certification process beginning in 2010. More recently, the use of point-of-care echocardiography and ultrasound has gained traction in multiple specialties including anesthesiology, emergency medicine, and critical care. The National Board of Echocardiography developed the newly established certification process for critical care echocardiography, thereby creating a standard of echocardiography and ultrasound knowledge requisite of certified critical care practitioners. This chapter will outline the utility of both modalities and include current details on the examination and certification processes for both basic perioperative transesophageal echocardiography and critical care echocardiography.

Transesophageal Echocardiography in Noncardiac Surgery and Intensive Care

There is broad application for the use of transesophageal echocardiography (TEE) as both a diagnostic and monitoring modality in noncardiac surgery. The notion that cardiac surgery is the only situation where perioperative care is improved using TEE is outdated. TEE has been used in noncardiac surgeries as well as in the intensive care unit (ICU) to identify myocardial ischemia, pericardial tamponade, left ventricular outflow obstruction, severe valvular abnormalities, hypovolemia, venous air embolism, intrapulmonary emboli, and a number of other causes

T. M. Maus (✉) · C. R. Tainter · S. T. Herway
Department of Anesthesiology, University of California San Diego Health, La Jolla, CA, USA
e-mail: tmaus@health.ucsd.edu

T. M. Maus, C. R. Tainter (eds.), *Essential Echocardiography*,
https://doi.org/10.1007/978-3-030-84349-6_1

of hemodynamic compromise of cardiac origin [1]. By providing direct visualization of cardiac structures and function, TEE can enable any trained practitioner to competently assess a patient who is experiencing hemodynamic compromise of cardiovascular origin in a way that no other monitor is able. As a provider gains experience in TEE, competency in transthoracic echocardiography (TTE) is readily acquired, and with this comes the ability to noninvasively assess the patient's cardiovascular status in pre- and postoperative settings.

For practitioners who have not pursued fellowship training in anesthesia for cardiac surgery or who have not had dedicated advanced training in the use of TEE, integrating TEE into clinical practice can be an intimidating proposition. However, a moderate amount of exposure to its use and knowledge of the principles of echocardiography contained in this text will enable the practitioner to make basic assessments of a patient's cardiac status and help guide initial management decisions. Additionally, the practitioner should also be able to determine when the nature of the surgery or the patient's cardiovascular status necessitates a comprehensive examination by an echocardiographer with an advanced echocardiography skill set.

This book is intended for practitioners with little to no previous experience with echocardiography seeking to employ this diagnostic modality in their clinical practice. The book also may serve as a review of basic echocardiography principles to those who do possess prior experience or training. Most graduates of US anesthesiology residency programs now receive an initial exposure to TEE during training. This book certainly fulfills the role as a guide during that initial exposure or as a framework for building upon the knowledge obtained during training. Echocardiography requires several skillsets: (1) Manual dexterity which is manifested as probe manipulation and image acquisition; (2) knowledge of normal anatomy; and (3) recognition of pathology or diseased states. For practitioners who have never had formal exposure to TEE, a basic introduction from a competent practitioner on safe probe insertion and manipulation and initial assistance with obtaining TEE views is important to get started. This topic will be discussed below; however, to become fluent with the TEE probe, repetition is key. Performing exams on a regular basis will begin to engrain certain subtleties of probe manipulation in order to display the structure of interest. Therefore, it is recommended to physically perform the exam as much as possible either through clinical indication or TEE simulation. Repetition is certainly the key to adult learning, and this is applicable to knowledge of normal anatomy. The more exams one visualizes or performs, the more data points one will have that represent normal anatomy. Similarly, the more exams performed, the more pathology one will observe and begin to develop patterns of recognition. In summary, when clinically indicated, performance of exams will increase manual dexterity as well as recognition of normal versus abnormal anatomy.

Initial attempts at performing a TEE exam can be frustrating and anxiety-ridden as the views can be challenging for the novice echocardiographer to obtain. Most practitioners notice that it takes roughly 20 to 30 performed exams before they can reliably find the basic views. Once able to obtain the basic views, they can then start recognizing pathology and abnormal findings. Like other clinical skills such as appreciating heart sounds with a stethoscope, a practitioner must be able to appreciate the normal findings before the pathologic exam becomes clear.

In addition to helping the practitioner seeking to implement the use of TEE into their clinical practice, this text is intended as an aid for those who are seeking basic certification in echocardiography including passing the Basic PTEeXAM®. This textbook includes chapters dedicated to general ultrasound principles, TEE imaging, and echocardiographic assessment of each of the major cardiac structures that are designed to address the core competencies that are tested in the basic exam and prepare the practitioner to obtain basic certification.

Certification in Basic Perioperative Transesophageal Echocardiography

As one becomes proficient in the use of perioperative echocardiography, they ultimately may seek certification to acknowledge the new skillset they have achieved. The National Board of Echocardiography, Inc. (www.echoboards.org) is a not-for-profit corporation that administers the examination in perioperative TEE as well as the board certification process. The purpose of certification is to recognize anesthesiologists who have demonstrated their competence in basic TEE. The NBE offers two levels of certification, Basic and Advanced, which differ primarily on their scope of practice and training requirements. Certification in Basic Perioperative Transesophageal Echocardiography is provided to recognize anesthesiologists utilizing TEE in a nondiagnostic or monitoring-only manner, except in emergency situations. The use of TEE as a diagnostic tool to direct medical or surgical interventions, particularly cardiac surgical interventions, is under the purview of anesthesiologists with Certification in Advanced Perioperative Transesophageal Echocardiography. This is an important distinction when considering the pathway and certification options for the individual practitioner.

The NBE offers two statuses in relation to basic perioperative TEE: Testamur and Certification. Testamur status indicates the successful completion of the Examination of Special Competence in Basic Perioperative Transesophageal Echocardiography (Basic PTEeXAM®). Certification also implies a passing score on the Basic PTEeXAM® in addition to meeting requirements that document proficiency. Readers are encouraged to visit the NBE's website for the most current requirements; however, the present requirements include a current license to practice medicine, current board certification in Anesthesiology, and specific training in basic perioperative TEE.

The specific training involves performing a certain number of exams and reviewing (but not performing) additional exams. There are several pathways to obtaining the specific training including a Supervised Training pathway, which is often suited to those still in a training institution, and the Extended Continuing Medical Education (CME) pathway which is more suited to those already in practice. Both pathways require the performance and interpretation of at least 50 basic perioperative TEE exams. The supervised training pathway involves reviewing (but not performing) additional exams with a supervising physician to a total of 150 basic TEE exams. The Extended CME pathway involves a review of 100 basic TEEs through the American Society of Anesthesiology (ASA)/Society of Cardiovascular Anesthesiologists (SCA) Basic Perioperative TEE Education Program to result in a total of 150 basic TEE exams. Lastly, there is an additional Practice Experience pathway for those who have previously completed residency and currently perform basic TEEs in their practice. Details of each of the pathways and the required documentation may be found on the NBE's website (www.echoboards.org).

Basic TEE Examination

The use of basic TEE in noncardiac surgery can be broadly categorized into two main areas: monitoring and diagnostic purposes. Monitoring uses of TEE occur during any type of surgery where preoperative evaluation suggests that either the nature of the surgery or the patient's cardiovascular status has the potential to result in hemodynamic compromise. Therefore, the TEE exam can be used to monitor for changes to the patients' hemodynamic status such as volume status, ischemia detection, and need for inotropy or vasopressor therapy. TEE is appropriate for any surgery ranging from common elective cases in patients with cardiovascular indications to large intra-abdominal, thoracic, or neurosurgical procedures where there is potential for hemodynamic compromise in otherwise healthy patients. The basic echocardiographer can also utilize TEE as a diagnostic modality in the situation of unexplained perioperative hemodynamic compromise, where the delay introduced in waiting for another imaging modality or an advanced echocardiographer may result in patient harm.

The ASA and the SCA have explained the use of basic TEE in monitoring and diagnostic capacities in their published practice guidelines [1]. In noncardiac surgery, the ASA and SCA recommend that TEE *may be used* when "the nature of the planned surgery or the patient's known or suspected cardiovascular pathology may result in severe hemodynamic, pulmonary, or neurologic compromise." The published guidelines also recommend TEE *should be used* when "unexplained life-threatening circulatory instability persists despite corrective measures." Considering any contraindications, TEE is therefore appropriate perioperatively when instability is either present or possible. The American Society of Echocardiography (ASE) and the SCA have created a consensus statement that further delineates indications and utility of basic perioperative TEE including evaluating ventricular function, valvular function, pericardial disease, embolism detection, and basic congenital heart disease in the adult [2].

Contraindications

Clinical judgment should be employed to determine the suitability of TEE for each individual patient. While prior practice guidelines divided contraindications by absolute and relative categories, current updated practice guidelines note that the use of TEE is a risk-versus-benefit evaluation even in the setting of potential contraindications [1, 3]. Absolute contraindications often involve pathology of the esophagus and include previous esophagectomy and esophagogastrectomy. Often included are a history of a tracheoesophageal fistula, esophageal trauma, esophageal surgery, esophageal stricture/mass, perforated viscus, and active upper gastrointestinal bleeding [1, 3]. Relative contraindications include pathologies of oral, esophageal, and gastric location, often with less severe presentations than those listed above as absolute contraindications. A suggested list of absolute and relative contraindications is provided in Table 1.1. However, it is noteworthy that current practice guidelines report TEE can be used even in patients with oral, esophageal, or gastric disease if the expected benefit outweighs the potential risk.

In such cases where there is some perceived additional risk, some precautions can be considered when TEE is used. Limiting the exam by either using only the views necessary or deferring to the most experienced provider will help avoid unnecessary probe manipulations and potentially avoid additional oropharyngeal, esophageal, or gastric trauma. For example, in the case of a patient with prior gastric surgery, limiting the exam to mid esophageal views will still provide excellent imaging and diagnostic information without the additional risk of gastric injury. As the echocardiographer becomes more familiar with the basic TEE views and the information that can be obtained from each view, it will become apparent that only one or two views are necessary to evaluate the aspect of cardiac function that is of interest. In these cases, leaving the probe in one location (i.e., mid esophageal) for monitoring purposes during the anesthetic may be the best course of action.

Table 1.1 Contraindications to transesophageal echocardiography

Absolute contraindications
Esophagectomy or esophagogastrectomy
Postesophageal surgery
Esophageal trauma, perforation, laceration
Esophageal obstruction (stricture, mass)
Tracheoesophageal fistula
Perforated viscus
Active upper gastrointestinal bleed
Relative contraindications
History of dysphagia
History of radiation to neck and mediastinum
Recent GI surgery
Barrett esophagus
Symptomatic hiatal hernia
Esophageal varices
Zenker diverticulum
Colonic interposition
Recent upper gastrointestinal bleed
Severe cervical arthritis with restricted mobility
Atlantoaxial joint disease with restricted mobility
Severe coagulopathy
Active esophagitis or peptic ulcer disease

In clinical scenarios where the potential risks outweigh the benefits of TEE probe placement, the use of other noninvasive imaging modalities that provide the same information (e.g., transthoracic echocardiography) should be considered [1]. Additionally, in an elective scenario, obtaining a gastroenterology consultation prior to probe placement may provide further insight into the patient's pathology and their risk-benefit ratio.

Complications

Perioperative TEE has been demonstrated to be a safe monitoring modality. The morbidity is often associated with a traumatic placement or manipulation of the probe. Careful attention to recognition of potential contraindications and gentle placement and manipulation of the probe are essential. The use of force is unnecessary in TEE imaging. A large study of 7200 cardiac surgical patients determined an intraoperative TEE-associated morbidity and mortality of 0.2% and 0%, respectively [4]. The majority of complications (86%) were associated with oropharyngeal, esophageal, or gastric trauma due to TEE probe insertion and manipulation (see Table 1.2). The reported morbidity of 0.2% in this study of intraoperative TEE correlates with a reported 0.18% complication rate in a large, multicenter survey of over 10,000 predominantly conscious adult patients undergoing TEE [5]. The low rates of morbidity and mortality have additionally been confirmed both in anesthetized and conscious adult patients [6, 7].

Table 1.2 Complications associated with intraoperative transesophageal echocardiography

Complication	Incidence (%)
Odynophagia	0.1
Swallowing abnormality	0.01
Esophageal abrasions	0.06
No associated pathology	0.03
Upper gastrointestinal hemorrhage	0.03
Esophageal perforation	0.01
Dental injury	0.03
Endotracheal tube malposition	0.03
Total	0.2

From Kallmeyer, et al. [4]

Using the TEE Probe

Insertion

In addition to consideration of contraindications to TEE prior to probe insertion, the mouth should be inspected for preexisting injuries including at-risk dental lesions. Limitations in cervical spine movement should also be considered.

The TEE probe can be inserted in a similar manner to an orogastric tube. Performing a jaw lift during insertion significantly facilitates insertion. This includes lifting the mandible with the left hand and utilizing the left thumb posterior to the lower incisors and the left fingers inferior to the mental protuberance. The right hand is used to advance the probe with constant gentle pressure. Lubrication of the probe facilitates advancement and reduces the incidence of trauma to soft tissues. Of note, nonsterile multiuse ultrasound transmission gel is not recommended as an oral lubricant for TEE procedures due to the risk of contamination and sepsis. Current FDA recommendations include the use of single-use sterile packets [8]. Ensure that the large and small knobs of the TEE probe are in the unlocked position as this will allow the distal end of the probe to remain flexible as it passes through the oropharynx. A loss of resistance is typically felt as the probe passes the upper esophageal sphincter. Again, excessive force is unnecessary. Anteflexion of the probe can help navigate the upper oropharynx, while once past the upper oropharynx, retroflexion aids in guiding the probe away from the glottis and toward the esophageal inlet. If blind insertion of the probe proves difficult, a laryngoscope or even a video laryngoscope can be used to identify the glottis and esophageal inlet and facilitate passage of the probe under direct visualization.

Manipulation

There are five primary movements of the TEE probe used to optimize the ultrasound image (Fig. 1.1). Some of these are analogous to the movement of a bronchoscope (familiar to most anesthesiologists and critical care physicians),

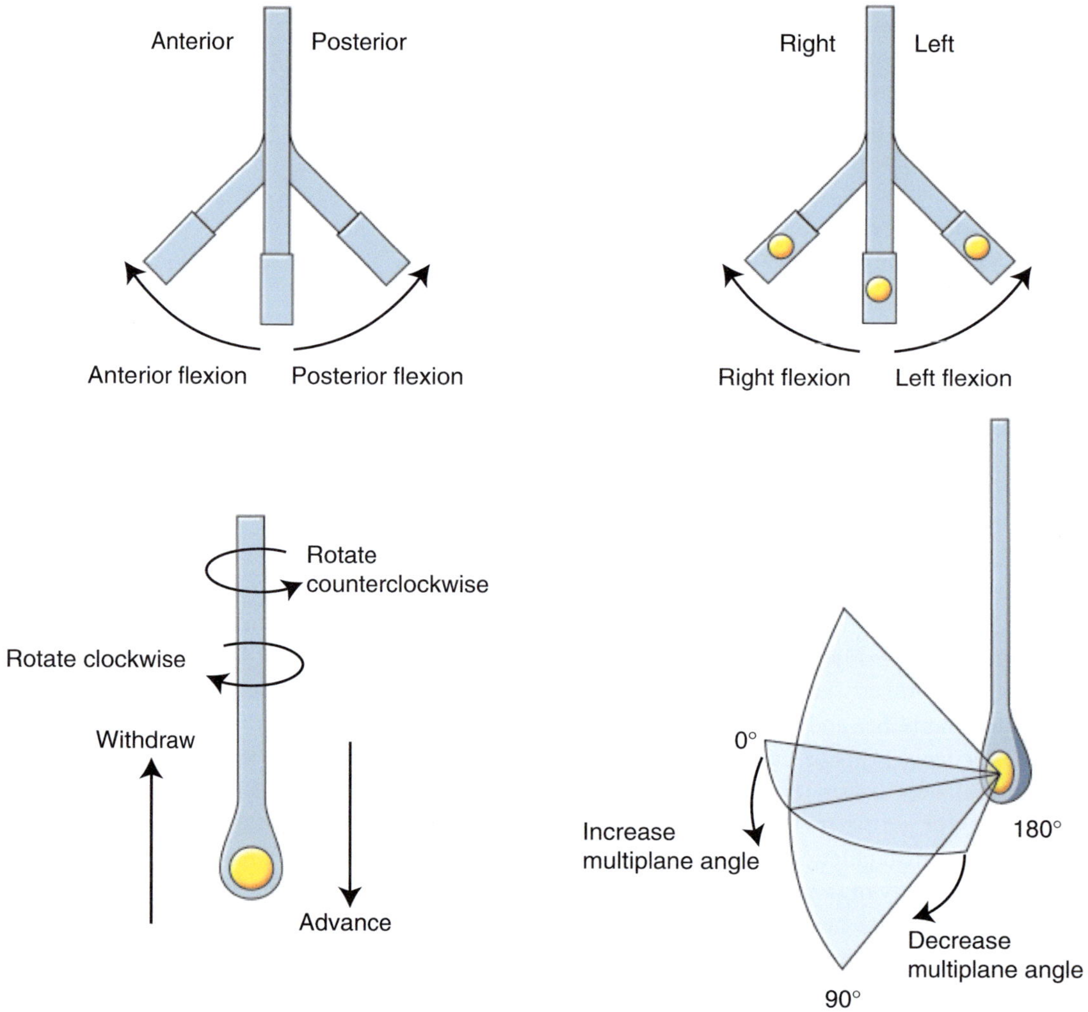

Fig. 1.1 Basic TEE probe manipulations

which include advance/withdrawal, anteflexion/retroflexion, and turning the probe to the left/right, while other functions are unique to TEE which include the image appearing perpendicular to probe tip (as opposed to in-line with the probe tip), flexion to the left/right, and the multiplane function. The movements in detail are:

1. *Advance and withdraw*. The probe can be advanced (and withdrawn) to more distal (and proximal) locations within the esophagus and stomach. The primary positions at which ultrasound images are obtained are, from proximal to distal, (1) upper esophagus, (2) mid esophagus, (3) transgastric, and (4) deep transgastric. In general, the tip of the transducer should be in the neutral position before advancing or withdrawing the probe. Brief recognition of depth can be determined by observing what is closest to the image transducer (closest to the top of the image): great vessels (high mid esophagus), left atrium (mid esophagus), and ventricle (transgastric) (Fig. 1.2).
2. *Anteflex and retroflex*. The large knob on the probe handle can be turned to move the tip of the probe anteriorly (anteflexion) or posteriorly (retroflexion). Again, this is analogous to the flexion on a bronchoscope.

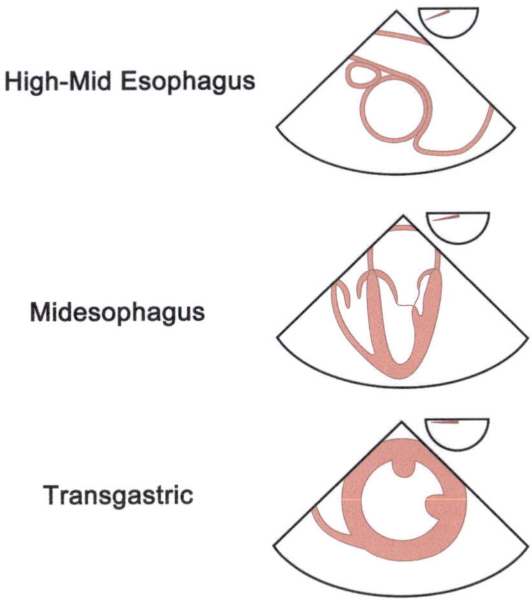

Fig. 1.2 Depth estimation via observation of what is nearest to the probe (apex of the image). (**a**) Great vessels – High-mid esophagus. (**b**) Left atrium – mid esophagus. (**c**) Ventricle – transgastric. (Illustrations adapted from Shanewise JS et al. *ASE/SCA guidelines for performing a comprehensive intraoperative multiplane transesophageal echocardiography examination: recommendations of the American Society of Echocardiography Council for Intraoperative Echocardiography and the Society of Cardiovascular Anesthesiologists Task Force for Certification in Perioperative Transesophageal Echocardiography*. J Am Soc Echocardiogr. 1999 Oct;12(10):884–900)

3. *Flexion to the left and right.* The small knob on the probe can be turned to flex the probe leftward or rightward. This motion is rarely utilized in basic TEE imaging as the esophagus is a relatively fixed structure. However, this motion is often necessary in the comprehensive examination for the deep transgastric five-chamber view to bring the tip of the probe toward the left-sided LV apex.
4. *Turn to the left and right.* The probe shaft can be rotated clockwise (called turning to the right) or counterclockwise (called turning to the left) to adjust the orientation of the ultrasound beam. This allows the imaging of the right- versus left-sided structures within the chest.
5. *Increase or decrease multiplane (omniplane).* Axial rotation of the multiplane angle from 0 to 180 degrees is called rotating forward and from 180 to 0 degrees is called rotating backward. This "movement" does not physically move the TEE probe; however, it moves the image produced by rotating the image in an axial direction relative to the transducer. This can be visualized by placing the right-hand palm face down in front of one's chest with the fingers spread out, imagining this as the imaging view from the esophagus. The thumb will be the right side of the image, while the small finger will be the left side of the image. Imagining a four-chamber view, the left atrium and left ventricle will be displayed on the right side of the image (near the thumb), while the right atrium and right ventricle will be displayed on the left side of the image (near the small finger). Increasing the multiplane can be demonstrated by rotating the hand clockwise. A 90-degree rotation will display a two-chamber view with the thumb directed over the anterior wall (on the right side of the image) and the small finger over the inferior wall (on the left side of the image). The use of the hand movement with either an imagined heart or a heart model will help understand the physical relationship of cardiac structures.

Orientation

By convention, the objects closest to the TEE transducer are displayed at the top of the screen, while the far field is displayed at the bottom. With a multiplane angle of 0 degrees and the TEE probe transducer angled anteriorly from the gastrointestinal tract toward the heart, the patient's right side is displayed on the left of the screen. When the multiplane is rotated toward 90 degrees, the left side of the screen is moved inferiorly toward the patient's feet. When the multiplane is increased to 180 degrees, the patient's right side is now displayed on the right of the screen, making it the mirror image of the display at 0 degrees (Fig. 1.3).

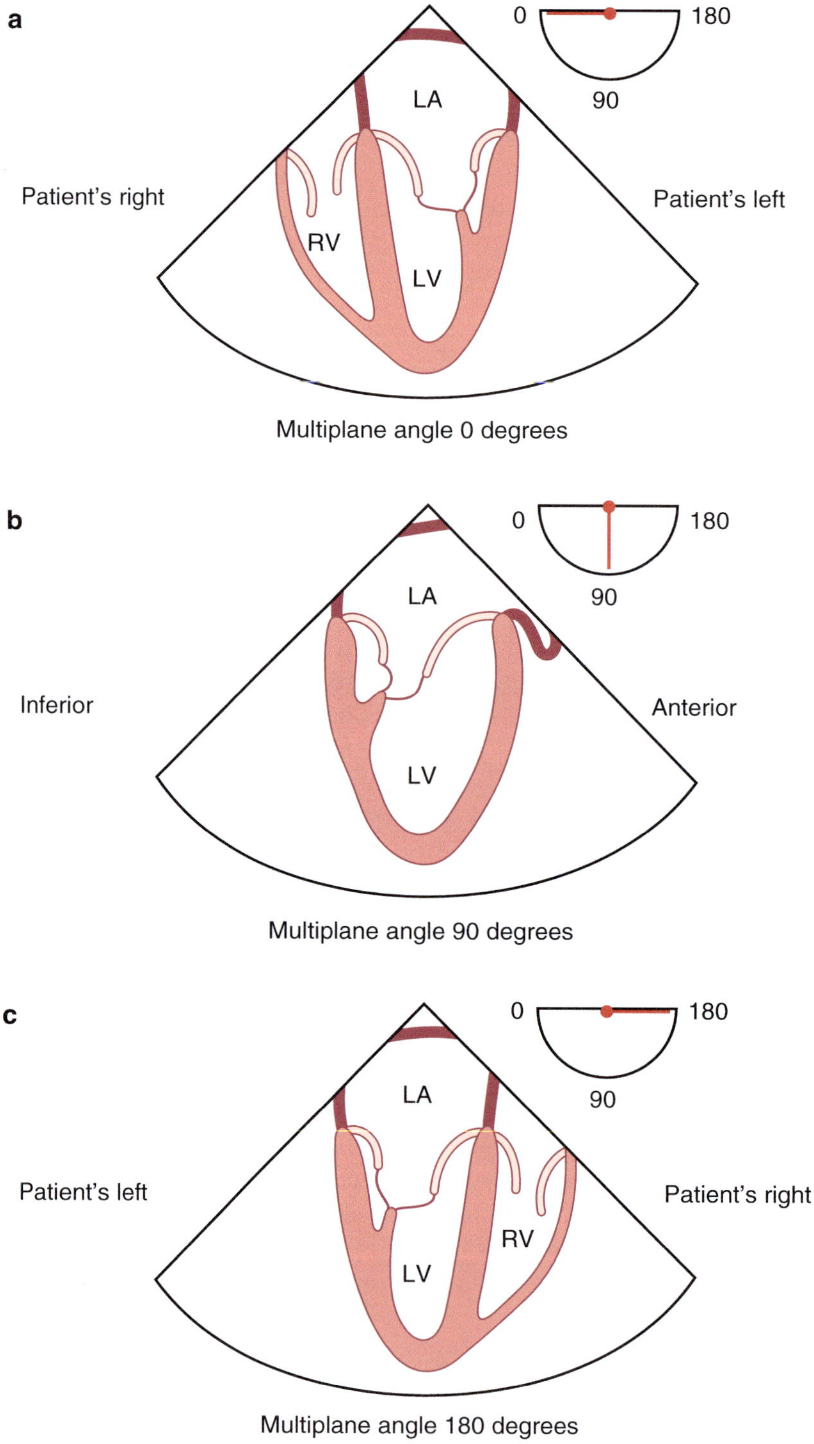

Fig. 1.3 Image orientation with multiplane angles 0 to 180 degrees. *LA* left atrium, *LV* left ventricle, *RV* right ventricle (Illustration adapted from Shanewise JS et al. *ASE/SCA guidelines for performing a comprehensive intraoperative multiplane transesophageal echocardiography examination: recommendations of the American Society of Echocardiography Council for Intraoperative Echocardiography and the Society of Cardiovascular Anesthesiologists Task Force for Certification in Perioperative Transesophageal Echocardiography.* J Am Soc Echocardiogr. 1999;12(10):884–900)

Point-of-Care Transthoracic Echocardiography and Ultrasound

Over the past decade, there has been an explosion of ultrasound imaging outside of the realm of cardiologists and radiologists, with a focus on point-of-care imaging as a tool to aid bedside decision-making. The notion that transthoracic echocardiography is overtly challenging and relegated only to cardiology departments is outdated. Point-of-care evaluations have demonstrated their utility from the emergency department, through the preoperative, intraoperative, and postoperative periods to the intensive care unit. Numerous professional societies, including the Society of Cardiothoracic Anesthesiologists, American College of Emergency Physicians, and the Society of Critical Care Medicine have supported the education, training, and application of transthoracic echocardiography among anesthesiologists, emergency medicine, and critical care providers, along with many other specialties. Similar to TEE, TTE has been used in noncardiac surgeries as well as in the intensive care unit to identify myocardial ischemia, pericardial tamponade, left ventricular outflow obstruction, severe valvular abnormalities, hypovolemia, venous air embolism, intrapulmonary emboli, and a number of other causes of hemodynamic compromise. Point-of-care TTE allows any trained practitioner to noninvasively assess a patient who is experiencing hemodynamic compromise in a way that no other monitor is able. The overall reduced cost, size, and the increasing ubiquity of ultrasound systems permit rapid deployment to the bedside, prompt image acquisition and interpretation, and immediate interventions to improve patient outcomes.

This book is intended for practitioners with little to no previous experience with echocardiography seeking to employ this diagnostic modality in their clinical practice. The book also may serve as a review of basic echocardiography principles to those who do possess prior experience or training. As expressed above, many disciplines now include point-of-care ultrasound training during residency education. This book certainly fulfills the role as a guide during that initial exposure or as a framework for building upon the knowledge obtained during training. Akin to TEE, transthoracic echocardiography requires several skillsets: (1) manual dexterity which is manifested as probe manipulation and image acquisition; (2) knowledge of normal anatomy; and (3) recognition of pathology or diseased states. For practitioners who have never had formal exposure to echocardiography, a basic introduction from a competent practitioner on probe placement and manipulation as well as initial assistance with obtaining TTE views is important to get started. This topic will be discussed below; however, to become fluent with the TTE probe, repetition is key. Performing exams on a regular basis will begin to ingrain certain subtleties of probe manipulation in order to display the structure of interest. Therefore, it is recommended to physically perform the exam as much as possible either through clinical indication, performance on patient models, or echocardiography simulation. Repetition is certainly the key to learning, and this is applicable to knowledge of normal anatomy. The more exams one visualizes or performs, the more data points one will have that represent normal anatomy. Similarly, the more exams performed, the more pathology one will observe and begin to develop patterns of recognition. In summary, when clinically indicated, performance of exams will increase manual dexterity as well as recognition of normal versus abnormal anatomy.

Again, very similar to TEE, initial attempts at performing a TTE exam can be frustrating and anxiety-ridden as the views and cardiac windows can be challenging for the novice echocardiographer to obtain. Unlike TEE which has an always open "window" to the heart from the esophagus, TTE image relies on finding "windows" in between rib spaces and lungs. Most practitioners notice that it takes roughly 20 to 30 performed exams before they can reliably find the basic views. Once able to obtain the basic views, they can then start recognizing pathology and abnormal findings. Like other clinical skills such as appreciating heart sounds with a stethoscope, a practitioner must be able to appreciate the normal findings before the pathologic exam becomes clear.

Point-of-care ultrasound extends beyond imaging of just the heart. At the bedside, a trained practitioner can evaluate the lung, pleura, abdominal vessels, peritoneal fluid, gastric and urinary bladder volumes among many other structures. While the use of ultrasound for some these organs has been utilized via the Focused Assessment with Sonography for Trauma (FAST) exam, the utility of each of these bedside interrogations has become apparent in the perioperative arena and much more so in the intensive care unit and the emergency department.

In addition to helping the practitioner seeking to implement the use of TTE and point-of-care ultrasound into their clinical practice, this text is intended as an aid for those who are seeking certification in critical care echocardiography including passing the CCEeXAM®. This textbook includes chapters dedicated to general ultrasound principles, TTE imaging, echocardiographic assessment of each of the major cardiac structures, as well as dedicated chapters to critical care ultrasonography that are designed to address the core competencies that are tested in the critical care echocardiography exam and prepare the practitioner to obtain critical care echocardiography certification.

Certification in Critical Care Echocardiography

As one becomes proficient in the use of critical care echocardiography, they ultimately may seek certification to acknowledge the new skillset they have achieved. The National Board of Echocardiography, Inc. (www.echoboards.org) is a not-for-profit corporation that administers the examination in critical care echocardiography as well as the board certification process. The purpose of certification is to recognize physicians who have demonstrated their competence in critical care echocardiography. Like basic perioperative TEE certification, the NBE offers two statuses in relation to critical care echocardiography: Testamur and Certification. Testamur status indicates the successful completion of the Examination of Special Competence in Critical Care Echocardiography (CCEeXAM®). Certification also implies a passing score on the CCEeXAM® in addition to meeting requirements that document proficiency. Readers are encouraged to visit the NBE's website for the most current requirements; however, the present requirements include a current license to practice medicine, current medical board certification, and specific training in critical care echocardiography.

The specific training involves performing 150 critical care exams which are defined as a transthoracic echocardiogram at the bedside in the management of a critically ill patient. There are two pathways to obtaining the specific training requirement, including a supervised training pathway which is often suited to those still in a training institution and the practice experience pathway which is more suited to those already in practice. Of note, the supervised training pathway ultimately requires completion of a 1-year fellowship in adult critical care, while the practice experience pathway requires a minimum of 750 hours of critical care experience over the preceding 3 years as well as the completion of 20 hours of CME related to echocardiography. Details of each of the pathways and the required documentation may be found on the NBE's website (www.echoboards.org).

Basic TTE Examination

While the American Society of Anesthesiologists have published practice guidelines on the use of perioperative transesophageal echocardiography, no such document exists regarding transthoracic echocardiography. Perioperative TEE is divided into monitoring and diagnostic capabilities with the focus of basic perioperative TEE on its monitoring usage. Similarly, TTE can be divided into similar arenas. The American Society of Echocardiography delineated the spectrum of bedside TTE from an ultrasound-assisted physical exam, point-of-care TTE, critical care echocardiography, to limited and comprehensive echocardiography [9]. Point-of-care TTE is not meant to supplant the comprehensive TTE performed by ultrasonographers and interpreted by cardiologists. In fact, a focused point-of-care TTE exam may subsequently prompt a more comprehensive echocardiography exam and cardiology consultation. Point-of-care TTE is intended as a rapidly deployable, focused assessment, guiding immediate therapeutic interventions. Therefore, the exam is often reduced in the number of views or tailored to the clinical situation at hand and involves qualitative or semi-quantitative analysis instead of comprehensive and quantitative evaluations.

Patient Positioning and Optimization

As previously mentioned, transthoracic echocardiography requires "windows" to the heart to avoid interference with ribs and lung, both dramatically limiting ultrasound transmission. The main "windows" used in a point-of-care transthoracic echocardiography exam include the left parasternal, apical, and subcostal windows, and occasionally the suprasternal window (Fig. 1.4). These windows will vary from person to person and may not be obtainable in all patients. Unlike transesophageal echocardiography, which benefits from the proximity of the heart to the esophagus, the transthoracic exam is achieved at a greater depth from the chest wall, and intercalated structures like lung tissue may impair image acquisition. Therefore, patient positioning and utilizing gravity to move the heart closer toward the chest wall can dramatically improve imaging. When imaging from the parasternal and apical windows, positioning the patient in the left lateral decubitus position will utilize gravity to bring the heart closer to the left chest wall thereby improving image acquisition. The subcostal windows benefit from a patient in the supine position.

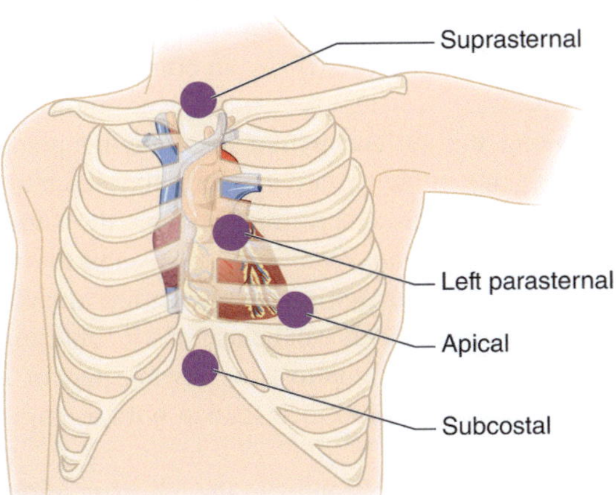

Fig. 1.4 Transthoracic echocardiography windows

Transesophageal echocardiography allows a near-continuous image of cardiac function, but transthoracic echocardiography is affected from ventilating lungs and therefore may have only an intermittent "window" to the heart. This necessitates a "timing" of the acquisition of images that is not present in transesophageal imaging. For example, as the patient inhales, there is significantly more air in the lung spaces which impedes imaging in the parasternal or apical views. This therefore requires a coordination of imaging to exhalation and/or breath holds. Subcostal views differ by benefiting from an inhalation which moves cardiac structures caudally toward the costal border. Therefore, coordination of imaging to inhalation will be beneficial. A recommended technique is the use of the acquisition button when obtaining and interpreting images. Instead of interpreting "on-the-fly," it is helpful to coordinate with the patient to hold in the desired part of the respiratory cycle and then acquire and store the image. The patient can then safely continue normal respiration while the stored image is interpreted.

The largest barrier to imaging may be patient positioning, body habitus, comorbidities, or the presence of incisions, bandages, or drains that impede adequate visualization. Often in the operating room or intensive care unit, achieving appropriate left lateral decubitus position for a parasternal or apical view is challenging or unsafe. Attempts at imaging in supine positions or the use of alternative views such as subcostal imaging can be utilized. A larger body habitus adds to the depth of visualization and may attenuate the image, while comorbidities such as chronic obstructive pulmonary disease or mechanical ventilation may increase the amount of aerated lung in the field of view, both which degrade image quality. Lastly, when imaging patients perioperatively, incisions and dressings such as in upper abdominal surgery may interfere with subcostal imaging. After cardiac surgery, subcostal views may be impeded by chest tube drains, while apical views may be impeded in patients with left ventricular assist devices. Again, it is important to be facile with multiple "windows" to allow imaging when a particular window is obstructed.

Contraindications and Complications

As opposed to TEE which is considered an invasive procedure, TTE is completely noninvasive and therefore does not carry the contraindications related to probe insertion and manipulation. The most important complication to be aware of with point-of-care ultrasound is misdiagnosis and the introduction of patient harm. While the previously described benefit of point-of-care ultrasound is the rapid diagnosis and immediate therapeutic guidance, it is important to realize that the information obtained in this fashion may be incomplete or limited. Inappropriate diagnoses due to inexperience or incomplete information which then is applied to inappropriate therapeutic intervention have the potential to introduce harm. As delineated above for transesophageal imaging, knowledge of a practitioner's own imaging limitations and when the clinical scenario dictates advanced imaging and interpretation is key to reducing potential patient harm.

Using the TTE Probe

Manipulation

There are several challenges inherent to image acquisition with transthoracic echocardiography that are not present with transesophageal imaging. While performing both imaging types relies on spatial reasoning, TTE allows for more range of movement of the transducer, because it is not contained within the relatively stable spaces of the esophagus and stomach. In addition, TTE does not benefit from the convenient juxtaposition of the esophagus immediately adjacent to the heart, and image availability may degrade from intervening structures like lungs and ribs. While this can be a challenge for new learners, it invariably improves with practice.

Like with TEE, TTE probe movement exists in three dimensions, and it can be manipulated along any of these three axes. To discuss imaging techniques, it is useful to have a consistent nomenclature for probe manipulation. Unfortunately, there is no accepted universal standard, as there is, for example, with the aviation industry, and some variation still exists [10]. If we use a conventional X, Y, and Z Cartesian coordinate system, these movements can be described in terms of these axes, as in Fig. 1.5. The movements in detail are:

1. **Sweeping.** This is linear movement along the X-axis. By physically moving the transducer footprint along this path, the imaging plane is moved to a new plane, parallel to the one prior. This can be used to image structures "out of plane" from a previous image, or to image with serial sections through a three-dimensional structure, like the left ventricle.
2. **Fanning.** Rotational movement within the X-axis (with the Y-axis as the pivot point) "fans" the imaging plane while keeping the transducer footprint in place. This can also be used to image adjacent structures, without disrupting the imaging window, and can also be necessary for image optimization, for example, if a longitudinal view of the ventricles is "foreshortened" by an oblique plane.
3. **Sliding.** Moving the transducer footprint along the surface within the imaging plane (Y-axis), either toward or away from the indicator, creates a new image along the same imaging plane, providing the ability to "extend" the imaging plane to the left or right of the screen. This can be useful for centering the structure of interest or viewing part of a structure too wide to visualize with a single image.
4. **Rocking.** Without moving the footprint of the transducer, changing the angle of the probe within the Y-axis (using the X-axis as the

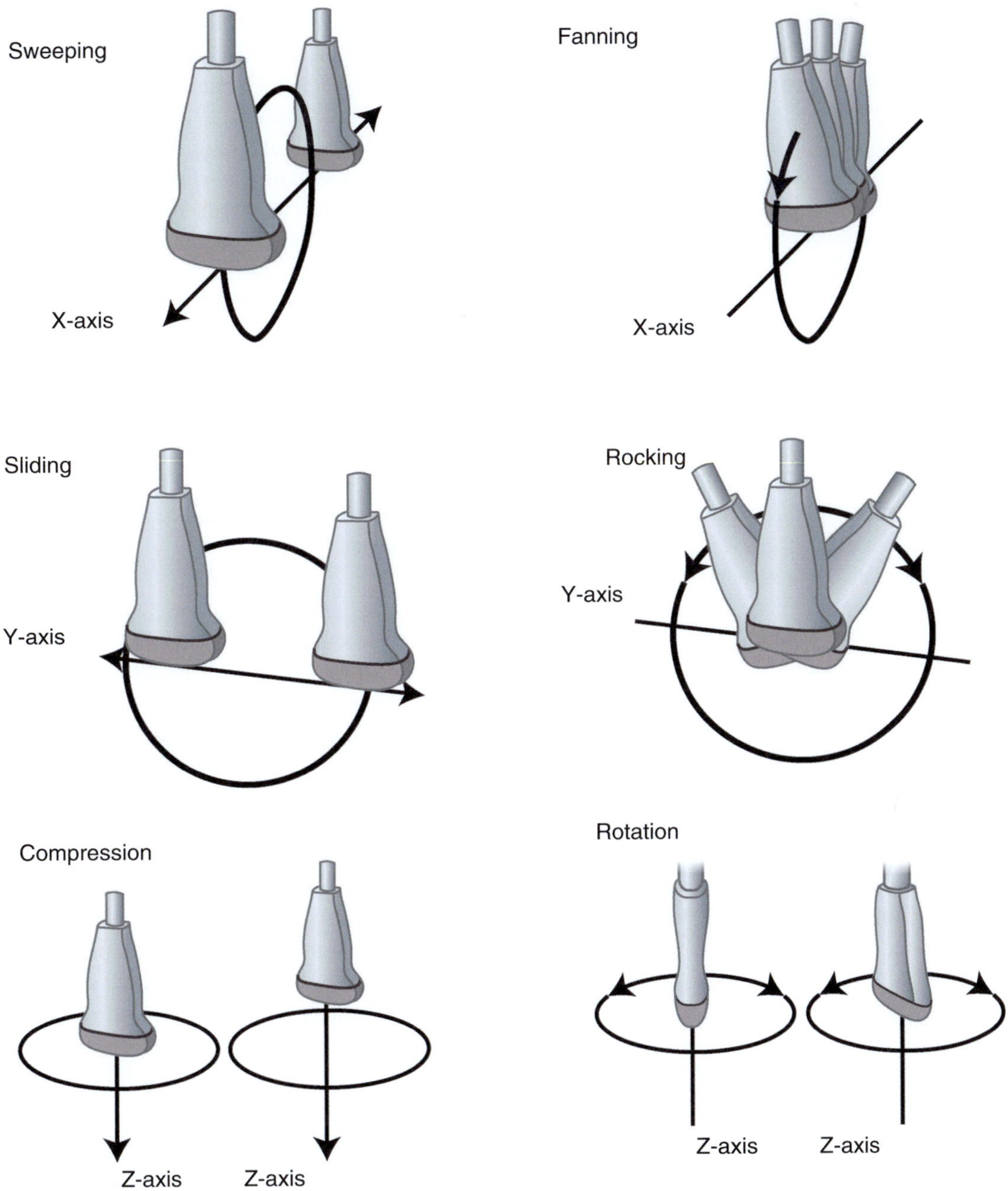

Fig. 1.5 Transthoracic echocardiography transducer manipulations. (Illustration adapted from Bahner DP et al. *Language of Transducer Manipulation: Codifying Terms for Effective Teaching*. J Ultrasound Med. 2016;35(1):183–8)

pivot point) will move the image toward or away from the indicator. This can be used to center a structure on the screen without moving the probe or finding a new imaging window.

5. **Compression.** This can be considered analogous to advancing/withdrawing the TEE probe; however, the imaging plane is along the same axis as the transducer, unlike TEE, which is perpendicular. Applying gentle, con-

tinuous pressure with the transducer into the Z-axis (into the patient) generally does not provide much physical movement, but may help optimize imaging by decreasing attenuation from soft tissues or moving competing structures like intestines out of the way.

6. **Rotation.** "Twisting" the transducer about the Z-axis rotates the imaging plane in much the same way that the multiplane works with TEE. The plane will pivot around the center of the image, which can be used to provide views perpendicular to each other, like the apical four-chamber and apical two-chamber views.

Orientation

By convention, the objects closest to the TTE transducer are displayed at the top of the screen, while the far field is displayed at the bottom. One side of the transducer is marked along the imaging plane with a reference point, the "indicator," or "probe marker." There is some variation in the orientation of this marker, but most sources agree that this corresponds with the top right corner of the imaging screen (in noncardiac ultrasound imaging, the convention is most commonly for this marker to appear on the left upper corner of the imaging screen). There is also some variation with the orientation of the transducer regarding left and right of the patient for some views, but the most important factor is that the provider interpreting the images is aware of the orientation.

Point-of-Care Echocardiography Reporting and Image Storage

Current basic perioperative TEE consensus statement recommends the image storage and reporting of all performed basic exams. Modern echocardiography machines can save exams digitally in a DICOM (Digital Imaging and Communications in Medicine) format, which allows retrieval and review when necessary. Older systems have allowed the storage of images and clips through VHS tapes or proprietary disc systems. Discussion with the echocardiography machine vendor and your information technology department is necessary to ensure proper storage and retrieval for your institution.

In addition to image storage, a documented report of the exam findings into the patient's chart is necessary. This may be performed as a written report or a clickable generated report in an electronic medical record. The report should include documentation of ventricular function, valvular function, chamber sizes, assessments of pericardium or pleura, and description of responses to interventions. The Society for Cardiovascular Anesthesiology website (www.scahq.org) hosts a template for a suggested adult TEE report. For a limited exam, a more brief description within a clinical note may be appropriate, depending on local practice patterns.

Conclusion

Transesophageal echocardiography (TEE) and transthoracic echocardiography (TTE) are safe monitoring modalities with broad applications in the perioperative and critical care arenas. A moderate amount of exposure to their use and knowledge of the principles of echocardiography can enable the practitioner to make basic assessments of a patient's cardiac status and help guide initial management decisions. The practitioner should also be able to determine when the nature of the surgery or the patient's cardiovascular status necessitates a comprehensive examination by a board certified advanced echocardiographer or when contraindications to an examination are present. Lastly, practitioners should be able to recognize the presence of complications.

Questions

1. Utilizing TEE to diagnose and guide surgical interventions is under the scope of practice of which of the following?

   a. Testamur status of the Examination of Special Competence in Basic Perioperative Transesophageal Echocardiography
   b. Certification in Basic Perioperative Transesophageal Echocardiography

c. Certification in Advanced Perioperative Transesophageal Echocardiography
d. Certification in Critical Care Echocardiography

2. Absolute contraindications to the use of transesophageal echocardiography include which of the following?

    a. History of unstable cervical spine
    b. Esophageal varices
    c. Esophageal stricture
    d. History of mediastinal radiation

3. Which of the following probe manipulations is correct?

    a. Turning the large knob clockwise results in anteflexion of the probe tip
    b. Turning the small knob counterclockwise results in left flexion of the probe tip
    c. The multiplane buttons increase and decrease from 0 to 180 degrees
    d. All the above are correct

4. At zero degrees of multiplane angle, which of the following is true?

    a. The right side of the screen displays the right side of the patient
    b. The right side of the screen displays the anterior portion of the heart
    c. The patient's left heart is on the right side of the screen
    d. The patient's posterior aspect of the heart is on the left side of the screen

5. Transthoracic echocardiography probe manipulations include which of the following?

    a. Sweeping, Fanning, Sliding, and Rocking
    b. Compression, Rotation, Anchoring, and Flexing
    c. Sweeping, Folding, Flexing, and Rocking
    d. Sliding, Rotation, Compression, and Pulsing

References

1. Practice Guidelines for Perioperative Transesophageal Echocardiography. Anesthesiology. 2010:1.
2. Reeves ST, Finley AC, Skubas NJ, et al. Basic perioperative transesophageal echocardiography examination: a consensus statement of the American Society of Echocardiography and the Society of Cardiovascular Anesthesiologists. J Am Soc Echocardiogr. 2013;26:443–56.
3. Hahn RT, Abraham T, Adams MS, et al. Guidelines for performing a comprehensive transesophageal echocardiographic examination. Anesthes Analgesia. 2014;118:21–68.
4. Kallmeyer IJ, Collard CD, Fox JA, Body SC, Shernan SK. The Safety of Intraoperative transesophageal echocardiography: a case series of 7200 cardiac surgical patients. Anesthes Analgesia. 2001:1126–30.
5. Daniel WG, Erbel R, Kasper W, et al. Safety of transesophageal echocardiography. A multicenter survey of 10,419 examinations. Circulation. 1991;83:817–21.
6. Min JK, Spencer KT, Furlong KT, et al. Clinical features of complications from transesophageal echocardiography: a single-center case series of 10,000 consecutive examinations. J Am Soc Echocardiogr. 2005;18:925–9.
7. Purza R, Ghosh S, Walker C, et al. Transesophageal echocardiography complications in adult cardiac surgery: a retrospective Cohort Study. Ann Thorac Surg. 2017;103:795–802.
8. O'Rourke M, Levan P, Khan T. Current use of ultrasound transmission gel for transesophageal echocardiogram examinations: a survey of cardiothoracic anesthesiology fellowship directors. J Cardiothoracic Vascul Anesthes. 2014;28:1208–10.
9. Kirkpatrick JN, Grimm R, Johri AM, et al. Recommendations for Echocardiography Laboratories Participating in Cardiac Point of Care Cardiac Ultrasound (POCUS) and Critical Care Echocardiography Training: Report from the American Society of Echocardiography. J Am Soc Echocardiogr. 2020;33:409–22. e4
10. Bahner DP, Blickendorf JM, Bockbrader M, et al. Language of transducer manipulation: codifying terms for effective teaching. J Ultrasound Med. 2016;35:183–8.

2 Transesophageal Echocardiography: Probe Manipulation and Essential Views

Timothy M. Maus and Sonia Nhieu

Abbreviations

PTE	Perioperative transesophageal echocardiography
ASE	American Society of Echocardiography
SCA	Society of Cardiovascular Anesthesiologists
TEE	Transesophageal echocardiography
2D	Two-dimensional
CFD	Color flow Doppler
TG	Transgastric
SAX	Short-axis
LV	Left ventricle
MV	Mitral valve
ME	Midesophageal
AV	Aortic valve
LVOT	Left ventricular outflow tract
RA	Right atrium
LA	Left atrium
RV	Right ventricle
TV	Tricuspid valve
WMA	Wall motion abnormality
LAA	Left atrial appendage
LAX	Long-axis
ASD	Atrial septal defect
PFO	Patent foramen ovale
RVOT	Right ventricular outflow tract
PV	Pulmonic valve

Supplementary Information The online version of this chapter (https://doi.org/10.1007/978-3-030-84349-6_2) contains supplementary material, which is available to authorized users.

T. M. Maus (✉)
Department of Anesthesiology, University of California San Diego Health, La Jolla, CA, USA
e-mail: tmaus@health.ucsd.edu

S. Nhieu
Department of Anesthesiology, Kaiser Permanente Santa Clara Medical Center, Santa Clara, CA, USA

Introduction

The goal of this chapter is for the echocardiographer to become familiar with the imaging views required to perform a basic perioperative transesophageal echocardiography (PTE) examination. Specific pathologies that can be appreciated in each view are discussed in subsequent chapters. As outlined by the consensus statement of the American Society of Echocardiography (ASE) and Society of Cardiovascular Anesthesiologists (SCA), the basic PTE examination focuses on acquiring the 11 most relevant views [1], while guidelines for performing a comprehensive PTE examination consist of acquiring 28 views [3]. While the 11 views of a basic PTE examination will provide the information needed to monitor patients perioperatively and diagnose general etiologies of hemodynamic instability (e.g., ventricular dysfunction, valvular abnormalities, volume status changes, and peri-

T. M. Maus, C. R. Tainter (eds.), *Essential Echocardiography*,
https://doi.org/10.1007/978-3-030-84349-6_2

cardial abnormalities), the basic PTE echocardiographer should also be familiar with how to acquire the comprehensive examination. Knowledge of the comprehensive exam will further refine the echocardiographer's skillset and comfort level with the transesophageal echocardiography probe. The basic PTE examination is designed to be complementary to a comprehensive transesophageal echocardiography (TEE) examination. Therefore, consultation with an advanced PTE echocardiographer should be requested when complex pathology is anticipated or when further investigation of abnormality is desired.

Beginning echocardiographers often exhibit anxiety and fear when learning the examination with a focus on the order of the exam. Each echocardiographer will have a different approach to the TEE examination, and the exact order of the examination is not critical. Completeness of the examination without missing important data is certainly the most important aspect. This text will offer a suggested order of views for both a basic and comprehensive examination based upon minimizing significant probe movement between views and maximizing the data obtained (Tables 2.1 and 2.2). The beginning echocardiographer is suggested to perform PTE exams as often as possible, when clinically indicated, in order to develop a comfort level moving from one view to the next as well as learning anatomical relationships.

In addition to obtaining the particular image, there are specific anatomical and physiologic interrogations that should occur within the image. These interrogations are divided into two-dimensional (2D) analysis, color flow Doppler (CFD), and spectral Doppler (pulsed-wave and continuous-wave) interrogation. It is recommended for the beginning echocardiographer to develop a systematic approach to the interrogations in addition to simply obtaining the images. For example, when obtaining the midesophageal four-chamber view, a 2D image is acquired, and color flow Doppler interrogation of the mitral valve and tricuspid valve is acquired, followed by a pulsed-wave or continuous-wave Doppler interrogation of mitral valve and tricuspid valve inflow and regurgitation. This approach of 2D > CFD > spectral evaluation allows an echocardiographer to develop an approach to the examination without missing data and prevents "bouncing around" the exam. Additionally, pathologies in this textbook will be summarized in the 2D > CFD > spectral format, highlighting important findings for each interrogation, as well as a method of remembering specific findings for each pathology.

Basic PTE Examination

The following are the 11 views as described by the ASE and SCA for performing a basic PTE examination. The additional 17 views that comprise the comprehensive exam will be subsequently discussed. Many practitioners will find that a complete 28-view examination is rarely necessary for a basic perioperative echocardiographic assessment. However, becoming familiar with all 28 views will allow the echocardiographer to become adept at choosing which views to obtain in a focused examination to evaluate for specific pathologies. The exam described below begins in the transgastric position (see Table 2.1). The aim of this sequence is to maximize the amount of information rapidly obtained in the exam while minimizing the amount of probe and multiplane manipulation between views, particularly the amount of probe insertion and withdrawal. The exam therefore begins with a transgastric view which often yields rapid information about the left ventricle (i.e., overall function, regional motion, and gross fluid status), withdraws to the mid-esophagus with attention to left and subsequently right heart structures, and completes the exam with views of the ascending and descending aorta. This exam sequence works particularly well in patients with hemodynamic compromise as the two initial views often identify the cause of instability allowing the prompt initiation of therapy. Please see Chap. 1 for image orientation, guides to probe manipulation, and multiplane use.

Table 2.1 Basic perioperative transesophageal echocardiography exam

Image order	Image name	Image depiction	2D > CFD > spectral
1	TG midpapillary SAX	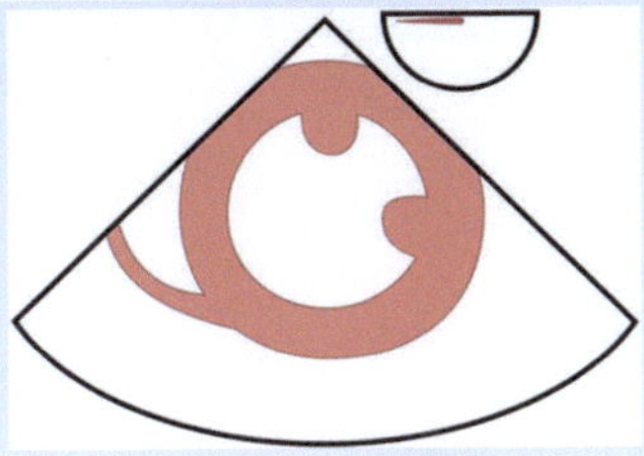	*2D* Chamber size: **LV** Ischemia detection: **LV (3 Coronaries) / RV** *CFD* Not typically utilized *Spectral* Not typically utilized
2	ME four-chamber	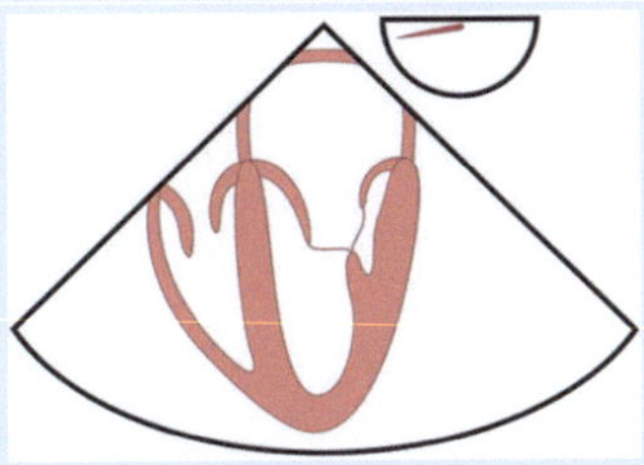	*2D* Chamber sizes: **RA/LA/RV/LV** Systolic function: **RV/LV** Ischemia detection: **RV / LV** Valvular anatomy/Motion: **TV/MV** *CFD* Valvular pathology: **TV/MV** Interatrial septum: **PFO/ASD** *Spectral* Inflow velocities: **TV/MV** Estimating PASP: **TV**
3	ME two-chamber	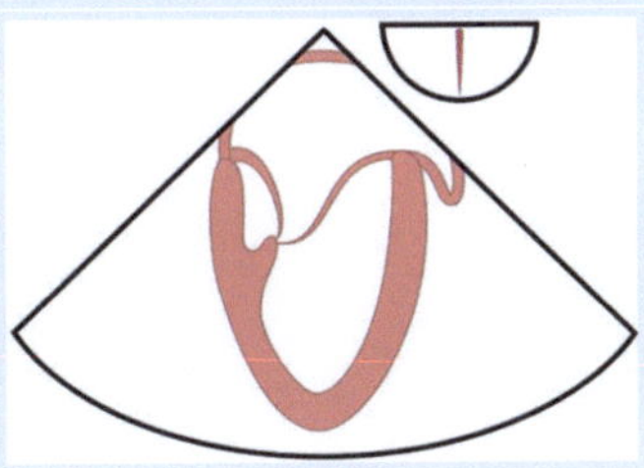	*2D* Chamber sizes: **LA/LV** Systolic function: **LV** Ischemia detection: **Anterior/inferior LV** Valvular anatomy/Motion: **MV** *CFD* Valvular pathology: **MV** Thrombus: **LAA** *Spectral* Inflow velocities: **MV; LUPV** Thrombus: **LAA**
4	ME long axis	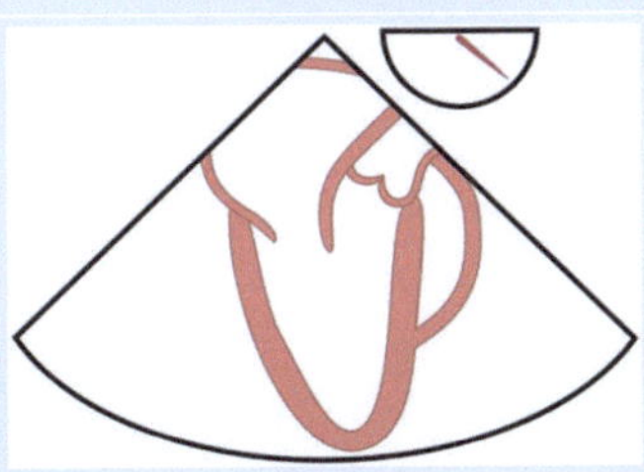	*2D* Chamber sizes: **LA/LV/LVOT/AV/Ao** Systolic function: **LV** Ischemia detection: **AntSept InfLat LV** Valvular anatomy/motion: **MV/AV** *CFD* Valvular pathology: **MV/AV** *Spectral* Inflow velocities: **MV**
5	ME AV short axis	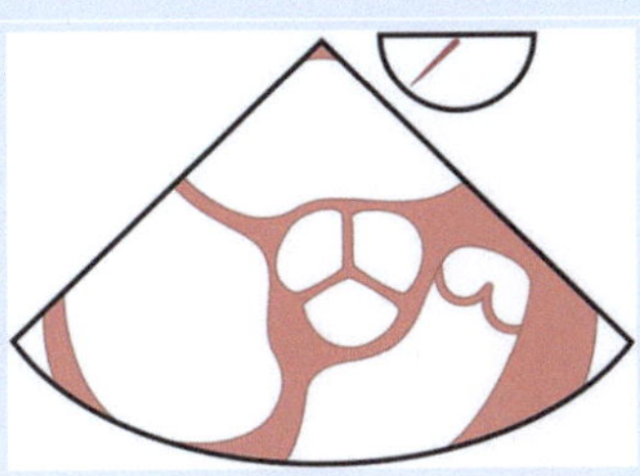	*2D* Chamber sizes: **LA** Valvular anatomy/motion: **AV** *CFD* Valvular pathology: **AV** Interatrial septum: **ASD/PFO** *Spectral* Not typically utilized

Table 2.1 (continued)

Image order	Image name	Image depiction	2D > CFD > spectral
6	ME RV inflow-outflow	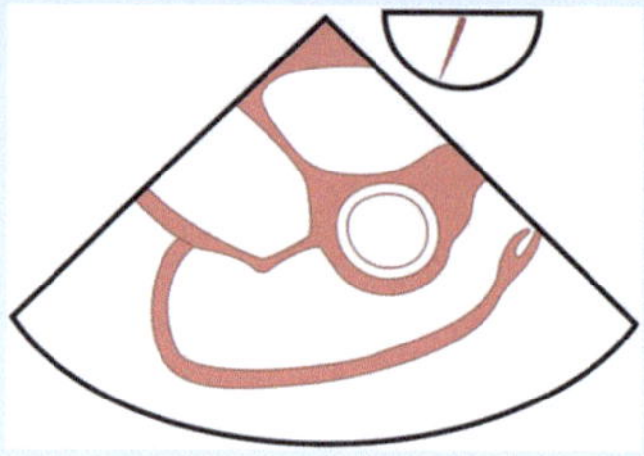	*2D* Chamber sizes: **RA/RV/PA/LA** Systolic function: **RV** Ischemia detection: **RV** Valvular anatomy/motion: **TV/PV** *CFD* Valvular pathology: **TV/PV** *Spectral* Estimating PASP: **TV**
7	ME bicaval	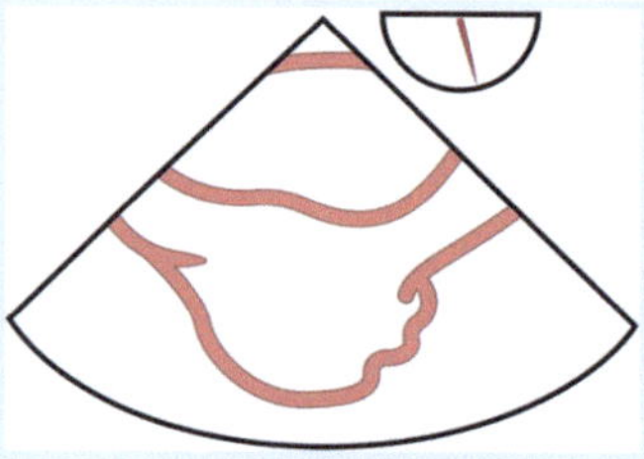	*2D* Chamber sizes: **LA/RA** Interatrial septum: competency *CFD* Interatrial septum: **ASD/PFO** *Spectral* Not typically utilized
8	ME ascending aortic SAX	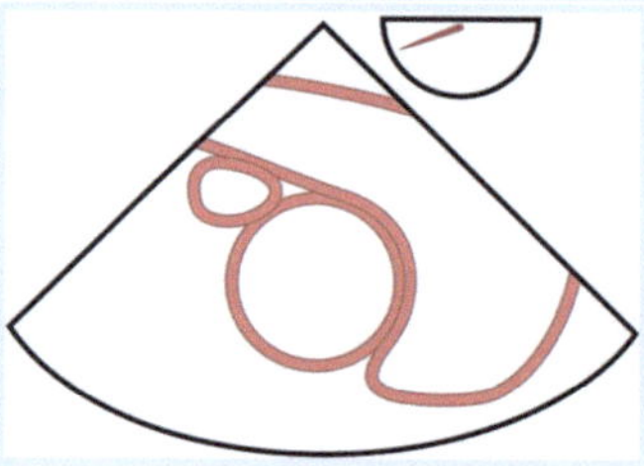	*2D* Vessel sizes: **Ao/PA/SVC** Dissection/plaque: **Ao** Thrombus: **PA/RPA** *CFD* Dissection: **Ao** *Spectral* Not typically utilized
9	ME ascending aortic LAX	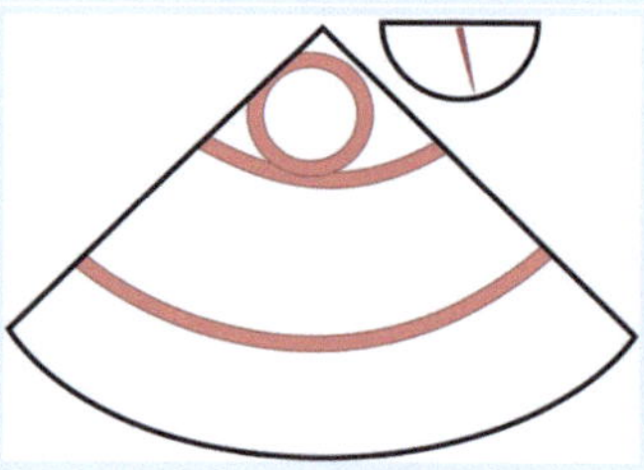	*2D* Vessel sizes: **Ao/RPA** Dissection/plaque: **Ao** Thrombus: **RPA** *CFD* Dissection: **Ao** *Spectral* Not typically utilized
10	Descending aortic SAX	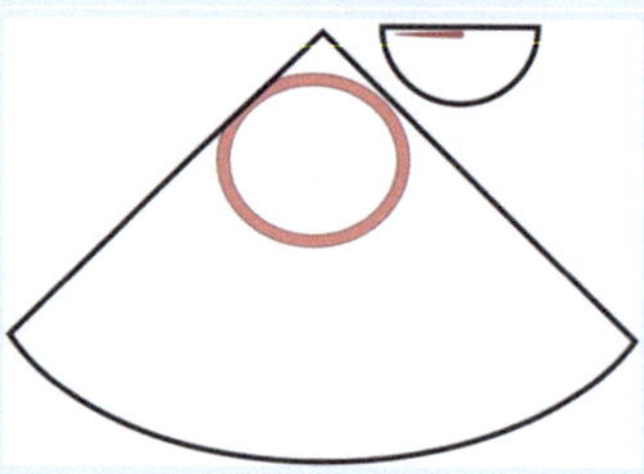	*2D* Vessel size: **Ao** Dissection/plaque: **Ao** *CFD* Dissection: **Ao** *Spectral* Not typically utilized

Table 2.1 (continued)

Image order	Image name	Image depiction	2D > CFD > spectral
11	Descending aortic LAX	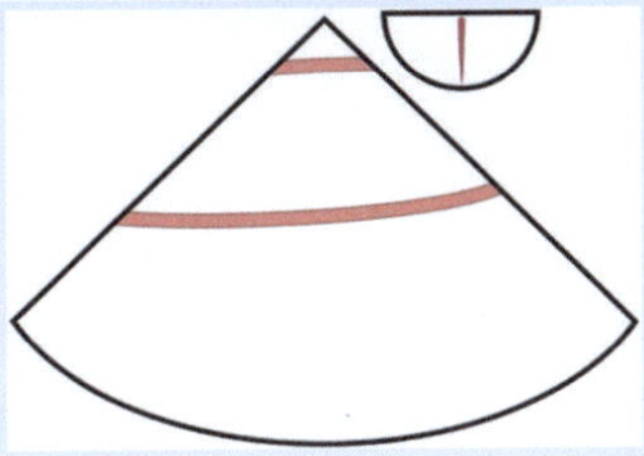	*2D* Vessel size: **Ao** Dissection/plaque: **Ao** *CFD* Dissection: **Ao** *Spectral* Not typically utilized

Abbreviations: ME Midesophageal; *TG* transgastric; *LAX* long axis; *SAX* short axis; *2D* two-dimensional; *CFD* color flow Doppler; *RA* right atrium; *LA* left atrium; *RV* right ventricle; *LV* left ventricle; *MV* mitral valve; *AV* aortic valve; *TV* tricuspid valve; *PV* pulmonic valve; *LVOT* left ventricular outflow tract; *PFO* patent foramen ovale; *ASD* atrial septal defect; *LAA* left atrial appendage; *LUPV* left upper pulmonary vein; *Ao* aorta; *PA* pulmonary artery; *RPA* right pulmonary artery; *AntSept* anterior septal wall; InfLat inferolateral wall; *SVC* superior vena cava
Adapted from: Shanewise et al. [2]

Table 2.2 Comprehensive perioperative transesophageal echocardiography exam

Image order	Image name	Image depiction	2D > CFD > spectral
Transgastric views			
1	Deep TG LAX	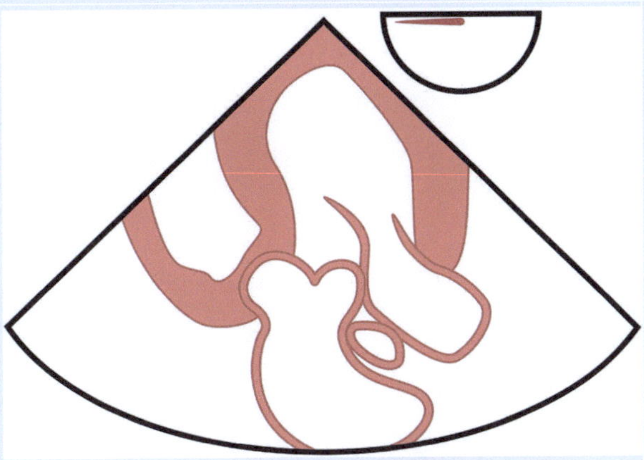	*2D* Chamber size: **LV** Ischemia detection: **Sept/Lat/Apex LV** Valvular anatomy and motion: **MV/AV** *CFD* Valvular pathology: **MV/AV** *Spectral* Outflow velocities: **LVOT/AV**
2	TG midpapillary SAX	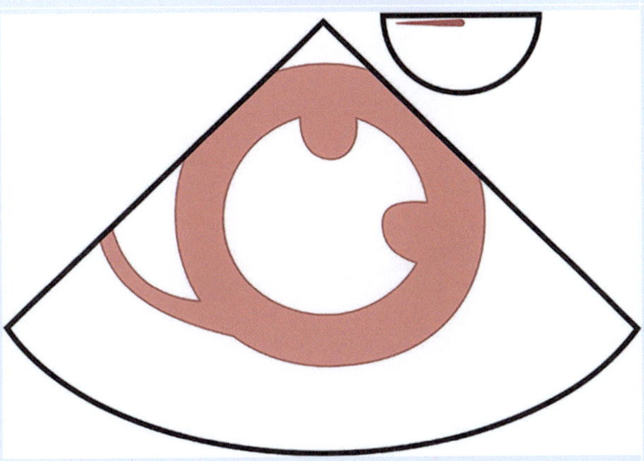	*2D* Chamber size: **LV** Ischemia detection: **LV (3 coronaries)/ RV** *CFD* Not typically utilized *Spectral* Not typically utilized

(continued)

Table 2.2 (continued)

Image order	Image name	Image depiction	2D > CFD > spectral
3	TG basal SAX	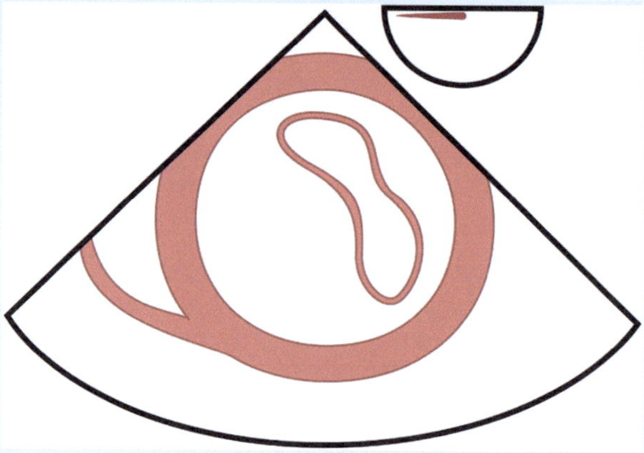	*2D* Chamber size: **LV** Ischemia detection: **Basal LV (3 coronaries)/RV** Valvular anatomy/motion: **MV** *CFD* Valvular pathology: **MV** *Spectral* Not typically utilized
4	TG apical SAX	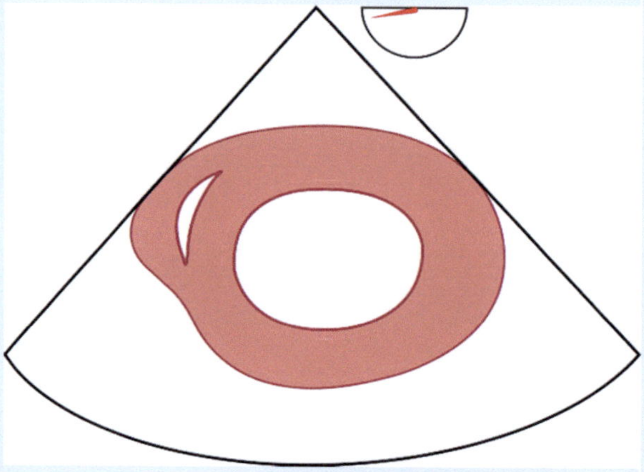	*2D* Chamber size: **LV** Ischemia detection: **Apical LV (3 coronaries)** *CFD* Not typically utilized *Spectral* Not typically utilized
5	TG two-chamber	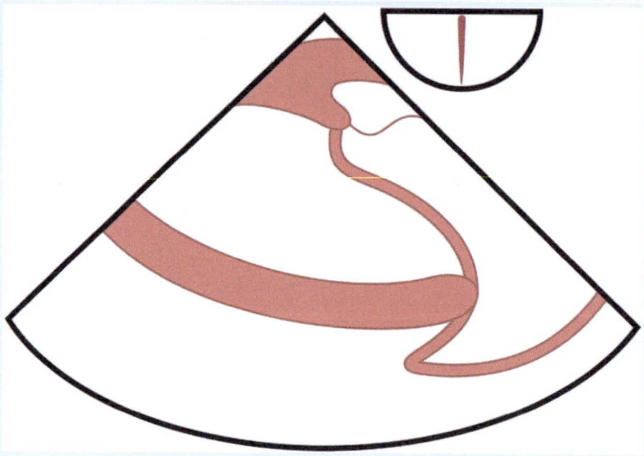	*2D* Chamber size: **LV** Ischemia detection: **Anterior/inferior LV** *CFD* Not typically utilized *Spectral* Not typically utilized

Table 2.2 (continued)

Image order	Image name	Image depiction	2D > CFD > spectral
6	TG LAX	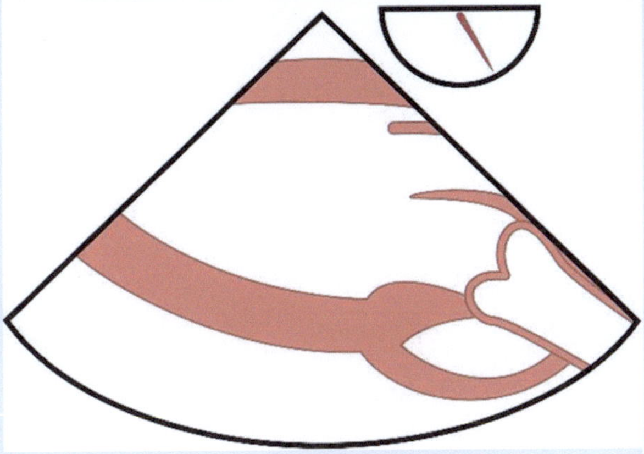	*2D* Chamber size: **LV** *CFD* Valvular pathology: **AV** *Spectral* Outflow velocities: **LVOT/AV**
7	TG RV basal SAX	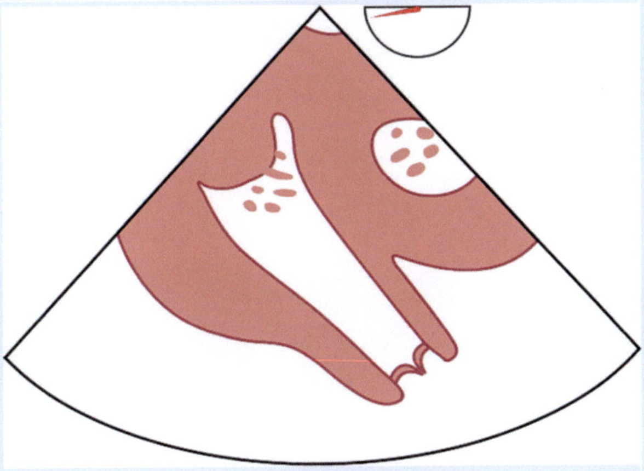	*2D* Chamber size: Ischemia detection: **RV** Valvular anatomy: **TV** *CFD* Valvular pathology: **TV** *Spectral* Typically not utilized
8	TG RV inflow-outflow	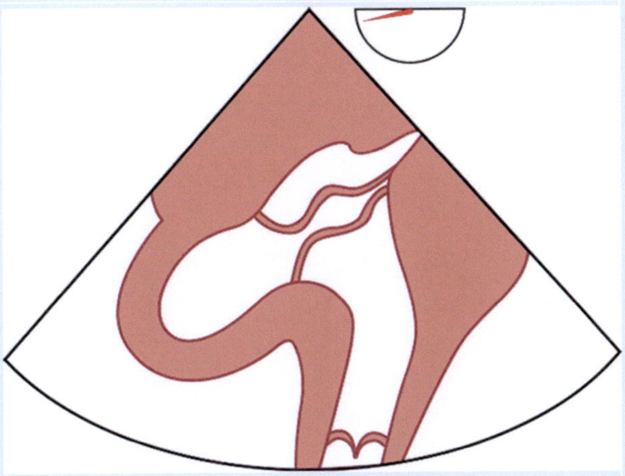	*2D* Chamber sizes: **RV/RA/RVOT** Valvular anatomy and motion: **TV, PV** *CFD* Valvular pathology: **TV, PV** *Spectral* Estimating PASP: **TV** Outflow velocities: **PV**

Table 2.2 (continued)

Image order	Image name	Image depiction	2D > CFD > spectral
9	TG RV inflow	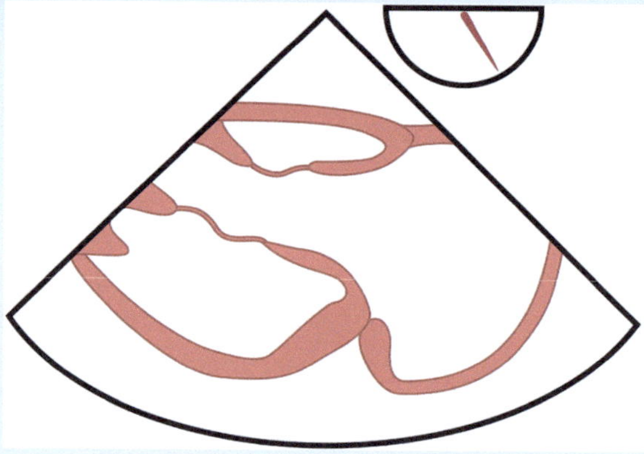	*2D* Chamber sizes: **RV/RA/TV annulus** Ischemia detection: **RV free wall** Valvular anatomy and motion: **TV** *CFD* Valvular pathology: **TV** *Spectral* Typically not utilized
Midesophageal views			
10	ME four-chamber	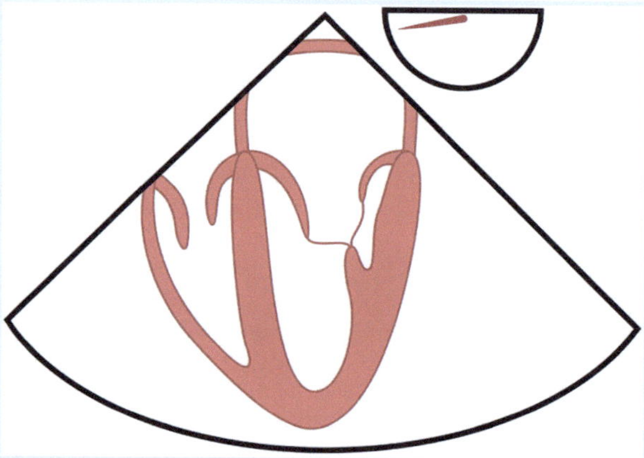	*2D* Chamber sizes: **RA/LA/RV/LV** Systolic function: **RV/LV** Ischemia detection: **RV/LV** Valvular anatomy/motion: **TV/MV** *CFD* Valvular pathology: **TV/MV** Interatrial septum: **PFO/ASD** *Spectral* Inflow velocities: **TV/MV** Estimating PASP: **TV**
11	ME five-chamber	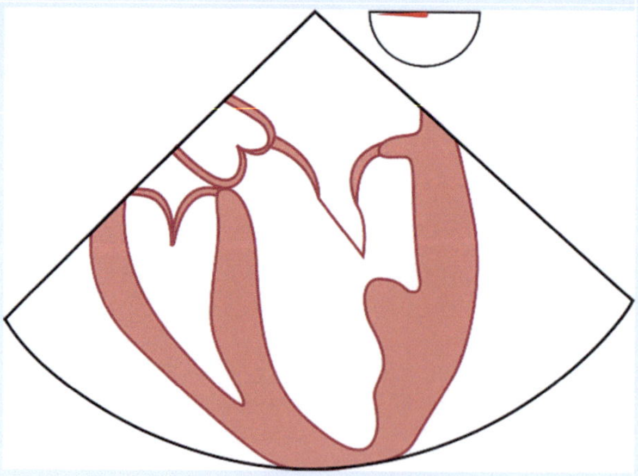	*2D* Chamber sizes: **RA/LA/RV/LV/LVOT** Systolic function: **RV/LV** Ischemia detection: **RV/LV** Valvular anatomy/motion: **TV/MV/AV** *CFD* Valvular pathology: **TV/MV/AV** *Spectral* Inflow velocities: **TV/MV** Estimating PASP: **TV**

(continued)

Table 2.2 (continued)

Image order	Image name	Image depiction	2D > CFD > spectral
12	ME mitral commissural	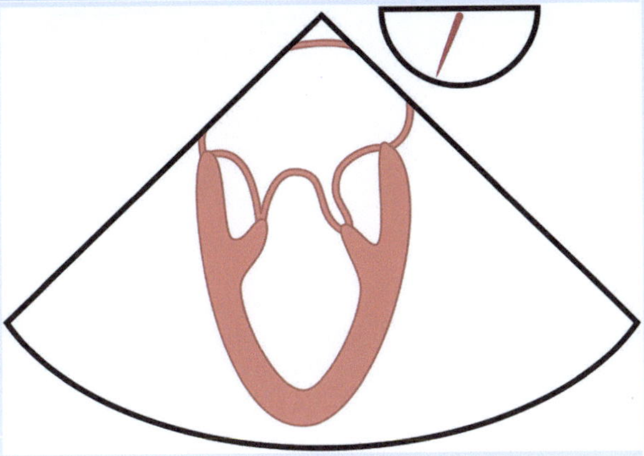	*2D* Chamber sizes: **LA/LV** Valvular anatomy/motion: **MV** *CFD* Valvular pathology: **MV** Thrombus: **LAA** *Spectral* Inflow velocities: **MV** Thrombus: **LAA**
13	ME two-chamber	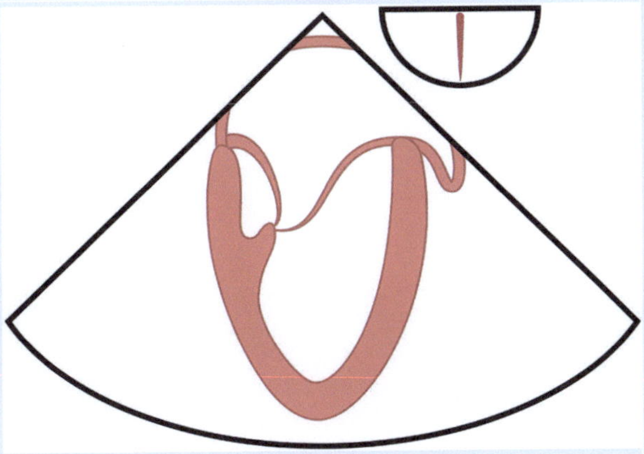	*2D* Chamber sizes: **LA/LV** Systolic function: **LV** Ischemia detection: **Anterior/Inferior LV** Valvular anatomy/motion: **MV** *CFD* Valvular pathology: **MV** Thrombus: **LAA** *Spectral* Inflow velocities: **MV; LUPV** Thrombus: **LAA**
14	ME LAA	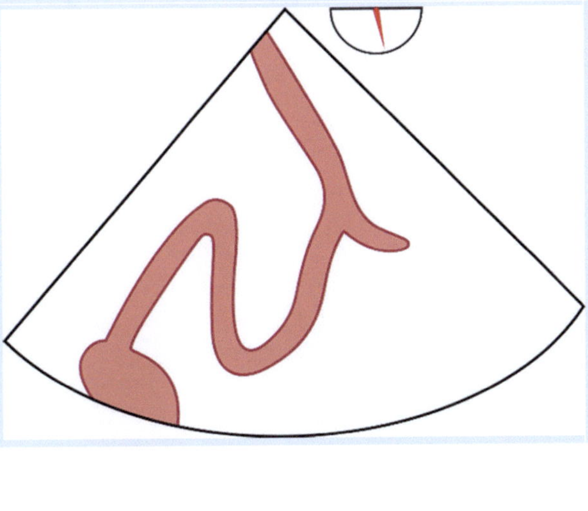	*2D* Anatomy: LAA *CFD* Thrombus: **LAA** *Spectral* Thrombus: **LAA**

(continued)

Table 2.2 (continued)

Image order	Image name	Image depiction	2D > CFD > spectral
15	ME LAX	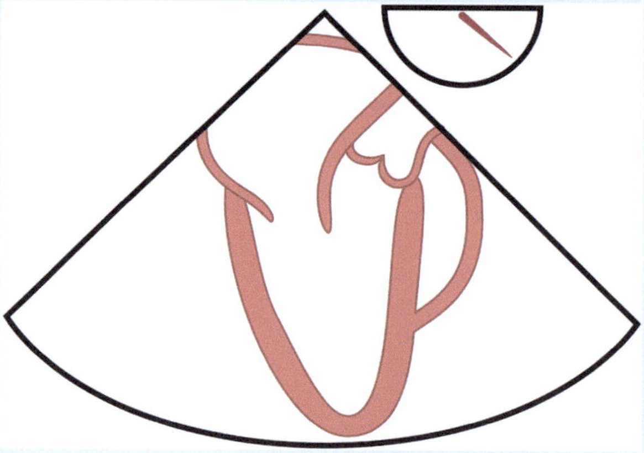	*2D* Chamber sizes: **LA/ LV/LVOT/AV/Ao** Systolic function: **LV** Ischemia detection: **AntSept/InfLat LV** Valvular anatomy/ motion: **MV/AV** *CFD* Valvular pathology: **MV/AV** *Spectral* Inflow velocities: **MV**
16	ME AV LAX	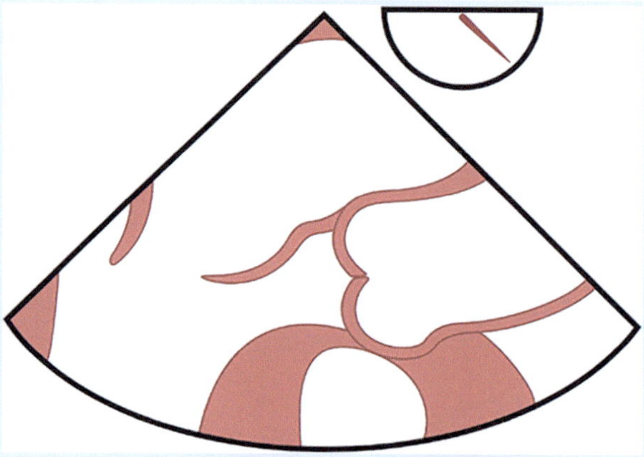	*2D* Chamber sizes: **LVOT/AV annulus/ Ao** Valvular anatomy/ motion: **AV** *CFD* Valvular pathology: **AV** *Spectral* Typically not utilized
17	ME AV SAX	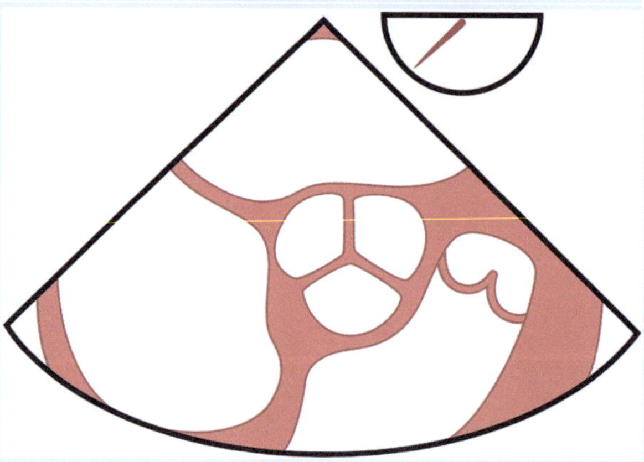	*2D* Chamber sizes: **LA** Valvular anatomy/ motion: **AV** *CFD* Valvular pathology: **AV** Interatrial septum: **ASD/PFO** *Spectral* Not typically utilized

Table 2.2 (continued)

Image order	Image name	Image depiction	2D > CFD > spectral
18	ME RV inflow-outflow	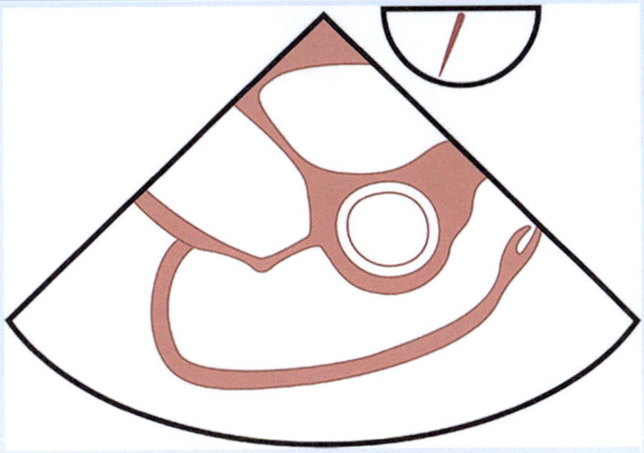	*2D* Chamber sizes: **RA/RV/PA/LA** Systolic function: **RV** Ischemia detection: **RV** Valvular anatomy/motion: **TV/PV** *CFD* Valvular pathology: **TV/PV** *Spectral* Estimating PASP: **TV**
19	ME bicaval	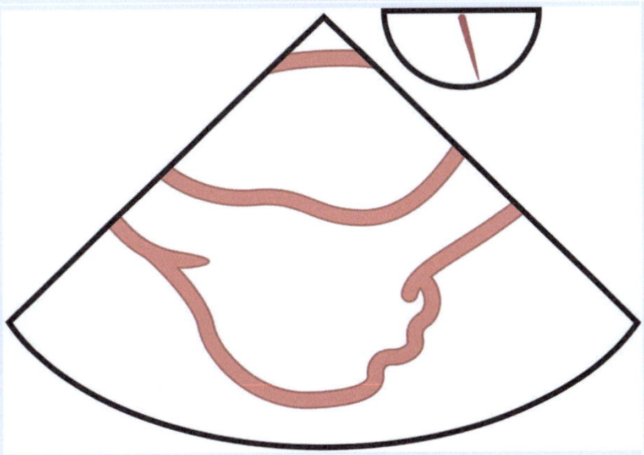	*2D* Chamber sizes: **LA/RA** Interatrial septum: **Competency** *CFD* Interatrial septum: **ASD/PFO** *Spectral* Not typically utilized
20	ME modified bicaval TV	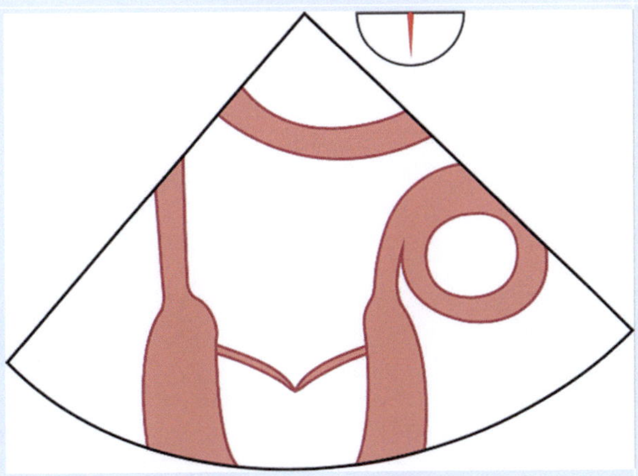	*2D* Chamber sizes: **LA/RA** Valvular anatomy: **TV** Interatrial septum: **Competency** *CFD* Interatrial septum: **ASD/PFO** *Spectral* Estimating PASP: **TV**

(continued)

Table 2.2 (continued)

Image order	Image name	Image depiction	2D > CFD > spectral
21	UE right and left pulmonary veins	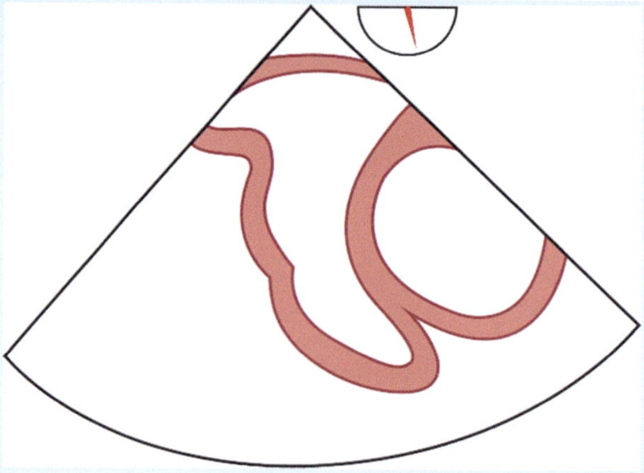	*2D* Anatomy: **RUPV/ LUPV** *CFD* Patency: **RUPV/ LUPV** *Spectral* Inflow velocities: **RUPV/LUPV**
22	ME right pulmonary vein	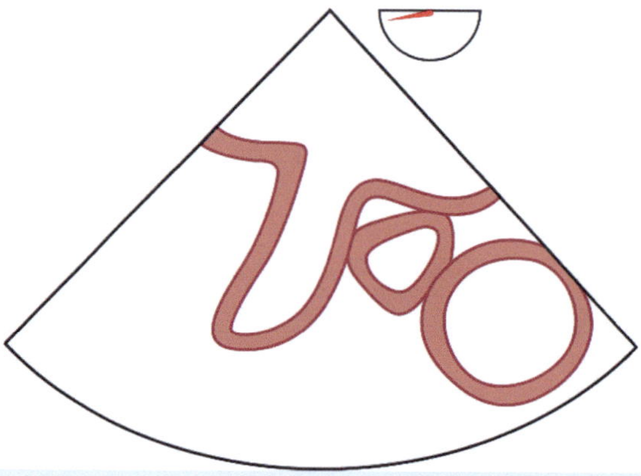	*2D* Anatomy: **RPV, SVC, ascending aorta** *CFD* Patency: **RPV** *Spectral* Inflow velocities: **RPV**
Aortic views			
23	ME ascending aortic SAX	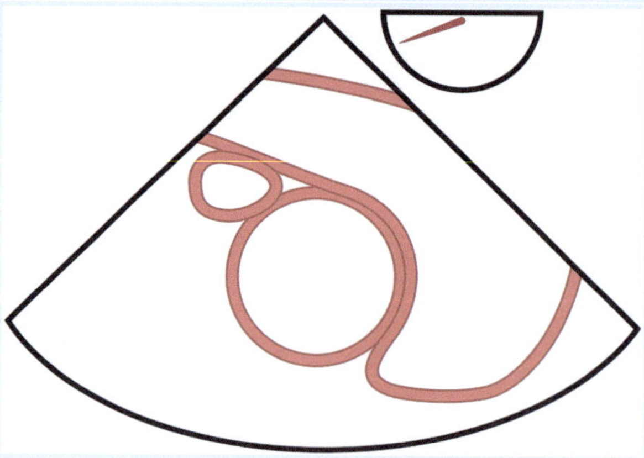	*2D* Vessel sizes: **Ao/PA/ SVC** Dissection/plaque: **Ao** Thrombus: **PA/RPA** *CFD* Dissection: **Ao** *Spectral* Not typically utilized

Table 2.2 (continued)

Image order	Image name	Image depiction	2D > CFD > spectral
24	ME ascending aortic LAX	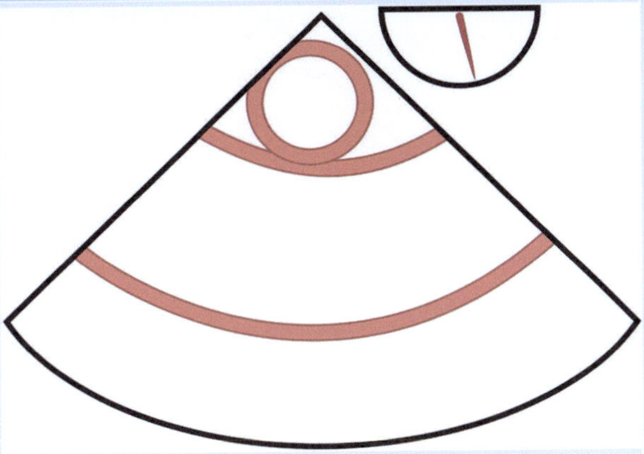	*2D* Vessel Sizes: **Ao/RPA** Dissection/plaque: **Ao** Thrombus: **RPA** *CFD* Dissection: **Ao** *Spectral* Not typically utilized
25	UE aortic arch LAX	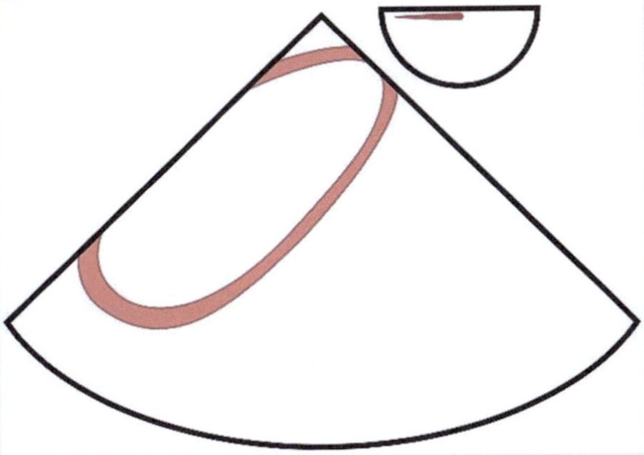	*2D* Vessel size: **Ao** Dissection/plaque: **Ao** *CFD* Dissection: **Ao** *Spectral* Not typically utilized
26	UE aortic arch SAX	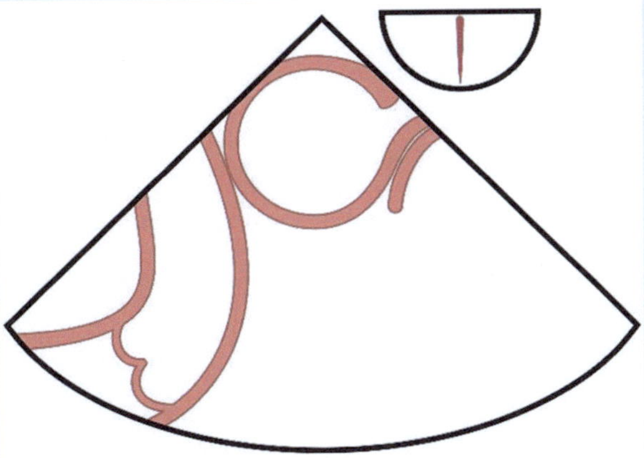	*2D* Vessel size: **Ao/PA** Dissection/plaque: **Ao** *CFD* Dissection: **Ao** Valvular pathology: **PV** *Spectral* Valvular/PA velocities: **PV/Main PA**

Table 2.2 (continued)

Image order	Image name	Image depiction	2D > CFD > spectral
27	Descending aortic SAX	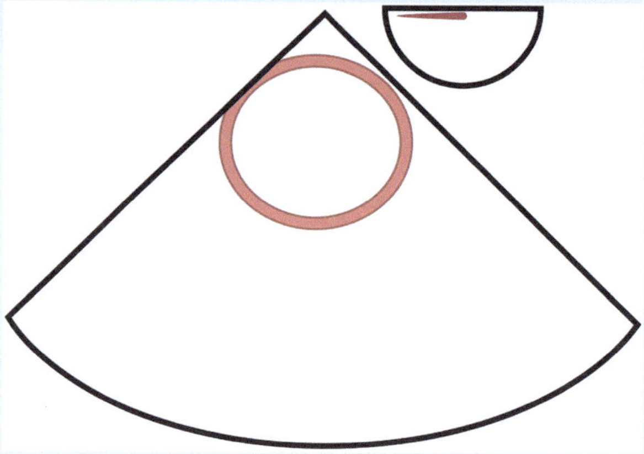	<u>2D</u> Vessel size: **Ao** Dissection/plaque: **Ao** <u>CFD</u> Dissection: **Ao** <u>Spectral</u> Not typically utilized
28	Descending aortic LAX	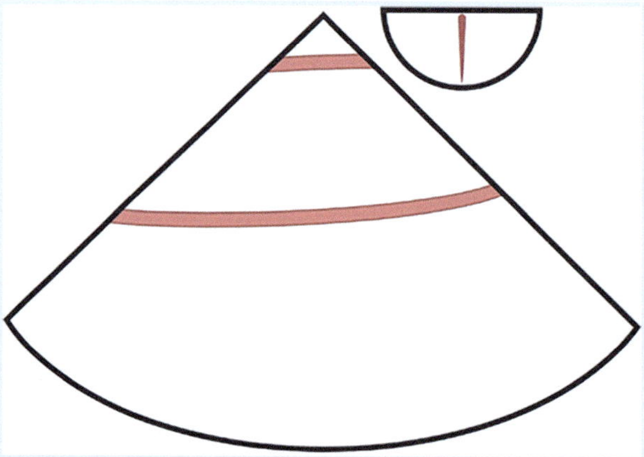	<u>2D</u> Vessel size: **Ao** Dissection/plaque: **Ao** <u>CFD</u> Dissection: **Ao** <u>Spectral</u> Flow pattern: **Ao**

Abbreviations: ME Midesophageal, *TG* transgastric, *UE* upper esophageal, *LAX* long-axis, *SAX* short-axis, *2D* two-dimensional, *CFD* color flow Doppler, *RA* right atrium, *LA* left atrium, *RV* right ventricle, *LV* left ventricle, *MV* mitral valve, *AV* aortic valve, *TV* tricuspid valve, *PV* pulmonic valve, *LVOT* left ventricular outflow tract, *PFO* patent foramen ovale, *ASD* atrial septal defect, *LAA* left atrial appendage, *LUPV* left upper pulmonary vein, *RUPV* right upper pulmonary vein, *RPV* right pulmonary veins, *Ao* aorta, *PA* pulmonary artery, *RPA* right pulmonary artery, *AntSept* anterior septal wall, *InfLat* inferolateral wall, *Sept* septal wall, *Lat* lateral wall, *SVC* superior vena cava

Adapted from: Shanewise JS, Cheung AT, Aronson S, Stewart WJ, Weiss RL, Mark JB, et al. ASE/SCA guidelines for performing a comprehensive intraoperative multiplane transesophageal echocardiography examination: recommendations of the American Society of Echocardiography Council for Intraoperative Echocardiography and the Society of Cardiovascular Anesthesiologists Task Force for Certification in Perioperative Transesophageal Echocardiography. J Am Soc Echocardiogr. 1999 Oct;12(10):884–900

Transgastric (TG) Midpapillary Short-Axis (SAX) View

To obtain the TG midpapillary SAX view, the probe is advanced into the stomach. When advancing, the image on the screen will often disappear when entering the stomach as the probe is no longer adjacent to tissue (free floating in the stomach). While keeping the multiplane angle at 0 degrees, the probe is gradually anteflexed while the depth is adjusted until the posteromedial and anterolateral papillary muscles are visualized. A proper TG midpapillary SAX view can be challenging to obtain since proper depth and anteflexion are required to obtain a true short-axis cross section of the left ventricle (LV). Since the posteromedial papillary muscle is closest to the TEE probe, the depth of the probe should first be adjusted until this papillary muscle is visualized. If the mitral valve (MV) chordae tendineae are visible, then the probe is too high and should be advanced. Once the depth is appropriate, small

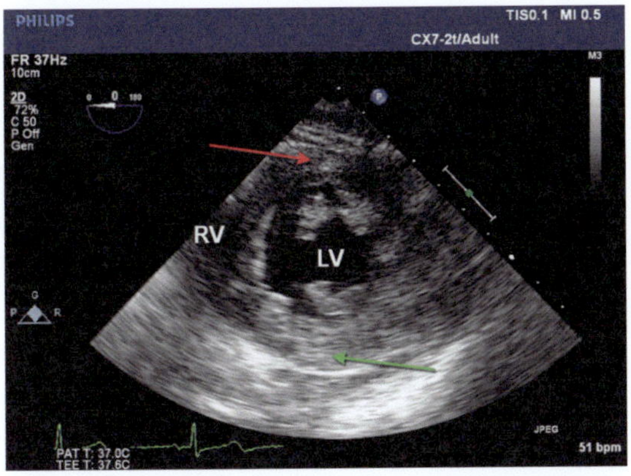

Fig. 2.1 TG midpapillary SAX view. The *green arrow* indicates the anterior wall of the left ventricle (LV), while the *red arrow* indicates the inferior wall of the LV. *RV* right ventricle

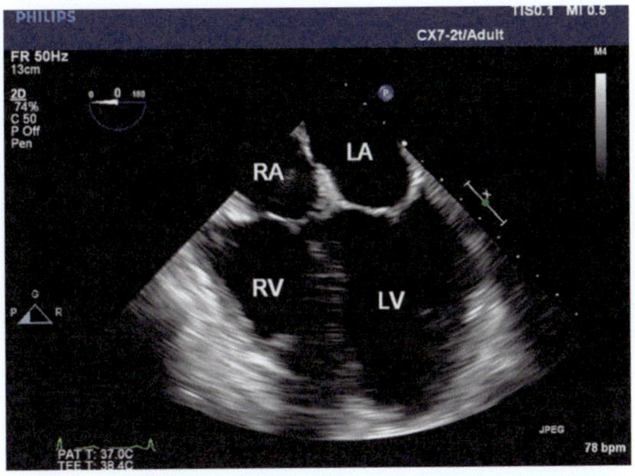

Fig. 2.2 ME four-chamber view. *RA* right atrium, *RV* right ventricle, *LA* left atrium, *LV* left ventricle

adjustments to the degree of anteflexion should be made until the anterolateral papillary muscle comes into view (Fig. 2.1; Video 2.1).

The TG midpapillary SAX view is commonly used during intraoperative monitoring and may frequently be the first view assessed during hemodynamic instability. Two-dimensional assessment includes volume status, LV systolic function, and regional wall motion. The TG midpapillary SAX view is especially useful because all three coronary artery branches that perfuse the different segments of the myocardium can be assessed simultaneously. However, it is important to remember that this view only provides a single cross section view of the LV and inadequate coronary perfusion to the base and apex of the LV will not be detected (see Chap. 7, "Regional Ventricular Function"). Color flow Doppler and spectral Doppler are typically not employed in this view.

Midesophageal (ME) Four-Chamber View

The ME four-chamber view is obtained by withdrawing the probe from the transgastric position to a depth of approximately 30–35 cm. A midesophageal position is identified by observing the left atrium at the apex of the imaging display. If the aortic valve (AV) and left ventricular outflow tract (LVOT) are visible (five-chamber view), then retroflexion of the probe and adjustment of the multiplane angle to 10 degrees may be necessary to obtain the ME four-chamber view. Structures that should be visible in this view include the right atrium (RA), interatrial septum, left atrium (LA), right ventricle (RV), interventricular septum, LV, tricuspid valve (TV), and MV. The image depth should be adjusted so that the apex of the LV is visible as well.

The ME four-chamber view is often a readily identified and very useful view to acquire that provides significant amounts of information, typically without any manipulation of the multiplane. Returning to this zero-degree view is recommended if the echocardiographer becomes disoriented during their TEE evaluation. The ME four-chamber view allows evaluation of chamber sizes, function, valvular function, and regional wall motion of the septal and lateral walls of the LV (Fig. 2.2; Video 2.2). Two-dimensional evaluation allows inspection of LV and RV systolic function; evidence of wall motion abnormalities (WMA); tricuspid and mitral valve anatomy and motion; chamber sizes of RA, LA, LV, and RV; and motion of the interatrial and interventricular septums. Color flow Doppler is utilized to interrogate the mitral and tricuspid valves for stenosis and regurgitation. Spectral Doppler is often utilized to measure mitral valve inflow in the evaluation of diastology and mitral stenosis.

ME Two-Chamber View

To obtain the ME two-chamber view, the multiplane angle is rotated to 80–100 degrees until the right-sided cardiac structures are no longer visi-

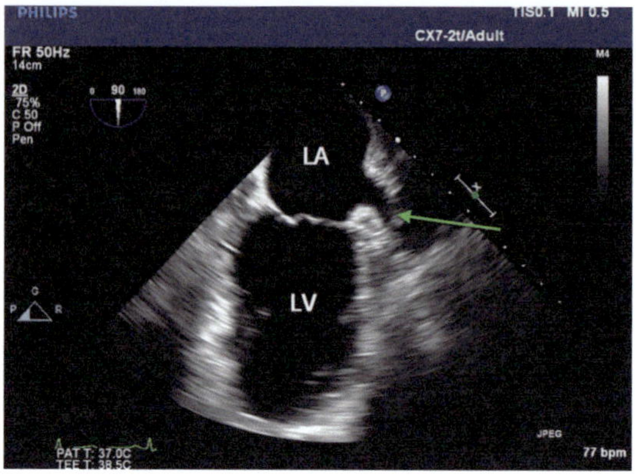

Fig. 2.3 ME two-chamber view with a *green arrow* indicating the left atrial appendage. *LA* left atrium, *LV* left ventricle

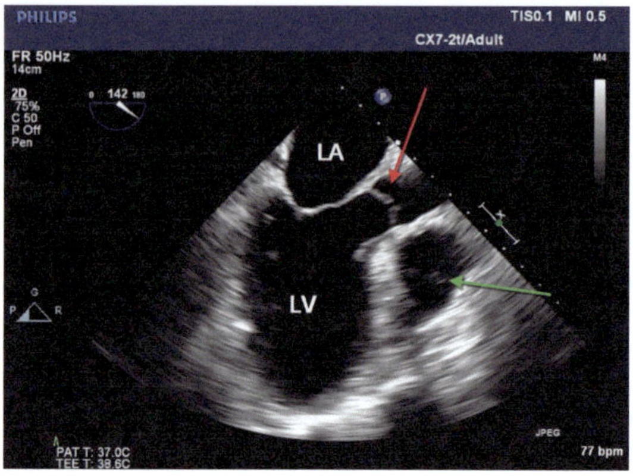

Fig. 2.4 ME LAX view with a *red arrow* indicating the aortic valve and a *green arrow* indicating the right ventricular outflow tract. *LA* left atrium, *LV* left ventricle

ble. It is easiest to center the LV in the imaging sector in the ME four-chamber view prior to increasing the multiplane angle. To optimize the view, the probe is turned to the left and right until the LV apex is visualized in the far field and the LV is not foreshortened. Structures that are visible in the ME two-chamber view are the left atrium, mitral valve, left ventricle, left atrial appendage (LAA), and left upper pulmonary vein (Fig. 2.3; Video 2.3). A short-axis view of the coronary sinus can also be appreciated in this view. Two-dimensional evaluation focuses on regional wall motion of the anterior and inferior walls of the LV, mitral valve motion, and thrombus in the LV apex or left atrial appendage. Color flow Doppler of the MV and LAA is helpful in evaluating for regurgitation and thrombus formation, respectively. Spectral Doppler can be helpful in evaluating mitral inflow and thrombus formation in the MV and LAA, respectively.

ME Long-Axis (LAX) View

From the ME two-chamber view, the multiplane angle is advanced to approximately 120 degrees when the LVOT is seen on the right-hand side of the imaging sector to obtain the ME LAX view. All patients are obviously different, and therefore, the multiplane degree is simply an estimate; this view may be developed in some patients as far out as 160 degrees of multiplane. The LA, MV, LV, LVOT, and AV should be visible in this view (Fig. 2.4; Video 2.4). This view is similar to the ME AV LAX (see "Additional Views" below). However, rather than focusing on the AV, the LV inflow and outflow tract as well as the entirety of the LV cavity can be seen in this view. 2D assessments that can be made in the ME LAX view include chamber sizes, regional wall motion of the anteroseptal and inferolateral walls of the LV, and mitral valve and aortic valve anatomy and motion. Color flow Doppler interrogation of the MV and AV and spectral Doppler interrogation of the mitral valve is possible as well. The AV is often positioned perpendicular to the probe in this view and is therefore not conducive to spectral Doppler interrogation.

ME AV SAX View

In TEE, when rotating a multiplane by 90 degrees, the object in the center of the image will be rotated from a long-axis to a short-axis orientation and vice versa. From the ME LAX view, centering the AV by slowly withdrawing the probe and then rotating the multiplane back to 30 degrees represent a 90-degree change. This will develop the ME AV SAX view with the cusps of the AV clearly seen (Fig. 2.5; Video 2.5). Two-dimensional assessment includes the general morphology of the AV (tricuspid versus bicuspid) as well as calcifications and mobility of the aortic leaflets. Color flow Doppler allows interrogation for aortic regurgitation. Again, the perpendicular orientation of the AV precludes spectral Doppler interrogation. Lastly, the interatrial septum can

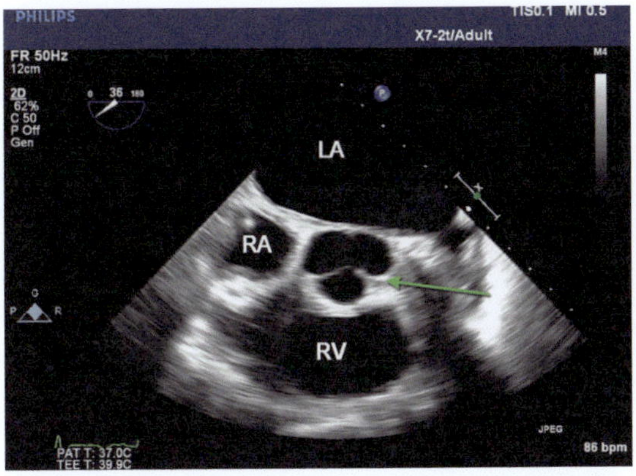

Fig. 2.5 ME AV SAX view with a *green arrow* indicating the aortic valve in short axis. *LA* left atrium, *RA* right atrium, *RV* right ventricle

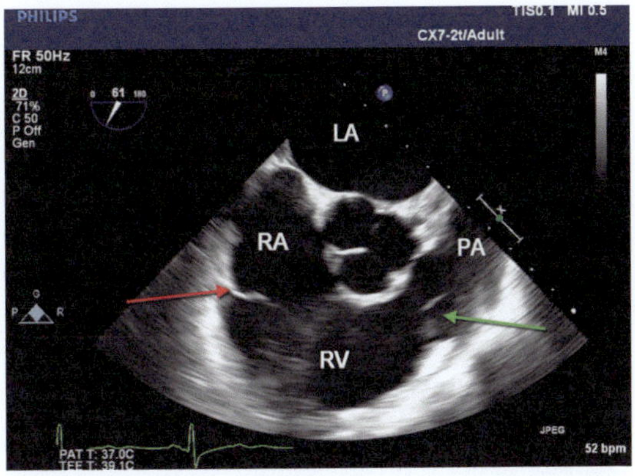

Fig. 2.6 ME RV inflow-outflow view with a *red arrow* indicating the tricuspid valve and a *green arrow* indicating the pulmonic valve. *LA* left atrium, *RA* right atrium, *RV* right ventricle, *PA* pulmonary artery

be identified proximal to the AV and can be evaluated for an atrial septal defect (ASD) or a patent foramen ovale (PFO).

ME RV Inflow-Outflow View

The initial views focus primarily on the left side of the heart including LV, AV, and MV, while the next two views transition the focus to the right side of the heart. The far field of the ME AV SAX view demonstrates the right ventricle (anterior to the aortic valve). Often the RA and part of the tricuspid valve (TV) may be visualized. Maintaining the RA, TV, and RV in view on the left side of the screen and increasing the multiplane to 60–90 degrees will bring the right ventricular outflow tract (RVOT) and pulmonic valve (PV) into view on the right side of the screen, constituting the ME RV inflow-outflow view (Fig. 2.6; Video 2.6). While some of the AV may still be in view, the focus of this view is the RA, TV, RV, RVOT, PV, and the proximal pulmonary artery. The "wrapping around" nature of the right heart is demonstrated by seeing the RA, RV, and pulmonary artery come around anteriorly to the AV. Two-dimensional assessment includes RV size and function, TV and PV anatomy and motion, and the position of the interatrial septum (the septum will bow away from the chamber with higher pressure). Color flow Doppler assessment focuses on the TV and PV for regurgitation and stenosis as well as the interatrial septum for a PFO or an ASD. Spectral Doppler interrogation

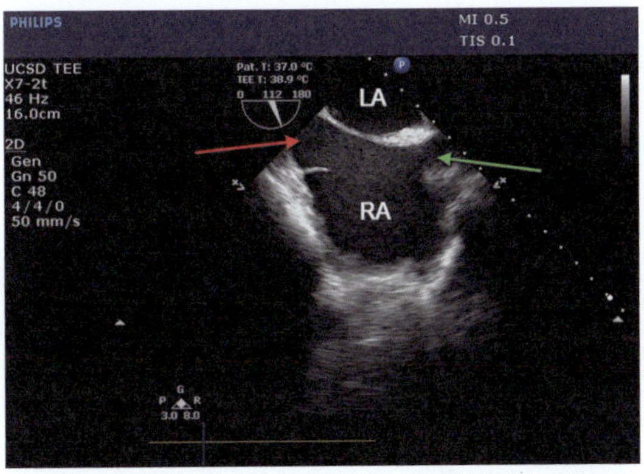

Fig. 2.7 ME bicaval view with a *red arrow* indicating the inferior vena cava and a *green arrow* indicating the superior vena cava. *LA* left atrium, *RA* right atrium

of the TV may prove helpful in estimating PA pressure (see Chaps. 4 and 10).

ME Bicaval View

The ME bicaval view is obtained by rotating the multiplane angle to 90–110 degrees and physically turning the probe clockwise. As a mid-esophageal view, the left atrium remains closest to the probe (apex of the imaging window); however, turning the probe clockwise moves the interatrial septum into the center of the image and the right atrium into the far field. The 90-degree orientation places the superior vena cava (SVC) on the right and the inferior vena cava (IVC) on the left of the RA (Fig. 2.7; Video

2.7). Two-dimensional assessment focuses on atrial size, interatrial septum competency and direction (the septum bows away from the chamber with higher pressure), and anatomical variants (see Chap. 16). Additionally, the ME bicaval view can aid in the placement of central venous catheters by observing the initial wire placement in the RA (see Chap. 23). Color flow Doppler interrogation aids in detection of an ASD or a PFO. An agitated saline study may also be utilized in this view to demonstrate a PFO. Spectral Doppler is not typically employed in a ME bicaval view.

ME Ascending Aortic SAX and LAX Views

Returning the multiplane to 0 degrees (approximately at the depth of the ME four-chamber view) and then withdrawing the probe allow the development of the ME ascending aortic SAX view which provides images of the proximal ascending aorta and bifurcation of the main pulmonary artery. Slight anteflexion of the probe and rotation of the multiplane angle from 0 to 45 degrees may be necessary to optimize the image (Fig. 2.8; Video 2.8). The right pulmonary artery in this view lies immediately posterior to the proximal ascending aorta in a long-axis orientation. The left pulmonary artery is typically not well visualized due to the interposed air-filled left main bronchus. Two-dimensional assessment is utilized for identification of aneurysms, plaque, and dissections of the ascending aorta as well as for identifying thrombus in the main or right pulmonary artery. Color flow Doppler may be helpful in the setting of aortic dissection (see Chap. 13). Spectral Doppler is often not employed in this view during a basic examination.

To obtain the ME ascending aortic LAX view, the aorta is centered in the image, and the multiplane angle is rotated to approximately 90 degrees until the right pulmonary artery is seen in the short axis, while the ascending aorta is seen in the long axis (Fig. 2.9; Video 2.9). Similarly, two-dimensional assessment is utilized for identifications of aneurysms, plaque, and dissections of the ascending aorta as well as for identifying thrombus in the right pulmonary artery. Color flow Doppler may be helpful in the setting of aortic dissection, while spectral Doppler is often not employed in this view during a basic examination.

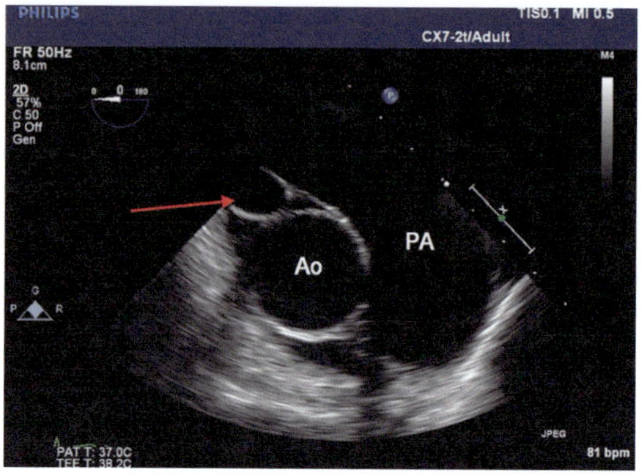

Fig. 2.8 ME ascending aortic SAX view with a *red arrow* indicating the superior vena cava. *Ao* ascending aorta, *PA* pulmonary artery

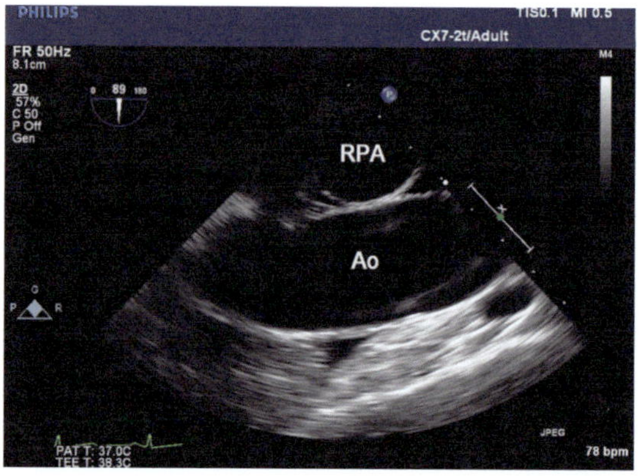

Fig. 2.9 ME ascending aortic LAX view. *Ao* ascending aorta, *RPA* right pulmonary artery

Descending Aortic SAX and LAX Views

To obtain the descending aortic SAX view, the probe is returned to the ME four-chamber view at 0 degrees and turned physically counterclockwise until the circular-shaped descending aorta appears in the apex of the image display. To enlarge and optimize the image, the image depth is decreased and the focus moved to the near field (Fig. 2.10; Video 2.10). The probe can then be withdrawn and

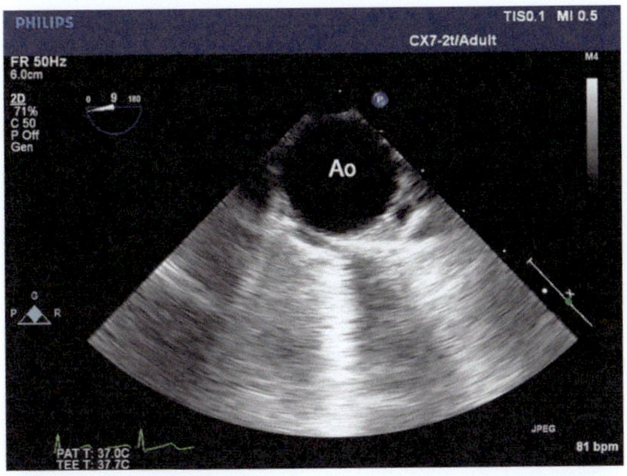

Fig. 2.10 Descending aortic SAX view. *Ao* descending aorta

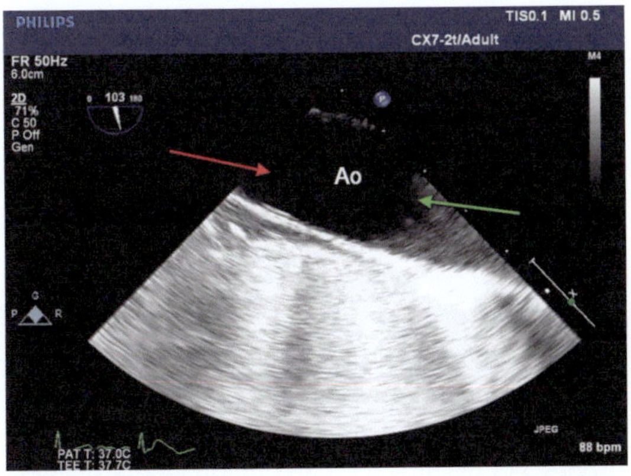

Fig. 2.11 Descending aortic LAX view. The *green arrow* indicates proximal, while the *red arrow* indicates distal aortic segments. *Ao* descending aorta

advanced, imaging the entire descending aorta in short axis. The probe will need to be slightly turned to the left or right as the probe is withdrawn and advanced to maintain the descending aorta in the center of the image. The aortic arch is reached when the aorta appears elongated at the apex of image display (see "Additional Views" below). At any point during the evaluation of the SAX of the descending aorta, the multiplane angle can be rotated to approximately 90 degrees to obtain the descending aortic LAX view (Fig. 2.11; Video 2.11). Two-dimensional assessment in these views includes aortic diameter, degree of atherosclerosis, and presence of a dissection. Color flow Doppler may be helpful in a dissection (see Chap. 13), while spectral Doppler of a descending aortic

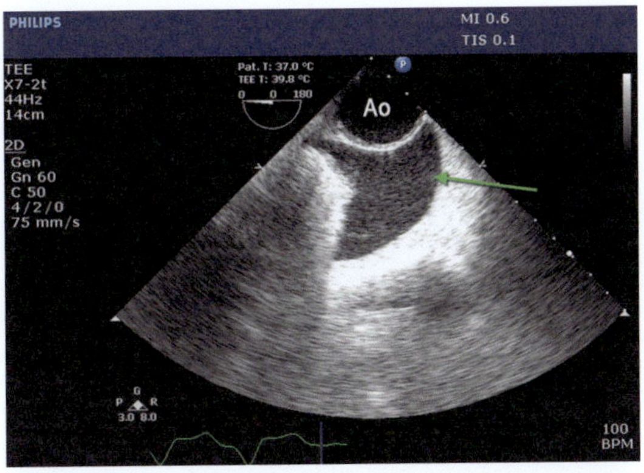

Fig. 2.12 Descending aortic SAX view with a left pleural effusion (*green arrow*). *Ao* descending aorta

LAX view may be helpful in assessing aortic valve regurgitation (see Chap. 9). In addition, the presence of a left pleural effusion (anterior to the descending aorta) can be identified in the descending aortic SAX view (Fig. 2.12; Video 2.12).

Additional Views

When added to the basic PTE exam, the following 17 additional views described below constitute a comprehensive TEE examination and are included for completeness. Again, the exact sequence of views is unimportant, while the comprehensiveness is the goal. The sequence of views described below and demonstrated in Table 2.2 is designed to acquire the views in quick succession with the least amount of probe manipulations between views. The sequence is organized into three major sections: transgastric views, midesophageal views, and aortic views. The transgastric and midesophageal views are subdivided such that left heart views are obtained followed by right heart views at each respective probe depth. Lastly, pulmonary vein views which occur in the transition between mid- and upper esophagus are placed in the exam between the transition from midesophageal to aortic views. These views can be challenging to obtain and may often be utilized in specific circumstances such as heart or lung transplantation. This organized approach to the exam reduces the time for acquisition as well as ensures completeness.

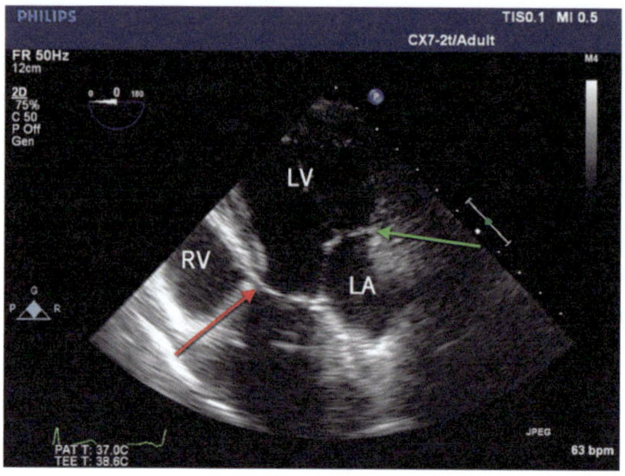

Fig. 2.13 Deep TG five-chamber view. The *green arrow* denotes the mitral valve, while the *red arrow* indicates the aortic valve. *LA* left atrium, *LV* left ventricle, *RV* right ventricle

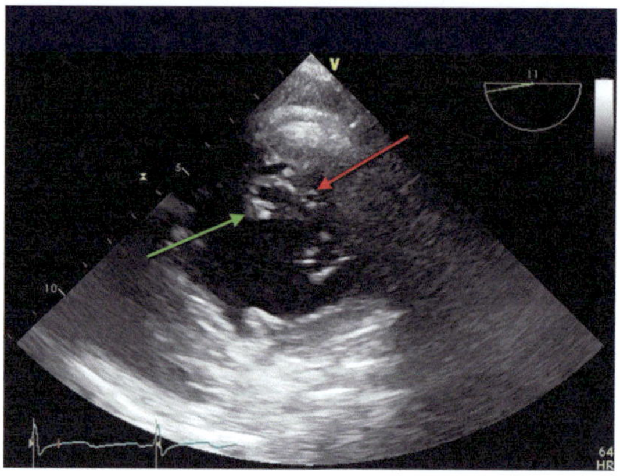

Fig. 2.14 TG basal SAX view with the *green arrow* indicating the edge of the anterior mitral valve leaflet and the *red arrow* indicating the posterior mitral valve leaflet

Deep TG Five-Chamber View

The examination begins with the deepest insertion of the probe. With the multiplane angle at 0 degrees, the probe is advanced deep into the stomach until an image disappears on the screen correlating with the probe "free-floating" in the stomach cavity. While anteflexed and left-flexed, the probe is slowly withdrawn until the deep TG five-chamber view is imaged (Fig. 2.13; Video 2.13). In this view, the LVOT and aortic valve are aligned parallel with the ultrasound beam. This parallel orientation allows for optimal spectral Doppler interrogation. Slow turning of the probe to the left or right or small multiplane increases may be needed for proper alignment. Two-dimensional interrogation focuses on the LV apex (at the apex of the image sector), the mitral and aortic valves, as well as the ventricular walls. Color flow Doppler interrogation focuses on the MV and AV. Spectral Doppler interrogation includes pulsed-wave Doppler evaluation of the LVOT as well as continuous-wave Doppler evaluation of the AV. This information will be helpful in determining aortic valve gradients, aortic valve area, and cardiac output (see Chap. 4).

TG Basal SAX View

Release of the left and anteflexion while withdrawing the probe until the left ventricle is visualized at the apex of the imaging sector allows development of additional transgastric level views. After visualization of the TG midpapillary SAX view as described above, the TG basal SAX view can be imaged through a combination of withdrawal of the probe and anteflexion. Withdrawal of the probe allows the development of the posterior portion of the mitral valve, while adjusting the anteflexion allows the development of the anterior portion of the mitral valve. A proper TG basal SAX view involves the viewing the mitral valve en face in a "fish mouth" perspective (Fig. 2.14; Video 2.14). This view can be used to evaluate calcifications of the mitral valve and estimate mitral valve area using planimetry for 2D assessment as well as localizing regurgitation using CFD (see Chap. 8). Additionally, the view allows evaluation for wall motion abnormalities at the basal ventricular level.

TG Apical SAX View

While the previous view involved withdrawing the probe above the TG midpapillary SAX view, the TG apical SAX view involves inserting the probe and utilizing anteflexion to obtain a cross section of the LV below papillary muscle insertion (Fig. 2.15; Video 2.15). Two-dimensional assessment is focused on wall motion of the apical ventricular segments. Color flow Doppler and spectral Doppler are not employed in this view.

TG Two-Chamber View

After returning to the TG midpapillary SAX view, the left ventricle is centered, and the multiplane angle is rotated to approximately 90 to 110 degrees to obtain the TG two-chamber view (Fig. 2.16; Video 2.16). This view provides a lengthwise view of the LV for evaluation of regional wall motion abnormalities of the basal, mid, and apical segments of the anterior and inferior walls. While CFD can be utilized on the mitral valve, its perpendicular orientation is suboptimal for Doppler interrogation.

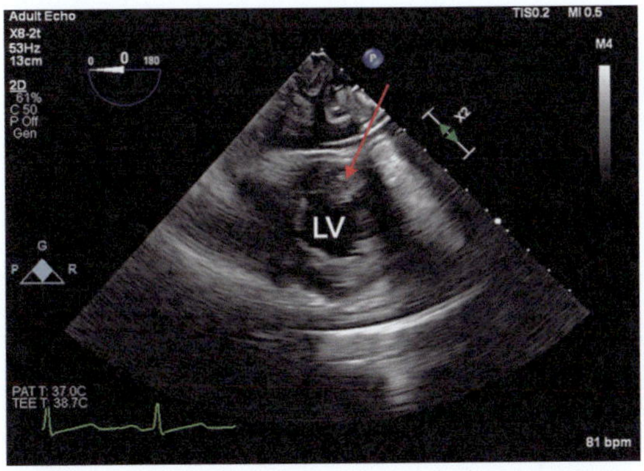

Fig. 2.15 TG apical SAX view with a *red arrow* indicating the insertion point of the posteromedial papillary muscle. *LV* left ventricle

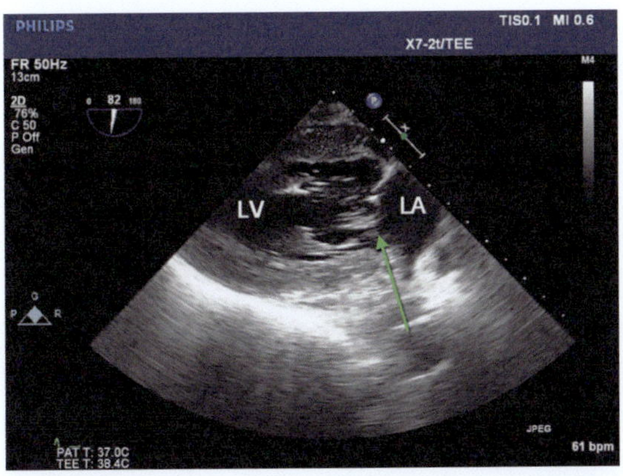

Fig. 2.16 TG two-chamber view with a *green arrow* indicating the mitral valve. Note the papillary muscles and chordae attached to the mitral valve. *LA* left atrium, *LV* left ventricle

TG LAX View

From the TG two-chamber view, the multiplane angle is rotated further to approximately 120 to 140 degrees until the LVOT and aortic valve come into view at the 4 o'clock position (Fig. 2.17; Video 2.17). In addition to the deep TG LAX view (see above), this view is useful for CFD and spectral Doppler interrogation of the LVOT and aortic valve. The TG LAX view serves as a second opportunity when the deep TG LAX proves difficult to obtain parallel alignment to the LVOT and aortic valve for Doppler interrogation.

TG RV Basal View

Returning the multiplane to zero degrees at the TG midpapillary SAX levels resets the echocardiographer to begin to examine the right-sided transgastric views. Turning the probe clockwise will center the RV on the screen, while small degrees of anteflexion and withdrawal of the probe will develop the tricuspid valve in short axis analogous to the TG basal SAX view of the mitral valve (Fig. 2.18; Video 2.18). The TG RV basal view allows evaluation of RV free wall and septal function, while CFD can be utilized to localize tricuspid regurgitation. With increased levels of anteflexion, the right ventricular outflow tract will come into view often with parallel

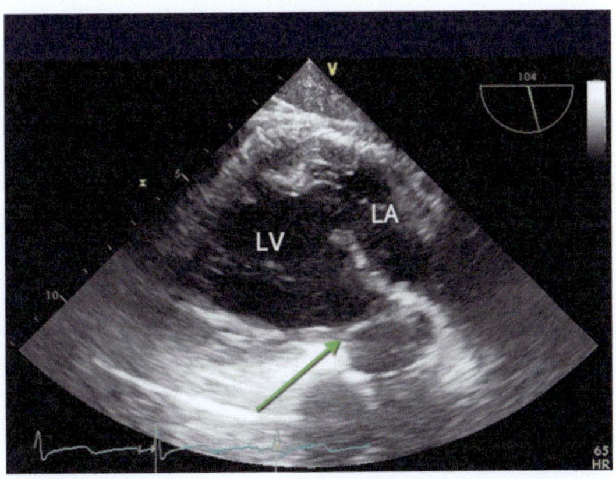

Fig. 2.17 TG LAX view with a *green arrow* indicating the aortic valve. *LA* left atrium, *LV* left ventricle

alignment permitting spectral Doppler interrogation of the RVOT and pulmonic valve.

TG RV Inflow-Outflow View

From the TG RV basal view, inserting the probe with anteflexion and right flexion (akin to obtaining the deep TG five-chamber view however with right flexion instead of left flexion) will develop the TG RV inflow-outflow view with the right atrium and tricuspid valve on the left side of the screen, the RV nearest to the probe and the RVOT and pulmonic valve to the right side of the screen (Fig. 2.19; Video 2.19). Two-dimensional evaluation focuses on RV free wall motion as well as valvular leaflet motion of the tricuspid and pulmonic valves. Color flow Doppler may be employed on the tricuspid and pulmonic valves, while spectral Doppler may be utilized on the TV, RVOT, and PV.

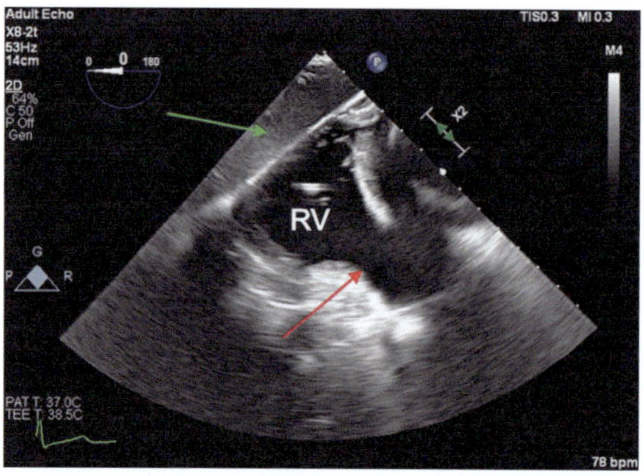

Fig. 2.18 TG RV basal view with a *red arrow* indicating the right ventricular outflow tract and a *green arrow* indicating the liver. *RV* right ventricle

TG RV Inflow View

Returning to the TG RV basal view, the probe is turned slightly clockwise until the RV is in the center of the image sector and the multiplane angle subsequently advanced to 90 to 110 degrees until the TG RV inflow view is seen (Fig. 2.20; Video 2.20). This view can be used to evaluate the function and thickness of the RV free wall as well as tricuspid valve leaflet motion. While CFD can be utilized on the tricuspid valve, its perpendicular orientation is suboptimal for Doppler interrogation.

ME Five-Chamber View

Transitioning to the esophageal views, the multiplane is returned to zero degrees and the probe withdrawn until the left atrium is noted nearest to the probe at the apex of the imaging sector. This probe position should develop the ME four-chamber view as described previously. The aortic valve is an anterior structure; therefore, either anteflexion or withdrawal of the probe will

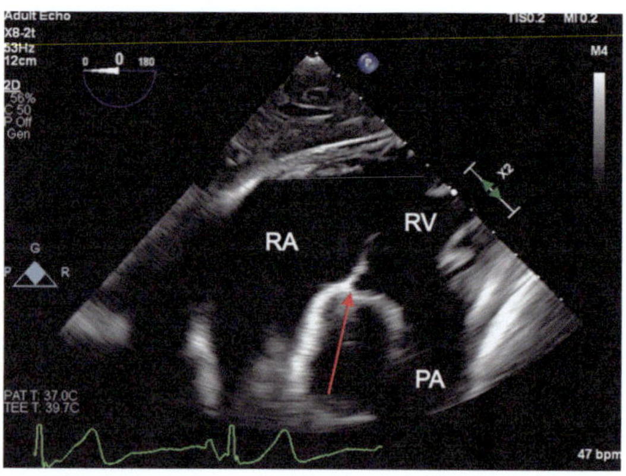

Fig. 2.19 TG RV inflow-outflow view with a *red arrow* indicating the tricuspid valve. *RA* right atrium, *RV* right ventricle, *PA* pulmonary artery

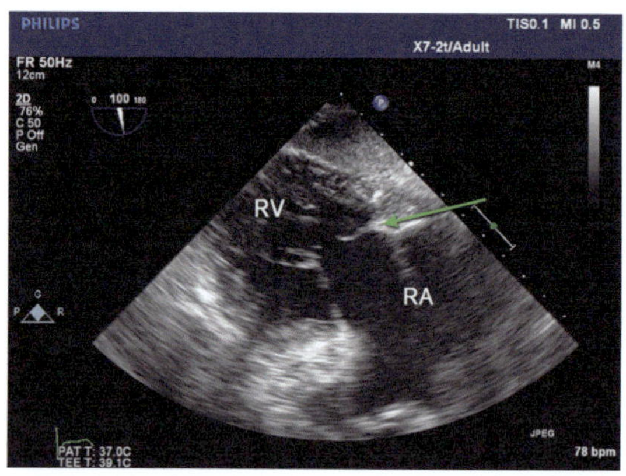

Fig. 2.20 TG RV inflow view. The *green arrow* indicates the tricuspid valve. *RA* right atrium, *RV* right ventricle

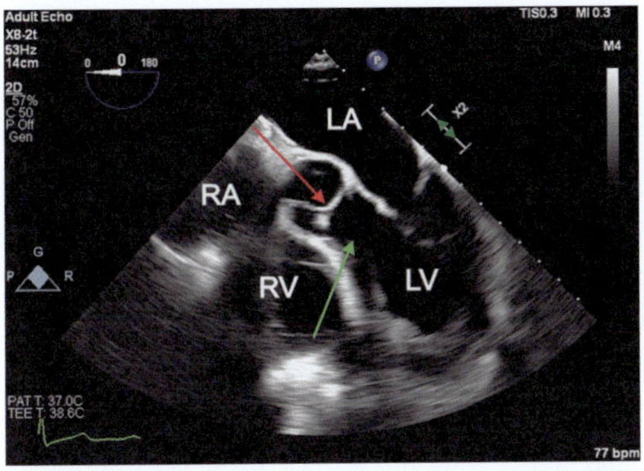

Fig. 2.21 ME five-chamber view. The *red arrow* indicates the aortic valve, and the *green arrow* indicates the left ventricular outflow tract. *RA* right atrium, *RV* right ventricle, *LA* left atrium, *LV* left ventricle

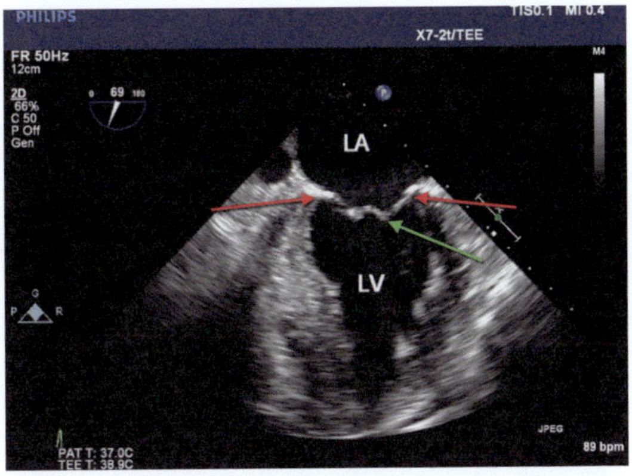

Fig. 2.22 ME mitral commissural view. The *red arrows* indicate the posterior mitral valve leaflet, while the *green arrow* indicates the anterior mitral valve leaflet. *LA* left atrium, *LV* left ventricle

develop the ME five-chamber view where the left ventricular outflow tract and aortic valve will be developed on the left side of the imaging sector (Fig. 2.21; Video 2.21). This view offers similar interrogation as the ME four-chamber view of the left ventricle for function and regional wall motion as well as the mitral valve. Additionally, the interaction of the anterior mitral valve and the left ventricular outflow tract can be observed. Color flow Doppler of the mitral and aortic valves may be employed, while the lack of parallel orientation precludes spectral Doppler interrogation of the aortic valve.

ME Mitral Commissural View

Returning to the ME four-chamber view with the mitral valve positioned in the center of the image, the multiplane angle is rotated to approximately 60 degrees to obtain the ME mitral commissural view. As the coaptation line of the MV is curved ("smile shaped"), the ME mitral commissural view will image through the coaptation line twice, giving the appearance of a posterior leaflet on the left and right with a central anterior leaflet portion. This view is helpful in evaluating the location of mitral valve pathology given that multiple scallops (P3-A2-P1) of the mitral valve can be seen (see Chap. 8). Other structures that can be seen include papillary muscles, chordae tendineae, and the coronary sinus (Fig. 2.22; Video 2.22). This view generally involves a 2D assessment of MV leaflet motion as well CFD for localizing regurgitation.

ME Left Atrial Appendage View

After increasing the multiplane to 90–110 degrees to develop the ME two-chamber view as described above, the left atrial appendage should be interrogated with closer inspection. This involves reducing the depth from the ME two-chamber view and a slight counterclockwise turning of the probe to center the LAA, resulting in the ME left atrial appendage view (Fig. 2.23; Video 2.23). Interrogation involves two-dimensional, color flow Doppler, and spectral Doppler interrogation of the LAA.

ME AV LAX View

The examination sequence continues to 120–140 degrees to obtain the ME LAX view as described previously. The ME LAX view will have the aortic valve on the right side of the imaging sector. A slow withdrawal of the probe will move the aortic valve from the right side of the screen toward the center of the imaging sector. A slight clockwise turn of the probe is often necessary to maintain the AV in view, ultimately providing an AV that is perpendicular to the probe. In this view, the LVOT, aortic valve, sinus of Valsalva, sinotubular junction, and proximal ascending aorta should be visualized well (Fig. 2.24; Video 2.24). Compared to the ME LAX view, the ME AV LAX view allows better evaluation of aortic valve function both structurally and, with color flow Doppler, measurements of structures from the annulus to the proximal ascending aorta, as well as appreciation of atherosclerotic plaques and dissections. The perpendicular orientation of blood flow precludes spectral Doppler interrogation. The evaluation of midesophageal left heart structures finishes with the ME AV SAX view (as described above). With the AV in the center of the imaging sector in the ME AV LAX view, the multiplane is reduced by 90 degrees moving the AV from long axis to short axis.

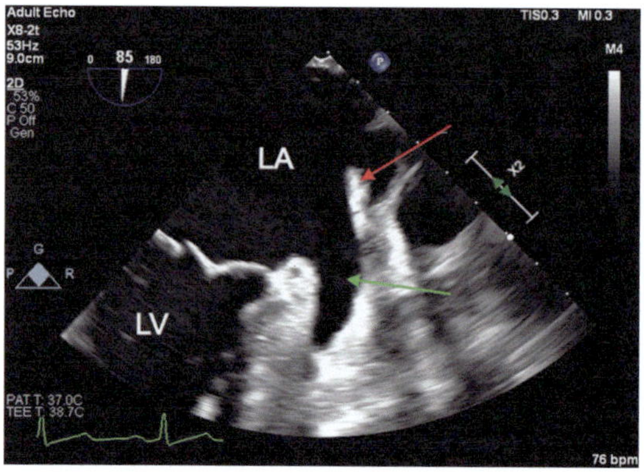

Fig. 2.23 ME left atrial appendage view with a *green arrow* indicating the left atrial appendage and a *red arrow* indicating the coumadin ridge (a normal finding). *LA* left atrium, *LV* left ventricle

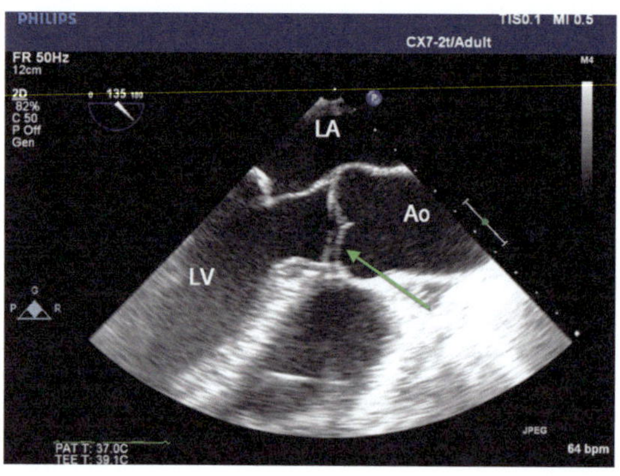

Fig. 2.24 ME AV LAX view with the aortic valve indicated by the *green arrow*. *LA* left atrium, *LV* left ventricle, *Ao* proximal ascending aorta

ME Modified Bicaval TV View

Transitioning the focus to right-sided midesophageal views, from the ME AV SAX, the multiplane is increased to 60–90 to obtain the ME RV inflow-outflow (as described above) and then increased to 90–110 to obtain the ME bicaval view (also described above). From the ME bicaval view, the multiplane is increased to 110–120 degrees while maintaining the superior vena cava on the right-hand side of the screen to obtain the ME modified bicaval TV view (Fig. 2.25; Video 2.25). This view replaces the inferior vena cava on the left-hand side of the screen with the TV at approximately the 7 o'clock position with the coronary sinus ostium adjacent to the TV annulus. Two-dimensional evaluation allows similar evaluation of the interatrial septum as the ME bicaval view; however, additional evaluation of the TV leaflet motion is possible. Tricuspid regurgitation is readily identifiable with CFD, and the orientation

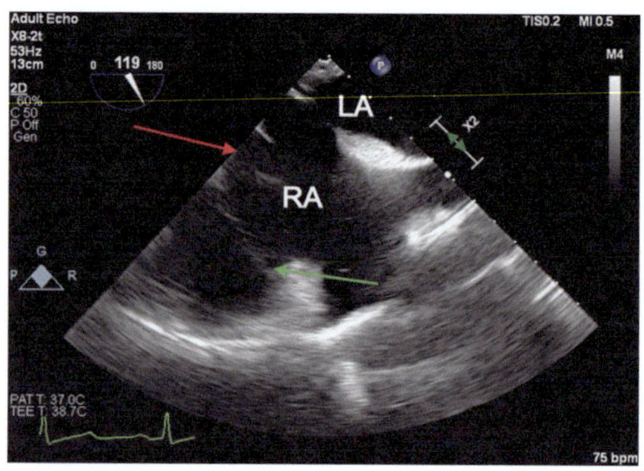

Fig. 2.25 ME modified bicaval TV view with a *green arrow* indicating the tricuspid valve and a *red arrow* indicating the ostium of the coronary sinus. *RA* right atrium, *LA* left atrium

of the jet toward the probe permits spectral Doppler interrogation and right ventricular systolic pressure estimation.

UE Right and Left Pulmonary Veins View

The pulmonary vein views are reserved for the end of the midesophageal views as they are obtained during the transition from midesophagus to upper esophagus. The UE right and left pulmonary vein view is a bit of a misnomer as no one view contains both right and left pulmonary veins. This is two separate views, one for the right and one for the left veins with both views obtained at 90 to 110 degrees of multiplane angle. From the ME bicaval view at 90–110 degrees, the probe is slowly withdrawn and slightly turned clockwise. The right upper pulmonary vein will come into view on the right-hand side of the screen and empty into the left atrium nearest the screen (Fig. 2.26; Video 2.26). From the ME LAA view also at 90–110 degrees, the probe is slowly withdrawn and slightly turned counterclockwise to reveal the left upper pulmonary vein immediately above the LAA and coumadin ridge (Fig. 2.27; Video 2.27). Identifying both the right and left pulmonary veins in these views can be aided by the addition of CFD. Additionally, spectral Doppler may be utilized to evaluate flow patterns in the veins as in evaluation of mitral regurgitation or diastology (see Chaps. 8 and 12).

ME Right Pulmonary Vein View

Returning the multiplane to the ME four-chamber view at 0 degrees, slowly withdrawing the probe, and turning slowly clockwise will develop an additional perspective of right-sided pulmonary veins, the ME right pulmonary vein view. As the probe is slowly withdrawn from the ME four-chamber view, the user will pass the ME five-chamber view and prior to encountering the ME ascending aorta short-axis view (as described above) will turn the probe rightward to identify the right pulmonary veins entering the left atrium (Fig. 2.28; Video 2.28). This view can be utilized to view both the right upper and right lower pul-

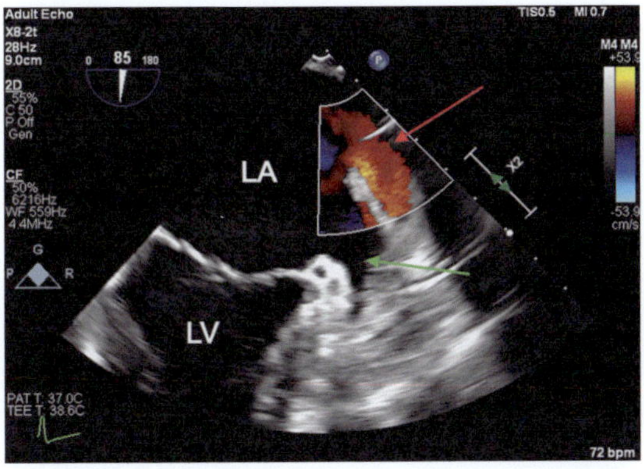

Fig. 2.27 UE left pulmonary vein view with a *red arrow* indicating the left upper pulmonary vein and a *green arrow* indicating the left atrial appendage. *LA* left atrium, *LV* left ventricle

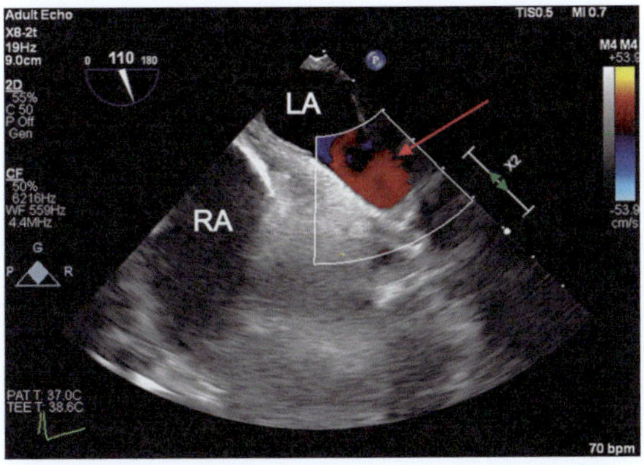

Fig. 2.26 UE right pulmonary vein view with a *red arrow* indicating the right upper pulmonary vein. *RA* right atrium, *LA* left atrium

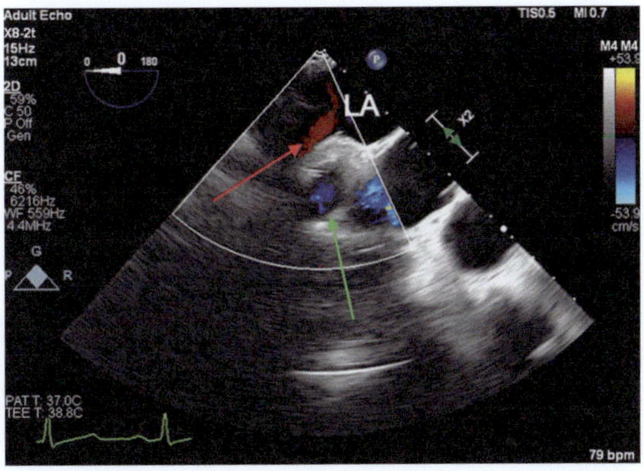

Fig. 2.28 ME right pulmonary vein view with a *red arrow* indicating the right pulmonary vein and a *green arrow* indicating the superior vena cava. *LA* left atrium

monary veins, with the right upper vein in a more parallel orientation for spectral Doppler interrogation. As described above, CFD can aid in identifying the pulmonary vein flow at its entrance to the left atrium.

Upper Esophageal (UE) Aortic Arch LAX and SAX Views

The remainder of the exam focuses on views of the three segments of the thoracic aorta: ascending, arch, and descending. As described above, withdrawal of the probe further from the pulmonary vein views will develop the ME ascending aortic SAX and LAX views at 0 and 90 degrees, respectively. While it is possible to further withdraw the probe to the arch level, the interposed trachea will impede visualization incurring the risk of withdrawing the probe from the patient. To safely visualize the arch without inadvertent probe removal, the descending aortic SAX view (as described above) is obtained by turning the probe counterclockwise. Once in view, the probe is slowly withdrawn and turned clockwise (to maintain the aorta in the center of the imaging sector) until the aorta begins to elongate. Once the aorta has elongated into an oval shape, the UE aortic arch LAX view has been developed (Fig. 2.29; Video 2.29). This view can be used to evaluate atherosclerotic plaques in the aortic arch as well as aneurysms and dissections. To obtain the UE aortic arch SAX view, the multiplane angle is rotated to 70 to 90 degrees. This places the aortic arch in a SAX view as well as brings the pulmonic valve and main pulmonary artery into view on the left-hand side of the screen. Because of the parallel alignment of the pulmonic valve and main pulmonary artery with the probe, Doppler interrogation of the pulmonary valve can be performed in this view. Other structures that can also be visualized include the left subclavian artery and the brachiocephalic vein (Fig. 2.30; Video 2.30). The exam concludes with following the descending aorta from the aortic arch to the diaphragm, providing both a short-axis and long-axis perspective. Below the diaphragm, the aorta dives into the retroperitoneum, while the probe enters the stomach, and visualization is difficult. At this depth, returning the probe clockwise to the patient's right with some anteflexion results in the TG midpapillary SAX view which serves as an excellent continuous monitoring view.

Conclusion

The individual views of the basic and comprehensive PTE exam are discussed above. Again, the performed order of the views is not essential.

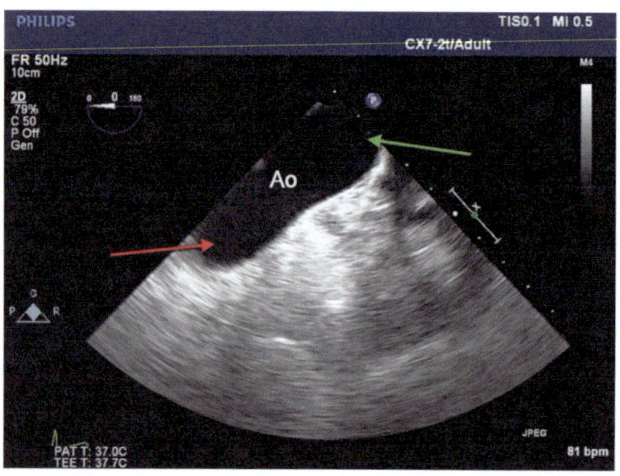

Fig. 2.29 UE aortic arch LAX view with a *green arrow* denoting the distal aortic arch (Ao) and a *red arrow* denoting the proximal aortic arch

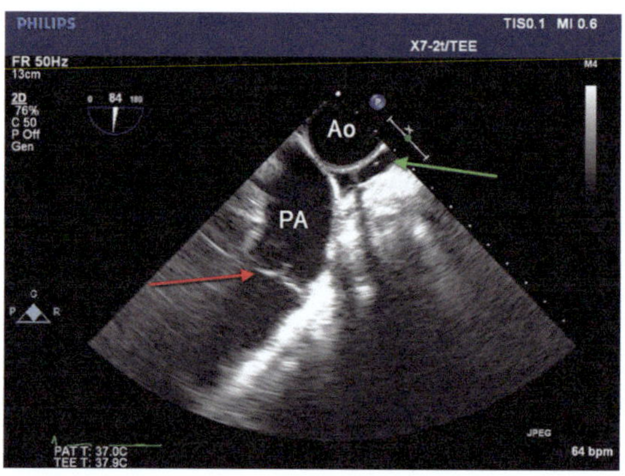

Fig. 2.30 UE aortic arch SAX view. The *red arrow* indicates the pulmonic valve, while the *green arrow* indicates the brachiocephalic vein. *PA* main pulmonary artery; *Ao* aortic arch

Developing a systematic approach to the order of the views as, well as modalities of interrogation, is important to develop a consistent approach to perioperative echocardiography. Tables 2.1 and 2.2 outline a suggested order of views for the basic and comprehensive PTE exams, respectively.

Questions

1. Which view allows evaluation of both atrioventricular valves as well as the septal and lateral walls of the LV?

   a. Midesophageal bicaval view
   b. Midesophageal four-chamber view
   c. Midesophageal two-chamber view
   d. Transgastric midpapillary view

2. Measurement of the left ventricular outflow tract and aortic valve annulus is best performed in which view?

   a. Midesophageal aortic valve short-axis view
   b. Deep transgastric five-chamber view
   c. Midesophageal aortic valve long-axis view
   d. Midesophageal two-chamber view

3. Doppler interrogation of the left ventricular outflow tract and aortic valve is best performed in which view?

   a. Upper esophageal aortic arch short-axis view
   b. Midesophageal long-axis view
   c. Deep transgastric five-chamber view
   d. Transgastric two-chamber view

4. Doppler interrogation of the pulmonic valve is best performed in which view?

   a. Upper esophageal aortic arch long-axis view
   b. Upper esophageal aortic arch short-axis view
   c. Midesophageal right ventricular inflow-outflow view
   d. Midesophageal aortic valve short-axis view

5. Which view allows evaluation of left ventricular territories supplied by all three coronary arteries?

   a. Transgastric midpapillary short-axis view
   b. Transgastric two-chamber view
   c. Midesophageal four-chamber view
   d. Midesophageal two-chamber view

6. Which view(s) can be helpful in the echocardiographic guidance of pulmonary artery catheter placement?

   a. Midesophageal modified bicaval tricuspid valve view
   b. Midesophageal right ventricular inflow-outflow view
   c. Midesophageal ascending aortic short-axis view
   d. All of the above

7. Which view gives the "fish mouth" appearance of the mitral valve?

   a. Transgastric basal short-axis view
   b. Transgastric midpapillary short-axis view
   c. Transgastric right ventricular inflow view
   d. Transgastric long-axis view

8. What is the difference between the midesophageal long-axis view compared to the midesphageal aortic valve long-axis view?

   a. Visualization of the left ventricular apex
   b. Visualization of the mitral valve
   c. Visualization of the aortic valve
   d. Visualization of the left atrium

9. Which view is useful for detection of an interatrial septal defect?

   a. Midesophageal mitral commisural view
   b. Midesophageal bicaval view

c. Transgastric midpapillary short-axis view
d. Transgastric two-chamber view

10. Which walls of the left ventricle can be evaluated in the midesophageal long-axis view?

    a. Anterior and lateral walls
    b. Anteroseptal and inferolateral walls
    c. Anterolateral and inferoseptal walls
    d. Lateral and septal walls

References

1. Reeves ST, Finley AC, Skubas NJ, Swaminathan M, Whitley WS, Glas KE, et al. Basic perioperative transesophageal echocardiography examination: a consensus statement of the American Society of Echocardiography and the Society of Cardiovascular Anesthesiologists. J Am Soc Echocardiogr. 2013;26(5):443–56.
2. Shanewise JS, Cheung AT, Aronson S, Stewart WJ, Weiss RL, Mark JB, et al. ASE/SCA guidelines for performing a comprehensive intraoperative multiplane transesophageal echocardiography examination: recommendations of the American Society of Echocardiography Council for Intraoperative Echocardiography and the Society of Cardiovascular Anesthesiologists Task Force for Certification in Perioperative Transesophageal Echocardiography. J Am Soc Echocardiogr. 1999;12(10):884–900.
3. Hahn RT, Abraham T, Adams MS, Bruce CJ, Glas KE, Lang RM, et al. Guidelines for performing a comprehensive transesophageal echocardiographic examination: recommendations from the American Society of Echocardiography and the Society of Cardiovascular Anesthesiologists. J Am Soc Echocardiogr. 2013;26(9):921–64.

3 Point-of-Care Transthoracic Echocardiography: Probe Manipulation, Positioning, and Essential Views

Christopher R. Tainter and Sonia Nhieu

Abbreviations

TTE	Transthoracic echocardiography
ASE	American Society of Echocardiography
ACEP	American College of Emergency Physicians
LLD	Left lateral decubitus
LAX	Long-axis
LA	Left atrium
LV	Left ventricle
LVOT	Left ventricular outflow tract
RVOT	Right ventricular outflow tract
TEE	Transesophageal echocardiography
ME	Midesophageal
RV	Right ventricle
SAX	Short-axis
TG	Transgastric
PMI	Point of maximal impulse
TAPSE	Tricuspid annular plane systolic excursion
PEEP	Positive end-expiratory pressure
IVC	Inferior vena cava

Supplementary Information The online version of this chapter (https://doi.org/10.1007/978-3-030-84349-6_3) contains supplementary material, which is available to authorized users.

C. R. Tainter (✉)
Department of Anesthesiology, University of California San Diego Health, La Jolla, CA, USA

S. Nhieu
Department of Anesthesiology, Kaiser Permanente Santa Clara Medical Center, Santa Clara, CA, USA

Introduction

Point-of-care transthoracic echocardiography (TTE) is an increasingly employed, noninvasive diagnostic tool for cardiac evaluation, particularly with unstable patients. The American Society of Echocardiography (ASE) and American College of Emergency Physicians (ACEP) emphasize the important role of point-of-care TTE in patient care and its complementary role to comprehensive echocardiography [1].

The goal of this chapter is to provide an overview of how to acquire the basic TTE views, as well as discussion of additional views, which may provide supplementary information when necessary. Evaluating the hemodynamically unstable patient focuses on identifying gross abnormalities and answering goal-directed questions, allowing the clinician to implement appropriate interventions. Subtle findings are typically not the cause of significant hemodynamic disturbances, so an exhaustive evaluation is not necessary for initial management in most patients. A comprehensive echocardiographic evaluation may be indicated to follow up and/or confirm preliminary findings from a point-of-care exam.

T. M. Maus, C. R. Tainter (eds.), *Essential Echocardiography*,
https://doi.org/10.1007/978-3-030-84349-6_3

Probe Manipulation

To describe probe manipulation, it is useful to have a consistent nomenclature, as described in Chap. 1. The probe (and resultant two-dimensional imaging plane) may be moved in either a linear or radial manner along any of the three-dimensional axes, creating six possible movements. If we use a conventional X, Y, and Z Cartesian coordinate system, these movements can be described in terms of these axes (see Chap. 1, Figure 1.5) [2]. Linear movement along the X-axis is "sweeping," while rotational movement is "fanning." Linear translation along the Y-axis is called "sliding," while rotational movement along this axis is "rocking." And movement along the length of the probe, or the Z-axis, is "compressing," while rotating along this axis is "rotation."

In addition, it is useful to note that one side of the probe along the imaging plane (Y-axis) is marked with a reference point, the "indicator," or "probe marker." Again, there is some variation in the orientation of this marker, but most commonly this corresponds with the top right corner of the imaging screen for echocardiographic examinations.

Positioning

When introducing TTE imaging into a practice, many practitioners may be discouraged by suboptimal image resolution. For a practitioner familiar with transesophageal imaging, the echocardiographer can rest assured that the ultrasound physics, cardiac structures, and cardiac physiology are unchanged. Adjustments to the machine or position changes can be helpful to improve resolution, but even with imperfect visualization, many important clinical questions can be answered. Commonly, not every piece of information is available from every view, but the visualization of structures from different views may still be able to answer the question at hand.

Unlike transesophageal imaging, where the esophagus remains near the heart despite patient position or respiration, transthoracic imaging requires interaction with the patient for optimal views. The optimal patient position for transthoracic imaging depends upon the specific imaging window and desired view and may be slightly different from patient to patient. Parasternal and apically located views often utilize the left lateral decubitus (LLD) position with the patient's left arm extended above the head. The purpose of this position is to bring the heart closer to the chest wall, as it displaces the lingula of the left lower lobe of the lung due to gravity. Raising the left arm also widens the intercostal spaces, decreasing shadowing from the ribs. However, this position is not always feasible, especially in the critically ill or perioperative patients.

Subcostal views often benefit from the patient remaining supine and therefore offer an alternative window in patients who are unable to be turned to a LLD position. Inspiration, or holding an inspired breath, may help visualization from the subcostal position, as the expansion of the lungs may help move the heart toward the transducer. In contrast, inspiration often obscures a parasternal window, as aerated lung tissue may reflect the ultrasound signal. Therefore, in addition to appropriate positioning, timing of ventilation or patient breath-holding can be manipulated to facilitate image optimization. Fortunately, in many cases, similar information may be obtained from different views, so it may not be necessary to have perfect visualization from every view to answer important clinical questions.

Essential TTE Views (Table 3.1)

Parasternal Long-Axis (LAX) View

The basic TTE examination generally begins with the parasternal long-axis view and proceeds in a clockwise fashion (Chap. 1, Fig. 1.4). With the ultrasound probe indicator pointing toward the patient's right shoulder, the transducer is placed in the second or third intercostal space just lateral to the left sternal border (Fig. 3.1). This view is often one of the easiest to obtain and simultaneously provides a significant amount of information. Structures that are seen from this view include the left atrium (LA), left ventricle

Table 3.1 Point-of-care transthoracic echocardiography views

Image order	Image name	Image example	2D > CFD > spectral
1	PS LAX	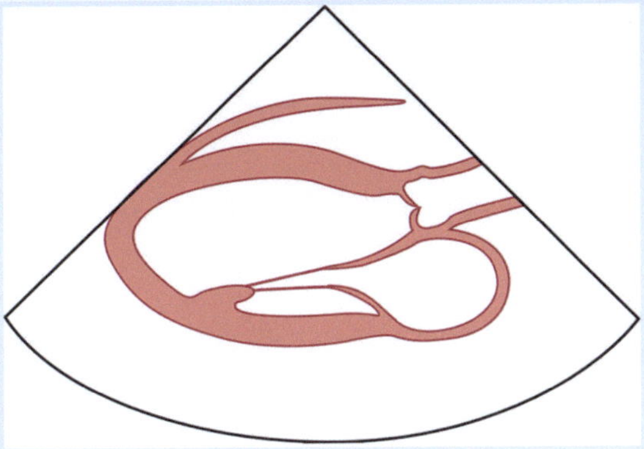	<u>2D</u> Chamber sizes: **LA/ LV/LVOT/AV/Ao/ RVOT** Systolic function: **LV** Ischemia detection: **AntSept/InfLat LV** Valvular anatomy/ motion: **MV/AV** <u>*CFD*</u> Valvular pathology: **MV/AV** <u>*Spectral*</u> Not typically utilized
2	PS RV inflow	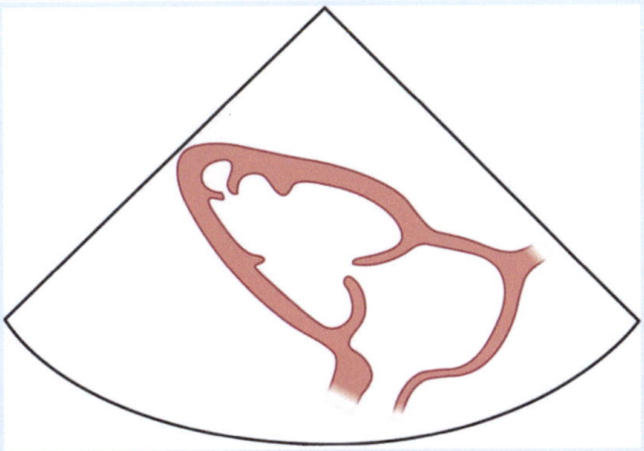	<u>2D</u> Chamber sizes: **RA/ RV** Valvular anatomy/ motion: **TV** <u>*CFD*</u> Valvular pathology: **TV** <u>*Spectral*</u> Inflow velocities: **TV** Estimating PASP: **TV**
3	PS SAX AV level	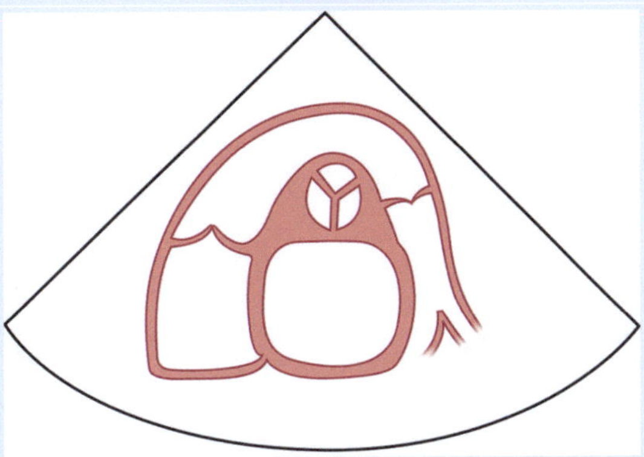	<u>2D</u> Chamber sizes: **LA/ RA/RV/PA** Valvular anatomy/ motion: **AV/TV/PV** <u>*CFD*</u> Valvular pathology: **AV/TV/PV** Interatrial septum: **ASD/PFO** <u>*Spectral*</u> Inflow velocities: **TV** Estimating PASP: **TV** Outflow velocities: **RVOT/PV**
4	PS SAX MV level	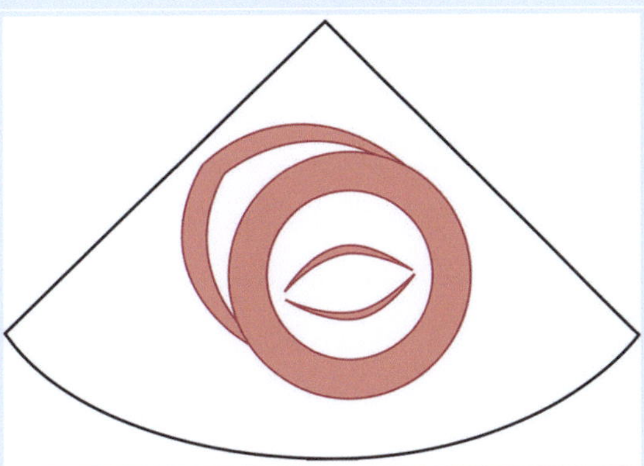	<u>2D</u> Chamber sizes: **LV/ RV** Systolic function: **LV** Ischemia detection: **basal segments** Valvular anatomy/ motion: **MV** <u>*CFD*</u> Valvular pathology: **MV** <u>*Spectral*</u> Not typically utilized

(continued)

Table 3.1 (continued)

Image order	Image name	Image example	2D > CFD > spectral
5	PS SAX midpapillary level	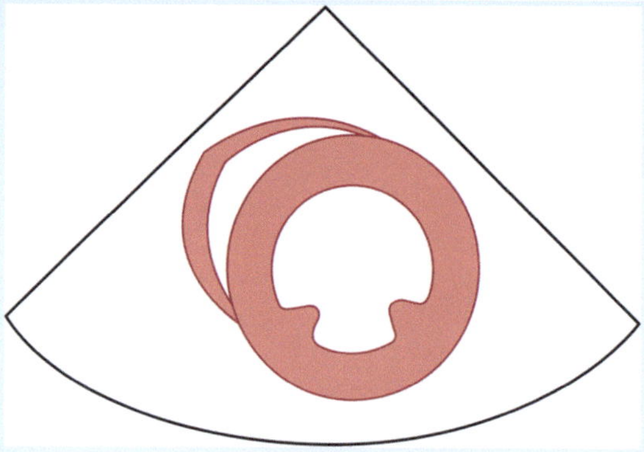	_2D_ Chamber sizes: **LV/RV** Systolic function: **LV** Ischemia detection: **midpapillary segments** _CFD_ Not typically utilized _Spectral_ Not typically utilized
6	PS SAX apical level	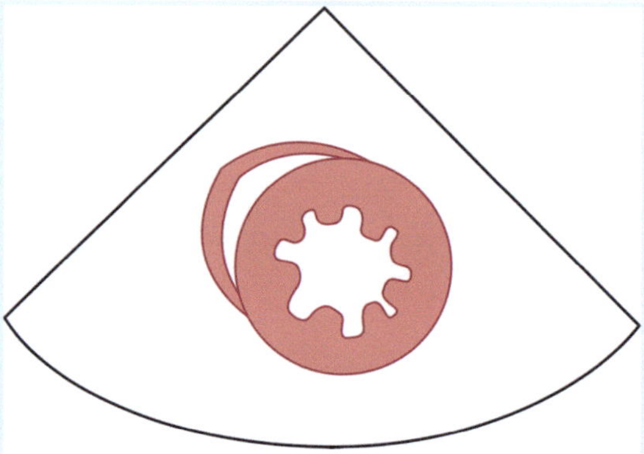	_2D_ Chamber sizes: **LV/RV** Systolic function: **LV** Ischemia detection: **apical segments** _CFD_ Not typically utilized _Spectral_ Not typically utilized
7	Apical four-chamber	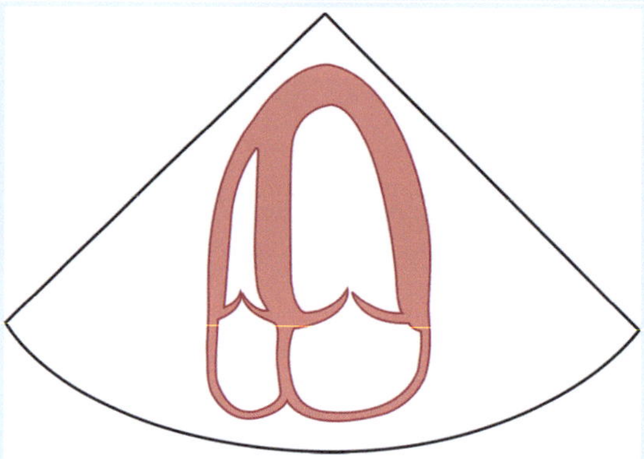	_2D_ Chamber sizes: **RA/LA/RV/LV** Systolic function: **RV/LV** Ischemia detection: **RV/LV** Valvular anatomy/motion: **TV/MV** _CFD_ Valvular pathology: **TV/MV** Interatrial septum: **PFO/ASD** _Spectral_ Inflow velocities: **TV/MV** Estimating PASP: **TV**

Table 3.1 (continued)

Image order	Image name	Image example	2D > CFD > spectral
8	Apical five-chamber	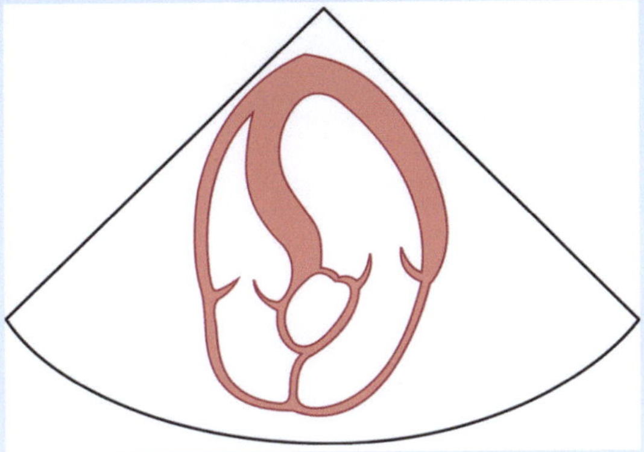	*2D* Chamber sizes: **RA/LA/RV/LV** Systolic function: **RV/LV** Ischemia detection: **RV/LV** Valvular anatomy/motion: **TV/MV/AV** *CFD* Valvular pathology: **TV/MV/AV** Interatrial septum: **PFO/ASD** *Spectral*
			Inflow velocities: **TV/MV** Outflow velocities: **LVOT/AV**
9	Apical two-chamber	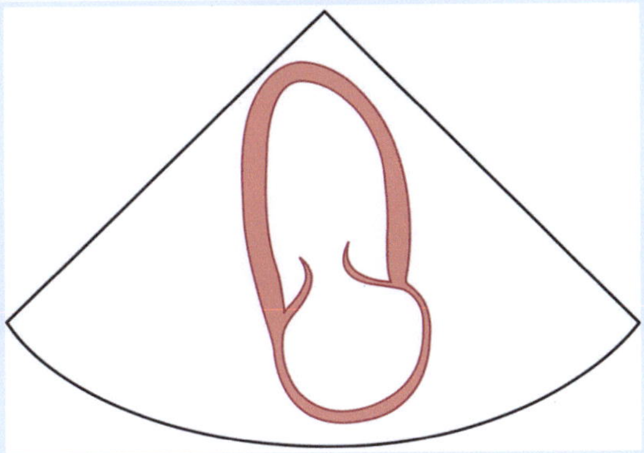	*2D* Chamber sizes: **LA/LV** Systolic function: **LV** Ischemia detection: **anterior/inferior LV** Valvular anatomy/motion: **MV** *CFD* Valvular pathology: **MV** *Spectral* Inflow velocities: **MV**
10	Apical LAX	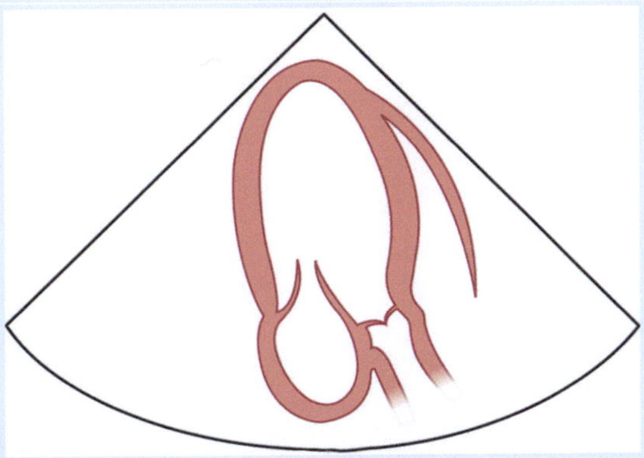	*2D* Chamber sizes: **LA/LV** Systolic function: **LV** Ischemia detection: **AntSept/InfLat LV** Valvular anatomy/motion: **AV/MV** *CFD* Valvular pathology: **AV/MV** *Spectral* Inflow velocities: **MV** Outflow velocities: **LVOT/AV**

(continued)

Table 3.1 (continued)

Image order	Image name	Image example	2D > CFD > spectral
11	Subcostal four-chamber	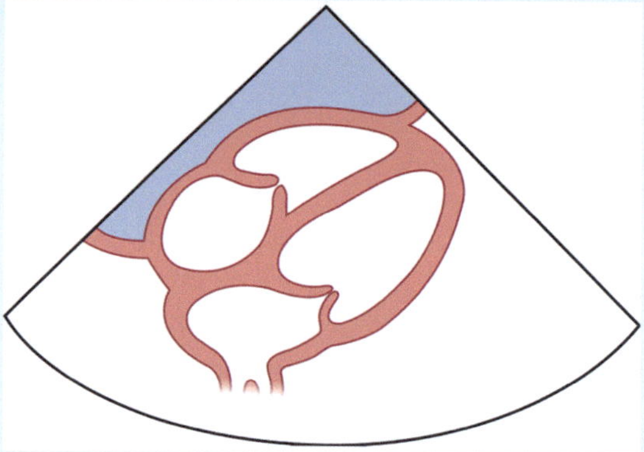	_2D_ Chamber sizes: **RA/ LA/RV/LV** Systolic function: **RV/ LV** Ischemia detection: **RV/LV** Valvular anatomy/ motion: **TV/MV** _CFD_ Valvular pathology: **TV/MV** Interatrial septum: **PFO/ASD** _Spectral_ Not typically utilized
12	Subcostal long-axis IVC	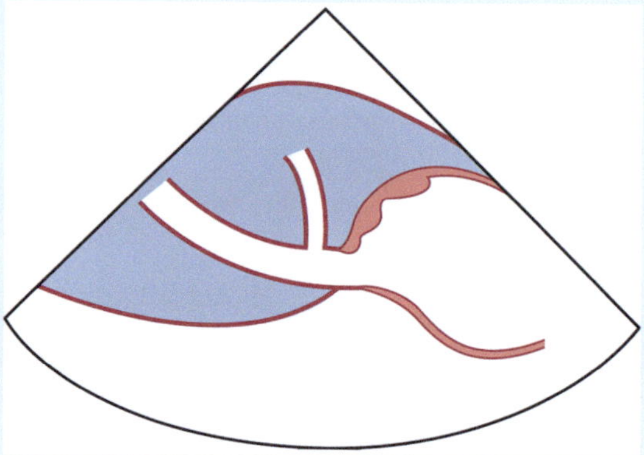	_2D_ Chamber sizes: **RA** Anatomy: **IVC size and collapsibility** _CFD_ Flow pattern: **IVC/ hepatic vein** _Spectral_ Inflow pattern: **hepatic vein flow**
13	Suprasternal	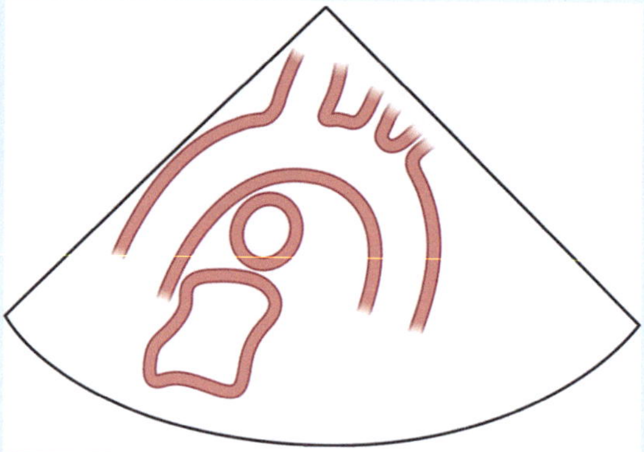	_2D_ Vessel sizes: **Ao, BC, LCA, LSC** Anatomy: **Ao, BC, LCA, LSC** _CFD_ Flow pattern: **Ao, BC, LCA, LSC** _Spectral_ Flow pattern: **Ao, BC, LCA, LSC**

Abbreviations: PS parasternal, *LAX* long-axis, *2D* two dimensional, *CFD* color flow Doppler, *LA* left atrium, *LV* left ventricle, *LVOT* left ventricular outflow tract, *AV* aortic valve, *Ao* Aorta, *RVOT* right ventricular outflow tract, *AntSept* anteroseptal wall, *InfLat* inferolateral wall, *MV* mitral valve, *RV* right ventricle, *TV* tricuspid valve, *SAX* short-axis, *PV* pulmonic valve, *ASD* atrial septal defect, *PFO* patent foramen ovale, *IVC* inferior vena cava, *BC* brachiocephalic artery, *LCA* left carotid artery, *LSC* left subclavian artery

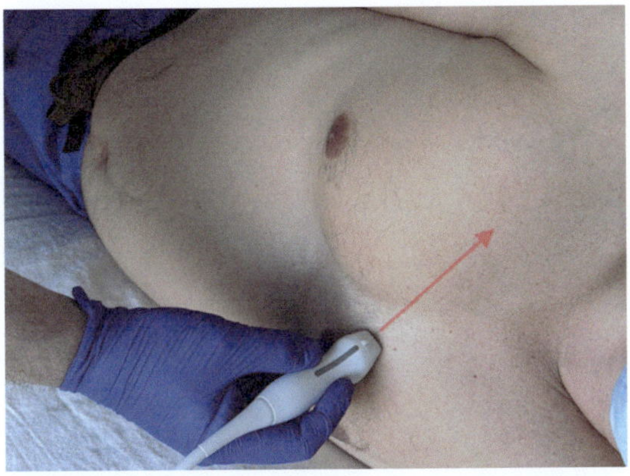

Fig. 3.1 Parasternal LAX probe position shown for a supine patient. The patient is turned to the left lateral decubitus position to optimize the viewing window. The probe is placed in the third intercostal space lateral to the sternum with the indicator pointed toward the patient's right shoulder

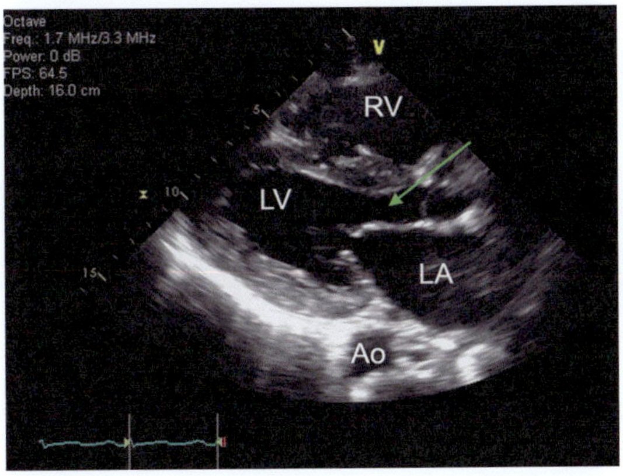

Fig. 3.2 Parasternal LAX view. *LA* left atrium, *LV* left ventricle, *green arrow* left ventricular outflow tract, *RV* right ventricle, *Ao* descending aorta

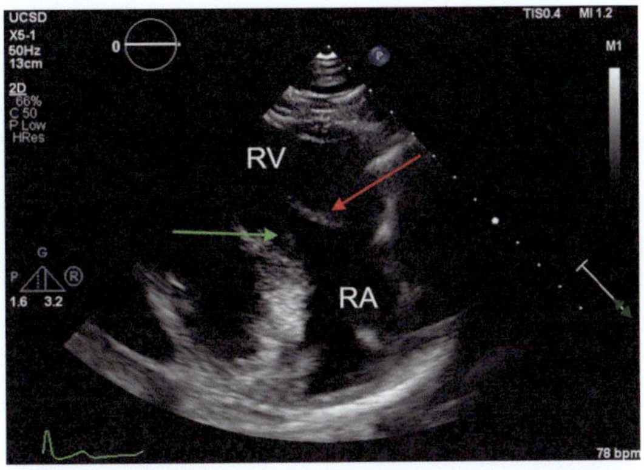

Fig. 3.3 RV inflow view. *RA* right atrium, *green arrow* posterior leaflet of the tricuspid valve, *red arrow* anterior leaflet of the tricuspid valve, *RV* right ventricle

(LV), left ventricular outflow tract (LVOT), right ventricular outflow tract (RVOT), the mitral and aortic valves, and the proximal ascending aorta (Fig. 3.2; Video 3.1). The descending aorta can be seen in cross section in the far field. When comparing to a similar TEE view, the parasternal long-axis view is nearly identical to a midesophageal long-axis view displayed on its side.

In this echocardiographic window, LV size and systolic function as well as regional wall motion of the anteroseptal and inferolateral walls can be assessed. In addition, significant stenosis or regurgitation of the mitral and aortic valves may be apparent, although they may be better quantified from other views. The parasternal LAX view can also be used to identify an anterior or a posterior pericardial effusion as a cause of hemodynamic instability. Often a pleural effusion may be identified posterior to the heart, which can be differentiated from a pericardial effusion if it does not continue past the descending aorta.

By fanning the probe more closely to the chest wall, the more anterior structures of the heart become visible, revealing the **RV inflow view** (Fig. 3.3; Video 3.2). This view provides direct visualization of the posterior and anterior leaflets of the tricuspid valve, the right atrium and base of the right ventricle, and may reveal the proximal portions of the superior vena cava and the inferior vena cava. It may be particularly useful for measuring the regurgitant velocity of flow across the tricuspid valve with Doppler echocardiography.

Parasternal Short-Axis (SAX) View

From the same transducer "footprint" as the parasternal LAX view, the transducer can be rotated 90 degrees clockwise on the skin to reveal the parasternal SAX view, now with the probe indicator pointed toward the patient's left shoulder (Fig. 3.4). This is analogous to rotating the multiplane with TEE imaging to obtain an orthogonal view. From this location, several important structures can be visualized via different axial planes through the heart.

By fanning the probe superiorly to inferiorly, a short-axis view of the aortic valve (Fig. 3.5;

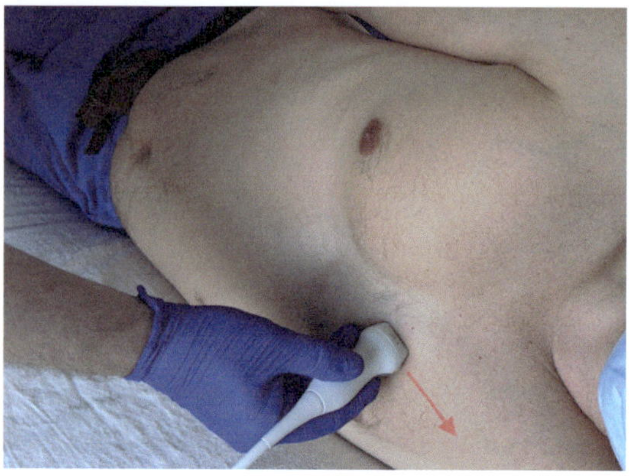

Fig. 3.4 Parasternal SAX probe position shown for a supine patient. The patient is turned to the left lateral decubitus position to optimize the viewing window. The indicator is pointed toward the patient's left shoulder. Fanning the probe superiorly to inferiorly allow short-axis imaging of the aortic valve, mitral valve, and LV

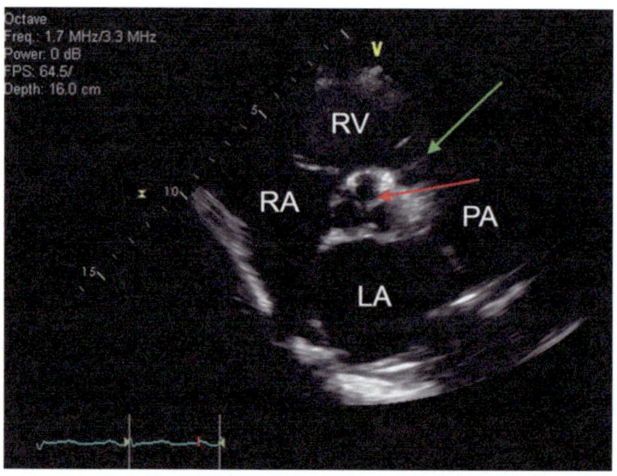

Fig. 3.5 Parasternal SAX view of the AV. *LA* left atrium, *RA* right atrium, *TV* tricuspid valve, *RV* right ventricle, *green arrow* pulmonic valve, *PA* pulmonary artery, *red arrow* aortic valve

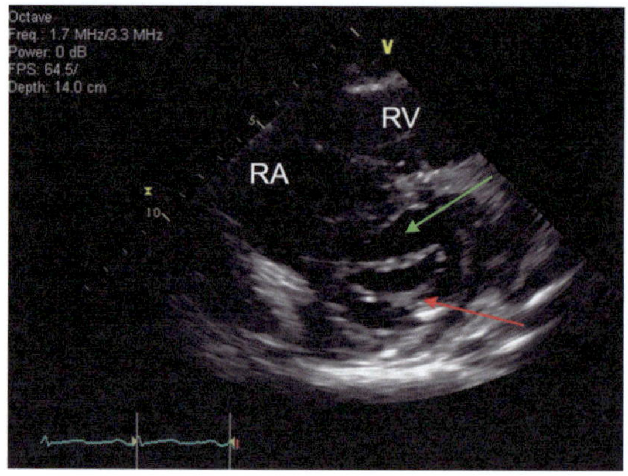

Fig. 3.6 Parasternal SAX basal view of the mitral valve with the leaflets open during diastole. *RA* right atrium, *RV* right ventricle, *green arrow* anterior leaflet, *red arrow* posterior leaflet

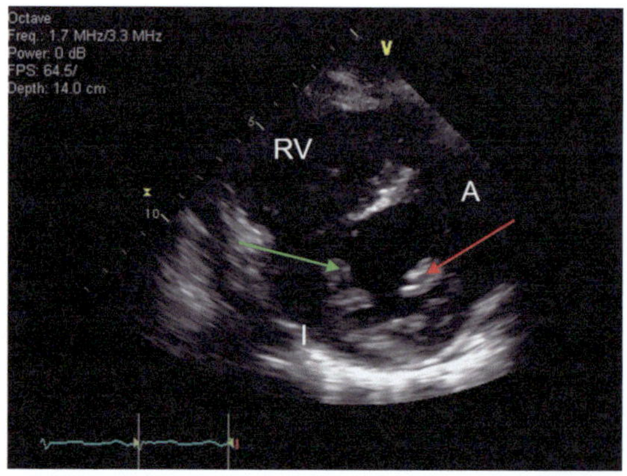

Fig. 3.7 Parasternal SAX mid-papillary view of the LV. *RV* right ventricle, *A* anterior LV wall, *I* inferior LV wall, *green arrow* posteromedial papillary muscle, *red arrow* anterolateral papillary muscle

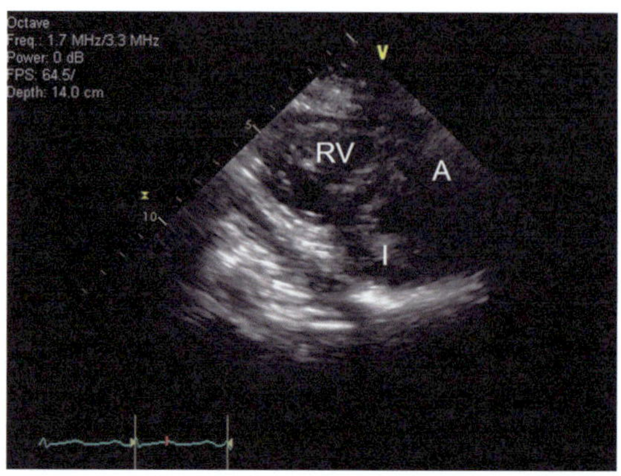

Fig. 3.8 Parasternal SAX apical view of the LV. *RV* right ventricle, *A* anterior apical LV wall, *I* inferior apical LV wall

Video 3.3), mitral valve (Fig. 3.6; Video 3.4), and LV (Fig. 3.7; Video 3.5) can be assessed, continuing through all of the segments of the LV to the apex (Fig. 3.8; Video 3.6). This angling of the probe can be analogous to anteflexion and retroflexion of the TEE probe to obtain superior to inferior structures.

In the parasternal SAX view of the aortic valve, overall chamber sizes of the left atrium, right atrium, and right ventricle can be appreciated. This view is analogous to the ME RV inflow-outflow view from TEE. It often has near parallel alignment with the tricuspid and pulmonic valves, allowing accurate Doppler assessments. The aortic valve can be evaluated in terms of calcifications and morphology. Continuing to fan the probe inferiorly, the basal short-axis view of the LV with the mitral valve will be imaged (akin to the TG basal short-axis view from TEE). With a continuation of the inferiorly-directed fanning, the mid-papillary SAX view of the LV will be imaged (akin to the TG mid-papillary short-axis view from TEE) and, even further inferiorly, the apical segment of the left ventricle (akin to the TG apical short-axis view from TEE). Each of these views will appear like their comparable TEE views except from an anterior perspective, such that the anteroseptal wall of the LV is closest to the probe (top of the image), as opposed to the inferior wall of the LV. Each of these views allows for evaluation of regional wall motion, degree of LV hypertrophy, and the presence of hypovolemia.

Apical Four-Chamber View

Similar to the ME four-chamber view from TEE, a transthoracic four-chamber view can image both atria and ventricles, however from the aspect of the LV apex. To obtain the apical four-chamber view, with the patient in LLD position and the left arm extended above the head, the transducer is placed at the apex of the heart identified by the point of maximal impulse (PMI). This is often found in the 4th or 5th intercostal space, anterior axillary line, or just below the nipple. The indicator is pointed toward the patient's left axilla, while slight angle adjustments should be made to align the septum in the center of the imaging sector (Fig. 3.9). The four chambers of the heart should be visible, with the left atrium and LV on the right side of the imaging sector and the right atrium and RV on the left side of the imaging sector (Fig. 3.10; Video 3.7).

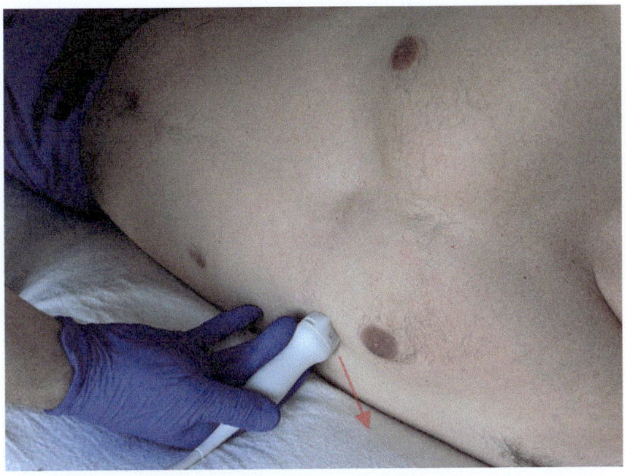

Fig. 3.9 Apical four-chamber probe position shown for a patient in a left lateral decubitus position. The probe is placed at the apex of the heart (point of maximal impulse), and the indicator is pointed toward the patient's left side. The patient is turned to the left lateral decubitus position to optimize the viewing window

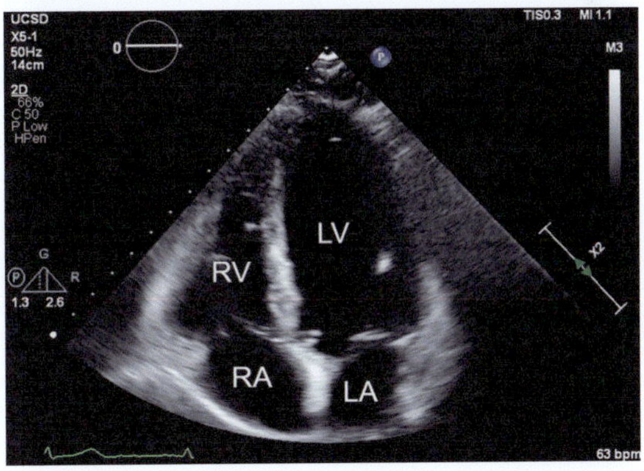

Fig. 3.10 Apical four-chamber view. *RA* right atrium, *RV* right ventricle, *LA* left atrium, *LV* left ventricle

Though this view can be more difficult to consistently obtain than parasternal views, it yields a large amount of helpful information. All four chambers of the heart can be evaluated for size, systolic function of the RV and LV can be assessed, Doppler interrogation of the mitral and tricuspid valves can be performed, and pericardial effusions can be appreciated in the apical four-chamber view. Mitral valve inflow and lateral wall tissue Doppler imaging can also be performed from this view to provide insight into diastolic function (see Chap. 12), and tricuspid annular plane systolic excursion (TAPSE) may be measured with M-mode (see Chap. 10).

Without moving the footprint of the transducer, fanning the ultrasound plane anteriorly from the apical four-chamber view, the left ventricular outflow tract (LVOT) and aortic valve should become apparent. This is known as the **apical five-chamber view** (Fig. 3.11; Video 3.8). The fifth "chamber" referenced in the name is the LVOT, which may provide useful information

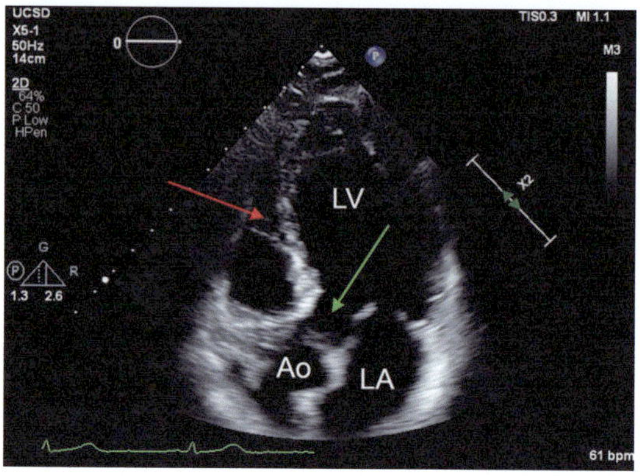

Fig. 3.11 Apical five-chamber view. *Red arrow* right ventricle, *LA* left atrium, *LV* left ventricle, *green arrow* left ventricular outflow tract, *Ao* proximal ascending aorta

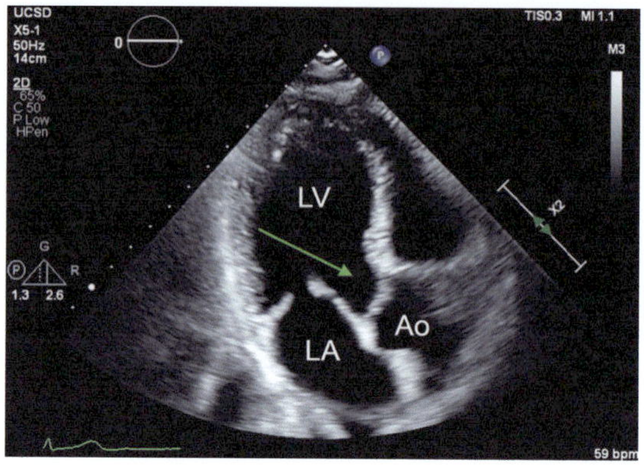

Fig. 3.13 Apical long-axis (three-chamber) view. *LA* left atrium, *LV* left ventricle, *green arrow* left ventricular outflow tract, *Ao* proximal ascending aorta

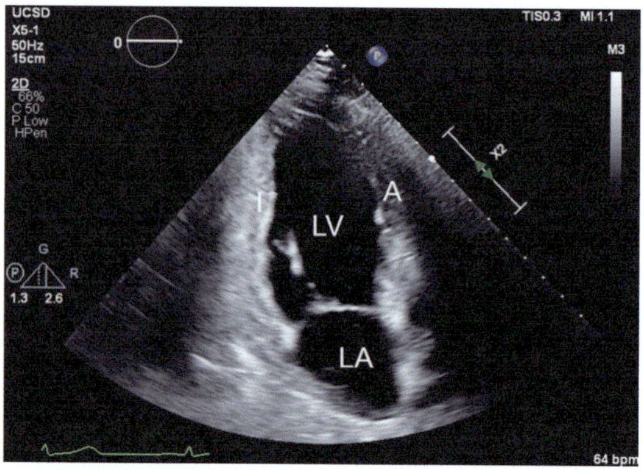

Fig. 3.12 Apical two-chamber view. *LA* left atrium, *LV* left ventricle, *A* anterior LV wall, *I* inferior LV wall

with Doppler evaluation provided its parallel alignment. This includes identification of aortic insufficiency with color flow Doppler and cardiac output determination with spectral Doppler techniques.

With transesophageal imaging and the use of multiplane, it is suggested to place the structure of interest in the middle of the imaging plane prior to adjusting the multiplane angle. This stabilizes the structure of interest as the angle changes. A similar approach can be provided with transthoracic imaging. From the apical four-chamber view after centering the LA and LV, a counterclockwise rotation of the probe on the skin will reveal the apical two-chamber view (Fig. 3.12; Video 3.9). From this view, the basal, mid, and apical segments of the anterior and inferior walls of the left ventricle can be evaluated for wall motion abnormalities. The view provides an additional imaging plane through the mitral valve.

By rotating counterclockwise an additional 30 degrees, the LVOT will come into view, creating the **apical long-axis view**, also called the apical three-chamber view (Fig. 3.13; Video 3.10). The third "chamber" in this case is again the LVOT, which may again provide a useful window for evaluation of cardiac output or aortic valve pathology, especially if the apical five-chamber view is insufficient.

Subcostal Views

In critically ill patients, especially those that are supine and receiving positive pressure ventilation and positive end-expiratory pressure (PEEP), aerated lung tissue may obscure the ability to obtain adequate parasternal or apical views. The subcostal (also called subxiphoid) four-chamber view can be particularly useful in this situation. The increased intrathoracic pressure may "push" the heart in a caudal direction improving subcostal imaging. In non-intubated patients, this may be replicated by asking the patient to perform an inspiratory breath hold. The subcostal four-chamber view is obtained by placing the probe just below the xiphoid process, with the indicator pointed toward the patient's left side and the ultrasound beam

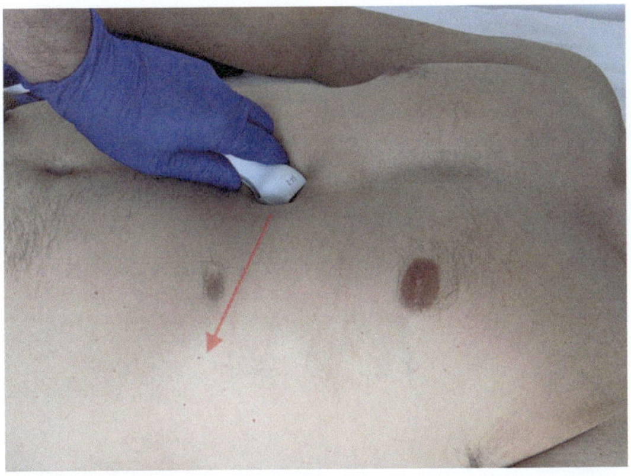

Fig. 3.14 Subcostal probe position shown for a supine patient. The probe is placed just below the xiphoid with the indicator pointed toward the patient's left. To view the IVC, the probe is rotated counterclockwise approximately 90 degrees

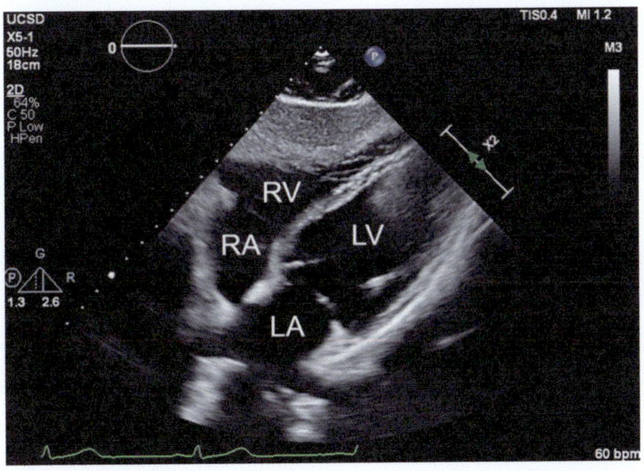

Fig. 3.15 Subcostal four-chamber view. *RA* right atrium, *RV* right ventricle, *LA* left atrium, *LV* left ventricle

directed superiorly toward the heart (Figs. 3.14 and 3.15; Video 3.11). Often, this view is obtained with the transducer almost flat against the patient's abdomen, pointing up under the rib cage.

The inferior vena cava (IVC) entering the RA can be developed from this subcostal window with counterclockwise rotation of the probe (Fig. 3.16). The diameter and collapsibility of the IVC can be used to aid in the prediction of fluid responsiveness and estimates of central venous pressure (see Chap. 20).

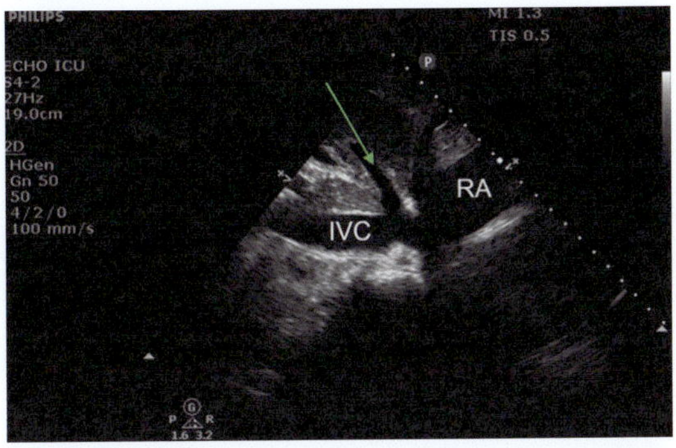

Fig. 3.16 Subcostal IVC view. *IVC* inferior vena cava, *RA* right atrium, *green arrow* hepatic vein

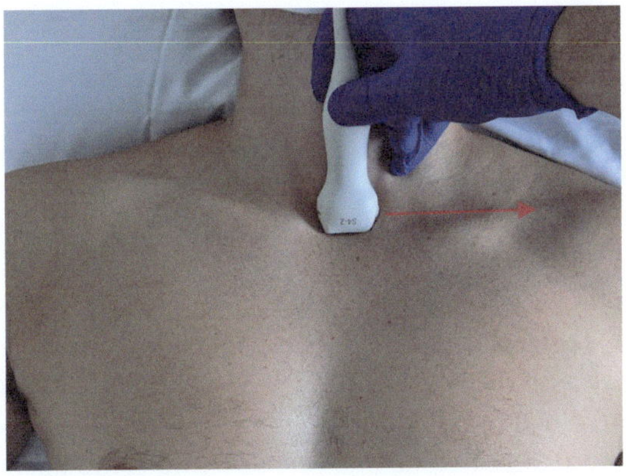

Fig. 3.17 Suprasternal probe positioning. The probe is placed in the suprasternal notch, directed into the thoracic cavity, with the probe indicator to the patient's left

Suprasternal View

While often not included in a point-of-care echocardiographic exam, an additional view that may help with visualization of the proximal and transverse aorta as well as the great vessels is the suprasternal view. From a supine or upright position, the patient's neck is extended, and the transducer is placed in the suprasternal notch with the indicator to the patient's left to obtain the suprasternal view of the distal ascending, transverse, and proximal descending aorta (Fig. 3.17). The origin of the great vessels can commonly be visualized from this view as well (Fig. 3.18; Video 3.12). In addition, it may be possible to visualize a cross-sectional view of the right pulmonary artery.

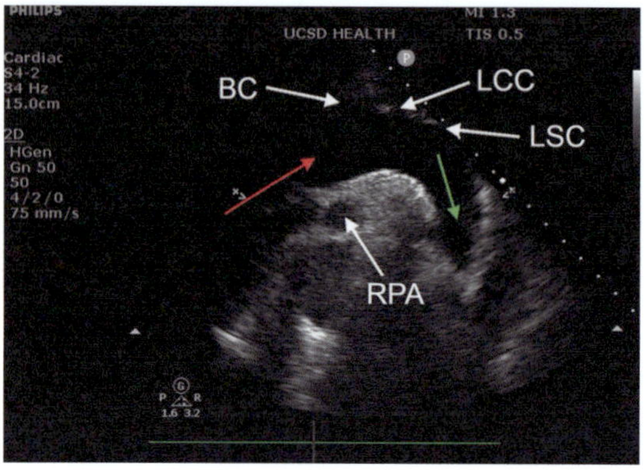

Fig. 3.18 Suprasternal view. *Red arrow* ascending aorta, *green arrow* descending aorta, *BC* brachiocephalic trunk, *LCC* left common carotid artery, *LSC* left subclavian artery, *RPA* right pulmonary artery

Conclusion

Point-of-care TTE is a valuable, noninvasive, and time-efficient diagnostic tool that has demonstrated its utility in hemodynamically unstable patients in a variety of clinical environments. Even for patients with limited ability to obtain all the standard views, important clinical questions can often be answered. While some basic technical skills are required for image acquisition and interpretation, point-of-care TTE can help quickly resolve many crucial goal-directed clinical questions.

Questions

1. Which anatomical structure is indicated by the arrow in the image below?

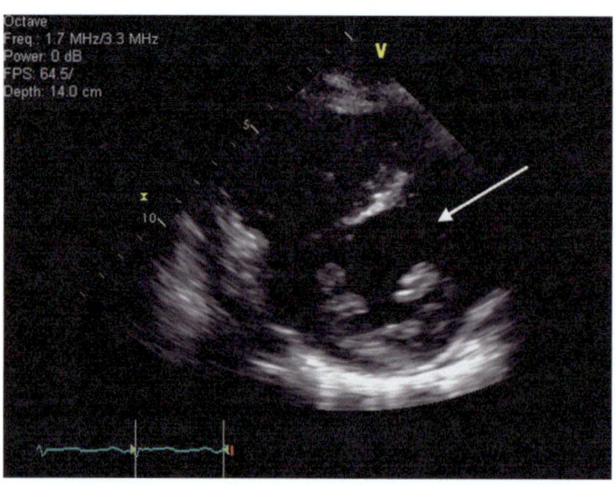

   a. Left ventricular mid-anterior wall
   b. Left ventricular mid-inferior wall
   c. Left ventricular mid-anterolateral wall
   d. Left ventricular mid-inferolateral wall

2. Which adjustment to the probe was made between the first and second image below?

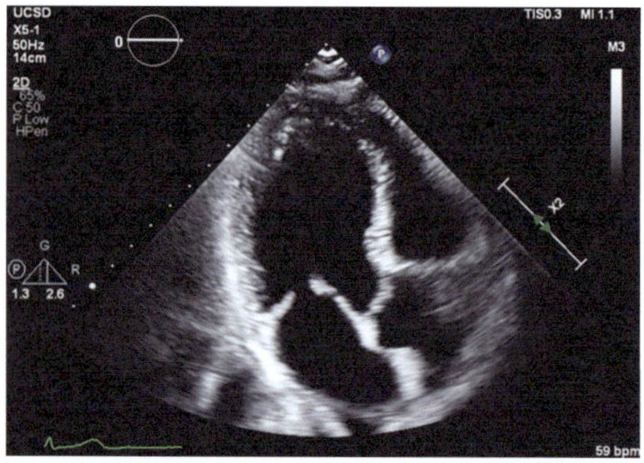

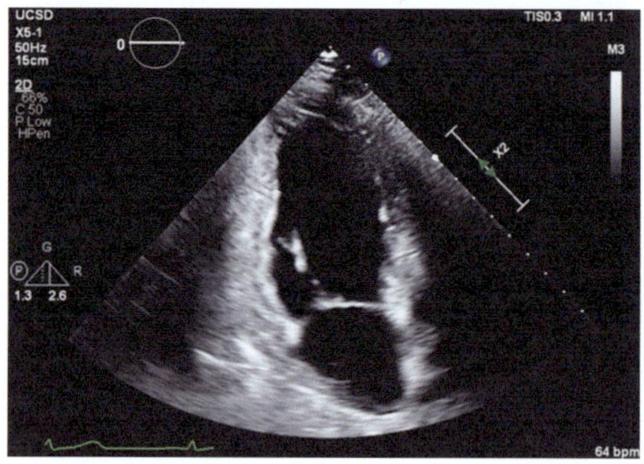

   a. Tilting medially
   b. Fanning inferiorly
   c. Twisting clockwise
   d. Twisting counterclockwise

3. In which of the following views is the aortic valve visible?

   a. Apical long-axis view
   b. Apical four-chamber view
   c. Subcostal four-chamber view
   d. None of the above

4. Which anatomical structure is indicated by the arrow in the image below?

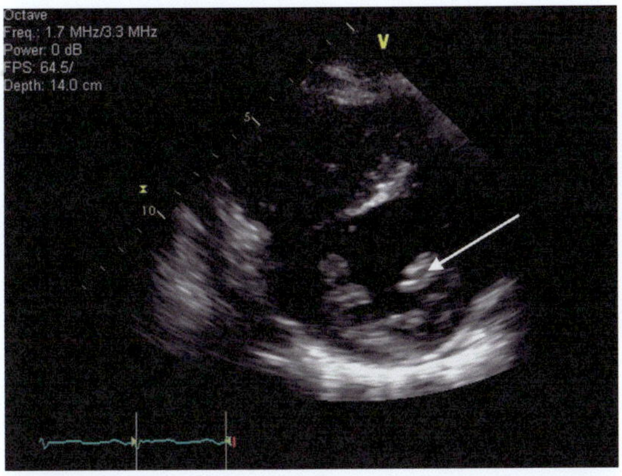

a. LV thrombus
b. Posteromedial papillary muscle
c. Inferolateral papillary muscle
d. Anterolateral papillary muscle

5. Which of the following images shows the correct orientation for a parasternal short-axis view?

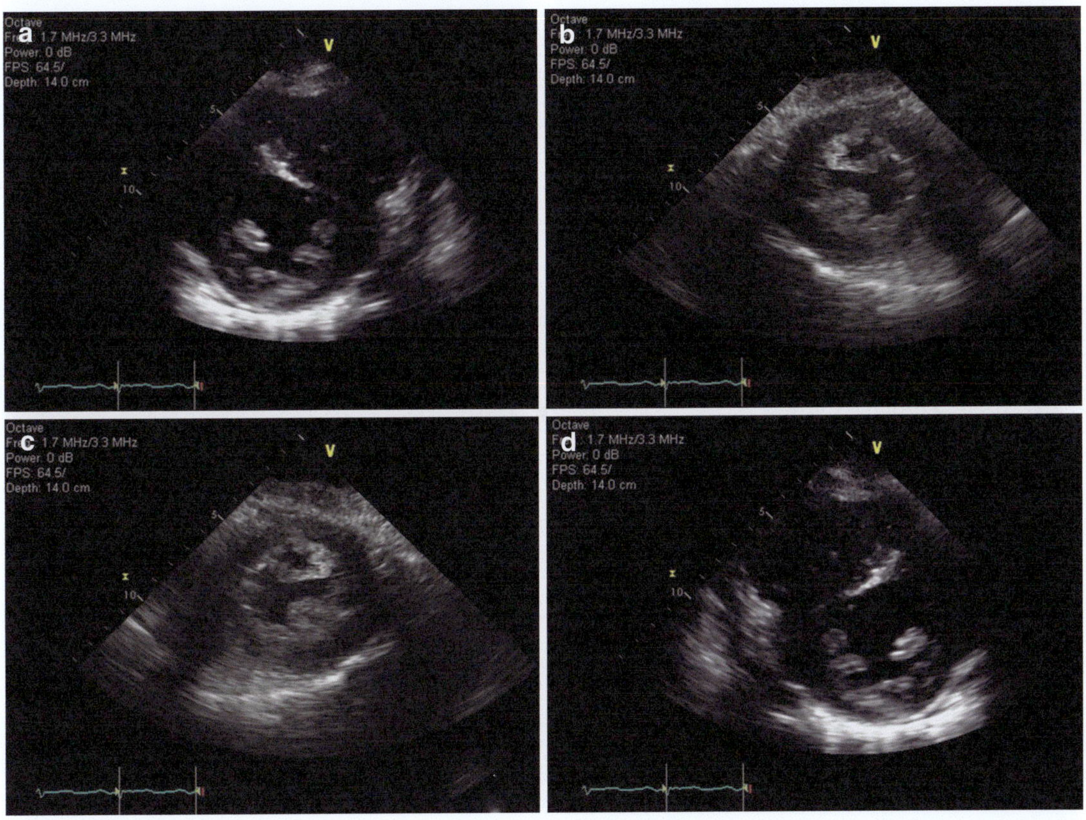

a. Image A
b. Image B
c. Image C
d. Image D

6. Which of the following most accurately describes the approximate position for the probe footprint to obtain a parasternal long-axis view?

a. 2nd or 3rd intercostal space, to the left of the sternum, with probe marker oriented toward the patient's right shoulder

b. 2nd or 3rd intercostal space, to the right of the sternum, with probe marker oriented toward the patient's right shoulder
c. 2nd or 3rd intercostal space, to the left of the sternum, with probe marker oriented toward the patient's left shoulder
d. 2nd or 3rd intercostal space, to the left of the sternum, with probe marker oriented toward the patient's left shoulder

7. From the following image, which structure is indicated by the arrow?

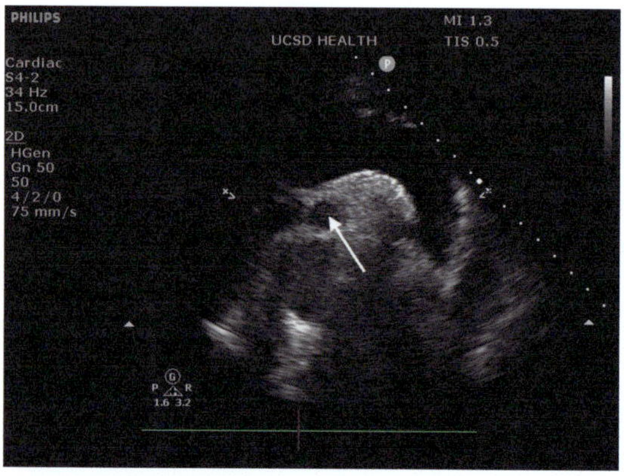

a. Main pulmonary artery
b. Left pulmonary artery
c. Right pulmonary artery
d. Superior vena cava

8. Which of the following statement is most true regarding the differences between transesophageal and transthoracic echocardiography?

a. Transthoracic echocardiography provides more accurate Doppler evaluation of the aortic valve
b. Transthoracic echocardiography provides more accurate Doppler evaluation of the mitral valve
c. Transthoracic echocardiography is not possible in mechanically ventilated patients
d. Transthoracic echocardiography is unable to visualize the aortic arch

9. Which of the following is most likely to improve visualization of an apical four-chamber view?

a. Having the patient hold in their breath
b. Laying the patient supine
c. Turning the patient to the left lateral decubitus position
d. Raising the head of the bed

10. Which adjustment to the probe was made between the first and second image below?

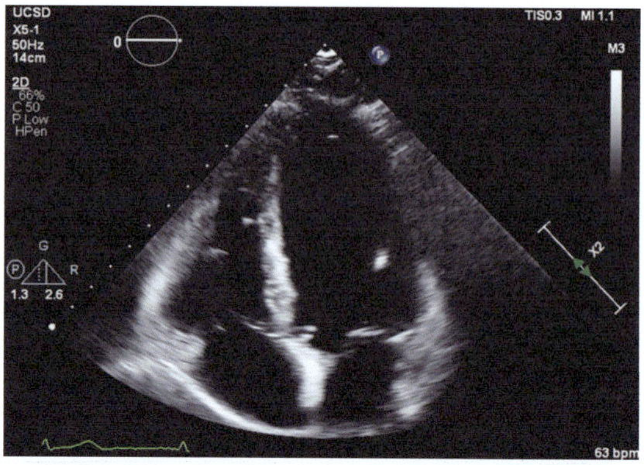

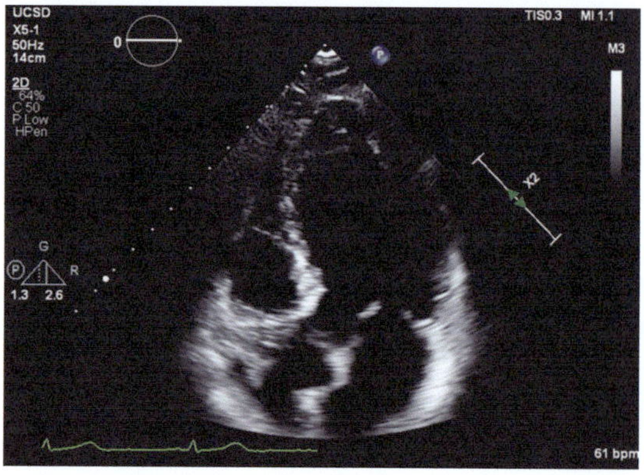

a. The probe footprint was moved anterior one rib space (swept)
b. The probe was angled anteriorly (fanned)
c. The probe was rotated clockwise
d. The probe was rotated counterclockwise

References

1. Labovitz AJ, Noble VE, Bierig M, et al. Focused cardiac ultrasound in the emergent setting: a consensus statement of the American Society of Echocardiography and American College of Emergency Physicians. J Am Soc Echocardiogr. 2010;23:1225–30.
2. Bahner DP, Blickendorf JM, Bockbrader M, et al. Language of transducer manipulation: codifying terms for effective teaching. J Ultrasound Med. 2016;35:183–8.

Basic Ultrasound Physics, Doppler Ultrasound, and Hemodynamic Assessment

4

Gerard Manecke and Patricia Guan

Introduction

Some animals make use of sound wave reflections to determine their position and direction of motion (echolocation) [1, 2]. Bats, despite their historic reputation, are not blind, and in fact, many actually have excellent eyesight, but they are especially known for their ability to transmit and receive ultrasonic signals used for echolocation [3, 4]. Visually impaired humans can develop similar capabilities using audible sound, resulting in an impressive ability to navigate surroundings [5, 6]. Dolphins are known to use a similar method of echolocation underwater, from which ultrasound in the form of *so*und *n*avigation *a*nd *r*anging (SONAR) was developed in the early twentieth century and was first employed for military purposes shortly after World War I [7]. Medical ultrasound was first introduced by George Ludwig in 1949 [8], and cardiac ultrasound was first employed in 1953 [9]. An explosion in computer technology in the 1980s allowed the development of two-dimensional (2D) ultrasound for continuous imaging and Doppler velocity measurements for blood flow and tissue movement. Further advances in computer technology provide the high-resolution three-dimensional imaging with continuous display we currently enjoy [10]. A timeline of the history of ultrasound is shown in Fig. 4.1.

G. Manecke (✉) · P. Guan
Department of Anesthesiology, University of California San Diego Health, La Jolla, CA, USA
e-mail: gmanecke@health.ucsd.edu

Physics of Ultrasound

Sound waves are longitudinal pressure waves: compressions and rarefactions of the molecules in the medium through which they are traveling. Like all waves, sound waves have amplitude (loudness) and frequency (Fig. 4.2). Humans can hear sounds within the range of 20–20,000 cycles per second (Hertz, Hz). Ultrasound is sound at frequencies above the audible range (> 20,000 Hz), and medical ultrasound is in the mega-Hz (MHz) range, or millions of Hz (Fig. 4.3).

Sound transmission depends upon the density of the medium, with higher density substances (e.g., liquid) transmitting sound more rapidly and efficiently than air. Ultrasound does not travel well through gas, so gas-filled spaces such as bronchi and gastric air result in "blackout" of the ultrasound image. Lower-frequency sound tends to propagate farther than high-frequency sound. One notices this when a storm is approaching. When the storm is distant, thunder sounds like a low-pitched "rumble." As the storm approaches, the sound of thunder includes higher frequencies, resulting in a "thunder clap." Ultrasound behaves similarly, so imaging objects far from the transducer requires lower frequencies than imaging near objects.

T. M. Maus, C. R. Tainter (eds.), *Essential Echocardiography*,
https://doi.org/10.1007/978-3-030-84349-6_4

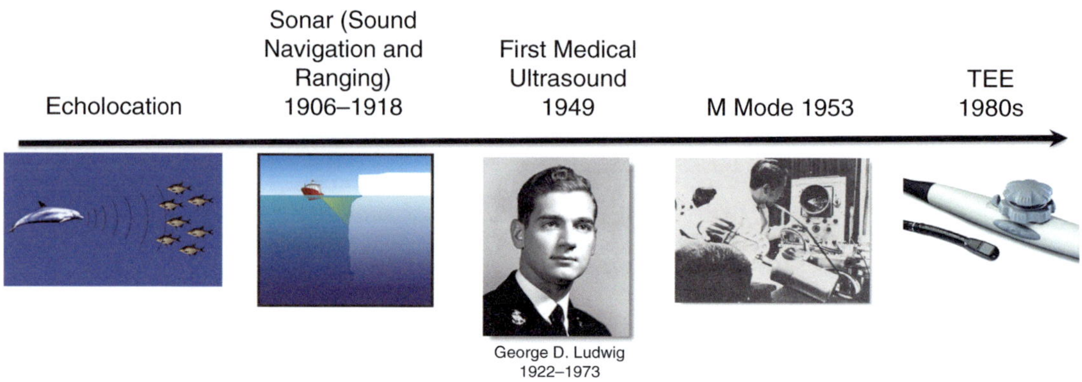

Fig. 4.1 Timeline of the history of ultrasound

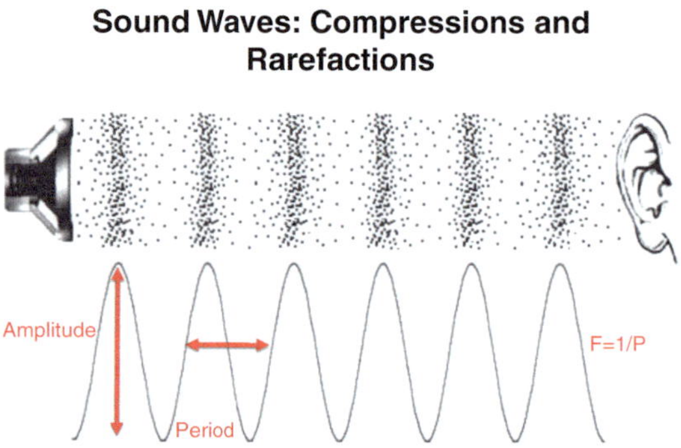

Fig. 4.2 Characteristics of sound waves. *F* frequency, *P* period

When sound waves strike an interface of a different density, they reflect off that interface. This is the principle upon which diagnostic ultrasound is based [11]. The ultrasound transducer emits an ultrasound wave, the wave bounces off a density interface (object) back to the transducer, and the time required in transit allows calculation of the distance between the object and the transducer. As demonstrated in Fig. 4.4, a cross-sectional image of the descending aorta shows ultrasound waves bouncing off of two density interfaces: a dissection intimal flap (A) and the distal wall of the aorta (B). A perpendicular orientation of the object to the ultrasound probe is optimal for return of echo signals. A parallel orientation may not provide a sufficient reflection of signals, leading to "drop out."

Ultrasound Probes

Most ultrasound probes contain a transducer with an array of pressure-electric (piezoelectric) crystals that convert electrical energy to pressure waves (for emitting ultrasound) and conversely, pressure waves to electricity (for sensing). Silicon micro-machining technology with a diaphragm sensor may also be used. The lateral resolution of the image depends upon the distance between the crystals aligned within the transducer, with a smaller distance associated with better resolution (Fig. 4.5). The lateral resolution may also be altered by focusing. Akin to utilizing a magnifying glass in the sunshine to focus the sunlight into a narrow beam, modern ultrasound machines have an adjustable focal point that represents the narrowest part of the beam (Fig. 4.6). Lateral resolution is best at the focal point, but is quite poor in the far field (distal to the focal point). Therefore, it is recommended to place the focal point at the level of the structure of interest.

The longitudinal or axial resolution depends on the pulse length, with shorter pulse length resulting in better resolution (Fig. 4.7). Pulse length can be decreased either by increasing the frequency of the probe (and thus decreasing the wavelength) or decreasing the cycles/pulse. Higher-frequency probes with shorter wavelengths have better resolution for nearby struc-

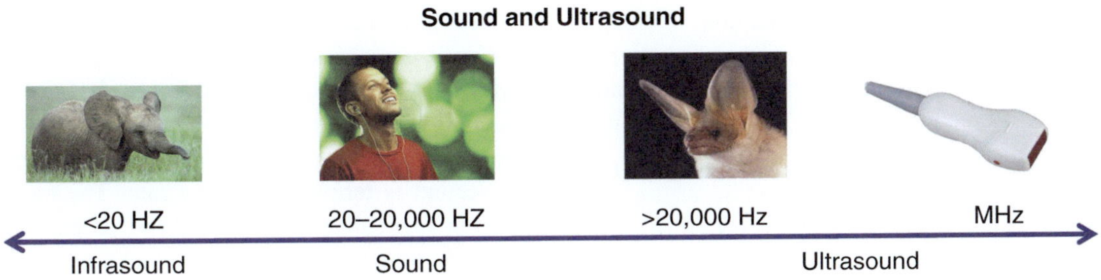

Fig. 4.3 Sound frequencies. Medical ultrasound is in the Mega-Hz (million Hz) range

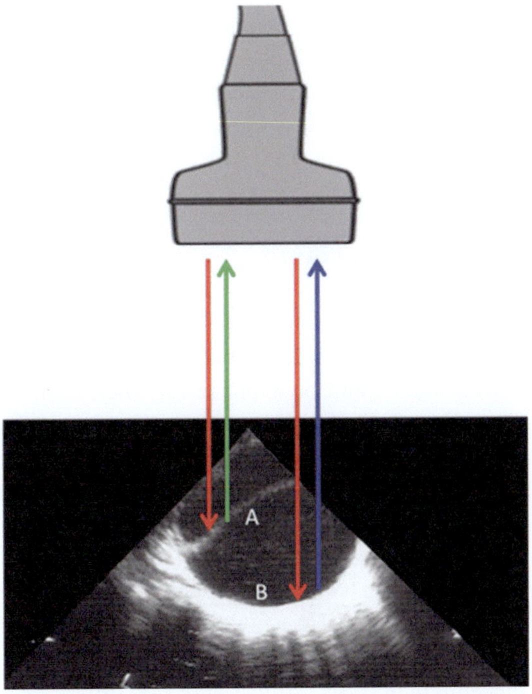

Fig. 4.4 "Specular echoes." Ultrasound waves bouncing off tissues of varying density. *A* is the intimal flap of an aortic dissection, *B* is the distal wall of the aorta

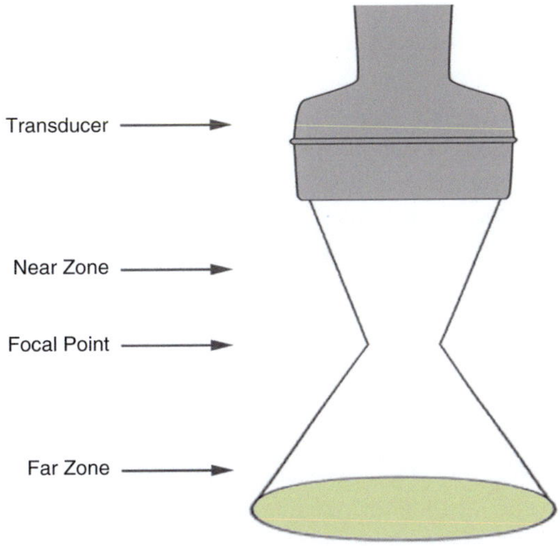

Fig. 4.6 Focus influence on beam width. The narrowest portion of the beam is at the focal point with poorer resolution in the far zone

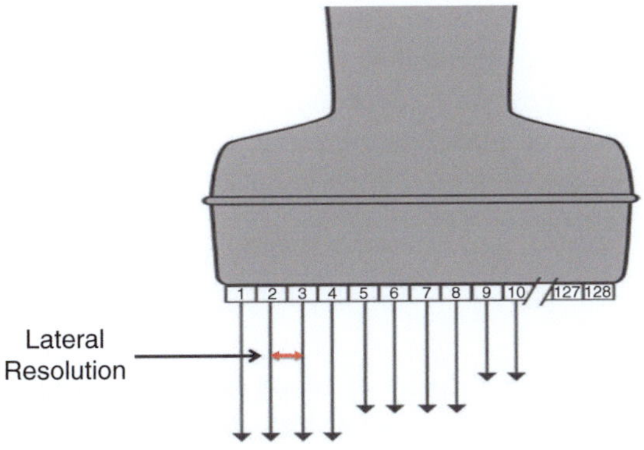

Fig. 4.5 Lateral resolution depends upon the distance between piezoelectric crystals in the probe

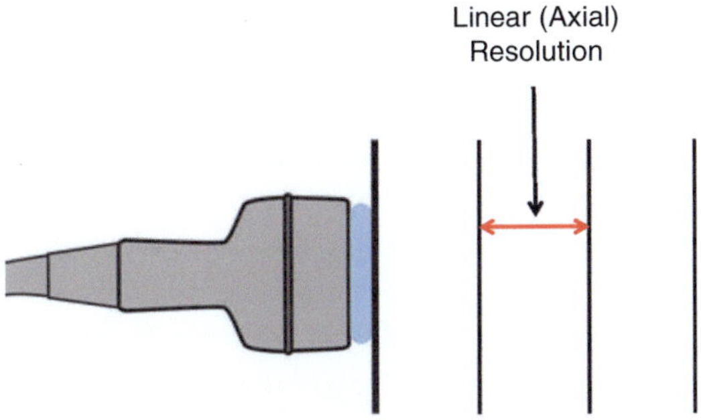

Fig. 4.7 Axial resolution depends upon the pulse length and the probe frequency

tures, but more signal attenuation, making it difficult to resolve structures through deeper tissue. Note that resolution is expressed as distance, so a *lower* number indicates *better* resolution.

$$\text{Frequency} = 1/\text{wavelength} \quad (4.1)$$

$$\text{Pulse length} = \text{wavelength} \times \text{cycles/pulse} \quad (4.2)$$

$$\text{Axial Resolution} = \frac{0.77 \times \frac{\text{cycles}}{\text{pulse}}}{\text{Frequency}} \quad (4.3)$$

The effects of transducer frequency on ultrasound imaging are summarized in Table 4.1. The general rule is that distant objects can be viewed best using a low-frequency transducer; however, the axial resolution will be poorer with the lower frequency. Likewise, small objects close to the probe, such as the radial artery, are best visualized using a high-frequency transducer because of the associated high resolution. The trade-off of high-frequency (and higher resolution) imaging is the inability to visualize deeper structures due to energy dissipation.

While lateral and axial resolution represent the spatial resolutions of ultrasound, cardiac ultrasound requires interpreting moving clips as opposed to still images. Therefore, one must also consider temporal resolution. This is similar to movie and television images where at an analog movie theater, one would note a flickering of the image when the movie begins; however, at home on a television and a higher frame rate, there is no longer a flickering of the image. With modern televisions, the high-definition frame rate is high enough such that even fast-moving objects (e.g., sporting events) appear smoothly. This is due to the increased frame rate moving from an analog movie theater to television to high-definition television.

Table 4.1 The effects of probe frequency on ultrasound imaging

High Frequency
More energy dissipation
Better linear resolution
Close objects with high resolution
Low Frequency
Less energy dissipation
Poor linear resolution
Far objects viewed but less resolution

With ultrasound, the machine has to produce numerous ultrasound pulses in a fan-like fashion to develop one single image. Repeating this process will provide subsequent images, yielding a moving clip. The number of images developed per second is termed the frame rate. The more imaging (e.g., deeper or wider) and processing (e.g., adding color flow Doppler) that a machine is requested to do, the longer it will take to generate a single image, subsequently reducing the frame rate. If the frame rate is too slow, the video will begin to appear choppy or like a flipbook, reducing the ability to detect fine movements. Therefore, only the minimum depth needed and the smallest color flow Doppler box size should be used to maintain the best frame rate.

Doppler Ultrasound

In 1842, Austrian physicist Christian Doppler postulated that the difference in color between double stars could be explained by their motion. The effect of an object's motion on the frequency of waves detected from it is known as the "Doppler effect." An example of the Doppler effect is the change in pitch of a train whistle as the train passes by an observer (a higher-pitched sound traveling toward the observer, then a lower-pitched sound as it travels away). This principle is applied in ultrasound with blood flow velocity measurements as illustrated in Fig. 4.8. Ultrasound at a known frequency (f_T) is transmitted from the probe and bounces off a moving object (blood cells), and the reflected sound is detected by the probe. The frequency of the returning ultrasound (f_r) is calculated, and the frequency shift between the transmitted and returning ultrasound wave (Δf) is used to calculate the velocity of blood flow (V):

$$v = \frac{C(\Delta f)}{2 f_T \cos\theta} \quad (4.4)$$

where v = velocity of blood flow, c = speed of sound, Δf = frequency shift (difference between transmitted and received frequency), and Θ = angle between blood flow path and Doppler beam.

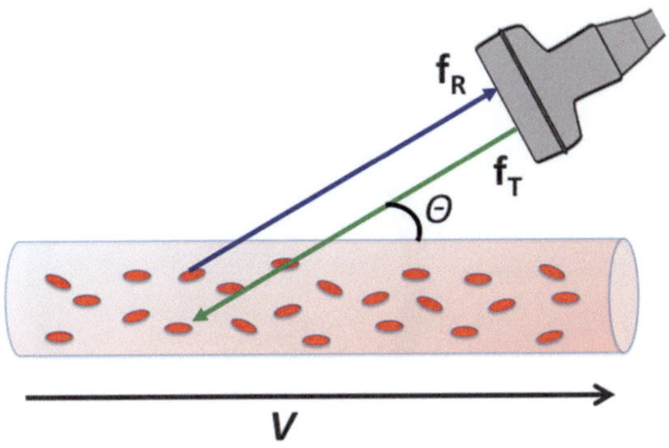

Fig. 4.8 Doppler assessment of blood flow velocity. The closer the alignment of blood flow with the Doppler beam (angle $\Theta = 0$), the more accurate the result. V is blood flow velocity, f_T is transmitted frequency (known), and F_R is the returning frequency (calculated). The difference between f_T and F_R is the frequency shift, Δf

Table 4.2 Characteristics and clinical use of Doppler techniques

	Color flow Doppler	Pulsed-wave Doppler	Continuous-wave Doppler
Color map	+	–	–
Assess flow at a discrete area	+	+	–
Assess flow along an axis	–	–	+
Qualitative assessment	Very useful	Useful	Less useful
Quantitative assessment high flow	Less useful	Less useful	Very useful
Aliasing	+	+	–

Closer alignment of the blood flow and the Doppler beam (Θ) yields a more accurate measurement (*cos* 0 = 1). Of note, *cos* 90 = 0, and therefore, measurement of flow completely perpendicular to the probe cannot be calculated. As opposed to 2D imaging, which prefers the object to be perpendicular to the probe, Doppler imaging prefers the object to be in parallel orientation.

The Doppler principle is used clinically in three ways: color flow Doppler (CFD), pulsed-wave Doppler (PWD), and continuous-wave Doppler (CWD). PWD determines the velocity at a discrete area in space ("sample volume"), and CWD determines flow velocity along an axis. PWD and CWD display as a spectrum of velocities along a time axis and are therefore referred to as spectral Doppler. CFD uses an array of PWD measurements to create a real-time color flow diagram. Tissue Doppler is another variation of PWD, used to determine the velocity of tissue movement (e.g., the mitral annulus), as opposed to blood movement. The characteristics, uses, and limitations of Doppler techniques are summarized in Table 4.2.

An important and sometimes useful artifact is *aliasing*. Aliasing is a false frequency wave or image resulting when the sampling rate of the sensor is too low to accurately detect the high frequency of the returning signal. The *Nyquist Theorem* states that the sampling rate must be at least twice the frequency of the wave being sampled. The *Nyquist Limit* is the highest frequency that can be accurately sampled at a given sampling rate. Aliasing is often called the "stroboscopic" or "wagon wheel" effect, in which rapidly moving spokes of a wheel in one direction appear as slow-moving blurred spokes (Fig. 4.9, https://www.youtube.com/watch?v=jHS9JGkEOmA). This results from either, in a video, the frame rate being too slow to pick up the actual speed of the spokes, or, in real time, the inability of the human central nervous system to process the fast spoke motion. If the "snapshots" (samples) of the moving spokes are not frequent enough, the spokes appear to be moving slowly, sometimes in the opposite direction.

After transmitting an ultrasound wave, the probe "samples" the returning wave. In CFD and PWD, the probe "waits" until a transmitted signal bounces off the target and is received, so the sampling rate is limited by this process. Aliasing results if the returning frequency is higher than half the sampling rate. In CWD, the sampling and transmission are simultaneous—the probe does not wait for the returning signal, so aliasing does not occur. CWD is thus preferred for measurement of high-velocity

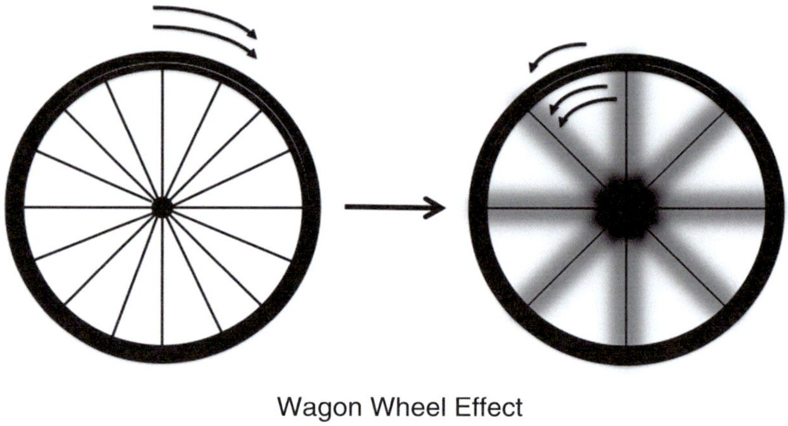

Fig. 4.9 "Wagon wheel effect." Rapid movement of spokes is interpreted as slow-moving, large "blurred" spokes, often in the opposite direction

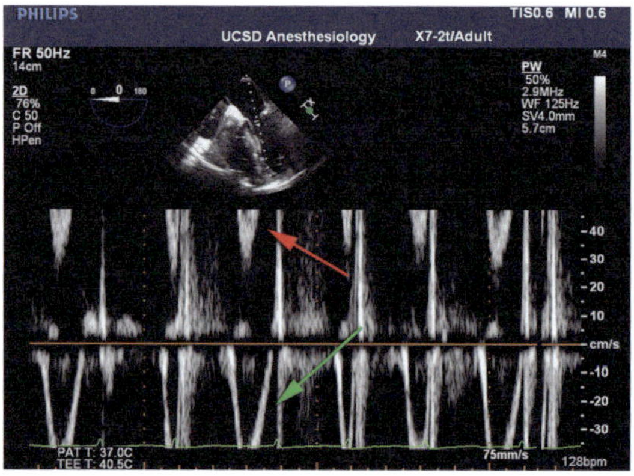

Fig. 4.10 Pulse wave Doppler of transmitral flow. Flow away from the transducer is displayed as below the zero line. Flow becomes so rapid (*green arrow*) that it is displayed as flow in the opposite direction (*red arrow*, "wraparound")

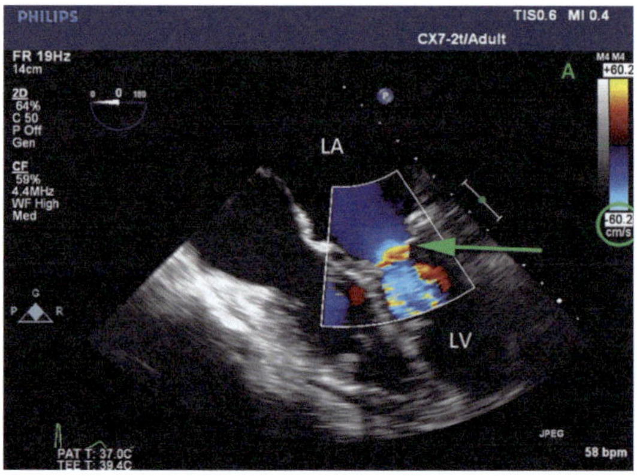

Fig. 4.11 Midesophageal four-chamber view with transmitral color flow Doppler demonstrating aliasing. The flow map (*A*) indicates that flow away from the probe is blue, flow toward the probe is yellow, and the limit below which aliasing does not occur is 60.2 cm/sec. The *green arrow* shows an aliasing line, where flow exceeds 60.2 cm/sec, and downward flow turns from blue to yellow. *LA* left atrium, *LV* left ventricle

(high returning frequency) flow, like flow through a stenotic valve. Aliasing results in the "wraparound" appearance of PWD tracings (Fig. 4.10) and the appearance of flow in the opposite direction of the actual flow in CFD (Fig. 4.11). The latter may be useful, since the velocity at which aliasing occurs is known and can be applied to calculations such as Proximal Isovelocity Surface Area (PISA) [12].

Hemodynamic Assessment

Echocardiography can be used for an accurate assessment of hemodynamics. The most common applications are quantifications of flow, valvular area, and pressure gradients.

Flow

Blood flow measurement is typically utilized in determining stroke volume and subsequently cardiac output. A stroke volume is determined by calculating the cross-sectional area of the blood vessel and multiplying it by the area under the Doppler velocity-time curve. The area under the Doppler velocity-time curve is called the "velocity time integral" (VTI), or the "stroke distance." Figure 4.12a explains how the area under the curve provides a distance by plotting velocity and time of a traveling car. In the example, a car trav-

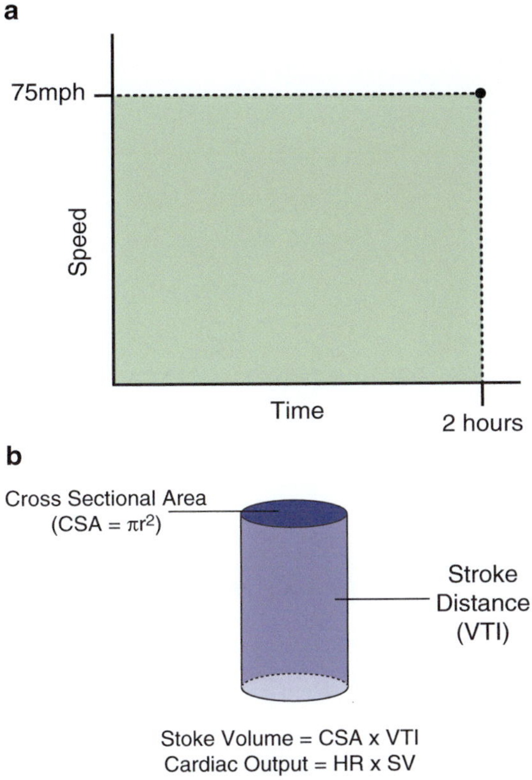

Fig. 4.12 (**a**) Graph of the speed of a car versus time. The area under the curve which is shaded green demonstrates the distance the car has traveled. (**b**) Depiction of the cross-sectional area of a cardiac structure multiplied by its velocity time integral ("stroke distance") will yield a stroke volume. *CSA* cross-sectional area, *VTI* velocity time integral, *HR* heart rate, *SV* stroke volume

eling at 75 miles per hour for 2 hours will have traveled a distance of 150 miles (analogous to "stroke distance"). The cross-sectional area of the blood vessel is estimated by determining the radius of the vessel (diameter divided by 2) and assuming the shape is circular (area = πr^2) (Fig. 4.12b).

$$\text{Stroke Volume} = \text{Area} \times \text{VTI} \tag{4.5}$$

For example, to calculate the left ventricular stroke volume, one can measure the diameter of the left ventricular outflow tract (LVOT) using the midesophageal aortic valve long-axis view via TEE (Fig. 4.13a), or parasternal long-axis view via TTE, with area = $\pi(\text{diameter}/2)^2$. Using the TEE deep transgastric five-chamber view or TTE apical five-chamber view, spectral Doppler can be used to obtain the LVOT systolic Doppler wave, and the VTI can be determined by tracing the area under the curve. Stroke volume is then calculated by multiplying the LVOT area by the VTI.

Valvular Area

In a closed fluid system, the amount of flow through one section is the same as the amount of flow through another. This conservation of mass principle is described by the *continuity equation.*

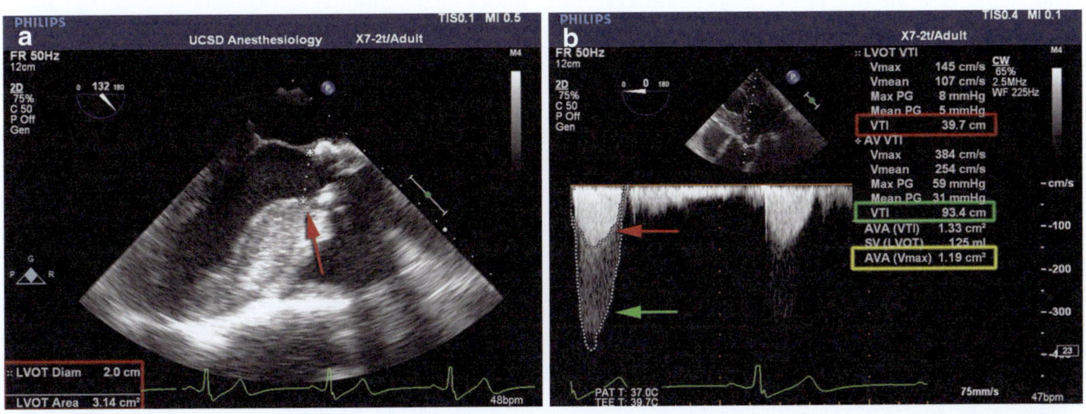

Fig. 4.13 (**a**) Measurement of the diameter (*red arrow*) of the left ventricular outflow tract (LVOT) using the mid-esophageal aortic valve long-axis view. (**b**) The "double envelope", showing a velocity envelope for the LVOT (*red arrow*, *red box*) and a higher velocity envelope for the aortic valve (*green arrow*, *green box*). Velocity time integrals (VTI) are used in the continuity equation for calculation of the aortic valve area (*yellow box*)

Most commonly utilized in the case of aortic stenosis (see Chap. 9, "Aortic Valve"), the flow through the aortic valve is the same as the flow through the LVOT, so the valve area of the stenotic valve can be determined:

$$A_1 \times V_1 = A_2 \times V_2 \tag{4.6}$$

In this example, $A_{LVOT} \times V_{LVOT} = A_{AV} \times V_{AV}$, where AV is the aortic valve and LVOT is the left ventricular outflow tract. One measures the area of the LVOT and the VTIs for the AV and LVOT (Figs. 4.13a and b). Solving for the area of the AV:

$$A_{AV} = \left(A_{LVOT} \times V_{LVOT}\right) / V_{AV}$$

Pressure Gradient Estimation

Clinically, practitioners often think in terms of pressure (mmHg), while echocardiography measures velocities (m/sec). Therefore, a relationship between velocity and pressure is necessary to provide appropriate clinical estimations. In physiologic conditions, the pressure gradient across a valve or orifice can be determined using the modified Bernoulli Equation:

$$\Delta P = 4v^2 \tag{4.7}$$

where ΔP is the pressure gradient and v is the peak velocity in m/sec. For example, the systolic right ventricular pressure gradient between right ventricle and right atrium during systole can be determined by CWD across the tricuspid valve. The peak velocity of the regurgitant jet, in m/sec, is used in Eq. 4.7. The right ventricular systolic pressure can then be estimated by adding the value of the gradient to the right atrial or central venous pressure (CVP). In the absence of pulmonic valve stenosis, right ventricular systolic pressure is equal to pulmonary artery systolic pressure. Therefore, the application of the modified Bernoulli equation to a tricuspid regurgitation jet in addition to CVP provides an estimation of pulmonary artery pressures (Fig. 4.14).

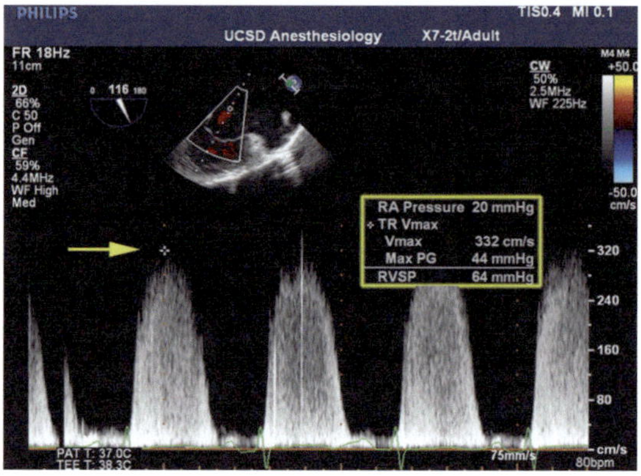

Fig. 4.14 A continuous-wave Doppler profile of a tricuspid regurgitation (TR) jet. The right ventricular systolic pressure (RVSP), which is an estimation of pulmonary artery systolic pressure, is determined by applying the modified Bernoulli equation to the peak regurgitant velocity in addition to the CVP (RA Pressure). *RA* right atrial, *Vmax* maximum velocity, *PG* pressure gradient

3D Echocardiography

Three-dimensional (3D) echocardiography allows improved spatial assessment of cardiac structures, both in real time and in retrospective measurement. The main difference between two-dimensional (2D) and three-dimensional imaging lies within the transducer. Two-dimensional transducer probes are composed of piezoelectric crystals arranged in a single row, whereas 3D imaging requires the use of a matrix array transducer that contains 2500–3000 (52 × 52) independent piezoelectric crystals arranged in rows and columns. Operating frequencies range from 2 to 4 MHz for transthoracic and 5 to 7 MHz for transesophageal transducers. While 2D echo scans sector planes in the vertical (or axial [y]) and lateral (or azimuthal plane [x]), 3D echo employs volume scanning by using an additional anteroposterior (or elevation plane [z]) to help produce a volumetric, pyramidal data set (Fig. 4.15). Technological advances have allowed for the individual activation and deactivation of these piezoelectric crystals both in transmission and reception. By selectively activating specific lines of piezoelectric crystals, the matrix array

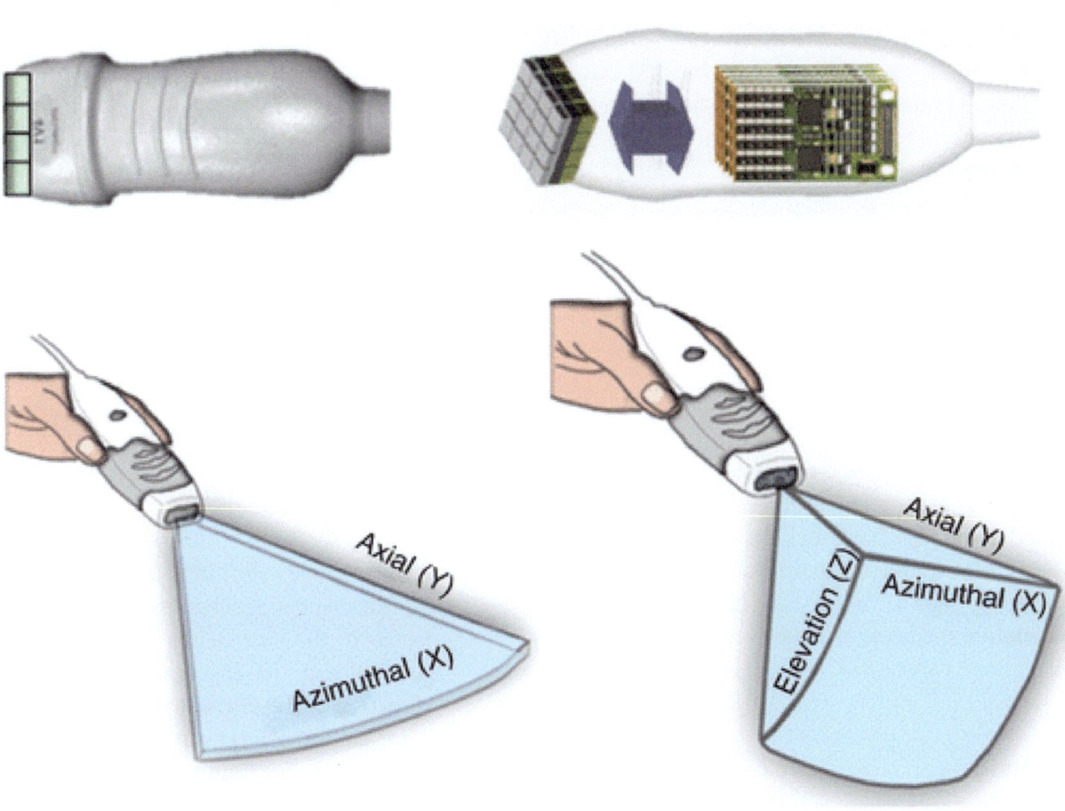

Fig. 4.15 Two- and three-dimensional transducers. A standard transducer (left panel) with an array of piezoelectric crystals allowing imaging in the x (azimuthal) and y (axial) planes, resulting in two-dimensional images, and a matrix transducer (right panel), with piezoelectric crystals in the x (azimuthal), y (axial), and z (elevation) planes providing the necessary data for creation of a three-dimensional image. (Reproduced with permission from Muraru D, Badano LP. Physical and Technical Aspects and Overview of 3D-Echocardiography in Rojo EC, et al. (eds.): Manual of 3D Echocardiography. Switzerland: Springer International Publishing AG, 2017, p. 2)

probe can perform 3D imaging while also providing real-time simultaneous 2D views.

Once data is acquired through one of the various scanning modes, it is then processed through conversion and interpolation. During conversion, all acquired raw data is assigned a point on the x-, y-, and z-axes of the coordinate plane to generate a three-dimensional image. Interpolation fills the gaps between all known charted points with data points of similar features to generate a volumetric pixel, also known as a voxel. This unit of graphic information defines a point in a three-dimensional space similar to how a pixel defines a point in a two-dimensional space. The larger the pixel size, the worse the spatial resolution of the image. Similarly, a larger voxel size creates a greater signal-to-noise ratio. The trade-off for increased voxel size is decreased spatial resolution. Displaying data as voxels allows the echocardiographer to visualize cardiac structures in different planes and rotations.

Bioeffects

Because ultrasound is an energy wave interfacing with the human body, it is important to note its potential to cause effects on the patient. While generally considered very safe, ultrasound imaging has the potential to cause tissue injury through temperature elevation (thermal injury) from agitation of the tissues or cavitation (nonthermal injury) from oscillation of small gas bubbles in the tissues. These effects are directly proportional to the energy delivered; thus, methods to minimize energy delivery are encouraged, known as the as low as reasonably achievable (ALARA) principle. This includes decreasing the continuous time spent on a single area and minimizing imaging modalities that increase the power of the ultrasound wave (see Chap. 5). In general, minimizing the field of view to the area of interest and saving clips for review, rather than continuous imaging, may help minimize these effects.

Conclusion

Understanding the basic principles of sound wave reflection, propagation, and frequency, as well as digital sampling, facilitates the effective clinical use of ultrasound technology. These principles can be applied to understand the anatomy and function of the heart, as well as the assessment of blood flow, valve areas, and pressure gradients.

Questions

1. Medical ultrasound is based on the same principle as which of the following?

   (a) Radio Detection and Ranging (RADAR)
   (b) Global Positioning Satellites (GPS)
   (c) Sound Navigation and Ranging (SONAR)
   (d) Cellular Triangulation

2. Which of the following is most true about ultrasound waves?

   (a) They do not propagate in a vacuum
   (b) They have a frequency > 1 kHz
   (c) They will not reflect off interfaces with different density
   (d) They are transverse waves

3. Lateral resolution of an ultrasound probe depends upon which of the following?

   (a) The amplitude of the transmitted wave
   (b) The frequency of the transmitted wave
   (c) The number of piezoelectric crystals in the transducer
   (d) The wavelength of the transmitted wave

4. The axial resolution of an ultrasound probe will improve with which of the following changes?

   (a) Increasing the number of piezoelectric crystals in the transducer
   (b) Increasing the wavelength of the transmitted wave
   (c) Decreasing the pulse length of the transmitted wave
   (d) Decreasing the frequency of the transmitted wave

5. Which of the following is most true regarding Doppler ultrasound?

   (a) The frequency shift between transmitted and received signals is inversely proportional to the sine of the angle between the velocity of the reflector and the direction of the ultrasound wave
   (b) The velocity of a reflector is directly proportional to the frequency shift between transmitted and received signals
   (c) The change in frequency of a reflected signal is inversely proportional to the speed of sound in the medium
   (d) The change in frequency of a reflected signal is directly proportional to the frequency of the transmitted wave

6. The regurgitant jet across the tricuspid valve is measured at 300 cm/sec. The patient's central venous pressure is 8 mmHg. What is the systolic pressure in the right ventricle during systole?

   (a) 28 mmHg
   (b) 36 mmHg
   (c) 44 mmHg
   (d) 104 mmHg

7. The LVOT diameter has been measured to be 2 cm. The LVOT VTI has been traced to be 25 cm. The patient's heart rate is 76 bpm. What is the patient's approximate cardiac output?

   (a) 4 L/min
   (b) 6 L/min

(c) 8 L/min
(d) 10 L/min

8. The patient's LVOT diameter has been measured to be 2 cm. The LVOT VTI has been traced to be 25 cm. The aortic valve VTI has been traced to be 100 cm. What is the area of the aortic valve?

(a) 0.79 cm^2
(b) 1.23 cm^2
(c) 1.56 cm^2
(d) 3.14 cm^2

9. In the absence of aortic stenosis, the left atrial pressure could be calculated knowing which of the following?

(a) Pulmonary arterial diastolic pressure and the velocity of mitral regurgitant flow
(b) Pulmonary arterial diastolic pressure and the diastolic peak mitral flow
(c) Systemic arterial pressure and the velocity of mitral regurgitant flow
(d) Systemic arterial pressure and the diastolic peak mitral flow

10. Which of the following is most true regarding the potential for ultrasound to cause tissue injury?

(a) Cavitation may lead to thermal injury of the tissues
(b) The ALARA principle encourages the use of alternative imaging strategies
(c) M-mode imaging has the highest potential for tissue injury
(d) Color Flow Doppler has a higher potential for tissue injury than B-mode imaging

References

1. Brinklov S, Fenton MB, Ratcliffe JM. Echolocation in oilbirds and swiftlets. Front Physiol. 2013;4:123.
2. Harmon K. Homing in on mammalian echolocation. Sci Am. 2010.
3. Ryckegham AV. How do bats echolocate and how are they adapted to this activity? Sci Am. 1998.
4. Ulanovsky N, Moss CF. What the bat's voice tells the bat's brain. Proc Natl Acad Sci U S A. 2008;105(25):8491–8.
5. Kolarik AJ, et al. A summary of research investigating echolocation abilities of blind and sighted humans. Hear Res. 2014;310:60–8.
6. Schornich S, et al. Psychophysics of human echolocation. Adv Exp Med Biol. 2013;787:311–9.
7. D'Amico A, Pittenger R. A brief history of active Sonar. Aquat Mamm. 2009;35(4):426–34.
8. Ludwig G, Struthers F. *Considerations Underlying the Use of Ultrasound to Detect Gallstones and Foreign Bodies in Tissue*. Naval Medical Research Institutes Reports, 1949. **Project 004001**(Report Number 4): p. 20.
9. Singh S, Goya A. The origin of echocardiography. Tex Heart Inst J. 2007;34(4):431–8.
10. Lang RM, et al. Three-dimensional echocardiography: the benefits of the additional dimension. J Am Coll Cardiol. 2006;48(10):2053–69.
11. Aldrich JE. Basic physics of ultrasound imaging. Crit Care Med. 2007;35(5 Suppl):S131–7.
12. Enriquez-Sarano M, et al. Effective mitral regurgitant orifice area: clinical use and pitfalls of the proximal isovelocity surface area method. J Am Coll Cardiol. 1995;25(3):703–9.

Knobology and Image Optimization

5

Byron Fergerson, Joshua Zimmerman, and Michele Curtis

Introduction

Obtaining quality echocardiographic images is essential for accurate assessment of function and improving diagnostic confidence. Adequate imaging depends on multiple factors including patient anatomy, the quality of the ultrasound system, echocardiographer experience, and the optimization of the ultrasound settings. This chapter will focus on knobology: the optimization of image quality through manipulation of the machine settings. It is important to understand that machine interfaces may appear to be different but have similar options (Fig. 5.1a-c). While illustrating each setting on every brand and model of ultrasound system is beyond the scope of this chapter, the remainder of the chapter will reference a commonly utilized perioperative ultrasound system, the Philips IE33 system (Phillips Medical Systems, Andover, MA). The system has both hard buttons, knobs, and a digital touch panel (Fig. 5.2a-c). Some newer portable or handheld devices may not be as comprehensive as the traditional machines, but the following principles still apply. Similar to keyboard panels, the visual display will differ between brands and models; however, the information displayed is often very similar.

Resolution

An initial review of a few physics concepts and how they apply to image optimization is necessary. More detail on these concepts may be found in Chap. 4. Simply stated, resolution is the ability of a system to distinguish two different points near each other as separate in space. Resolution is divided into three categories: spatial resolution, temporal resolution, and contrast resolution.

Spatial resolution is further categorized as axial, lateral, and elevational resolution (Fig. 5.3). Axial resolution – also referred to as longitudinal, depth, or linear resolution – is defined as the resolution in the direction parallel to the ultrasound beam. Axial resolution is generally the best resolution in the three categories. It is improved by increasing frequency (Fig. 5.4a-b). Lateral resolution is the ability to distinguish equidistant points perpendicular to the beam. Lateral resolution worsens at increasing depth and is improved by focusing the ultrasound beam at the depth of the structure of interest. Elevational resolution refers

B. Fergerson (✉)
Department of Anesthesiology, University of California San Diego Health, La Jolla, CA, USA
e-mail: bfergerson@health.ucsd.edu

J. Zimmerman · M. Curtis
Department of Anesthesiology, University of Utah School of Medicine, Salt Lake City, UT, USA

T. M. Maus, C. R. Tainter (eds.), *Essential Echocardiography*,
https://doi.org/10.1007/978-3-030-84349-6_5

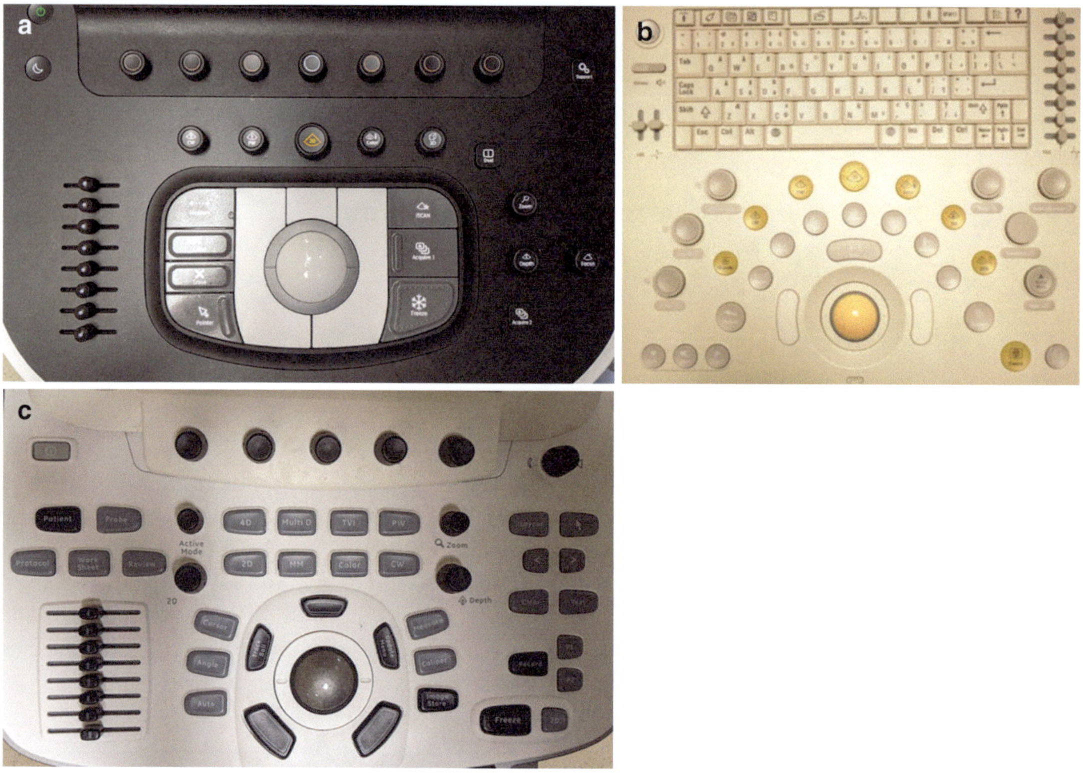

Fig. 5.1 Various ultrasound system keyboards. (**a**) Philips EPIC CVx; (**b**) Philips CX50; (**c**) GE Vivid E9

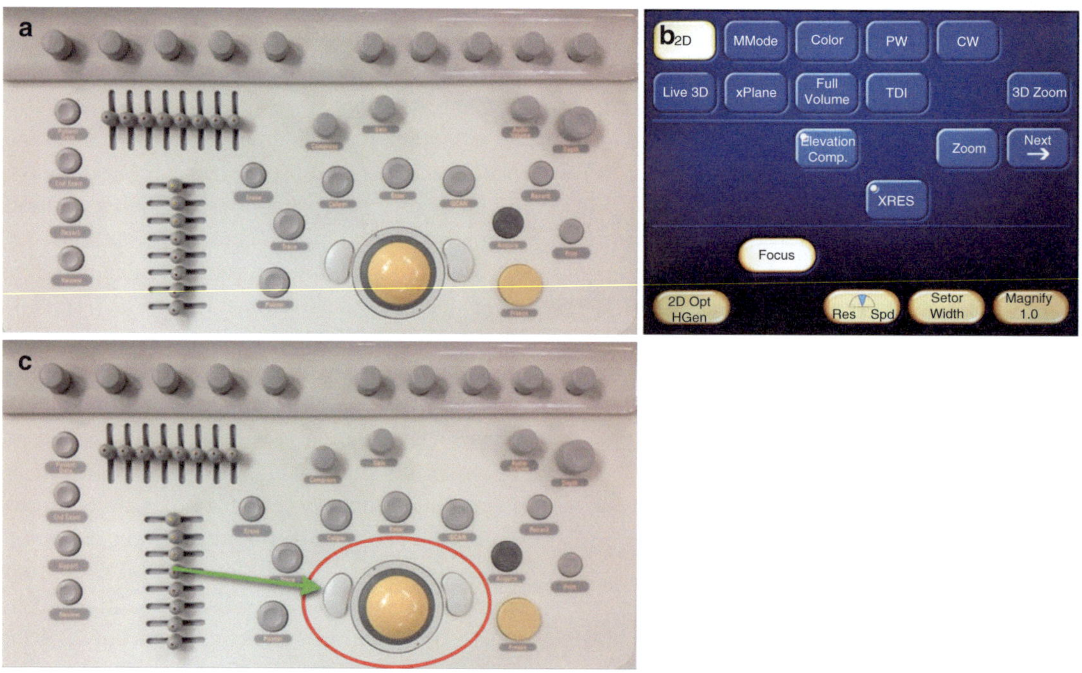

Fig. 5.2 (**a**) Philips IE33 ultrasound system keyboard. (**b**) Philips IE33 digital instrument panel. (**c**) Philips IE33 ultrasound system keyboard. The *red circle* indicates the trackball and selector buttons for utilizing and selecting menus and on-screen cursors. The *green arrow* indicates the kidney buttons that select options at the bottom of the on-screen display and confirm trace and caliper points (similar to mouse buttons)

to the ability to distinguish points above and below the imaging plane and can be thought of as the "thickness" of the imaging plane.

Temporal resolution is the "smoothness of motion" which is directly related to frame rate: the higher the frame rate, the better the movie (Fig. 5.5). Temporal resolution competes with spatial resolution because a high-resolution picture takes more time to acquire and thus decreases the frame rate. It is rare that you can improve one category of resolution without detracting from another.

Contrast resolution is the ability to differentiate between returning signal intensities of adjacent structures. Signal intensities are assigned differing values on the gray scale. Resolution – or the ability to distinguish two different signal intensities near each other – is dependent upon the number of bits per pixel in the image memory as well as the dynamic range of echo signals being evaluated. Simply, the more bits per pixel in the memory, the greater the number of gray shades available to display for different returning echo intensities.

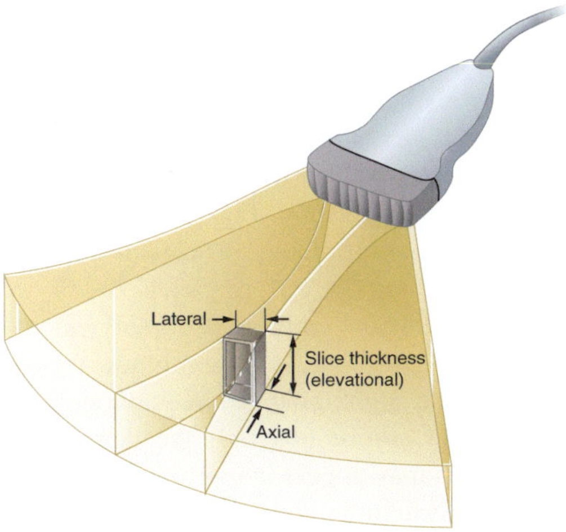

Fig. 5.3 Demonstration of the relationship of axial, lateral, and elevational planes in relation to transducer position

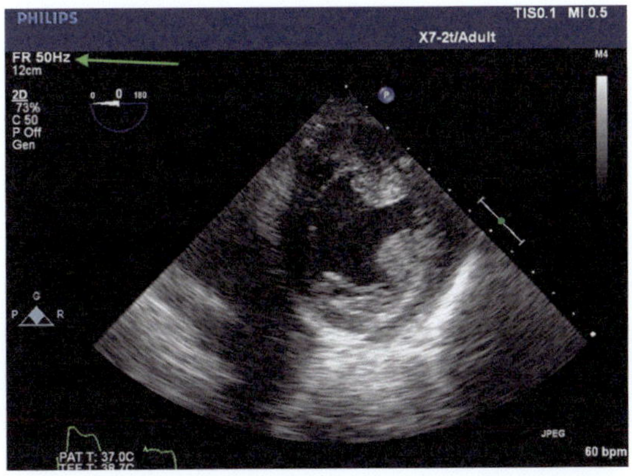

Fig. 5.5 The on-screen display notes the frame rate (*green arrow*) which represents the temporal resolution

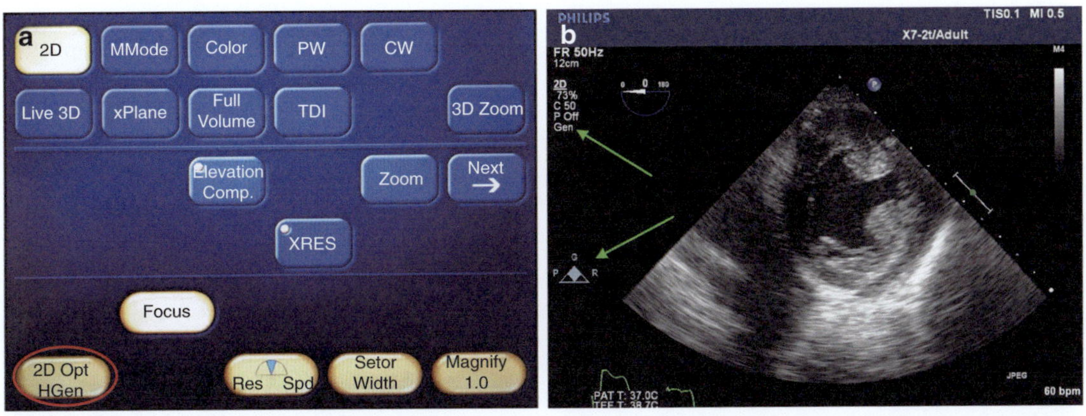

Fig. 5.4 (**a**) Frequency is adjusted with the knob below 2D Opt indicated by the *red circle*. Options include Pen, Gen, and Res corresponding to low-frequency (Penetration), mid-frequency (General), and high-frequency (Resolution) modes. Other brand systems may differ in selection and provide actual frequency settings, typically ranging from 3 to 8 MHz. (**b**) The on-screen display notes the current frequency setting in both word and figure form (*green arrows*)

2D Controls

Preprocessing Versus Postprocessing

Preprocessing controls affect the transmission and acquisition of the echo signals. Changing these preprocessing controls affects how the image is created and therefore must be done during image acquisition. Postprocessing controls affect how the formatted information is displayed on the screen and are performed after the ultrasound signal is received. Preprocessing optimizes the image, while postprocessing determines the "cosmetic appearance" of the images displayed. This chapter will focus on the preprocessing optimization.

Transmit Power

Transmit power controls the acoustic energy, or amplitude, of the ultrasound signal. Simply stated, the power is how loud the transducer "shouts." Higher power creates more tissue compression and rarefaction and thus has increased risk of tissue injury, which is more of a concern with fetal ultrasound. While still preserving adequate image quality, power should be kept as low as possible to decrease this risk and also to mitigate some types of artifacts such as reverberation, side lobe, and beam width (see Chap. 16). Federal standards have been set to limit the maximal intensities for ultrasound studies, and most commercial systems typically default to these settings. Also, most commercial systems have presets for different ultrasound applications, for example, lung, cardiac, abdominal, fetal, and vascular. These presets will automatically change many settings including transmit power and frequency for the type of examination to be done. Most of the time, the default settings will be adequate for imaging. The most common reason to adjust transmit power is for studies utilizing ultrasound contrast agents; however, those studies are beyond the scope of this chapter.

Gain

Gain is the sensitivity of the transducer to receiving a reflected ultrasound signal, or, simply, how well the machine "listens." Gain should be set as high as possible without showing "noise" on echo-free portions of the image, such as anechoic blood or fluid (Fig. 5.6a-b). Optimal gain should allow for the gray scale to differentiate tissues using the differing echo density of those tissues. Low-amplitude signals should appear dark gray, and high-amplitude signals should appear light gray, while cavities with blood should appear black. If the gain is too high, images may appear inappropriately white, and linear structures appear thicker than they actually are, both of which make it difficult to differentiate structures. Conversely, if the gain is too low, only bright or "echodense" structures are visualized, and the ability to differentiate structures is also lost (Fig. 5.7a-c).

Optimal imaging is most easily accomplished in a darker room. In bright ambient light, the

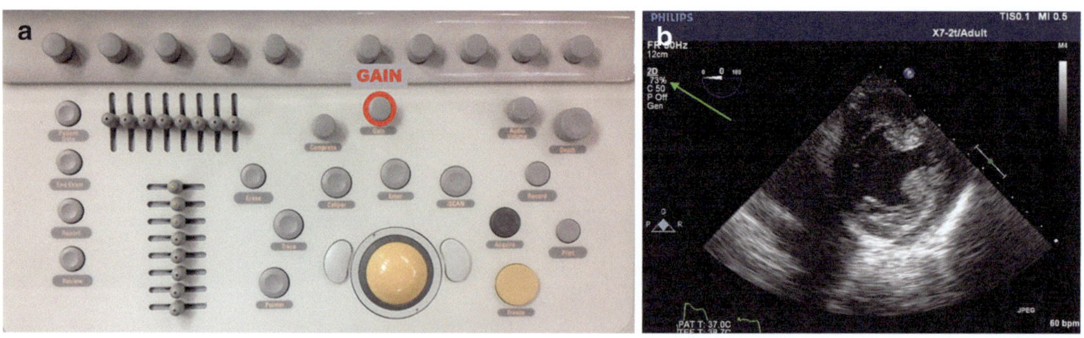

Fig. 5.6 (**a**) The gain knob on the ultrasound keyboard panel is indicated by the *red circle*. Turning the knob clockwise increases gain, while turning counterclockwise decreases the image's gain. (**b**) The on-screen display notes the current gain setting indicated by the *green arrow*

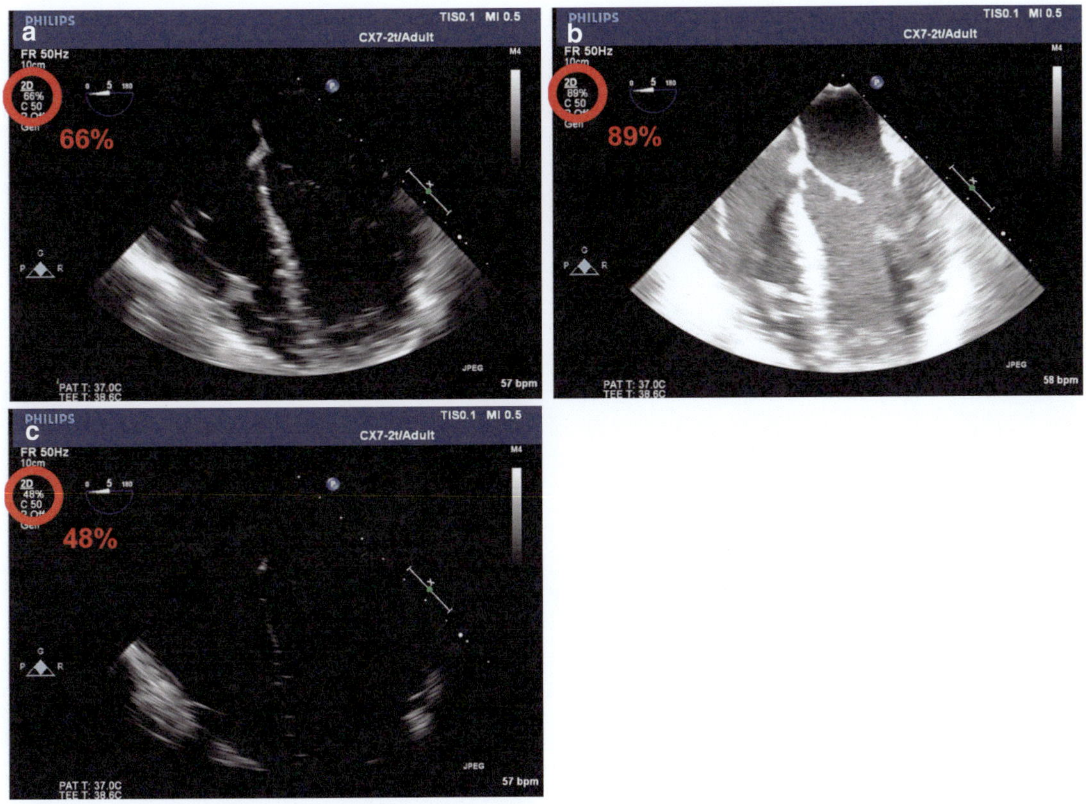

Fig. 5.7 (**a**) Midesophageal four-chamber view with appropriate gain settings; note that blood is dark black, while myocardium is appropriately bright. The gain setting is 66% (*red circle*). (**b**) The same image over-gained with the setting increased to 89% (*red circle*). (**c**) The same image under-gained with the setting decreased to 48% (*red circle*). Note the lack of delineation of the myocardium when the gain is inappropriate

echocardiographer is more likely to increase the gain beyond what is necessary, making the image appear "over-gained." In practice, ambient light should first be reduced, and then gain should be altered if necessary.

Time Gain Compensation and Lateral Gain Compensation

Time gain compensation (TGC) allows optimization of gain at depth, allowing the echocardiographer to compensate for attenuation, which is the loss of ultrasound energy as it travels through a medium. Attenuation is the absorption of energy into the tissues as the ultrasound wave travels from the transducer, leaving less energy available to reflect back and be received for imaging. The echocardiographer needs to be cognizant of the position of the TGC dials as they can greatly impact imaging quality. Typically, the dials should be set midrange in all fields, or slightly higher in the far field (Fig. 5.8a-d). Lateral gain compensation (LGC) is similar to TGC but allows for gain compensation across the field. This can compensate for changes in reflectivity or attenuation. Some machines will have LGC, but many will not. Typically, only experienced echocardiographers make changes in LGC.

Autoscan/iScan

Autoscan or iScan (the name may vary among different ultrasound manufacturers) is an option on many machines that allows the software to

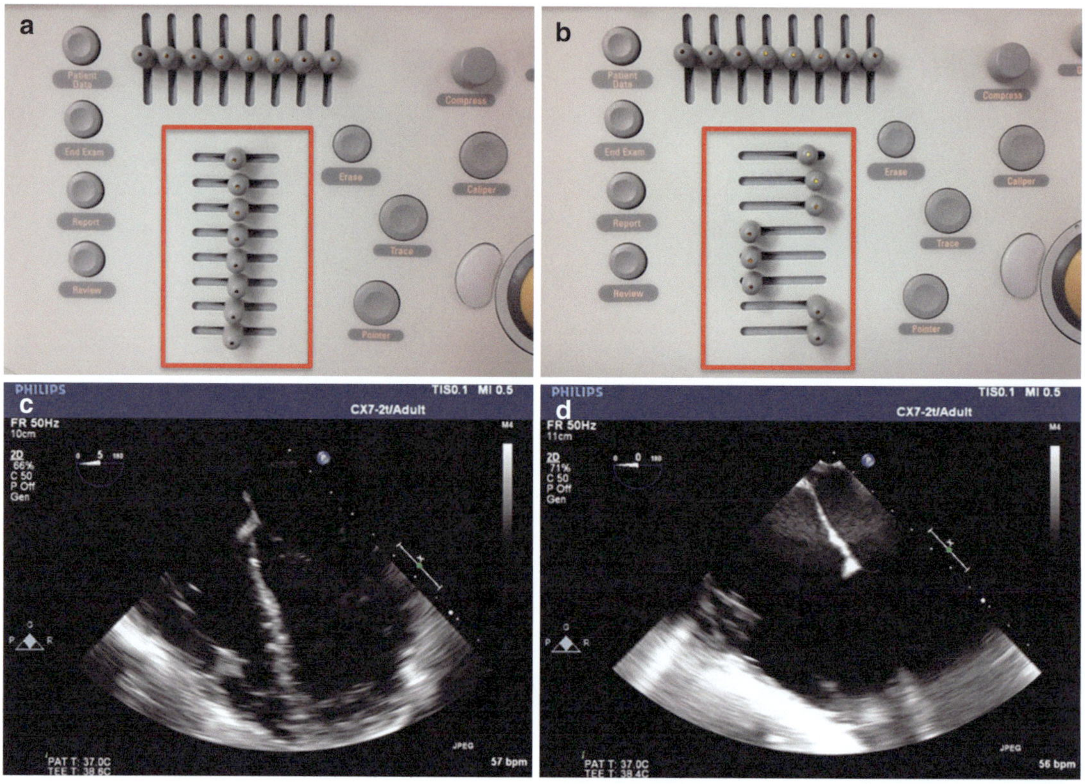

Fig. 5.8 The effect of the time gain compensation (TGC) is demonstrated. (**a**) The TGC is adjusted to a middle setting at all sliders (*red box*). (**b**) The TGC is adjusted with the middle sliders reduced completely (*red box*). (**c**) Midesophageal four-chamber view corresponding to TGC settings in Image **a**. (**d**) Midesophageal four-chamber view corresponding to TGC settings in Image **b**; note the lack of image definition corresponding to the reduced middle TGC sliders

optimize gain across the image with minimal manipulation by the user (Fig. 5.9). It is essentially an "auto-TGC," where a computer algorithm detects the brightness across the ultrasound field and automatically adjusts the TGC to an even level of brightness. In practice, all of the TGC sliders (if present) should be in mid-position prior to pressing the Autoscan button. Adjustments in TGC can then be made, if necessary, but often the Autoscan function alone is sufficient.

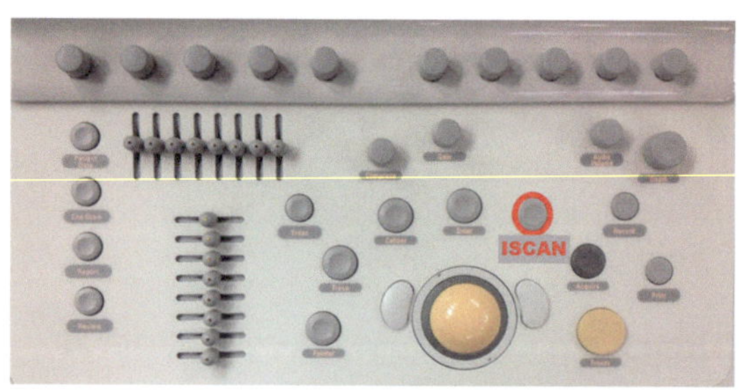

Fig. 5.9 The ultrasound keyboard with the iScan button marked by the *red circle*

Depth

Depth controls the maximum distance to be imaged. Depth markers typically appear on the side of the display to help estimate size and calibrate the eye to the image. The markers are generally 1 centimeter apart, sometimes with smaller gradations present, depending on the scale (Fig. 5.10a-b). Depth directly controls the frame rate: the machine needs to "wait longer" for the ultrasound waves to be received if they have further to travel. With increasing depth, the frame rate decreases, as does temporal resolution.

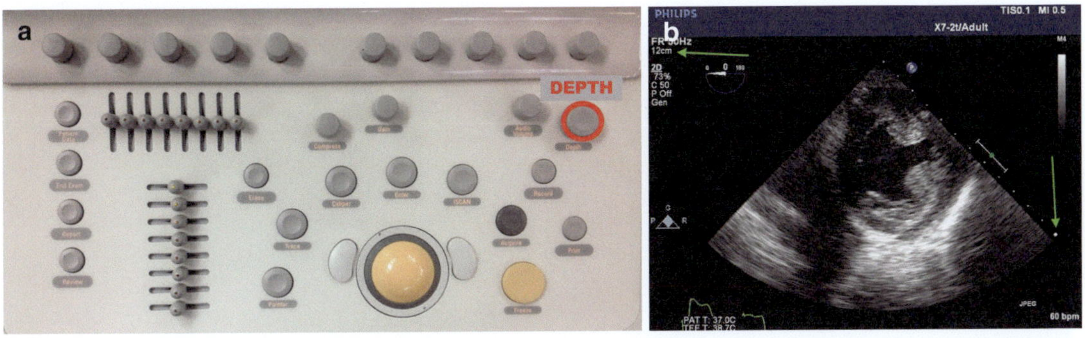

Fig. 5.10 (**a**) The ultrasound keyboard panel with the depth knob indicated by the *red circle*. Turning the knob clockwise increases depth, while turning the knob counterclockwise decreases the depth. (**b**) The on-screen display with the depth setting indicated by the *green arrows*. The dots along the right side of the image indicate the depth typically in 1 centimeter increments

To optimize an image, use the shallowest depth possible to see the structure of interest. This is beneficial for two reasons. First, the screen size is fixed, and by imaging only the structure of interest, it will appear larger on the screen allowing for better evaluation. Second, decreasing the depth will increase temporal resolution. An exception to this reasoning is that, for some structures, it is best to calibrate one's eye to a specific depth. For example, when imaging the LV in the TEE transgastric midpapillary short-axis view or TTE parasternal midpapillary short-axis view, a standard depth should be used for qualitatively assessing LV size. It is easy to make a normal LV appear enlarged or small simply by changing the depth (Fig. 5.11a-c).

Focus

The ultrasound beam progressively narrows until it reaches its smallest diameter and then widens again (see Chap. 4). The smallest diameter is the focal point and has the best lateral resolution. Distal to the focal point, the beam rapidly diverges worsening lateral resolution in the far field. Most machines will allow the operator to move the focal point to optimize lateral resolution at different parts of the image. The focus should be positioned at, or just beyond, the structure of interest for the best lateral resolution (Fig. 5.12a-b).

Sector Width/Sector Steer

The sector width allows the echocardiographer to manipulate the sector angle, thereby changing the number of scan lines and consequently the frame rate and temporal resolution (Fig. 5.13a-b). A larger sector angle allows more information to be included in the picture, but at the cost of a decreased frame rate. For the best temporal resolution, the sector width should be decreased to include only the structure of interest (Fig. 5.14a-c). Decreasing the sector width will decrease the number of scan lines on both sides of the screen equally, allowing visualization of only images in the middle of the original sector angle, which may be problematic if the structure of interest is on the left or right of the original sector angle. Sector steer allows movement of the narrowed sector angle to the other areas within the original sector without moving the transducer.

Freeze

The freeze button stops ultrasound transmission (Fig. 5.15). The display will maintain the image stored immediately before the freeze control was engaged, allowing the echocardiographer to scroll through the cardiac cycle slowly to take measurements and make annotations. Freeze stops transmit power, so if the ultrasound is currently not needed, it decreases the risk of tissue injury. This is particularly important if TEE is being used during surgery

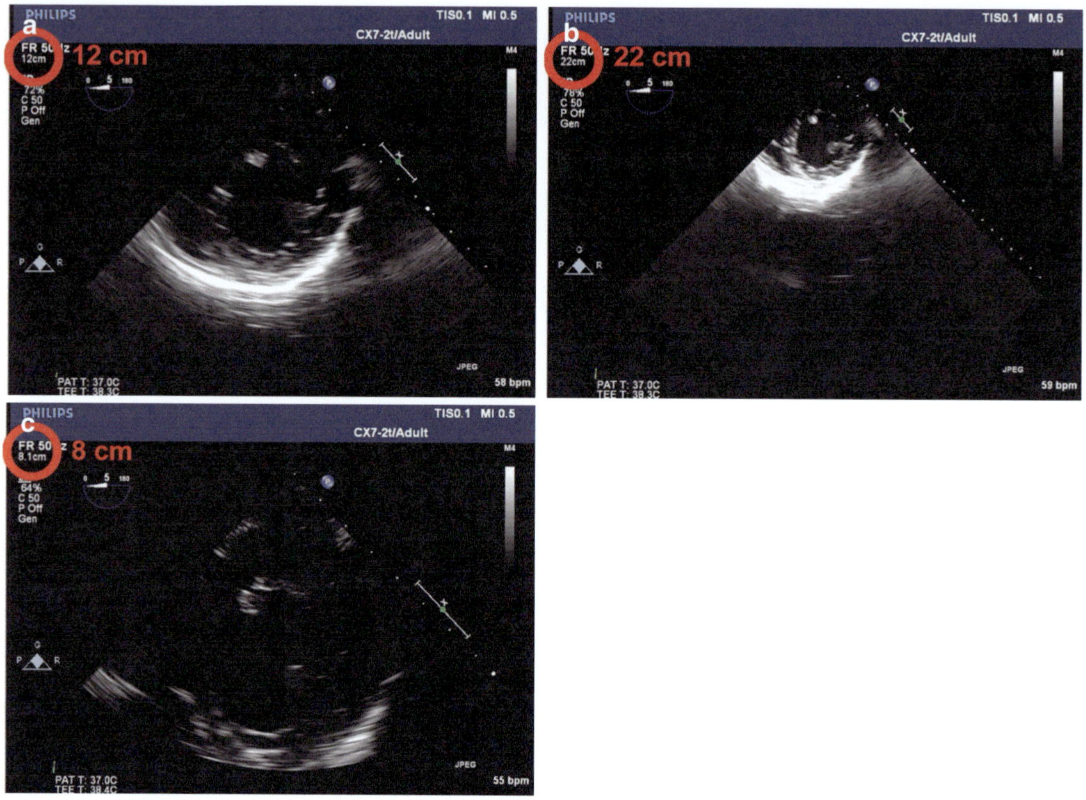

Fig. 5.11 Transgastric midpapillary short-axis view demonstrating the effect of depth setting on imaging. (**a**) Appropriate depth setting of 12 centimeters (*red circle*) displays the left ventricle entirely within the image sector. (**b**) Excessive depth setting of 22 centimeters (*red circle*) displays the left ventricle as small and potentially misdiagnosed as hypovolemic. (**c**) Reducing the depth setting to 8 centimeters (*red circle*) incompletely displays the left ventricle

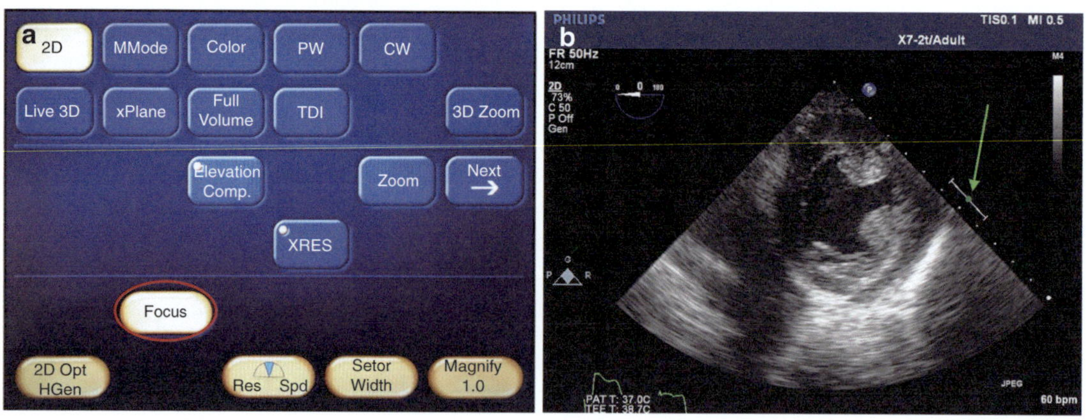

Fig. 5.12 (**a**) The digital panel indicating the focus setting (*red circle*). The knob immediately below the digital focus setting allows adjustment of the ultrasound focus. Turning the knob clockwise moves the focus toward the far field, while turning the knob counterclockwise moves the ultrasound focus toward the near field. (**b**) The on-screen display notes the location of the focus setting as indicated by the *green arrow*

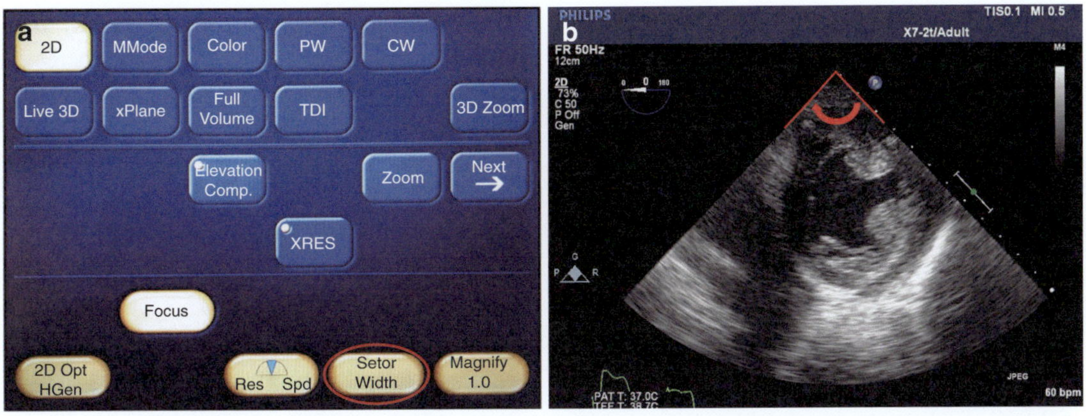

Fig. 5.13 (**a**) The digital panel indicating the sector width setting (*red circle*). The knob immediately below the digital sector width setting allows adjustment of the sector width size. Turning the knob clockwise increases the sector width size, while turning the knob counter-clockwise decreases the sector width size. (**b**) The on-screen display with a maximum sector width size of 90 degrees (*red arrow*)

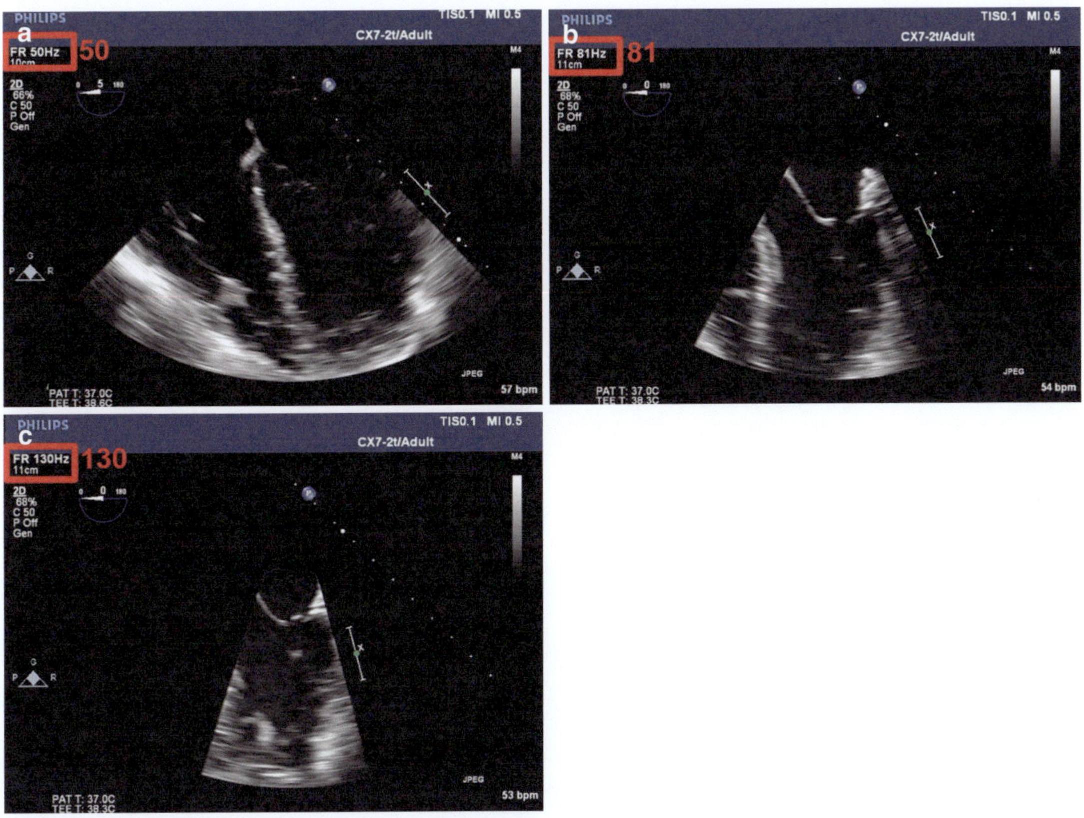

Fig. 5.14 Midesophageal four-chamber view demonstrating the temporal resolution effect of reducing the sector width size (*red boxes*). (**a**) Maximum sector width demonstrates a frame rate of 50 frames per second (Hz). (**b**) Reduced sector width increases the frame rate to 81 frames per second. (**c**) Further reduction in sector width increases the frame rate to 130 frames per second

for intermittent imaging. A practical tip is that when imaging is paused (such as when on cardiopulmonary bypass), the freeze button should be used to prevent overheating of the probe and potential tissue injury.

M-Mode

M-Mode (Motion-Mode) is an imaging modality in which returning echo signals from a single vertical scan line are plotted over time in a dynamic, real-time display. Thousands of ultrasound pulses are repeated per second, increasing temporal resolution along that particular scan line, but at the expense of visualizing adjacent areas. A 2D image is typically displayed on the screen to help orient the viewer to the line being scanned, and the EKG is superimposed to help correlate the image with the cardiac cycle. M-mode is the method of choice for measuring distances of structures perpendicular to the beam as well as visualizing rapidly moving structures because of the greatly increased temporal resolution (Fig. 5.16a-b).

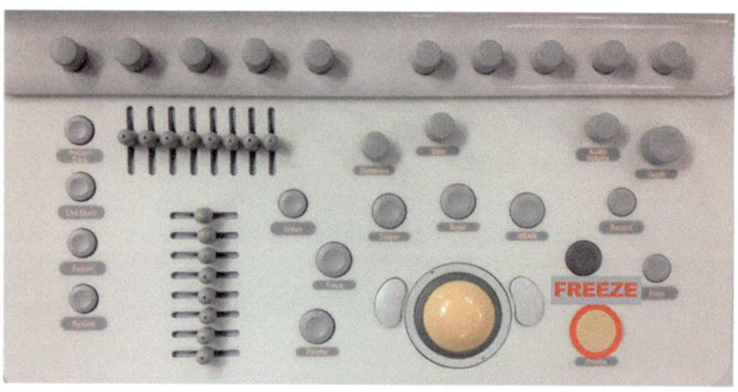

Fig. 5.15 The ultrasound keyboard with the Freeze button marked by the *red circle*

Doppler Controls

Doppler Effect

To understand spectral Doppler (pulsed-wave and continuous-wave Doppler) and color flow Doppler, it is helpful to review the Doppler effect and how it relates to image optimization (see Chap. 4). Simply stated, the Doppler effect is the change in frequency of a wave as the object and the source move toward or away from each other. When an object is moving toward the receiver, the reflected frequency increases, and the wavelength decreases, and when it moves away, the reflected frequency decreases, and the wavelength increases. The ultrasound machine uses this principle to determine the velocity of a moving object such as blood or tissue (velocity is a measure of speed and direction). It is important to remember that the Doppler equation takes into the account the angle at which the objects are moving relative to one another. The velocity calculation will be most accurate when the objects and the ultrasound wave are moving along the same path. Because ultrasound pulses are sent down a particular scan line, objects that are moving parallel to the scan line will have their velocities more accurately assessed. As the angle between ultrasound

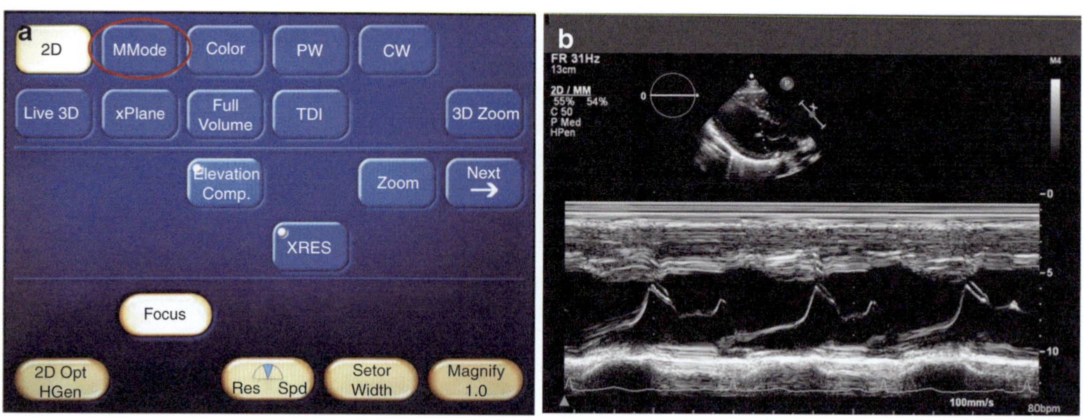

Fig. 5.16 (**a**) The digital panel indicating the digital button to switch to M-mode imaging (*red circle*). (**b**) Parasternal long-axis M-mode imaging of mitral valve motion. Note the depth on the y-axis and time as indicated by the EKG tracing on the x-axis

scan line and direction of object get larger, the velocity of the object will be underestimated.

Pulsed-Wave Doppler

Pulsed-wave Doppler (PWD) uses a single crystal to emit ultrasound pulses along a scan line toward a predetermined target. The crystal then switches to receiving mode to "listen" to and interpret the returning echo signals. The changes in frequency of the returning ultrasound pulses are used to determine the velocity of the object at a specified location using the Doppler equation. The target or sample gate is set by the echocardiographer. Because the speed of sound is constant in tissue, the receiving time delay (or listening time) is based solely on the distance from the transducer to the target before sending another pulse. The farther the target is from the transducer, the longer the "listening" time and the lower the pulse repetition frequency (PRF) will be (this is analogous to frame rate in 2D imaging). The transducer will only interpret returning ultrasound signals received during a predetermined period of time set by the target distance, so only signals associated with that specific depth are interpreted. This principle is called time gating and is the reason that PWD has range resolution (i.e., is able to measure in a specific area).

After the echo signals are received, each of the individual velocities is then plotted on the Y-axis of the graph with the corresponding time on the X-axis with the EKG superimposed. By convention, objects travelling toward the transducer will be above the baseline, while objects moving away from the transducer will be below the baseline. The display for pulsed-wave Doppler typically has an "outlined" rather than a "filled-in" appearance because there is a limited range of velocities within the sample range. The application of PWD is limited to slower maximum velocities because of the intermittent data collection. The maximal frequency that can be evaluated is known as the Nyquist limit. At velocities above the Nyquist limit, they become ambiguous and uninterpretable, which presents a "wrap-around" effect on the display.

Pulsed-wave Doppler should be used when evaluating lower velocities and when range resolution is important. Some examples include measurement of velocities of blood in the left ventricular outflow tract (LVOT) and pulmonary veins, as well as measuring mitral inflow and tissue velocities for diastology (see Chap. 12). The view with the transducer closest to the target, while preserving alignment of flow to the Doppler signal, should be utilized, decreasing the "listening time" and increasing PRF (and, thereby, the Nyquist limit). The sample gate, or target, should be placed at the location where velocities are to be measured (Fig. 5.17a-b). The baseline should be shifted to maximize the range of velocities in the direction of interest. The scale should be adjusted to the range of velocities on the graph for a more accurate evaluation. Gain can be

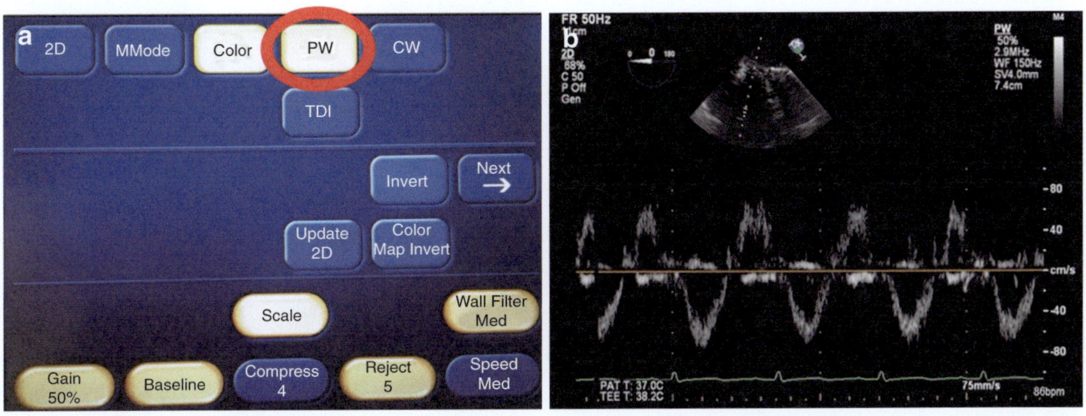

Fig. 5.17 (**a**) The digital panel indicating the digital button to switch to pulsed-wave Doppler imaging (*red circle*). (**b**) An example of pulsed-wave Doppler imaging in the deep transgastric five-chamber view. Note the sample volume placed within the left ventricular outflow tract

increased to amplify the signal, which can pick up weaker reflections, although it will also increase noise (Fig. 5.18a-g).

Continuous-Wave Doppler

Continuous-wave Doppler (CWD) is another form of spectral Doppler, like PWD, with a few key differences. Unlike PWD, which uses a single crystal to alternate transmitting and receiving pulses, CWD uses two separate transducer crystals: one continuously transmits ultrasound waves, while the other continuously receives them (Fig. 5.19a-c). The transducers are oriented so their beam patterns overlap, resulting in all of the returned ultrasound waves along the same scan line superimposed on the graph. Since these ultrasound waves will be a spectrum of velocities, the waveform appears "filled in." Compared to PWD, which is limited by PRF, continuous-wave Doppler can measure higher velocities. The cost, however, is range ambiguity (i.e., you cannot discern at what depth the various velocities are measured), since the velocities being sampled are being collected from along the entire scan line. Continuous-wave Doppler is most useful in evaluating high velocities in valvular pathology, such as aortic stenosis (AS) or mitral regurgitation (MR), or in evaluating velocities in obstructive lesions, like systolic anterior motion of the mitral valve (SAM) or hypertrophic obstructive cardiomyopathy (HOCM). A simple rule of thumb is that CWD is used for "fast" things (i.e., flow through a valve or obstruction) and PWD is used for "slow" things (i.e., everywhere else).

Image optimization for CWD is similar to that for PWD. The CWD should be aligned with the direction of flow. The baseline can be adjusted to present the full range of velocities in the direction of interest. The scale should be optimized to maximize the spectral signal. Spectral gain can amplify weak signals, but at the cost of increasing noise.

Color Flow Doppler

In basic terms, color flow Doppler (CFD) shows a real-time color display of blood flow information superimposed on 2D images. It takes a tremendous amount of computational power, and therefore, the scan lines within the color flow box are typically ½ to ¼ of the line density of the 2D image. The mean sample velocities are assigned colors, with the convention that maximal velocities directed toward the transducer are red, and similar velocities directed away are blue (consider the mnemonic BART: Blue Away, Red Toward). Because CFD is a pulsed technique like PWD, it has similar limitations. Aliasing occurs when the mean maximal velocity exceeds the Nyquist limit. When velocities surpass the Nyquist limit, the color appears turbulent and may appear to flow in the opposite direction (Fig. 5.20a-b). This is often used to suggest high-velocity situations, such as left ventricular outflow tract obstruction or valvular regurgitation, which may be evaluated more precisely with continuous-wave Doppler.

Color flow Doppler can be optimized in several ways. The frame rate can be increased by (1) narrowing the sector width, (2) decreasing the color flow box size, and (3) imaging structures closer to the transducer. Gain can be optimized using the proper dial. "Over-gained" CFD will result in color speckles within tissues where there should be no flow. The Nyquist limit can also be adjusted in CFD. Adjusting the Nyquist limit allows visual assessment of both lower-velocity flow, such as flow through a patent foramen ovale (PFO), or higher-velocity flow such as regurgitation or stenosis. The "scale" dial can be used to adjust the Nyquist limit with lower limits showing

Fig. 5.18 (**a**) The digital panel indicating the settings of gain, baseline, and scale (*green circles*) that are displayed once the pulsed-wave Doppler (PWD) mode (*red circle*) is selected. Turning the knobs immediately below gain, baseline, and scale indicators adjusts the respective settings. Deep transgastric five-chamber view with the PWD sample volume placed in the left ventricular outflow tract (LVOT) demonstrates various settings of baseline, gain, and scale. (**b**) Adjusted baseline away from the probe; note the aliasing velocities (wrap around) of flow through the LVOT. (**c**) Optimized baseline appropriately displaying LVOT velocities below the baseline. (**d**) Reduced scale settings impair the ability to accurately measure LVOT velocities, resulting in aliasing artifact. (**e**) Appropriate scale and gain settings allow accurate measurement of LVOT velocities. (**f**) Reduced spectral gain settings impair the ability to detect LVOT velocities. (**g**) Excessive gain settings lead to potentially inaccurate or excessive velocity measurements

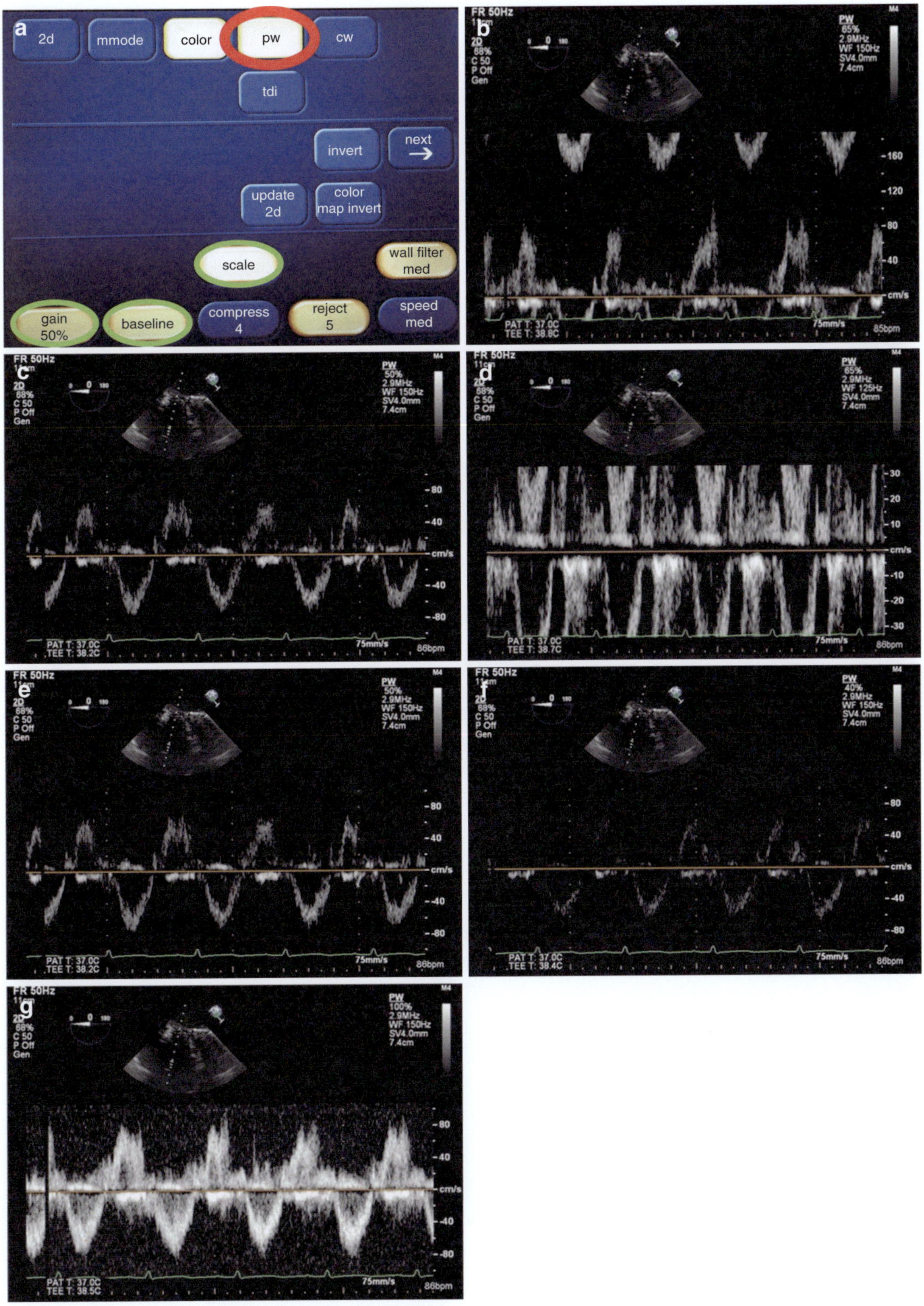
a
2d
mmode
color
pw
cw
tdi
invert
next
update 2d
color map invert
scale
wall filter med
gain 50%
baseline
compress 4
reject 5
speed med
b
c
d
e
f
g

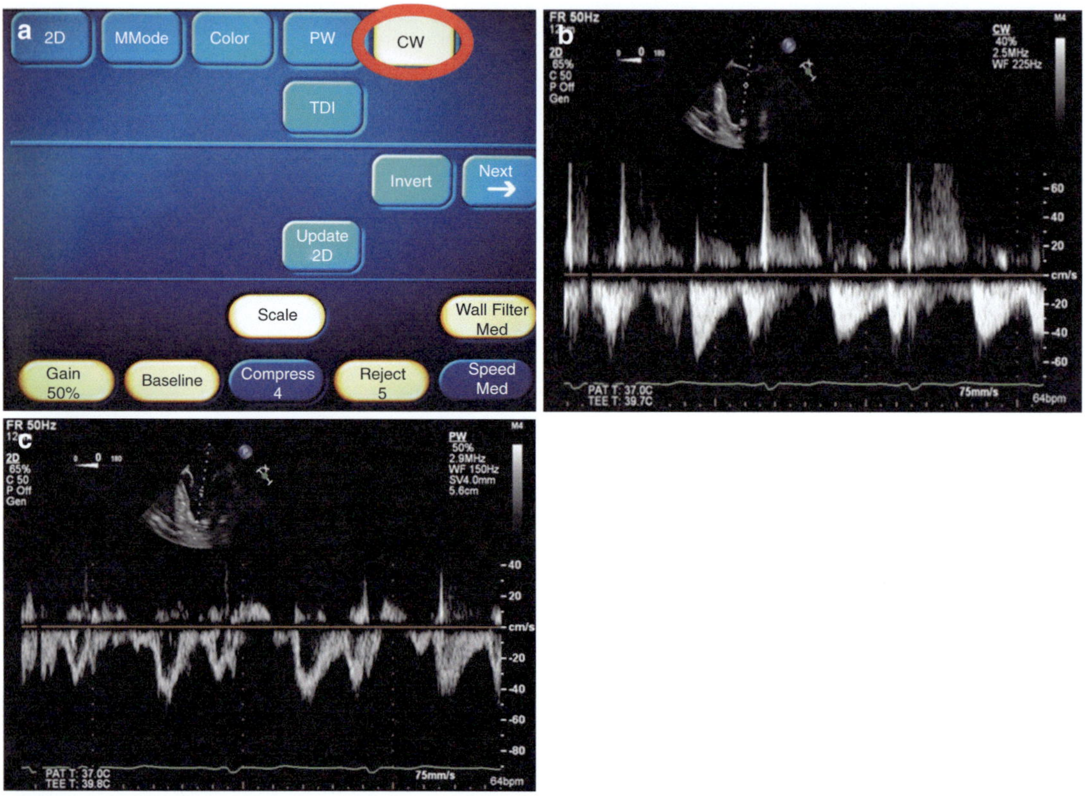

Fig. 5.19 (**a**) The digital panel indicating the digital button to switch to continuous-wave Doppler imaging (*red circle*). Note similar settings of gain, baseline, and scale at the bottom of the image. (**b**) An example of continuous-wave Doppler imaging of mitral valve inflow in the mid-esophageal four-chamber view. Note the "filled-in" appearance of the spectral Doppler signal as the beam measures velocities along the entire ultrasound beam. (**c**) In comparison, pulsed-wave Doppler imaging demonstrates the lack of a "filled-in" profile as velocities are only measured at the sample volume in the mitral inflow

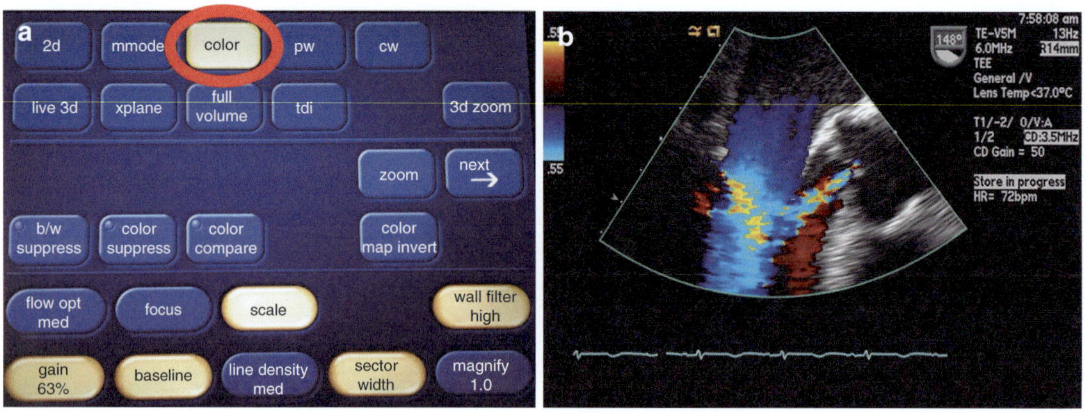

Fig. 5.20 (**a**) The digital panel indicating the digital button to switch to color flow Doppler imaging (*red circle*). (**b**) An example of color flow Doppler imaging in a mid-esophageal long-axis view. Note the flow away from the probe (blue) in diastole through the mitral valve and the speckled appearance of turbulent flow of aortic regurgitation

slow flow better and higher limits removing noise in high-flow situations. However, changing the Nyquist limit can also be a source of misinterpretation and misdiagnosis. If the Nyquist limit is set at a low velocity, the amount of regurgitation may seem much larger than it is, because the appearance of turbulence will occur at lower velocities. Conversely, in evaluating the interatrial septum for a PFO, the flow may be missed if the Nyquist limit is set too high. In general, it is advisable initially to evaluate all valves with a similar Nyquist limit to "calibrate" your eye (Fig. 5.21a-e).

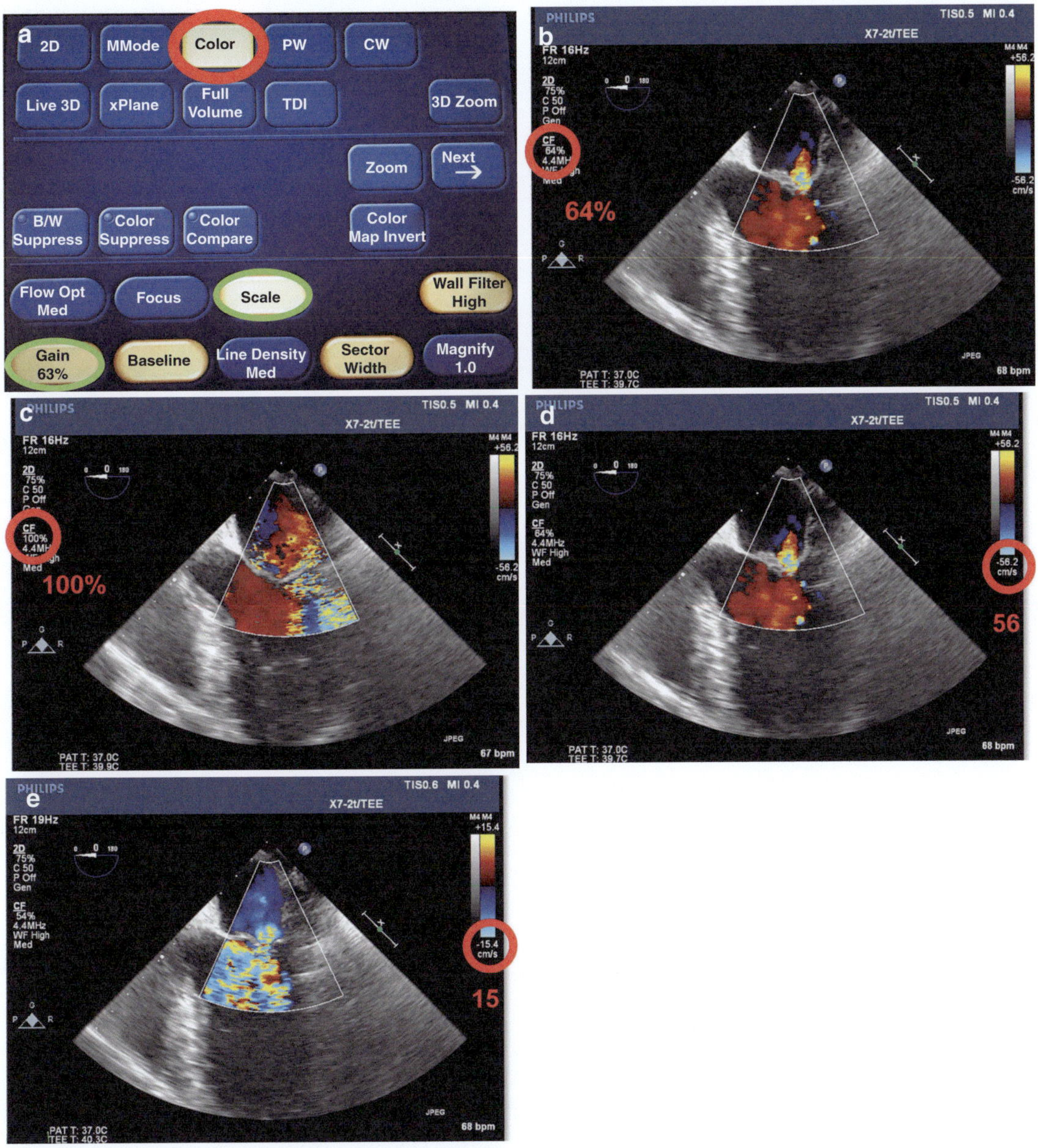

Fig. 5.21 (**a**) The digital panel indicating the settings of gain and scale (*green circles*) that are displayed once the color flow Doppler (CFD) mode (*red circle*) is selected. Midesophageal five-chamber view of a patient with mitral regurgitation demonstrating the effects of gain and scale settings. (**b**) Appropriate spectral gain of 64% (*red circle*) demonstrates laminar flow exiting the left ventricular outflow tract and turbulent flow through the mitral valve. (**c**) Excessive gain (*red circle*) leads to a speckled appearance where there is no expected blood flow (within the myocardium) and difficulty identifying the mitral regurgitation. (**d**) Appropriate scale settings (*red circle*) allow the grading of mitral regurgitation. (**e**) Inappropriately reduced color flow scale (*red circle*) leads to aliasing at lower velocities, obscuring the mitral regurgitation and causing the inappropriate appearance of turbulent flow in the LVOT

Conclusion

There are many factors that contribute to obtaining quality echo imaging, including patient variability, ultrasound technology, and echocardiographer experience. There are also many knobs and buttons provided on the ultrasound machine to facilitate the optimization of image quality and structural assessment. Understanding the various processing technologies available will help the echocardiographer create quality images essential to accurate diagnosis and optimal management.

Questions

1. Which of the following best describes the optimal gain settings?

   a. Blood filled spaces appearing gray
   b. Reduced gain so that only the brightest structures are apparent
   c. Low amplitude reflections appearing dark gray and high amplitude reflections appear light gray
   d. Adjustment to ensure a wider range of amplitude displayed

2. Time gain compensation involves which of the following?

   a. Utilizing the sliders that move left and right on the keyboard
   b. Adjustment of the focus knob
   c. Manipulation of dynamic range
   d. Adjustment of the depth of the pulsed-wave Doppler sampling gate

3. Autoscan or iScan buttons perform which of the following functions?

   a. Computer algorithm-based adjustment of dynamic compression
   b. Computer algorithm-based adjustment of ultrasound power
   c. Computer algorithm-based adjustment of beam focusing
   d. Computer algorithm-based adjustment of time gain compensation

4. Optimal focal knob adjustment should include which of the following?

   a. Focal point positioning at the far end of the screen to allow all cardiac structures to reside within the near field
   b. Focal point positioning at the near end of the screen to allow all cardiac structures to reside within the far field
   c. Focal point positioning near or just beyond the structure of interest
   d. Focal point positioning does not affect the resolution of the ultrasound image

5. Narrowing the sector width of the image results in which of the following changes?

   a. Increased temporal resolution
   b. Increased spatial resolution
   c. Increased elevational resolution
   d. Increased contrast resolution

6. Which imaging modality has the highest temporal resolution?

   a. B-mode imaging
   b. Tissue Doppler imaging
   c. M-mode imaging
   d. Three-dimensional imaging

7. Pulsed-wave Doppler involves which of the following?

   a. Two crystals; one to emit and one to receive
   b. A sample gate to detect velocities at a specific location
   c. Near limitless accurate measurement of blood flow velocities
   d. Range ambiguity of detected velocities

8. Which of the following statements apply to color flow Doppler (CFD)?

   a. CFD is based on continuous-wave Doppler
   b. An enlargement of the selected CFD box leads to a decrease in temporal resolution
   c. An enlargement of the selected CFD box leads to an increase in spatial resolution
   d. CFD does not result in aliasing

9. Continuous-wave Doppler involves which of the following?

   a. Two crystals; one to emit and one to receive
   b. A sample gate to detect velocities
   c. Susceptibility to aliasing at high velocities
   d. Being best-suited for measurement of low velocities at a specific location

10. Thermal injury from transesophageal echocardiography imaging can be reduced by which of the following?

    a. Utilization of the freeze button when not actively imaging (e.g., while on cardiopulmonary bypass)
    b. Increased use of three-dimensional imaging over two-dimensional imaging
    c. Increased use of color flow Doppler over two-dimensional imaging
    d. Avoiding the ALARA principle

Part II

Echocardiographic Assessment

Left Ventricular Systolic Function

6

Swapnil Khoche and Timothy M. Maus

Abbreviations

TEE	Transesophageal echocardiography
TTE	Transthoracic echocardiography
EF	Ejection fraction
LV	Left ventricle
LVEDV	Left ventricular end-diastolic volume
LVESV	Left ventricular end-systolic volume
PSAX	Parasternal short-axis (view)
A4C	Apical four-chamber (view)
LVIDd	LV internal diameter at end-diastole
LVIDs	LV internal diameter at end-systole
LVEDA	Left ventricular end-diastolic area
LVESA	Left ventricular end-systolic area
dP/dt	Change in pressure over time
TDI	Tissue Doppler imaging
S'	Mitral annular velocity (systole)

Supplementary Information The online version of this chapter (https://doi.org/10.1007/978-3-030-84349-6_6) contains supplementary material, which is available to authorized users.

S. Khoche (✉) · T. M. Maus
Department of Anesthesiology, University of California San Diego Health, La Jolla, CA, USA
e-mail: skhoche@health.ucsd.edu

Introduction

Echocardiography has long been used for the assessment of left ventricular function and the diagnosis of heart failure [2]. However, because there is no gold standard to measure the true efficacy of cardiac contraction (adequate blood propulsion that leads to adequate tissue perfusion), surrogates such as ejection fraction (EF) are employed [3].

The ejection fraction is a measure of the left ventricle's (LV) ability to project forward a portion of the volume it contains at the end of diastole. End-diastole is noted by mitral valve closure and correlates with the onset of the QRS complex on the electrocardiogram (EKG). End-systole immediately precedes the mitral valve opening and correlates with the end of the T-wave on EKG [4]. The American Society of Echocardiography (ASE) defines normal ejection fraction as greater than 52% for men and 54% for women [5]. As the amount of blood ejected is the difference between end-diastolic and end-systolic volumes, the EF is mathematically represented as:

$$EF(\%) = \left[\left(LVEDV - LVESV\right) / LVEDV\right] x 100\%$$

LVEDV = LV end-diastolic volume, LVESV = LV end-systolic volume

T. M. Maus, C. R. Tainter (eds.), *Essential Echocardiography*,
https://doi.org/10.1007/978-3-030-84349-6_6

Several other echocardiography-derived parameters, like fractional area change or fractional shortening, use the same formula structure with other measurements substituted for the volumes:

$$EF = \frac{(\text{LV ED parameter} - \text{LV ES parameter})}{\text{LV ED parameter}} x100$$

These provide estimations of EF or surrogate measures of left ventricular systolic function (Highlight Box 6.1). Methods that should be familiar to the basic echocardiographer include visual estimation of EF, fractional shortening, fractional area change, the modified Simpson's method, the rate of rise of ventricular pressure, and mitral annular motion utilizing tissue Doppler imaging. Advanced techniques such as three-dimensional (3D) EF measurement and global longitudinal strain analysis will be briefly mentioned but are beyond the scope of this text.

Highlight Box 6.1

LV systolic function	
2D	• Reduced FS, FAC, EF • EF determination: Modified Simpson's method or visual estimation • Secondary changes – LAE, biventricular dysfunction
CFD	• Typically not utilized
Spectral	• dP/dt determination • S' – tissue Doppler imaging

LV left ventricle, *FS* fractional shortening, *FAC* fractional area of change, *EF* ejection fraction, *LAE* left atrial enlargement, *dP/dt* rise in pressure over time, *S'* lateral mitral annular velocity

Visual Estimation of Ejection Fraction

The most basic way to determine a patient's ejection fraction is to qualitatively estimate it based on visual evaluation of 2D echocardiography. Although objective measures of LV function result in reduced inter-observer variability and better reproducibility, visual estimation of ejection fraction by skilled echocardiographers can approach objective measurements, even after relatively little training [6, 7]. For the basic echocardiographer, a simple qualitative estimate of poor, moderate, or good ventricular function is often all that is needed. Over time, as experience is gained in obtaining objective measurements of EF, the practitioner will be better able to calibrate their visual estimate of the patient's EF with the actual quantitative estimate. For TEE, the mid-esophageal four-chamber and the transgastric midpapillary short-axis windows are excellent views for visual estimation of EF, visually comparing the size of the chamber at end-diastole versus end-systole. For TTE, comparable views are the parasternal short-axis (PSAX) view and the apical four-chamber (A4C) view. Subcostal views can also provide reasonable LV views for visual estimation of LV function.

It is important to note that both quantitative and qualitative estimates of EF can be prone to error in cases of arrhythmia, extremes of heart rate, and presence of significant wall motion abnormalities. Most two-dimensional (2D) measurements rely heavily on adequate endocardial border definitions, which requires gain optimization to improve the blood-tissue interface. Contrast agents may be used to better delineate LV volumes, but their use in basic perioperative and critical care echocardiography is not routine [5].

Fractional Shortening

Fractional shortening is a linear measurement of changes in the LV cavity diameter, expressed as a percentage. To calculate the percentage of fractional shortening, a transgastric midpapillary short-axis view is obtained, and endocardial border-to-border measurements of the LV cavity during systole and diastole are acquired. Measurements of the endocardial borders can be made directly from the transgastric midpapillary short-axis window or by using M-mode with the interrogation line along the inferior and anterior wall. When utilizing TTE, a parasternal short-axis or parasternal long-axis view provides adequate visualization of the LV cross-sectional dimensions for this purpose. Fractional shortening is calculated as a percentage of the difference between the internal diameters of the LV at end-systole and end-diastole. Care should be taken to exclude the papillary muscles from the measurement to avoid error. Normal values for fractional shortening are 25–45% [5] (Figs. 6.1a & b and 6.2).

$$\text{Fractional shortening of the LV } (\%) = \left[\left(\text{LVIDd} - \text{LV IDs} \right) / \text{LV IDd} \right] \text{x } 100\%$$

LVIDd = LV internal diameter at end-diastole, LVIDs = LV internal diameter at end-systole

Whether it is from traditional 2D imaging or M-mode, fractional shortening can provide an estimate of LV systolic function; however, it is the least representative of overall global function, especially with regional abnormalities or distorted LV geometry. This limitation results from the fact that fractional shortening is a measurement of just one dimension along two isolated points of the LV, rather than each wall segment. This measurement does not consider septal and lateral wall motion, nor basal or apical function. Another source for error is the need for appropriate beam orientation, since an off-axis ultrasound beam orientation can result in inappropriate measurements of LV internal diameters [5]. It is also vital to remember that most reference values for fractional change, in either ventricular dimensions or area, are different than the reference values for EF (Table 6.1). For example, a fractional shortening of 30%, while "appearing" as a low percentage, actually represents normal systolic function [1]. However, most machines will provide a corresponding estimated EF extrapolated from the values measured.

Fractional Area Change

Fractional area change extends the principle of fractional shortening into two dimensions, evaluating the change in the cross-sectional area of the LV between systole and diastole to estimate LV systolic function, rather than just the change in the LV cavity along a straight line (single dimension). Fractional area change is easy to perform and reproducible and provides a more accurate surrogate for EF than fractional shortening. Although multiple methods have been devised to put this principle into practice, measuring fractional area change at the transgastric midpapillary short-axis view from TEE is the quickest, since it requires just one view to be obtained. This equates to using the parasternal short-axis view from TTE at the level of the papillary muscles (Fig. 6.3). However, it should be noted that

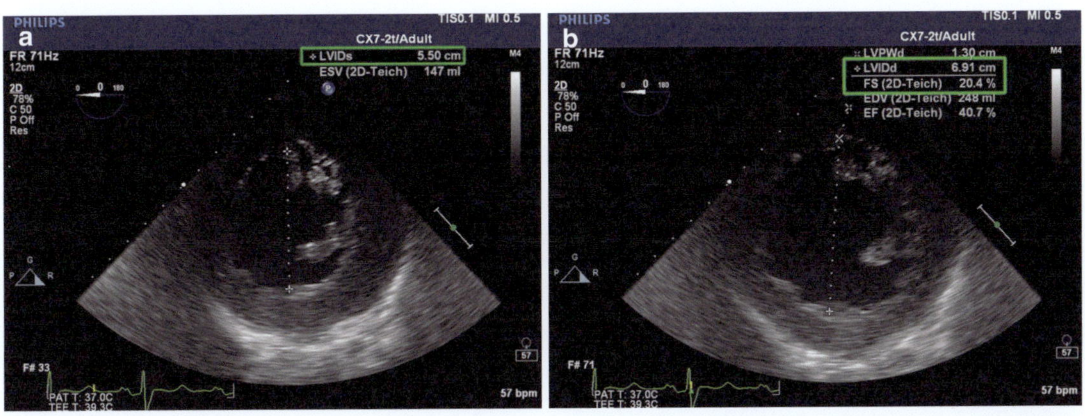

Fig. 6.1 (**a**) Transgastric midpapillary SAX view in systole, where the endocardium-to-endocardium measurement is obtained. The machine calculates an end-systolic volume based on a pre-determined algorithm. (**b**) The acquisition of an end-diastolic dimension results in a calculation of fractional shortening (FS), as well as estimations of end-diastolic volume and EF, based on pre-determined algorithms. The LV systolic function shown here is poor, (low FS)

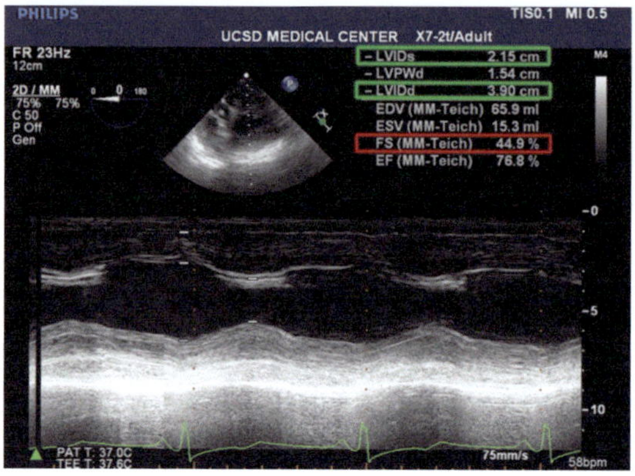

Fig. 6.2 Fractional shortening calculation based on M-mode, along a one-dimensional axis from the inferior to anterior wall. The dark portions denote the LV cavity, while the echogenic lines indicate inferior and anterior wall motion over time. Note that care has been taken to exclude the papillary muscles, which encroach on the LV cavity during systolic measurement. Fractional shortening is obtained by noting the internal diameter in systole and diastole

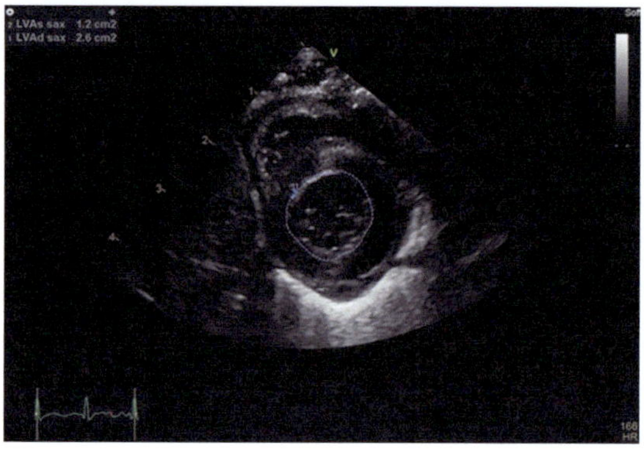

Fig. 6.3 Parasternal midpapillary short-axis view of the LV with TTE. The LV cavity has been traced in systole and diastole (measured in a previously acquired separate frame), resulting in a fractional area change of (2.6–1.2)/2.6 = 0.53 or 53 %

Table 6.1 Values for grading left ventricular function

	Normal	Mild dysfunction	Moderate dysfunction	Severe dysfunction
Fractional shortening	25–45%	20–24%	15–19%	< 15%
Fractional area of change	56–62% (male) 59–65% (female)			
EF	52–72% (male) 54–74% (female)	41–51% (male) 41–53% (female)	30–40% (male) 30–40% (female)	< 30% (male) < 30% (female)
dP/dt (mmHg/sec)	> 1200	800–1200	< 800	< 500
S'	> 10 cm/s			< 5 cm/s

EF Ejection fraction, *dP/dt* rate of rise of ventricular pressure, *S'* peak systolic velocity via tissue Doppler imaging of the lateral mitral annulus

calculating fractional area change in a single plane is still not a global representation of LV function and can become very inaccurate in the setting of wall motion abnormalities or LV distortion. In particular, simply utilizing the TG midpapillary short-axis view will not account for wall motion of the basal and apical LV segments.

To calculate the fractional area change, the internal area of the LV cavity can be traced out manually at end-systole and end-diastole, carefully excluding the papillary muscles from the tracing. The difference in the area of the LV is then calculated as a percentage, according to the equation below:

$$\text{Fractional Area Change of the LV}(\%) = \left[(\text{LV EDA} - \text{LV ESA}) / \text{LV EDA}\right] \text{x}\, 100\%$$

LV EDA = End-diastolic area of the left ventricle,
LV ESA = End-systolic area of the left ventricle

Some machines have algorithms that automate this process using semi-automatic endocardial border detection. Normal values are defined as 56–62% for males and 59–65% for females [8].

Left Ventricular Volumes

Determination of ejection fraction requires calculation of ventricular volumes at end-diastole and end-systole. While volume is a three-dimensional measurement, performing this calculation from two-dimensional images can be challenging and often requires geometric assumptions of the left ventricular shape. Multiple methods exist (ellipsoid method, bullet method, etc.) to provide this estimation of the left ventricle; however, the modified Simpson's method described below is the most often utilized.

The ellipsoid method recognizes the nonspherical shape of the LV and attempts to calculate its volume as a symmetrical ellipsoid (Fig. 6.4). A line connecting the insertion points of the mitral leaflets (the mitral annulus) forms the base of the ellipsoid. In a ME four-chamber, ME two-chamber, or a TG two-chamber view, the LV is divided into two axes along its length and width, and its volume using the single plane ellipsoid method is calculated using a formula involving the left ventricular area in the long-axis view and the diameter of the left ventricle. To further increase the accuracy of the estimation, the biplane ellipsoid method also uses the minor-axis and short-axis area measurements.

Another form of LV volume estimation is the bullet, or hemisphere-cylinder formula (Fig. 6.5). It assumes that the LV is shaped like a hemisphere sitting on top of a cylinder [9]. This can be performed using TTE or TEE, but like with any of these methods, LV foreshortening can plague the result. These methods have not gained popularity in LVEF estimation, likely related to the complexity of the techniques, introduction of errors in measurement of the LV area, and inter-observer variability.

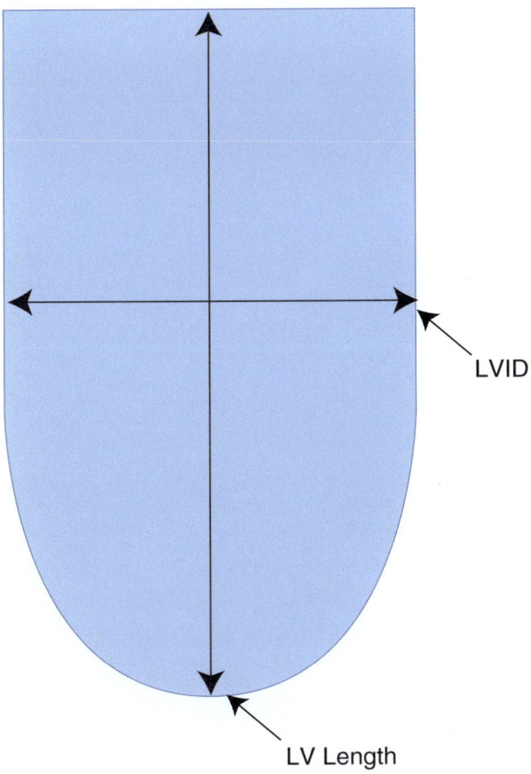

Fig. 6.4 The ellipsoid method for determining LV volume, which is based on the LV internal diameter (LVID) and the LV length

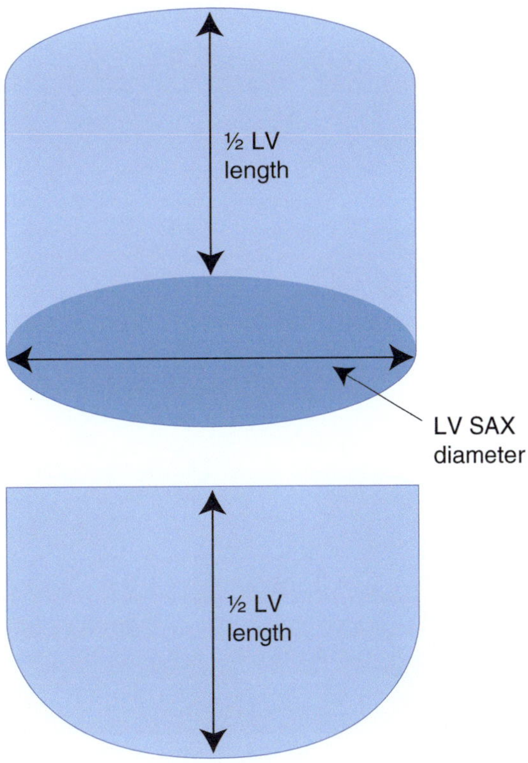

Fig. 6.5 Description of LV volume as a "bullet" shape, where part is cylindrical, while the remainder is hemispheric

Modified Simpson's Method

The modified Simpson's method is the preferred technique of two-dimensional echocardiography-based LV volume estimation and EF determination, per the American Society of Echocardiography [5]. This method is an extension of the previously discussed fractional area change method, except the fractional area change is now calculated at multiple points across the LV instead of a single "slice," more closely approximating a measure of fractional volume change. The modified Simpson's method divides the LV into a series (typically 20) of symmetrical discs. The area of each disc is calculated based on the height and the diameter of the disc and summated to obtain an LV volume. This is analogous to calculating the volume of a stack of coins with different diameters, where the diameter of the coins corresponds to the diameter of that particular segment of the left ventricle. Using TEE, the midesophageal four-chamber and two-chamber views are commonly used for this method [9]. Using TTE, the apical four- and two-chamber views are used. Although it can be done using either single view, combining the two views increases accuracy. The endocardium is either manually or automatically traced in both the four-chamber and two-chamber views at end-diastole and end-systole. The ultrasound machine software splits the designated area into 20 discs, calculates the volume of each disc, and then summates all the discs to generate estimates for end-diastolic and end-systolic volumes in both views (i.e., septal-lateral in the four-chamber view and anterior-posterior in the two-chamber view), thus generating a biplane EF (Figs. 6.6a–d and 6.7a–b).

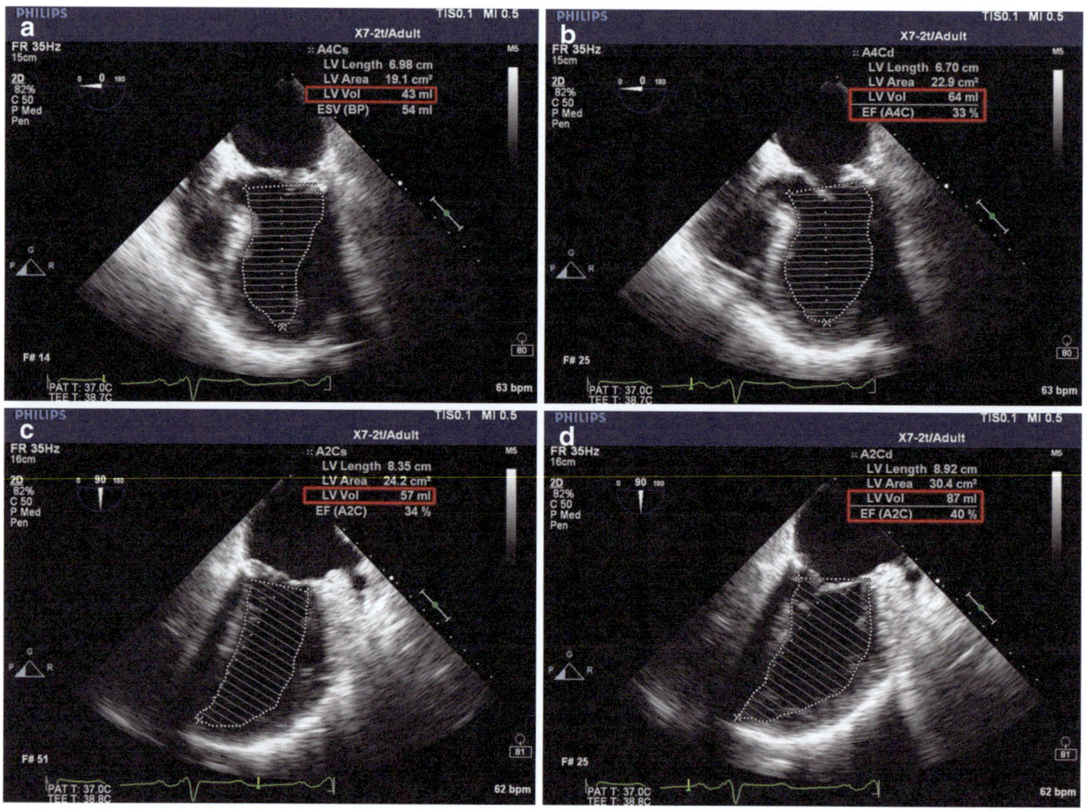

Fig. 6.6 The modified Simpson's method of EF calculation using a midesophageal window via TEE. The dotted line from the mitral valve annulus measures the length of the LV, while the numerous horizontal lines depict the stack of "discs" from which the volume of the LV is calculated. (**a**) ME four-chamber view in systole. (**b**) ME four-chamber view in diastole. (**c**) ME two-chamber view in systole. (**d**) ME two-chamber view in diastole

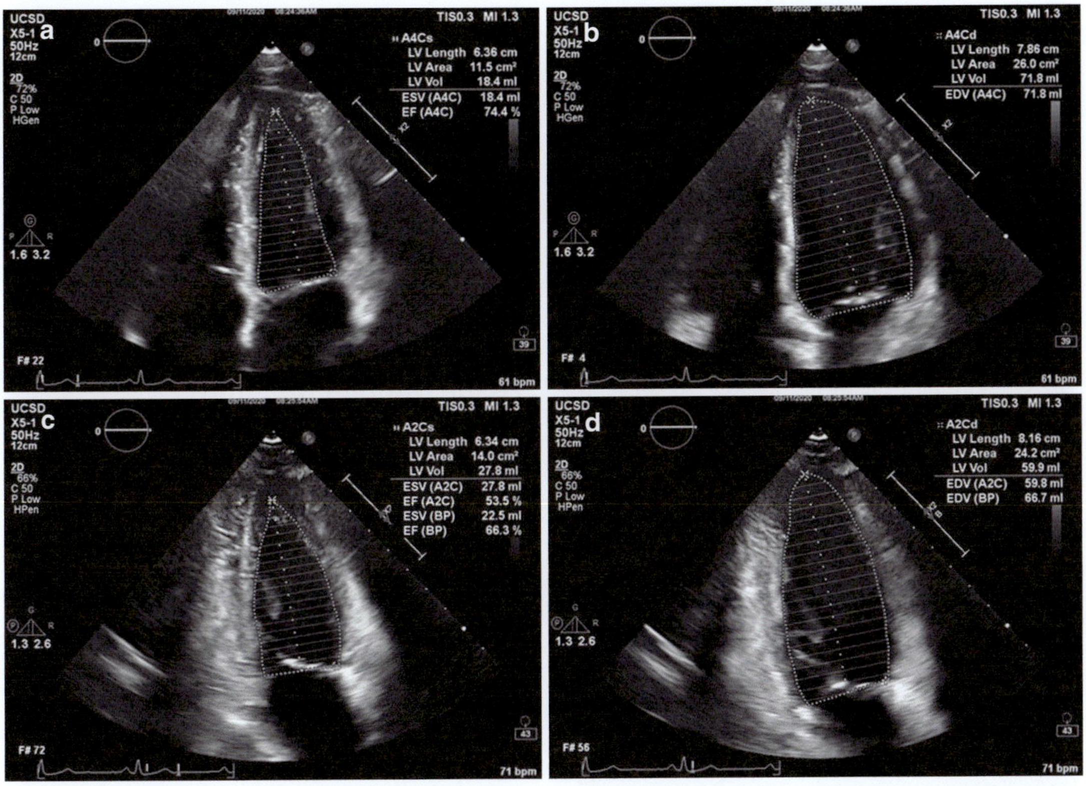

Fig. 6.7 The modified Simpson's method of EF calculation using an apical window via TTE. The dotted line from the mitral valve annulus measures the length of the LV, while the numerous horizontal lines depict the stack of "discs" from which the volume of the LV is calculated. (**a**) Apical four-chamber view in systole. (**b**) Apical four-chamber view in diastole. (**c**) Apical two-chamber view in systole. (**d**) Apical two-chamber view in diastole

The modified Simpson's method is easy to perform, and has been shown to have low interobserver variability [10]. Although this technique overcomes some of the difficulties in estimating EF in patients with altered LV geometry and segmental dysfunction, it is important to remember that only two views of the LV are used to predict global function. Therefore, it is still possible to miss dysfunction of segments not visualized and therefore may not truly be representative of the entire LV. Adequate 2D imaging is essential to reduce foreshortening, which results in reduced volume estimation and errors in EF estimation [11]. To ensure that foreshortening of the LV is not causing errors in calculation, there should be less than a 10% discrepancy between the measurements in the four-chamber view and the two-chamber view for both phases of the cardiac cycle [5].

Rate of Rise of Ventricular Pressure (dP/dt)

The rate of rise of left ventricular pressure (dP/dt) is used as a single measure to evaluate left ventricular systolic function. The left atrial (LA) pressure changes during systole are negligible, and therefore using a mitral regurgitant velocity to estimate the pressure gradient that forms is primarily a result of the rise in LV pressure only. LV contractility determines how swiftly the pressure gradient develops between the LV and LA, making dP/dt an appropriate surrogate for measurement of left ventricular systolic function.

The basis of this method is the modified Bernoulli equation, $P = 4v^2$, discussed in Chap. 4. The midesophageal or apical four-chamber view is used with a focus on the mitral valve and the mitral regurgitant (MR) jet. Other views of the mitral valve from the midesophageal or apical positions can be considered if alignment of the jet is improved with the Doppler interrogation line. The cursor is placed over the MR jet during systole, and a continuous-wave Doppler waveform is obtained, ensuring the scale is appropriately set to at least 5 m/s. The display will differ based upon TEE or TTE imaging; TEE will demonstrate the parabolic shaped MR curve above the baseline, while TTE imaging will demonstrate the MR Doppler curve below the baseline. The caliper is placed on the initial edge of the MR jet envelope at 1 m/s and 3 m/s, and the time needed for this transition is measured and converted to seconds (*t*) [12] (Fig. 6.8a–b).

The pressure gradient that drives the mitral jet changes from 4 mmHg when the velocity is 1 m/s ($4v^2 = 4 \times (1)^2 = 4$) to 36 mm Hg when the velocity is 3 m/s ($4v^2 = 4 \times (3)^2 = 36$). The pressure gradient change (dP) is therefore 32 mm Hg, which remains constant for the calculation [13]. The time to change (dt) from 4mm Hg to 36 mm Hg is determined from the Doppler tracing. The following equation is used to measure the rate of change in the pressure gradient:

$$dP/dt = [4\,(3)^2 - 4\,(1)^2]\,/\,t = (36 - 4)/\,t = 32/t;$$

therefore,

$$dP/dt = 32/t, \text{ with t in seconds}$$

A value greater than 1000–1200 mmHg/sec is considered normal. The advantages of this technique include ease of performance and relative load independence. The measurement also correlates well with other parameters of systolic function. However, it requires the presence of a well-aligned mitral regurgitation jet and is prone to error with significant alterations in left atrial pressure.

Tissue Doppler Imaging

During systolic contraction, the piston-like contraction of the LV pulls the mitral annulus downward toward the LV apex and the speed of this displacement can be used as a surrogate for left ventricular systolic function. Utilizing tissue Doppler imaging, the peak velocity that the mitral annulus attains can be measured. Tissue Doppler imaging uses an inverted filter to measure the velocity of low-speed high-intensity signals (i.e., myocardium), filtering out high-speed, low-intensity signals (i.e., blood). Mitral annular velocity (S') reflects the longitudinal motion of the left ventricle and correlates well with global systolic function, analogous to the use of the tricuspid annular motion for the right ventricle (see Chap. 10). Mitral annular velocity has also been

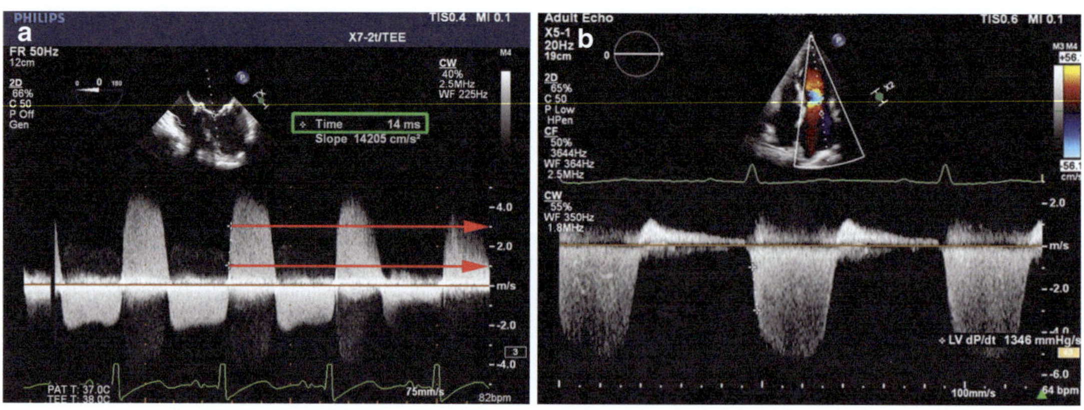

Fig. 6.8 (**a**) The measurement for the rate of ventricular pressure rise (dP/dt) from a midesophageal four-chamber view. The determination of dP/dt = 32mmHg / 0.014s = 2285 mmHg/s, which indicates normal systolic function. The *red arrows* indicate the pressure gradient determinations at 1 m/s and 3 m/s. The time required to increase pressure to this degree is calculated as 14 ms (*green box*). (**b**) The measurement of dP/dt from an apical four-chamber view of 1346 mmHg/s also denotes normal left ventricular systolic function

shown to be predictive of cardiac mortality in patients over time [14].

A midesophageal four-chamber view (TEE) or an apical four-chamber view (TTE) is used, with a focus on the lateral mitral annulus. Tissue Doppler imaging (TDI) is used, which generates a color-coded image on the screen, reflecting tissue motion toward and away from the ultrasound probe. A pulsed-wave Doppler sample volume cursor is placed over the lateral mitral annulus. The height of the S' wave, the deflection below (TEE) or above (TTE) the baseline during systole, is measured and represents the peak systolic velocity of the lateral mitral annulus. Healthy subjects generally have a velocity of more than 7.5 cm/s, though using a cutoff of 10 cm/s makes this measurement even more specific [15] (Fig. 6.9). In LV failure, this velocity is almost always below 5 cm/s. This method offers ease of performance, reliability, and relative load independence as its advantages [9]. Additionally, no endocardial tracing is needed [16]. However, a calcified or artificial mitral valve can confound the measurement, since the lack of movement of a calcified annulus can underestimate LV function. In addition, getting the lateral mitral annulus into view using TTE can be challenging in cases with difficult thoracic windows.

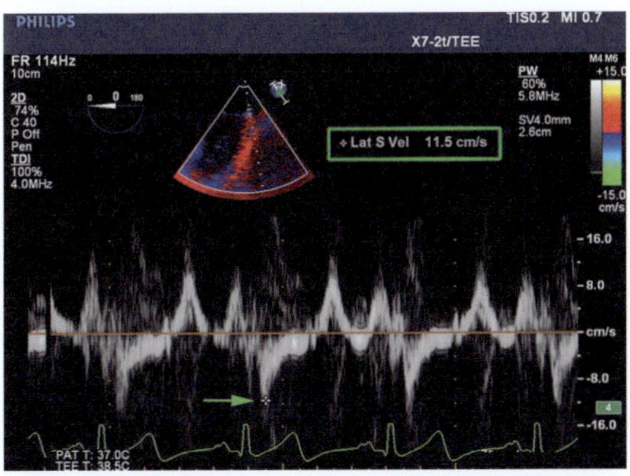

Fig. 6.9 Tissue Doppler-based calculation of the lateral mitral annular velocity during systole (*green arrow*). The measurement is obtained below the baseline since during systole the annulus movement is downward toward the apex

Advanced Methods

Three-Dimensional (3D) EF Calculation

This modality correlates well with the gold standard, cardiac MRI and with recent improvements in technology and can be carried out relatively quickly [17]. It involves post-capture processing of a full volume dataset, typically with multi-beat acquisition (Fig. 6.10; Video 6.1). Since it involves visualization of the entire LV, wall motion abnormalities and altered LV geometry typically do not make the results less accurate. It is, however, technically difficult and time-consuming and relies heavily on excellent 2D visualization in all segments. In the presence of arrhythmias, multi-beat acquisition is not possible, degrading the temporal resolution, as well as the accuracy of the results. The details of this methodology are outside the scope of this text, but can be found elsewhere [17]. Data regarding its efficacy continues to emerge, and this may become the preferred modality in the future, as the workflow becomes less complicated [18].

Global Longitudinal Strain (GLS)

Strain measurement is a load-independent variable that uses the analysis of individual bright spots on the ultrasound image (speckles) and calculates the myocardial deformation and strain based on the separation or approximation of individual speckles during the cardiac cycle. Strain can be calculated using tissue Doppler as well, but speckle tracking is becoming the preferred modality [3]. Midesophageal LV views are used in TEE, while apical LV views are used in TTE to visualize myocardial segments (Fig. 6.11; Videos 6.2, 6.3, 6.4, and 6.5). The complete methodology of this technique is outside the scope of this text, but it is important to note that normal strain values are reported as negative numbers, since systolic myocardial length is shorter than diastolic (due to the contraction). Scant prospectively validated data and time-consuming

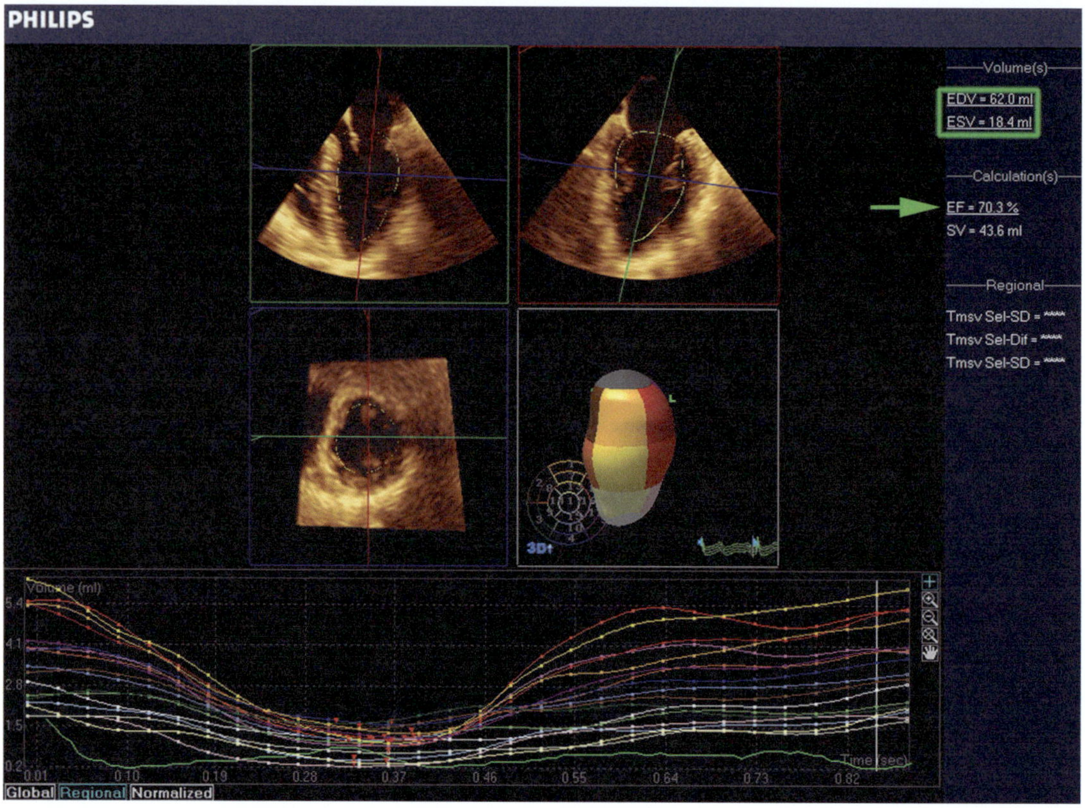

Fig. 6.10 Calculation of EF using 3D echocardiography. The individual lines represent contribution from all LV segments. The global EF is displayed on the panel to the right (*green arrow*)

calculations have prevented widespread use, and it remains primarily a research tool [5].

Measurements of Left Ventricular Geometry

Left Ventricular Wall Thickness

The wall thickness of the LV during diastole is a measure of its hypertrophy, and is generally measured from the transgastric short-axis view at the level of the papillary muscles. Using TTE, the parasternal long-axis view can provide similar measurements of the posterior and septal walls. Both 2D and M-mode can be utilized for this measurement. The septal wall is measured from the endocardium to the endocardium, whereas the inferolateral wall is measured from the endocardium to the epicardium. Sources of error can include measurement of an oblique section of the wall, a regional aneurysm, and inclusion of pericardial structures or papillary muscles. While LV hypertrophy does not contribute directly to abnormal systolic function, its identification may indicate the presence of LV diastolic dysfunction. Normal values for LV wall thickness are 0.6–1.0 cm and 0.6–0.9 cm for males and females, respectively [5].

LV Mass Calculation

While not typically utilized in noncardiac surgery, LV mass is a strong predictor of adverse cardiovascular events and can be calculated from M-mode or 2D or 3D images. M-mode is generally used for screening large population samples, whereas 2D methodology is used in cases of altered LV geometry and for serial measurements

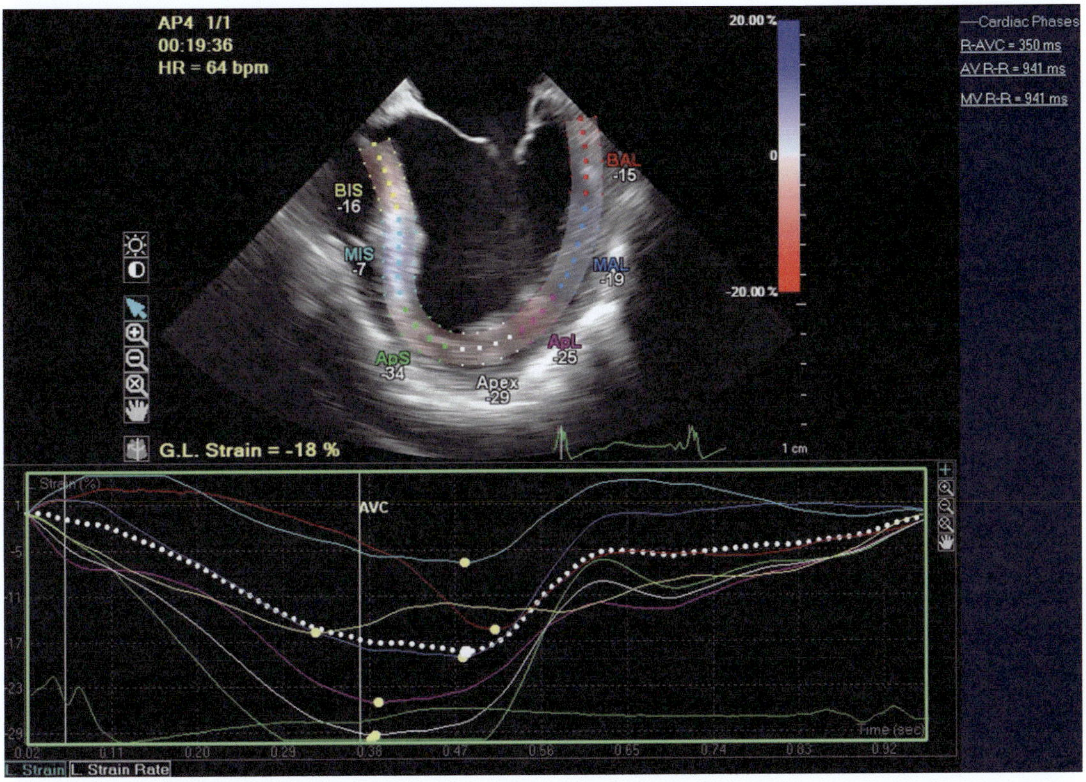

Fig. 6.11 Measurement of global longitudinal strain using speckle tracking in 2D echocardiography. The individual lines represent individual segments, while the white dotted line represents the global summation of individual strain measurements

in one patient. All measurements are done in diastole, and the myocardial volume calculated is then multiplied by its density (1.05 grams/ml) to calculate the mass. The 2D measurements are made from the transgastric midpapillary short-axis view or a parasternal long-axis view, with the LV mass calculated by the formula recommended by the ASE [1]:

$$\text{LV mass} = 0.8 \text{ x } 1.04 \text{ x}\left[\left(\text{LVIDd} + \text{PWT} + \text{IVS}\right)^3 - \text{LVIDd}^3\right] \text{ x } 0.6 \text{ grams}$$

LVIDd = LV internal diameter in diastole, PWT = Inferolateral (posterior) wall thickness, IVS = Interventricular septum thickness

The ASE recommends the 2D modality for this purpose, since 2D is easier and the most studied technique, but 3D estimation of LV mass has been validated as well [5, 17]. This technique suffers from the fault of overestimating the LV mass and the need for good beam alignment. The normal values range from 67 to 162 g for women and 88 to 224 g for men [1]. A calculation of relative wall thickness (based on the ratio of posterior wall thickness and the diastolic LV diameter) can help differentiate between concentric and eccentric hypertrophy.

Conclusion

For the basic echocardiographer, the main use of echocardiography is to identify causes or potential causes of hemodynamic instability.

Identifying changes in LV systolic function and being able to quantify changes in EF can be valuable for management in the perioperative or critical care setting. While there are many methods available to evaluate LV systolic function, it is important to remember the limitations of each method. The modified Simpson's method may give a more accurate result because it considers two planes of the LV, but it can be time-consuming and tedious. It also requires distinct endocardial borders. Simpler methods, such as fractional shortening, fractional area change, the rate of rise of ventricular pressure, and tissue Doppler imaging, may be easier to acquire in time-sensitive situations, but may not consider altered LV geometry and regional wall motion. The results also do not directly equate to an EF and may simply tell you whether LV systolic function is normal or abnormal. With experience over time, visual estimation of EF can approximate the calculated EF and may be all that is needed to guide management in an emergent situation.

Questions

1. Which of the following is a relatively load-independent measure of LV systolic function?

    a. Mitral annular systolic velocity measured by TDI
    b. Lateral E/e'
    c. Color flow propagation velocity
    d. Fractional area change

2. Which of the following is most true regarding the rate of pressure increase in the left ventricle (dP/dT)?

    a. It requires the presence of an AI jet
    b. It can be measured from the transgastric midpapillary short-axis view
    c. It is expressed in seconds
    d. It assumes the pressure in the left atrium is negligible

3. In a patient with suboptimal LV imaging, it was found that the velocity of a mitral regurgitant jet increased from 1 to 3 m/s over 20 msec. Which of the following is most likely true?

    a. LV systolic function is preserved
    b. LV systolic function is reduced
    c. LV diastolic function is preserved
    d. LV diastolic function is reduced

4. Which of the following is an advantage of calculating the ejection fraction using 3D echocardiography?

    a. Systolic and diastolic function can be measured simultaneously
    b. It is easier than 2D estimation
    c. It is reliable in altered LV geometry
    d. It requires the presence of a mitral regurgitation jet

5. Fractional area change can be accurately applied to which of the following views?

    a. Midesophageal aortic valve short-axis view
    b. Deep transgastric five-chamber view
    c. Transgastric midpapillary short-axis view
    d. None of the above

6. Which of the following is most true about strain measurement?

    a. It is useful to assess valvular abnormality
    b. It requires the use of color flow Doppler
    c. It can be applied using continuous-wave spectral Doppler
    d. It can be applied using tissue Doppler

7. Which of the following is most true about the Simpson's biplane method of EF calculation?

    a. It cannot be used in the four-chamber view
    b. It uses a "stacked disc" model to calculate EF
    c. It is load-independent
    d. It does not require precise endocardial border definition

8. Which of the following is most true about the measurement of LV fractional shortening?

    a. It is accurate in the presence of altered LV geometry
    b. It can be calculated from spectral Doppler
    c. It provides values that are lower than, but correlate with, the EF
    d. It is the recommended technique for 2D EF estimation per the ASE

9. Left ventricular wall thickness should be measured at which of the following?

    a. Septal wall
    b. Anterior wall
    c. Lateral wall
    d. Anterolateral wall

10. The Simpson's biplane method of ejection fraction measurement involves:

    a. Systolic and diastolic frames of transthoracic four- and three-chamber views
    b. Systolic and diastolic frames of transthoracic parasternal short-axis and long-axis views
    c. Systolic and diastolic frames of transesophageal four- and two-chamber views
    d. Systolic and diastolic frames of transesophageal transgastric short-axis and midesophageal long-axis views

References

1. Lang R, Bierig M, Devereux R, et al. Recommendations for chamber quantification☆. Eur J Echocardiogr. 2006;7:79–108.
2. Parameshwar J, Keegan J, Sparrow J, et al. Predictors of prognosis in severe chronic heart failure. Am Heart J. 1992;123:421–6.
3. Thomas JD, Popović ZB. Assessment of left ventricular function by cardiac ultrasound. J Am Coll Cardiol. 2006;48:2012–25.
4. Fukuta H, Little WC. The cardiac cycle and the physiologic basis of left ventricular contraction, ejection, relaxation, and filling. Heart Fail Clin. 2008;4:1–11.
5. Lang RM, Badano LP, Mor-Avi V, et al. Recommendations for Cardiac Chamber Quantification by Echocardiography in Adults: An Update from the American Society of Echocardiography and the European Association of Cardiovascular Imaging. J Am Soc Echocardiography. 2015;28:1–39.e14.
6. Foster E, Cahalan MK. The search for intelligent quantitation in echocardiography: "Eyeball," "trackball" and beyond. J Am Coll Cardiol. 1993;22:848–50.
7. Unlüer EE, Karagöz A, Akoğlu H, et al. Visual estimation of bedside echocardiographic ejection fraction by emergency physicians. West J Emerg Med. 2014;15:221–6.
8. Skarvan K, Lambert A, Filipovic M, et al. Reference values for left ventricular function in subjects under general anaesthesia and controlled ventilation assessed by two-dimensional transoesophageal echocardiography. Eur J Anaesthesiol. 2001;18:713–22.
9. Gottdiener J, Bednarz J, Devereux R, et al. American Society of Echocardiography recommendations for use of echocardiography in clinical trials A report from the American society of echocardiography's guidelines and standards committee and the task force on echocardiography in clinical trials. J Am Soc Echocardiogr. 2004;17:1086–119.
10. Nijland F. Early prediction of improvement in ejection fraction after acute myocardial infarction using low dose dobutamine echocardiography. Heart. 2002;88:592–6.
11. McGowan JH, Cleland JGF. Reliability of reporting left ventricular systolic function by echocardiography: A systematic review of 3 methods. Am Heart J. 2003;146:388–97.
12. Bargiggia GS, Bertucci C, Recusani F, et al. A new method for estimating left ventricular dP/dt by continuous wave Doppler-echocardiography. Validation studies at cardiac catheterization. Circulation. 1989;80:1287–92.

13. Kolias TJ, Aaronson KE, Armstrong WF. Doppler-Derived dP/dt and −dP/dt predict survival in congestive heart failure. J Am Coll Cardiol. 2000;36:1594–9. ACC Curr J Rev. 10:43-44, 2001.
14. Yu C-M, Sanderson JE, Marwick TH, et al. Tissue Doppler imaging. J Am Coll Cardiol. 2007;49:1903–14.
15. Kadappu KK, Thomas L. Tissue Doppler imaging in echocardiography: value and limitations. Heart Lung Circulat. 2015;24:224–33.
16. Marwick TH. Techniques for comprehensive two dimensional echocardiographic assessment of left ventricular systolic function. Heart. 2003;89:2iii–8.
17. Kühl HP, Bücker A, Franke A, et al. Transesophageal 3-Dimensional Echocardiography: In vivo determination of left ventricular mass in comparison with magnetic resonance imaging. J Am Soc Echocardiogr. 2000;13:205–15.
18. Monaghan MJ. Role of real time 3D echocardiography in evaluating the left ventricle. Heart. 2006;92:131–6.

Regional Ventricular Function

7

Tariq Naseem, Timothy M. Maus,
and Ramon Sanchez

Abbreviations

AV	Atrioventricular (node)
CFD	Color flow Doppler
EKG	Electrocardiogram
IVS	Interventricular septum
LCA	Left coronary artery
RCA	Right coronary artery
LAD	Left anterior descending (coronary) artery
LCx	Left circumflex (coronary) artery
LVEDV	Left ventricular end-diastolic volume
LVESV	Left ventricular end-systolic volume
LVOT	Left ventricular outflow tract
OM	Obtuse marginal (artery)
PDA	Posterior descending (coronary) artery
RI	Ramus intermedius (artery)
RVOT	Right ventricular outflow tract
SA	Sinoatrial (node)
TEE	Transesophageal echocardiography
TTE	Transthoracic echocardiography
WMA	Wall motion abnormality

Supplementary Information The online version of this chapter (https://doi.org/10.1007/978-3-030-84349-6_7) contains supplementary material, which is available to authorized users.

T. Naseem
Department of Anesthesiology, Cedars-Sinai Medical Center, Los Angeles, CA, USA

T. M. Maus · R. Sanchez (✉)
Department of Anesthesiology, University of California San Diego Health, La Jolla, CA, USA
e-mail: rsanchez@health.ucsd.edu

Introduction

One of the most useful applications of echocardiography in perioperative and critically ill patients is qualitative assessment of myocardial function. Both transesophageal echocardiography (TEE) and transthoracic echocardiography (TTE) can serve as adjuncts to other modalities in diagnosing or ruling out myocardial ischemia. In fact, compared to arterial blood pressure, EKG changes, and pulmonary artery catheter measurements, regional wall motion abnormality (WMA) observed on echocardiography is the most sensitive method for early detection of ischemic changes in the heart [1–3]. This chapter will describe the normal coronary anatomy and distribution including echocardiography correlates, as well as describe normal and abnormal regional myocardial function. Lastly, caveats of regional wall motion abnormalities and complications of ischemic events are discussed.

T. M. Maus, C. R. Tainter (eds.), *Essential Echocardiography*,
https://doi.org/10.1007/978-3-030-84349-6_7

Coronary Anatomy

A basic understanding of the vascular anatomy of the heart is key to interpreting echocardiographic images of ventricular wall function (Fig. 7.1). There is significant variability in the normal coronary circulation; however, the most common anatomic presentations are discussed here. The heart is supplied by two major arteries: the left coronary artery (LCA) and the right coronary artery (RCA). They arise from just above the left and right coronary cusps of the aortic valve, respectively. The LCA bifurcates into the left anterior descending (LAD) and the left circumflex (LCx) arteries. Less commonly, the LCA trifurcates into an LAD, LCx, and ramus intermedius (RI) arteries. The LAD descends anteriorly toward the apex traveling within the anterior interventricular groove. Its major branches are the diagonal branches that supply the free wall of the left ventricle and the septal branches that feed into the interventricular septum. Therefore, the LAD is commonly responsible for blood flow to the apex as well as the anterior, anterolateral, and anteroseptal walls of the left ventricle.

The LCx takes a path along the atrioventricular groove toward the left side after emerging from the LCA and travels posteriorly toward the crux, the meeting point of the interventricular septum (IVS) and atrioventricular groove. In 15–20% of patients, the LCx supplies the posterior descending artery (PDA), resulting in "left-

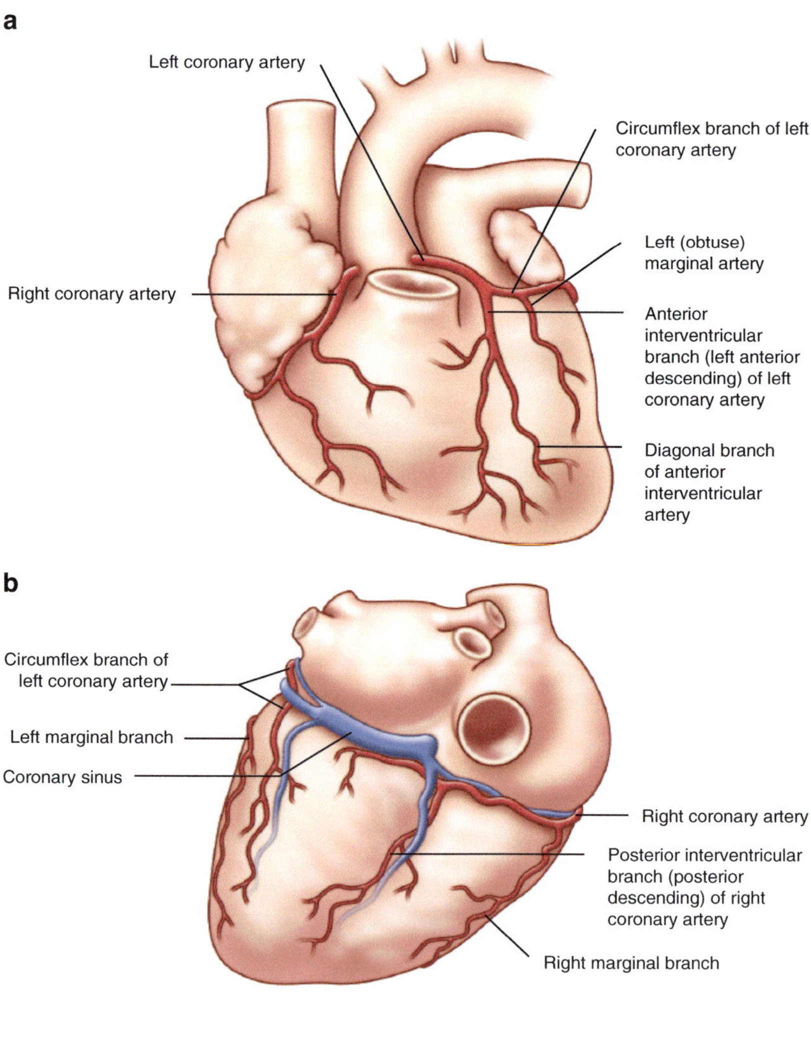

Fig. 7.1 Coronary artery anatomy. (**a**) Anterior aspect; (**b**) posterior aspect

dominant" circulation. In these patients, the left coronary circulation supplies the interventricular septum (IVS) and often the atrioventricular (AV) node. Along its path toward the crux, the LCx provides branches termed the obtuse marginal (OM) arteries, which supply the lateral wall of the left ventricle (LV). Therefore, the LCx is commonly responsible for the blood flow to the lateral aspect of the left ventricle, and the infero-apical aspect in patients with left-dominant circulation.

The RCA travels in the right atrioventricular groove and turns posteriorly toward the crux. The RCA provides branches, termed acute marginal arteries, supplying the right ventricle free wall and the sinoatrial (SA) and AV nodes. In 80–85% of patients, the RCA terminates as the PDA, supplying the inferior IVS. This constitutes a "right-dominant" circulation. About 5% of patients have a "co-dominant" circulation, where the PDA is equally supplied from the LCx and RCA. The RCA is also responsible for providing blood flow to the inferior wall of the left ventricle. Therefore, the RCA is commonly responsible for the blood flow to the right ventricle and inferior wall of the left ventricle, as well as the infero-apical aspect of the left ventricle in patients with right-dominant circulation.

The segmentation of the heart is intended to match that of the coronary blood supply. While several segmentation models exist, recent guidelines suggest the use of a 17 segment model [4] (Fig. 7.2). The purpose of the model is to improve communication between specialties (e.g., cardiologists, intensivists, anesthesiologists, emergency physicians.) as well as between imaging modalities (e.g., echocardiography, nuclear medicine imaging). In this model, the LV is broadly divided into basal, mid-cavitary, and apical areas, which are then divided into segments. The basal and mid-cavitary areas are divided into anterior, inferior, anteroseptal, inferoseptal, anterolateral, and inferolateral segments. The apical area is divided into four segments, anterior, inferior, septal, and lateral, with the apical cap comprising the 17th segment. The echocardiographic correlation of which segments are perfused by certain coronary arteries is discussed below.

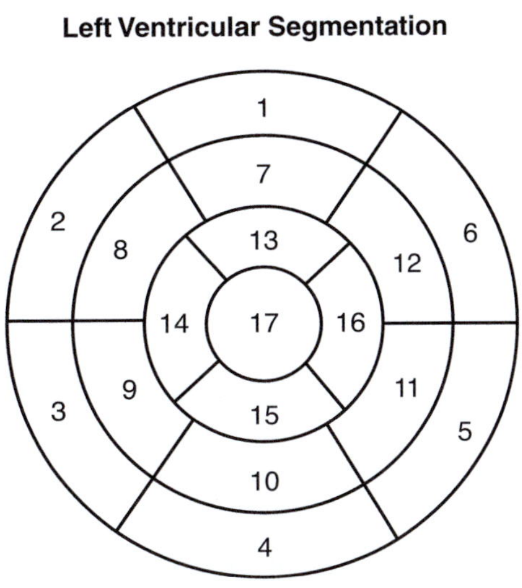

1. basal anterior
2. basal anteroseptal
3. basal inferoseptal
4. basal inferior
5. basal inferolateral
6. basal anterolateral
7. mid anterior
8. mid anteroseptal
9. mid inferoseptal
10. mid inferior
11. mid inferolateral
12. mid anterolateral
13. apical anterior
14. apical septal
15. apical inferior
16. apical lateral
17. apex

Fig. 7.2 The seventeen-segment model of the left ventricle (Reprinted from Douglas [14])

Application of Coronary Topography to Echocardiography

Coronary perfusion to the myocardium can be assessed qualitatively with echocardiography, with attention to the coronary blood flow distribution to each segment as described. This concept is depicted in Fig. 7.3a and b, which describes the common coronary anatomy of the heart utilizing transesophageal and transthoracic echocardiography views, respectively. The overlap in the depicted coronary supply is explained by normal anatomic variation in coronary perfusion (e.g., the inferolateral wall may be supplied by the LCx in some patients, but by the RCA in others). This can present as variability in the appearance of the wall motion abnormality during an ischemic event. In one patient, an LAD lesion may lead to a WMA of just the anterior and anteroseptal wall, while in another patient, the WMA may extend to cover the entire anterior half of the LV (inclusive of the anterolateral wall). Therefore, it is important when assessing for WMAs in a busy perioperative or critical care setting to not become overfocused on interpretation of the "normal" coronary distribution.

Transesophageal Echocardiography Correlation

The transesophageal echocardiography examination for ischemia involves transgastric and midesophageal imaging. The transgastric midpapillary short-axis view is particularly useful, as in that one view, all three coronary distributions are represented: the LAD covers the anterior and anteroseptal segments, the LCx covers the anterolateral and inferolateral segments, and the RCA typically covers the inferior segment and the right ventricle (Fig. 7.4). While it is convenient that all three coronary distributions

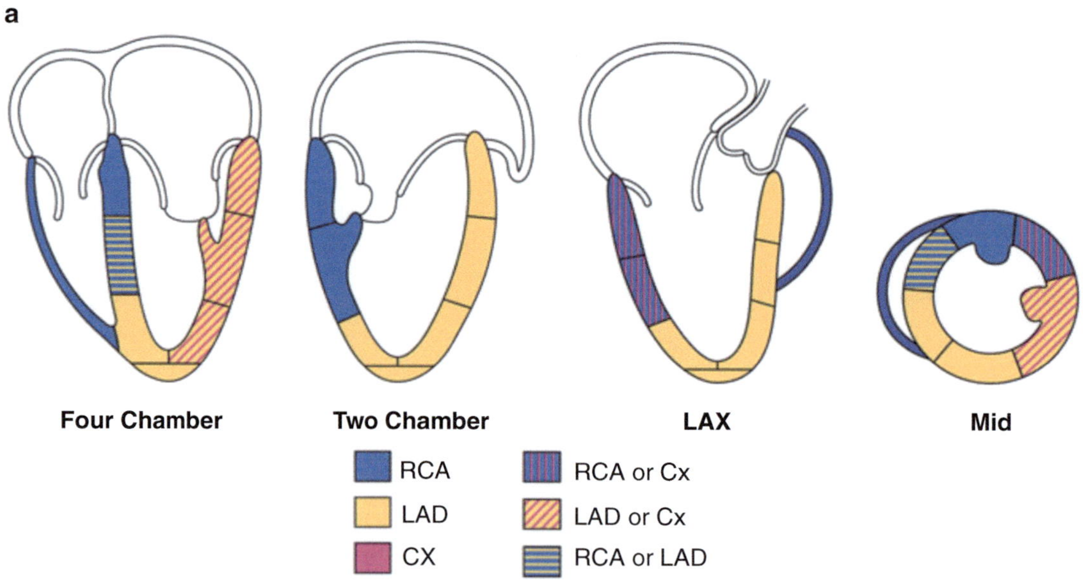

Fig. 7.3 (**a**) Transesophageal views with the representative coronary blood supply and segmentation. The views are the midesophageal (ME) four-chamber, ME two-chamber, ME long-axis (LAX), and transgastric midpapillary short-axis (Mid). (**b**) Transthoracic views with representative coronary blood supply and segmentation. The views are the apical four-chamber, apical two-chamber, apical long-axis (LAX), and parasternal short-axis at the basal (base), midpapillary (mid), and the apical (apex) levels. *RCA* right coronary artery, *LAD* left anterior descending artery, *Cx* left circumflex artery

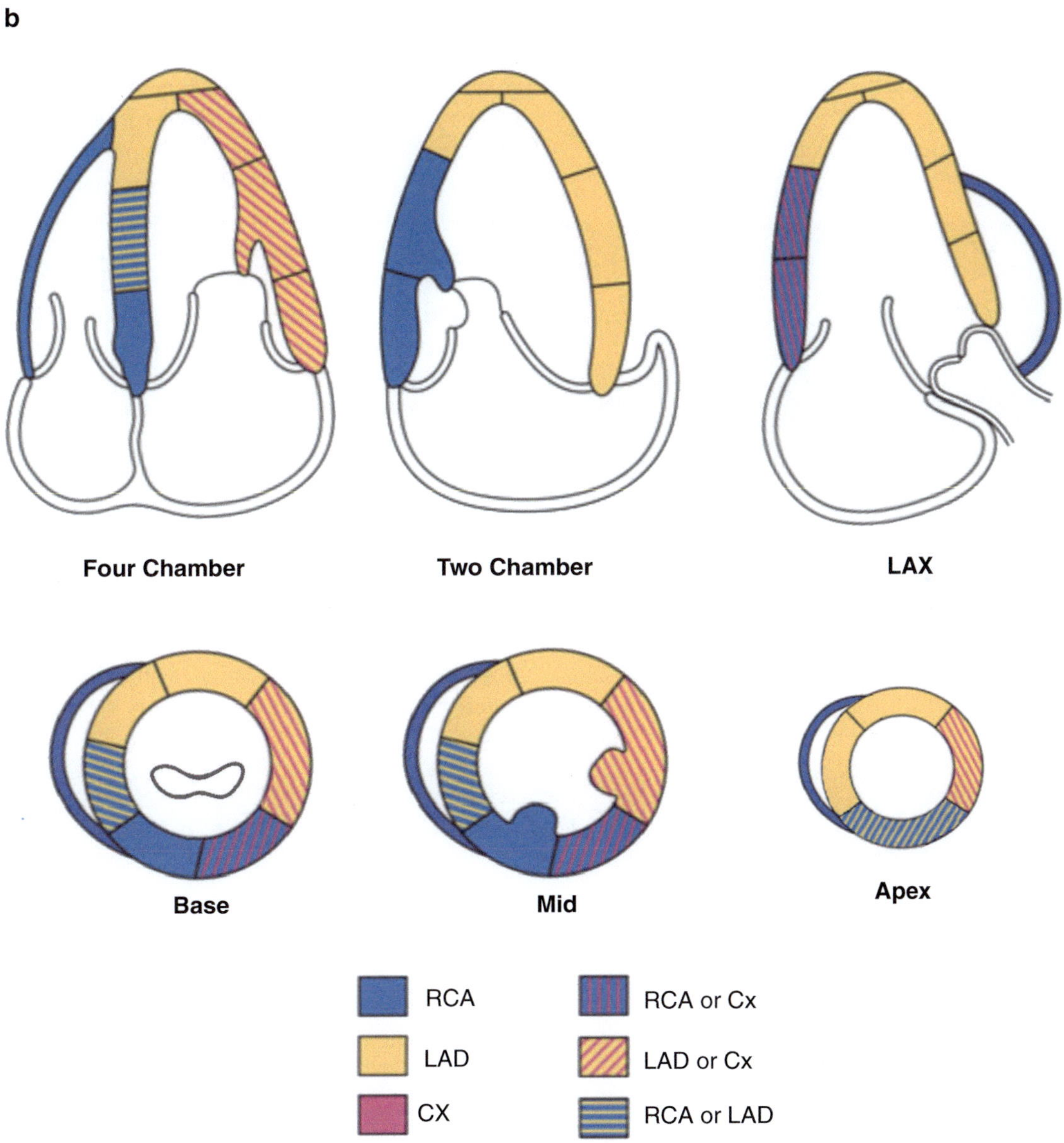

Fig. 7.3 (continued)

are observed in one view, it is important to recognize that this view may not detect all wall motion abnormalities (e.g., basal and apical segments). One study noted that the midpapillary short-axis view only recognized 17% of wall motion abnormalities, while adding other short-axis orientations as well as long-axis imaging significantly increased the recognition of WMAs. Therefore, midesophageal imaging with various multiplane orientations is necessary and complementary to imaging of the transgastric midpapillary short-axis view.

When envisioning the myocardial walls in the midesophageal views, it is helpful to think of the direction of the multiplane "slice" through a transgastric view (Fig. 7.5). The ME four-chamber view will present the septal and lateral walls, the ME two-chamber view will present the anterior and inferior walls, and the ME long-axis view will present the anteroseptal and inferolateral walls. The advantage of the midesophageal views is the ability to display basal, mid-cavitary, and apical segments of a particular wall at once, allowing detection of abnormalities beyond just the mid-cavitary segments.

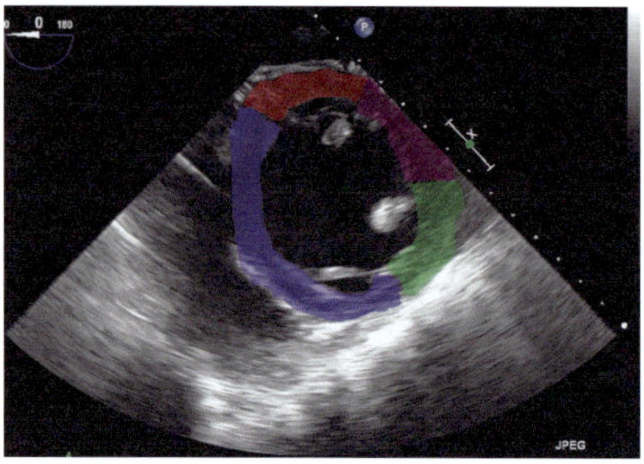

Fig. 7.4 Transgastric midpapillary short-axis view with overlying color representation of coronary perfusion. *Blue* = left anterior descending artery (LAD), *red* = right coronary artery (RCA), *purple* = RCA or left circumflex artery (LCx), *green* = LAD or LCx

The midesophageal four-chamber view allows for observation of all three coronary distributions in one view, including observation of basal, mid-cavitary, and apical function (Fig. 7.6). Depending upon the flexion of the probe, the septum is most commonly perfused by the LAD, the lateral wall is perfused by the LCx, and the RV is perfused by the RCA. Flexion or retroflexion of the probe in a midesophageal four-chamber view allows the observation of anteroseptal/anterolateral and inferoseptal/inferolateral segments, respectively.

Rotation of the multiplane to roughly 90 degrees develops the ME two-chamber view (Fig. 7.7). This view nicely displays the basal, mid-cavitary, and apical segments of the anterior and inferior walls. In the majority of patients, the anterior wall and LV apex will be covered by the LAD, while the inferior wall will be perfused by the RCA.

The ME long-axis view, at approximately 120 degrees of multiplane rotation, will develop the anteroseptal and inferolateral walls of the LV

Fig. 7.5 Transgastric midpapillary short-axis representation with indications of the walls visualized in respective midesophageal views

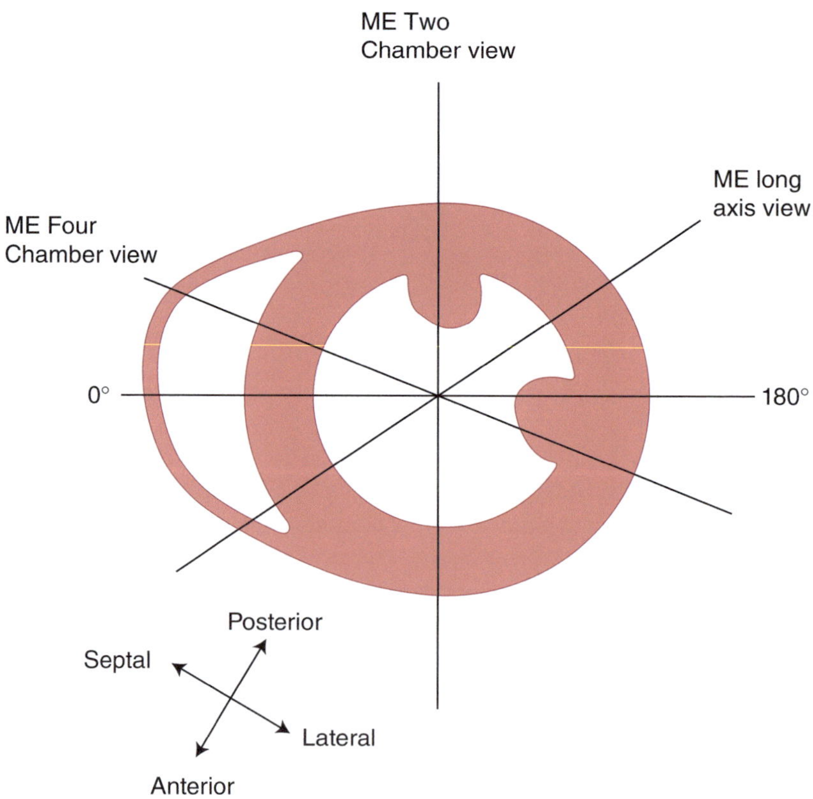

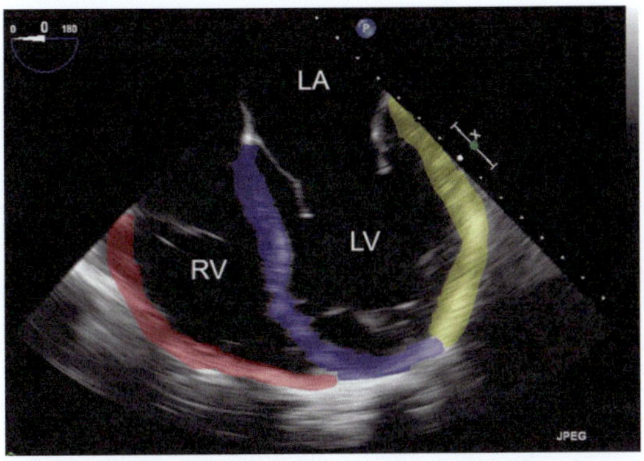

Fig. 7.6 Midesophageal four-chamber view with overlying color representation of coronary perfusion. *Blue* = left anterior descending artery (LAD), *red* = right coronary artery (RCA), *yellow* = left circumflex artery (LCx). *LA* left atrium, *LV* left ventricle, *RV* right ventricle

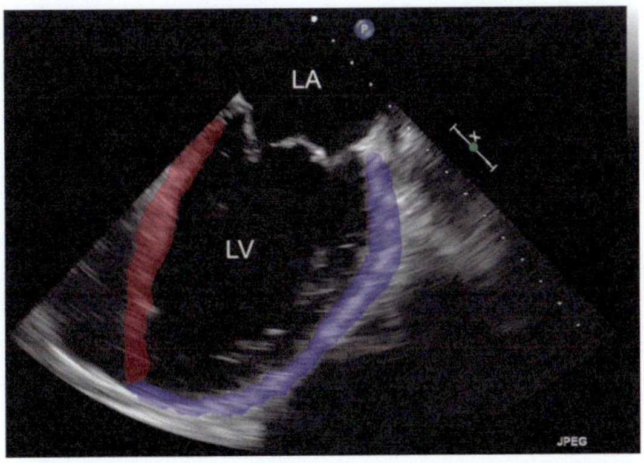

Fig. 7.7 Midesophageal two-chamber view with overlying color representation of coronary perfusion. *Blue* = left anterior descending artery (LAD), *red* = right coronary artery (RCA). *LA* left atrium, *LV* left ventricle

while also displaying a portion of the right ventricular outflow tract (RVOT) (Fig. 7.8). The wall motion of basal, mid-cavitary, and apical segments should be assessed. The LAD typically covers the anteroseptal wall and apex, while the RCA or LCx perfuses the inferolateral wall. The RVOT is perfused by the RCA. Again, the combination of midesophageal and transgastric imaging allows the echocardiographer to provide a composite analysis of wall motion throughout all segments of the LV and RV.

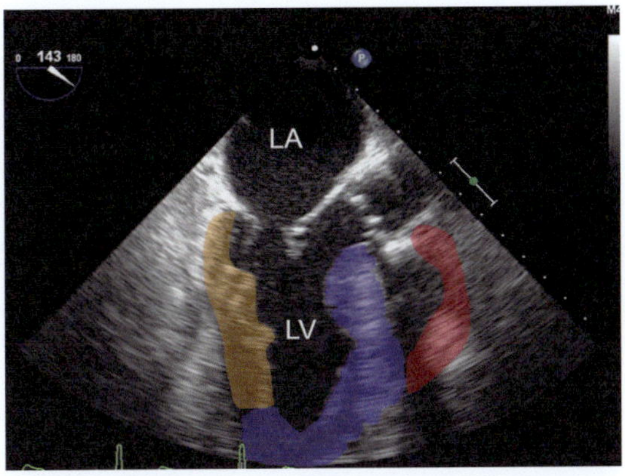

Fig. 7.8 Midesophageal long-axis view with overlying color representation of coronary perfusion. *Blue* = left anterior descending artery (LAD), *red* = right coronary artery (RCA), *orange* = RCA or left circumflex artery (LCx). *LA* left atrium, *LV* left ventricle

Transthoracic Echocardiography Correlation

The transthoracic echocardiography examination for ischemia involves parasternal and apical imaging. Similar to the transgastric midpapillary short-axis view with TEE, the parasternal midpapillary short-axis view is useful, as in one view, all three coronary distributions are represented: the LAD covers the anterior and anteroseptal segments, the LCx covers the anterolateral and inferolateral segments, and the RCA typically covers the inferior segment and the right ventricle (Fig. 7.9). While it is convenient that all three coronary distributions are observed in one view, again, it is important to recognize that this view may not detect all wall motion abnormalities (i.e., basal and apical segments). Apical imaging, like midesophageal imaging in TEE, is necessary for complete evaluation of all segments and coronary territories. The advantage of apical views is the ability to display basal, mid-cavitary, and apical segments of a particular wall, allowing detection of abnormalities beyond just the mid-cavitary segments.

The apical four-chamber view allows for observation of all three coronary distributions in

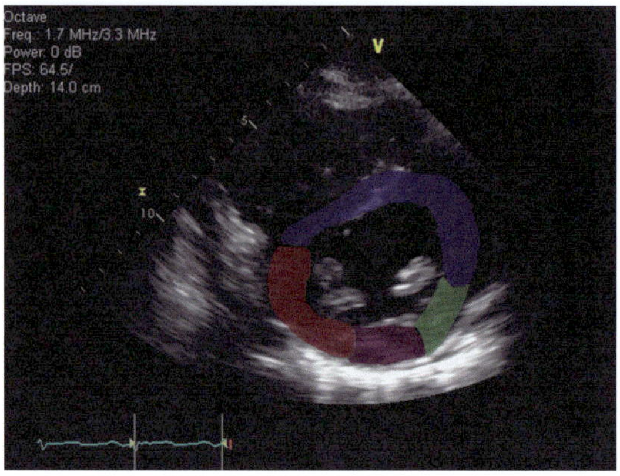

Fig. 7.9 Parasternal midpapillary short-axis view with overlying color representation of coronary perfusion. *Blue* = left anterior descending artery (LAD), *red* = right coronary artery (RCA), *purple* = RCA or left circumflex artery (LCx), *green* = LAD or LCx

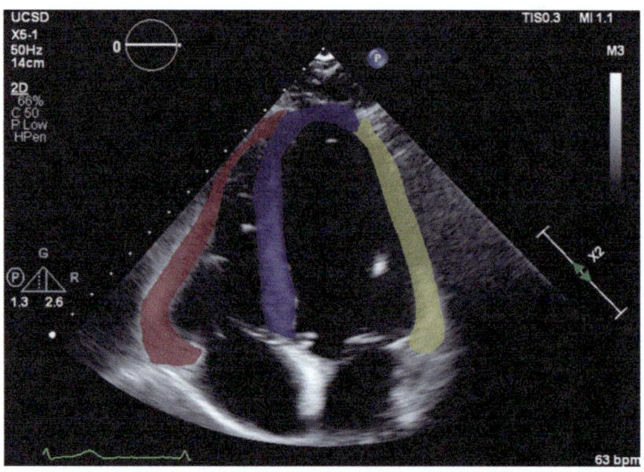

Fig. 7.10 Apical four-chamber view with overlying color representation of coronary perfusion. *Blue* = left anterior descending artery (LAD), *red* = right coronary artery (RCA), *yellow* = left circumflex artery (LCx)

one view, including observation of basal, mid-cavitary, and apical function (Fig. 7.10). Depending upon the angle of the probe, the septum is most commonly perfused by the LAD, the lateral wall is perfused by the LCx, and the RV is perfused by the RCA. Similar to flexion or retroflexion of the TEE probe in a midesophageal four-chamber view, fanning the TTE place anteriorly and posteriorly allows the observation of anteroseptal/anterolateral and inferoseptal/inferolateral segments, respectively.

Rotation of the probe counterclockwise develops the apical two-chamber view (Fig. 7.11). This

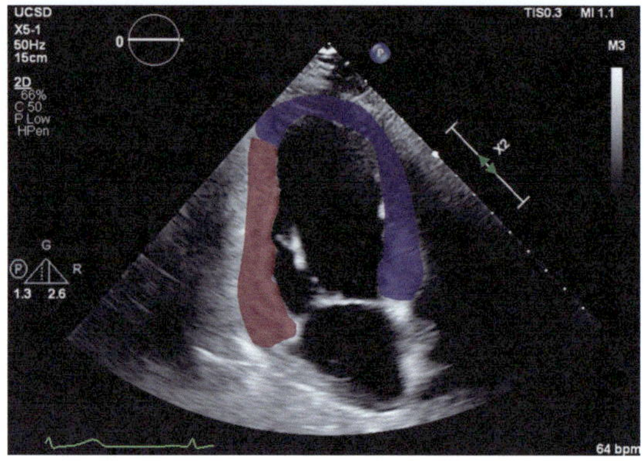

Fig. 7.11 Apical two-chamber view with overlying color representation of coronary perfusion. *Blue* = left anterior descending artery (LAD), *red* = right coronary artery (RCA)

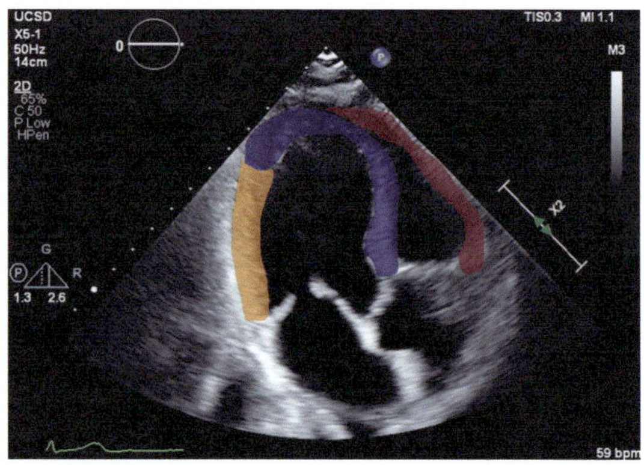

Fig. 7.12 Apical long-axis view with overlying color representation of coronary perfusion. *Blue* = left anterior descending artery (LAD), *red* = right coronary artery (RCA), *orange* = RCA or left circumflex artery (LCx)

view nicely displays the basal, mid-cavitary, and apical segments of the anterior and inferior walls. In the majority of patients, the anterior wall and LV apex will be covered by the LAD, while the inferior wall will be perfused by the RCA.

The apical long-axis (three-chamber) view, obtained with further counterclockwise rotation, will develop the anteroseptal and inferolateral walls of the LV while also displaying the LVOT and a portion of the RVOT (Fig. 7.12). The wall motion of basal, mid-cavitary, and apical segments should be assessed. The LAD typically covers the anteroseptal wall and apex, while the RCA or LCx perfuses the inferolateral wall. The

RVOT is perfused by the RCA. Again, the combination of parasternal and apical imaging allows the echocardiographer to provide a composite analysis of wall motion throughout all segments of the LV and RV.

Grading of Regional Wall Motion Abnormalities (Highlight Box 7.1)

Highlight Box 7.1

Regional ventricular function	
2D	• Left ventricular systolic assessment (Chap. 6)
	• Regional wall motion abnormalities o Systolic wall thickening o Concentric myocardial movement o M-mode assessment o Dilated LV with chronic ischemic changes
CFD	• New onset mitral regurgitation
Spectral	• Worsening diastolic function (Chap. 12) • Worsening pHTN

LV left ventricle, *pHTN* pulmonary hypertension

Regional myocardial function can be quantified based on both observed wall thickening and endocardial motion of the myocardial segment. These two measurements can be graded separately, and each segment should be analyzed in multiple views, ensuring that an appreciation of thickening and motion be obtained for all 17 segments. During systolic contraction, normal myocardial tissue should thicken and move concentrically toward the center of the left ventricular cavity by more than 30 percent. A reduction in thickening or excursion constitutes as hypokinesis, which usually indicates ischemia (Video 7.1) (Table 7.1). Akinesis is the near-complete cessation of any wall movement, along with absent or minimal thickening of the wall (Figure 7.13a, b; Video 7.2 & Video 7.3). Significant ischemia or frank infarction can lead to akinesia (Figure 7.14a, b; Video 7.4). Lastly, dyskinesis is seen when the myocardial wall moves in the opposite (outward) direction during

Table 7.1 Grading of Regional Wall Motion Abnormalities

Grade	Endocardial motion (%)	Wall thickening (%)
Normal or hyperkinetic	> 30%	30–50%
Hypokinesis	10–30%	< 30%
Akinesis	None	Absent or Minimal thickening
Dyskinesia	Outward movement	Systolic stretching or thinning (e.g., aneurysm)

contraction, with thinning of the myocardium, which is usually seen with long-standing infarction and scarring (Video 7.5). Recent American Society of Echocardiography (ASE) guidelines have classified an LV aneurysm (i.e., focal LV dilation) under the category of akinesis or dyskinesis [4] (Fig. 7.15; Video 7.6).

There are some caveats to interpreting WMAs, in that all that does not move is not necessarily ischemia. There may be regional differences in wall motion due to anatomic location. For example, the basal portion of the anteroseptal wall often contracts toward the left ventricular outflow tract (LVOT), as opposed to directly concentric contraction. This may give the appearance of a hypokinetic segment. Additionally, there is interventricular septal dependence between the LV and RV, such that RV dysfunction may cause septal WMA (see Chap. 10). This septal flattening may be interpreted as septal akinesis or dyskinesis. Other causes of non-ischemic WMAs include abnormal conduction (e.g., pacing or bundle branch block), post-pericardiotomy (e.g., abnormal septal bounce), and hemodynamic changes (e.g., acute loading changes and anesthetic-induced myocardial depression). Lastly, since the myocardium is contiguous, and not 17 discrete segments, abnormal motion in one segment can "tether" additional segments. This can cause the interpretation of WMA in segments that may have normal perfusion. Therefore, it is imperative to integrate the echocardiographic findings clinically before instituting therapy for an abnormal myocardial wall motion.

With the understanding of coronary blood supply and its echocardiographic correlation, it is important to have an approach to the exam when

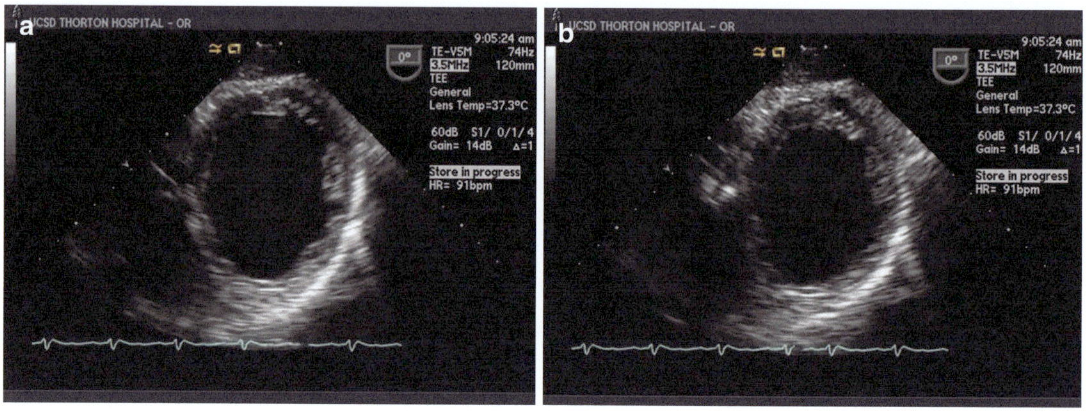

Fig. 7.13 Transgastric midpapillary short-axis view in a patient with an akinetic anterior wall secondary to a left anterior descending lesion (LAD). Note the lack of thickening and central wall excursion in the anterior portion of the left ventricle. (**a**) Diastole; (**b**) systole

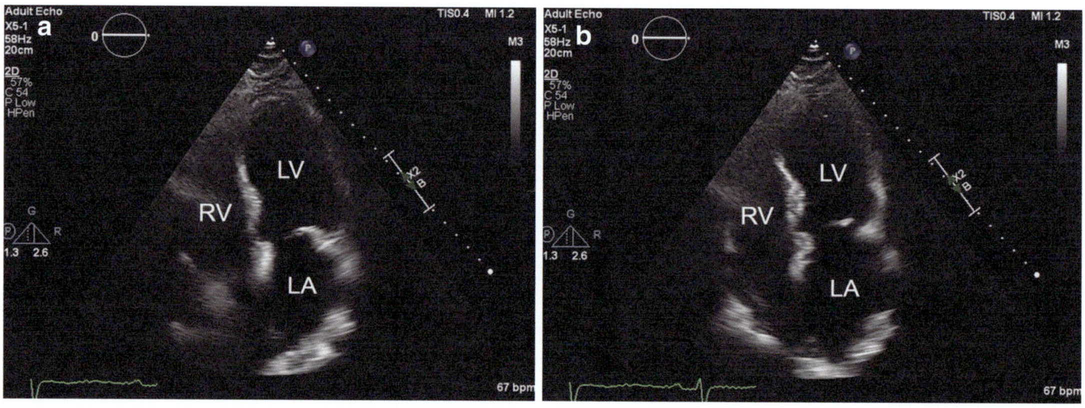

Fig. 7.14 Apical four-chamber view in a patient with akinetic mid- and apical- septal and lateral walls secondary to a large left anterior descending (LAD) obstruction. Note the lack of thickening and central wall excursion in the mid- and apical- segments as opposed to basal septal and lateral segments of the left ventricle. (**a**) Diastole; (**b**) systole. *RV* right ventricle, *LV* left ventricle, *LA* left atrium

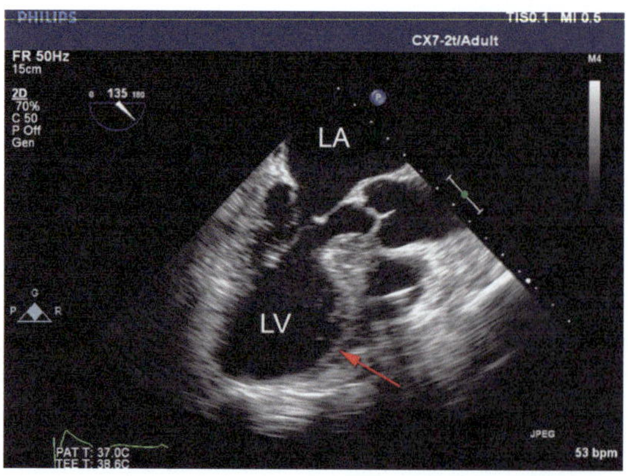

Fig. 7.15 Midesophageal long-axis view in a patient with a prior anterior myocardial infarction, now with a resultant anteroseptal left ventricular aneurysm (*red arrow*). *LA* left atrium, *LV* left ventricle

focusing on ischemic changes. A standard approach of evaluating the basal, mid-cavitary, and apical segment in each midesophageal view, as well as transgastric short-axis imaging, is helpful. Unlike other pathologies, wall motion abnormalities generally do not benefit from color flow Doppler (CFD) or spectral Doppler interrogation, and detection largely rests upon two-dimensional interrogations. However, the implementation of M-mode two-dimensional imaging can prove quite helpful; M-mode provides a single ultrasound pathway displayed on a graph format with depth on the Y-axis and time on the X-axis. A transgastric midpapillary short-axis view with the

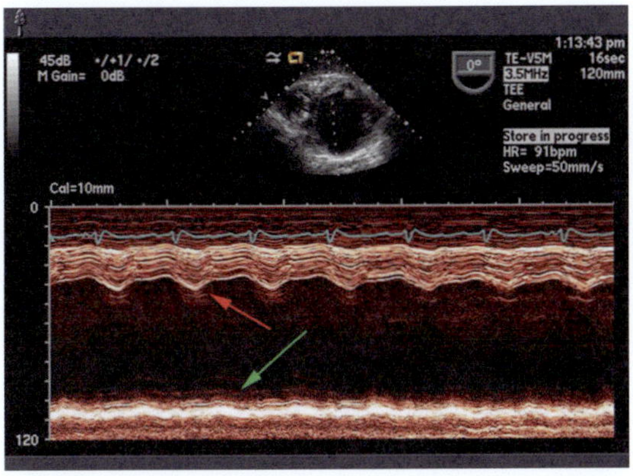

Fig. 7.16 M-mode imaging in a transgastric midpapillary short-axis view. The *red arrow* indicates the systolic thickening and wall excursion of the inferior wall. The *green arrow* indicates the akinetic anterior wall

M-mode cursor through the inferior and anterior walls will demonstrate wall motion with excellent temporal resolution (Fig. 7.16).

Complications from Myocardial Ischemia

While ischemia typically manifests on echocardiography as a regional wall motion abnormality, ischemic damage can lead to other complications which may be detected echocardiographically. These can largely be categorized into reversible changes, which will resolve with return of coronary blood flow, and irreversible changes, which are typically related to infarction and result in permanent structural damage.

Reversible secondary changes include diastolic dysfunction, stunned myocardium, and mitral regurgitation. As diastolic relaxation is an energy-dependent function, diastolic dysfunction is a common occurrence with new ischemia. As explained further in Chap. 12, diastolic relaxation is a dynamic process, and patients may shift between varying degrees of diastolic function. For example, a patient with normal diastology experiencing an acute ischemic event will progress to impaired relaxation. With restoration of coronary blood flow, their diastolic profile may improve back to normal.

Stunned myocardium refers to cardiac tissue that has experienced an ischemic insult and, despite restoration of blood flow, still has transient persistent dysfunction. This is commonly seen after coronary artery bypass grafting surgery, where an aortic cross clamp and a cardioplegic state has resulted in a brief ischemic insult that requires inotropic support until the reperfused myocardium recovers. Stunned myocardium differs from hibernating myocardium, which is a portion of cardiac tissue that is chronically underperfused (e.g., long-term coronary artery disease). In an attempt to preserve structural integrity, the contractility in hibernating myocardium is reduced [5]. Stunned myocardium benefits from exogenous inotropy and time, while hibernating myocardium will benefit from revascularization [6].

As discussed in Chap. 8, the mitral apparatus consists of not just the mitral valve itself, but also the supporting annulus, the left atrium, papillary muscles, and the ventricular walls to which the papillary muscles attach. There are two supporting papillary muscles, the anterolateral and posteromedial muscles, which attach to the mitral valve via multiple chordae. Myocardial ischemia can lead to the cessation of blood flow supplying the papillary muscles or to the myocardial segments underlying those papillary muscles. Dysfunction of either the papillary muscle or underlying segment will lead to abnormal motion of the papillary muscle, chordae, and attachments to the mitral valve leaflets. This leaflet restriction leads to malcoaptation and mitral insufficiency (Fig. 7.17; Video 7.7). The posteromedial papillary muscle is at greater risk due to its single blood supply from the RCA (in right dominant patients), as opposed to the anterolateral papillary muscle which has a dual blood supply from the LAD and LCx circulations. It is therefore especially prudent to evaluate the mitral valve in the setting of ischemic insult to the RCA territory (e.g., when inferior and/or inferoseptal wall motion abnormalities are evident). The converse is also true: new mitral insufficiency should prompt the search for evidence of ischemia (e.g., WMAs).

Irreversible secondary changes, which do not immediately recover with restoration of blood flow, include papillary muscle rupture, ischemic ventricular septal defects, ventricular free wall rupture, ventricular dilation, and aneurysm formation. Papillary muscle rupture is an extension

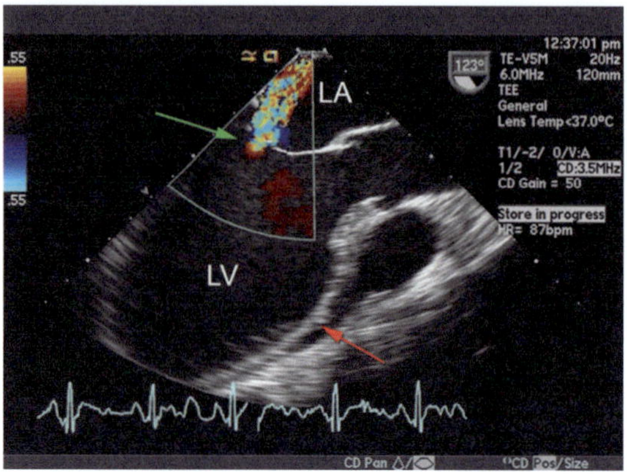

Fig. 7.17 Midesophageal long-axis view in a patient with an acute LAD ischemic event and significant ischemic MR (*green arrow*). Note the lack of thickening during systole of the anteroseptal wall (*red arrow*). *LA* left atrium, *LV* left ventricle

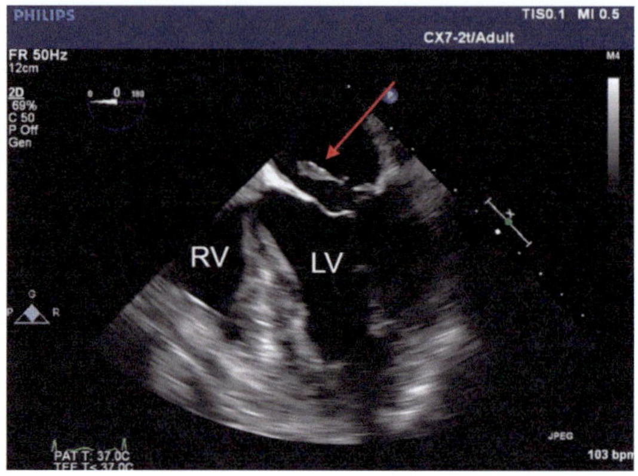

Fig. 7.18 Midesophageal four-chamber view in a patient with a ruptured papillary muscle (*red arrow*). *LV* left ventricle, *RV* right ventricle

of the papillary muscle dysfunction previously described, with significant hemodynamic and functional consequences. As mentioned above, this is most commonly seen with the posteromedial papillary muscle that has the RCA as a single feeding vessel, as opposed to the anterolateral papillary muscle that is supplied by both LAD and LCx [7]. Frank infarction of the territory including the papillary muscle may lead to rupture and separation of the papillary head. Papillary muscle rupture is a surgical emergency, requiring an urgent evaluation for possible mitral valve replacement [8] (Fig. 7.18; Video 7.8).

The most serious complication of myocardial infarction may be ventricular rupture, which includes both septal and ventricular free wall rupture. Ventricular free wall rupture is more common and is one of the most fatal complications of an acute myocardial infarction [9–11]. Both pathologies can be diagnosed effectively with echocardiography with the addition of CFD. Using CFD, turbulent blood flow can be seen moving from the ventricular cavity into the pericardial space in the case of free wall rupture. Likewise, in the setting of septal rupture, blood flow can be seen moving from the left ventricle into the right ventricle, creating a left-to-right shunt. If there is preexisting pulmonary hypertension or elevated right-sided pressures, the septal rupture can then cause a right-to-left shunt, and hypoxia and cyanosis may ensue (Fig. 7.19; Video 7.9).

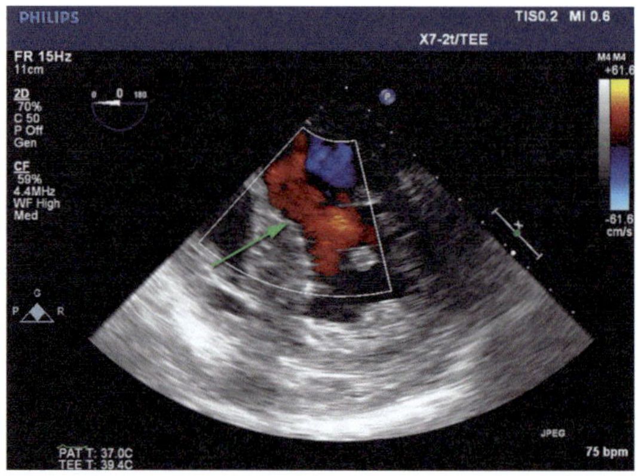

Fig. 7.19 Transgastric midpapillary short-axis view with color flow Doppler in a patient after an inferior myocardial infarction and inferior wall rupture (*green arrow*). Note the contained rupture with flow exiting the ventricular cavity

Left ventricular remodeling and dilatation resulting in myocardial dysfunction is frequently observed after an acute myocardial infarction [12]. With chronic ischemia, the dilation and loss of contractile function lead to an echocardiographic presentation similar to non-ischemic cardiomyopathy. This can be evaluated using echocardiography by looking at parameters such as left ventricular end-diastolic and end-systolic volumes (LVEDV, LVESV), ejection fraction (LVEF), and myocardial strain models (see Chap. 6).

The incidence of aneurysm formation has decreased in recent years with the evolution of improved therapy. However, up to 15% of patients may suffer from a left ventricular aneurysm after an acute myocardial infarction [13]. Over 70% of aneurysms are seen in the anterior wall and apex due to an LAD infarct. Another 10–15% of patients may show involvement of the inferior wall due to RCA disease. On echocardiography, an outpouching of the myocardial segment is seen, with no contraction or systolic contribution. See Fig. 7.15; Video 7.6.

Conclusion

The interpretation of myocardial function and detection of an ischemic event is a fundamental application of echocardiography. In a busy clinical setting that demands a quick and definitive diagnosis, the echocardiography's ability to detect regional wall motion abnormalities before other diagnostic tools makes it an indispensable resource. Recognizing the attributes of a wall motion abnormality, such as decreased wall excursion or decreased wall thickening, helps to detect ischemia, but not all wall motion abnormalities are ischemic (e.g., pacing effect). Additionally, echocardiography allows the interrogation of secondary changes, both reversible and irreversible.

Questions

1. Which of the following is the most sensitive for detecting myocardial ischemia?

   A. Increase in pulmonary capillary wedge pressure (PCWP)
   B. Wall motion abnormality
   C. Electrocardiographic changes
   D. Decrease in arterial blood pressure

2. What are the three most common major coronary arterial branches?

   A. Left main coronary artery, posterior descending artery, and right coronary artery
   B. Left main coronary artery, first diagonal artery, and right posterolateral artery
   C. Left anterior descending artery, left circumflex artery, and right coronary artery
   D. Left anterior descending artery, left circumflex artery, and posterior descending artery

3. Which of the following coronary artery to myocardial territory matches are correct?

   A. Left anterior descending artery : inferolateral wall
   B. Left circumflex artery : anterolateral wall
   C. Posterior descending artery : anterior wall
   D. Right coronary artery : anteroseptal wall

4. The midesophageal two-chamber view visualizes the territory of which two coronary arteries?

   A. Left circumflex and right coronary arteries
   B. Left circumflex and left anterior descending arteries
   C. Posterolateral and ramus intermedius arteries
   D. Left anterior descending and right coronary arteries

5. Which of the following is a concern with only utilizing a transgastric midpapillary short-axis view for monitoring for ischemia?

   A. Visualization of only one coronary artery territory
   B. Visualization of only left-sided circulation
   C. Lack of visualization of basal and apical segments
   D. Lack of visualization of the left anterior descending artery territory

6. Wall motion abnormalities are graded upon which two criteria?

   A. Wall excursion and change in wall thickness during diastole
   B. Wall excursion and change in wall thickness during systole
   C. Wall thickening during systole and wall tension
   D. Wall excursion and myocardial wall mass

7. Which of the following can mimic an ischemic wall motional abnormality?

   A. Ventricular pacing
   B. Acute hemodynamic or volume changes
   C. Profound bradycardia
   D. All of the above

8. Which of the following reversible changes may be associated with ischemia in addition to wall motion abnormalities?

   A. Tissue Doppler imaging lateral mitral annulus velocity greater than 10 cm/s
   B. Posteromedial papillary muscle rupture
   C. Impaired relaxation on diastolic assessment
   D. Ventricular septal rupture

9. Which of the following is most true regarding stunned myocardium?

   A. It necessitates revascularization.
   B. It does not respond to increasing doses of inotropic agents.
   C. It possess normal coronary blood flow.
   D. None of the above.

10. Which of the following is most true regarding left ventricular aneurysm formation?

   A. It may be due to reversible demand ischemia.
   B. It appears as a dyskinetic wall motion abnormality.
   C. It most common appears at the basal anterolateral wall.
   D. It presents within minutes of an acute ischemic episode.

References

1. Beaupre PN, Kremer PF, Cahalan MK, et al. Intraoperative detection of changes in left ventricular segmental wall motion by transesophageal two-dimensional echocardiography. Am Heart J. 1984;107:1021.
2. van Daele ME, Sutherland GR, Mitchell MM, et al. Do changes in pulmonary capillary wedge pressure adequately reflect myocardial ischemia during anesthesia? A correlative preoperative hemodynamic, electrocardiographic, and transesophageal echocardiographic study. Circulation. 1990;81:865.
3. Akchurin RS, Tkachuk LM, Lepilin MG, et al. Intraoperative transesophageal echocardiography for detection of myocardial ischemia. Herz. 1993; 18:372.
4. Lang RM, Badano LP, Mor-Avi V, et al. Recommendations for Cardiac Chamber Quantification by Echocardiography in Adults: An Update from the American Society of Echocardiography and the European Association of Cardiovascular Imaging. J Am Soc Echocardiogr. 2015;28:1–39.
5. Braunwald RA. Kloner: the stunned myocardium: prolonged, postischemic ventricular dysfunction. Circulation. 66:1146–9. 1982 tmn
6. Kloner RA, Jennings RB. Consequences of brief ischemia: stunning, preconditioning, and their clinical implications, part I. Circulation. 2001;104:2981.
7. Otsuji Y, Handschumacher MD, Kisanuki A, et al. Functional mitral regurgitation. Cardiologia. 1998;43:1011–6.
8. Russo A, Suri RM, Grigioni F, Roger VL, Oh JK, Mahoney DW, et al. Clinical outcome after surgical correction of mitral regurgitation due to papillary muscle rupture. Circulation. 2008;118:1528–34.
9. Reeder GS. Identification and treatment of complications of myocardial infarction. Mayo Clin Proc. 1995;70:880.
10. López-Sendón J, González A, López de Sá E, et al. Diagnosis of subacute ventricular wall rupture after acute myocardial infarction: sensitivity and specificity of clinical, hemodynamic and echocardiographic criteria. J Am Coll Cardiol. 1992;19:1145.
11. Figueras J, Alcalde O, Barrabés JA, et al. Changes in hospital mortality rates in 425 patients with acute ST-elevation myocardial infarction and cardiac rupture over a 30-year period. Circulation. 2008; 118:2783.
12. Giannuzzi P, Temporelli PL, Bosimini E, et al. Heterogeneity of left ventricular remodeling after acute myocardial infarction: results of the Gruppo Italiano per lo studio della Sopravvivenza nell'Infarto Miocardico-3 Echo substudy. Am Heart J. 2001;141:131.
13. Glower DG, Lowe EL. Left ventricular aneurysm. In: Edmunds LH, editor. Cardiac surgery in the adult. New York: McGraw-Hill; 1997. p. 677.
14. Douglas PS, et al. ACCF/ACR/AHA/ASE/ASNC/HRS/NASCI/RSNA/SAIP/SCAI/SCCT/SCMR 2008 Health Policy Statement on Structured Reporting in Cardiovascular Imaging. Circulation. 2009 Jan 6;119(1):187.200.

Mitral Valve

8

Liem Nguyen and Neal Gerstein

Abbreviations

TEE	Transesophageal echocardiography
TTE	Transthoracic echocardiography
LA	Left atrium
LV	Left ventricle
MR	Mitral regurgitation
MS	Mitral stenosis
ME	Midesophageal (window)
TG	Transgastric (window)
LAX	Long-axis (view)
SAX	Short-axis (view)
PSAX	Parasternal short-axis (view)
PLAX	Parasternal long-axis (view)
A4C	Apical four-chamber (view)
A2C	Apical two-chamber (view)
LUPV	Left upper pulmonary vein
PISA	Proximal isovelocity surface area
EROA	Effective regurgitant orifice area

Supplementary Information The online version of this chapter (https://doi.org/10.1007/978-3-030-84349-6_8) contains supplementary material, which is available to authorized users.

L. Nguyen (✉)
Department of Anesthesiology, University of California San Diego Health, La Jolla, CA, USA
e-mail: liem@ucsd.edu

N. Gerstein
Department of Anesthesiology and Critical Care Medicine, University of New Mexico School of Medicine, Albuquerque, NM, USA
e-mail: NGerstein@salud.unm.edu

Introduction

The mitral valve apparatus consists of the annulus, leaflets, chordae tendineae, papillary muscles, myocardium, and its attendant chambers, the left atrium (LA) and left ventricle (LV) (Fig. 8.1). The coordinated actions of the entire left heart contribute to the normal functioning of the mitral valve. The complex design of the mitral valve is a consequence of its ability to perform two critical yet divergent functions: the unobstructed opening of the valve leaflets with passage of blood into the LV during diastole followed by a reduction in area to prevent retrograde flow back into the LA during systole. To achieve this duality, the function and competency of the mitral valve apparatus is intimately dependent on the structural integrity and precise coordination of each of its components [1–8].

Anatomy and Function

The shape of the bicuspid mitral valve provides the origin of its name, from the Latin *mitre* (bishop's hat). It is composed of two anatomically distinct leaflets, the anterior leaflet and posterior leaflet (Fig. 8.2). The anterior leaflet is located in

T. M. Maus, C. R. Tainter (eds.), *Essential Echocardiography*,
https://doi.org/10.1007/978-3-030-84349-6_8

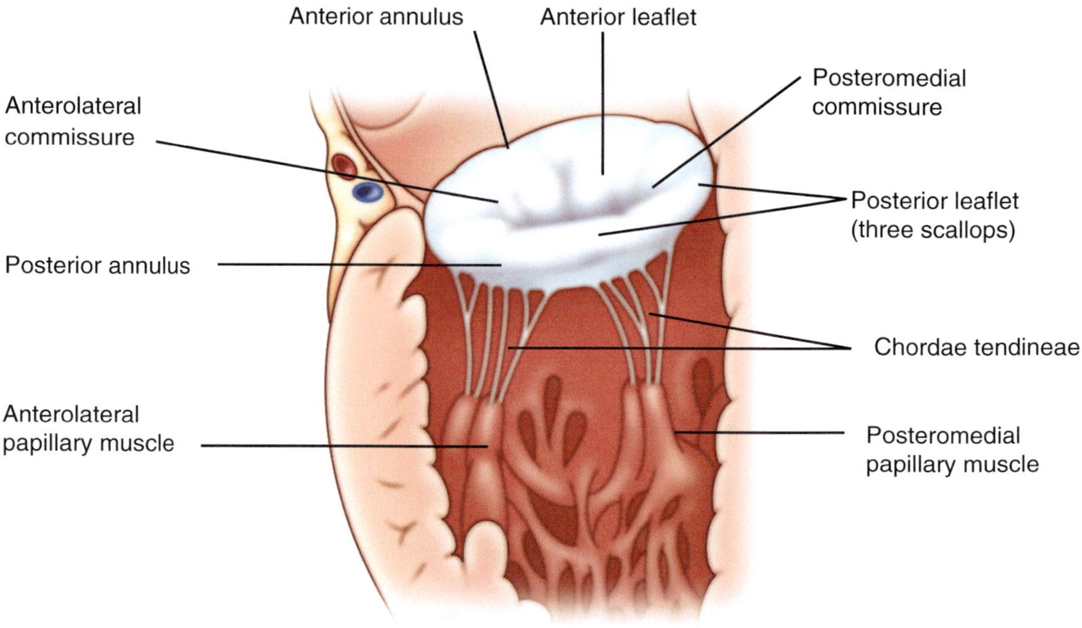

Fig. 8.1 Components of the mitral valve apparatus, as viewed from a posterior perspective

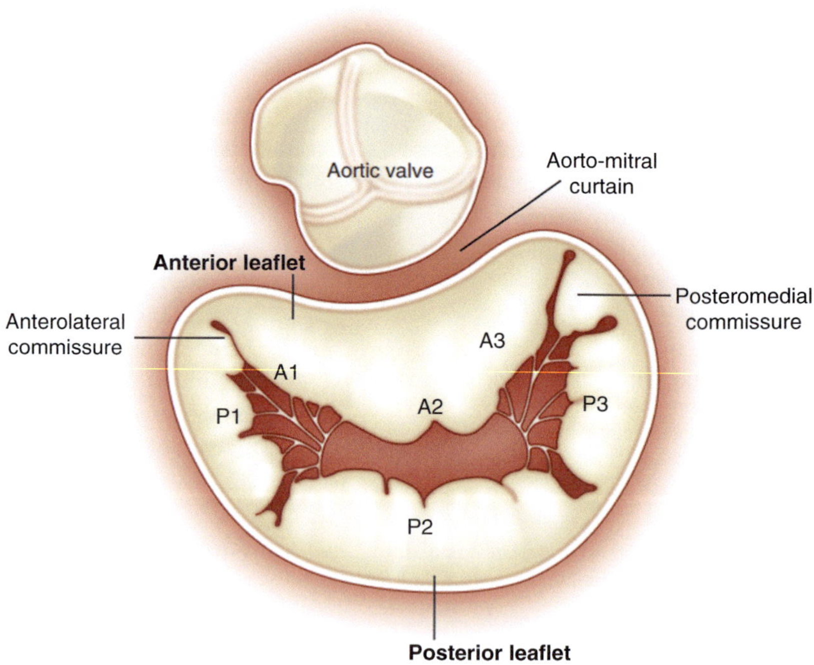

Fig. 8.2 Leaflets of the bicuspid mitral valve, according to the standard Carpentier nomenclature, as viewed from a superior perspective ("Surgeon's view")

close proximity to the left and noncoronary cusps of the aortic valve, separated by a thin piece of tissue termed the aorto-mitral curtain. Distinct from the anterior leaflet, the posterior leaflet contains three identifiable subunits called scallops. In the commonly utilized Carpentier description of mitral valve anatomy, these individual scallops are labeled from anterior to posterior as P1, P2, and P3. The posterior leaflet subtends approximately two thirds of the circumference of the annulus [3–5]. By contrast, the anterior leaflet encompasses about one-third of the circumference of the annulus. The anterior leaflet is devoid of individually distinct scallops, providing a smooth surface designed to promote systolic ejection of blood into the left ventricular outflow tract. Despite lacking discrete scallops, the Carpentier description divides the anterior leaflet into three analogous segments, A1, A2, and A3, which coincide with the corresponding posterior scallops (i.e., P1 coapts with A1, P2 with A2, P3 with A3). The anterior and posterior leaflets adjoin at two distinct points near the edges of the annulus, which are termed the anterolateral and posteromedial commissures [3–5] (Fig. 8.2).

As an interdependent unit, the anterior and posterior leaflets come together during systole to form a coaptation line resembling a semicircle during closure [3–5] (Fig. 8.3). The mitral leaflets are circumferentially supported by a fibrous tissue-reinforced ring, referred to as the mitral annulus. The mitral annulus geometrically resembles a hyperbolic paraboloid, or saddle shape, and anatomically serves as the attachment points for both mitral leaflets. While a saddle has two high points (the front and back of a saddle) and two low points (the sides of the saddle), the mitral valve is similarly shaped with analogous high and low points. The anterior-posterior (front to back) axis of the annulus defines the higher peak to peak dimension, whereas the lateral axis (side-to-side or commissure-to-commissure) defines the trough-to-trough dimension, which is positioned at a lower point (Fig. 8.4).

The posterior aspect of the mitral annulus is structurally thinner and contains less fibrous support, causing it to be more prone to dilation and flattening compared to the more reinforced anterior portion. Overall, the unique geometry of the saddle-shaped annulus serves to reduce the tension on both of the mitral leaflets during systole [2, 3, 5, 7]. Inferiorly, on the ventricular aspect, the mitral leaflets connect to a complex network of chordae tendineae, which are attached to the anterolateral and posteromedial papillary muscles. During systole, the papillary muscles contract in concert with the ventricular walls to prevent prolapse of the mitral leaflets into the atrium [4–7]. The coordinated movement of the entire mitral valve apparatus results in the closure

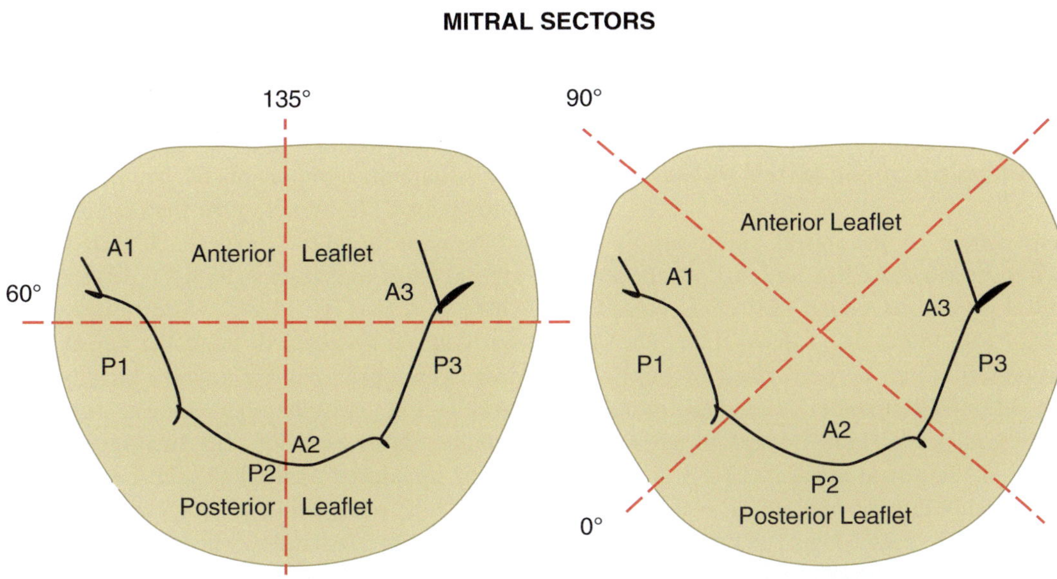

Fig. 8.3 Mitral sectors with representative leaflet segments expected from the midesophageal (ME) transesophageal views

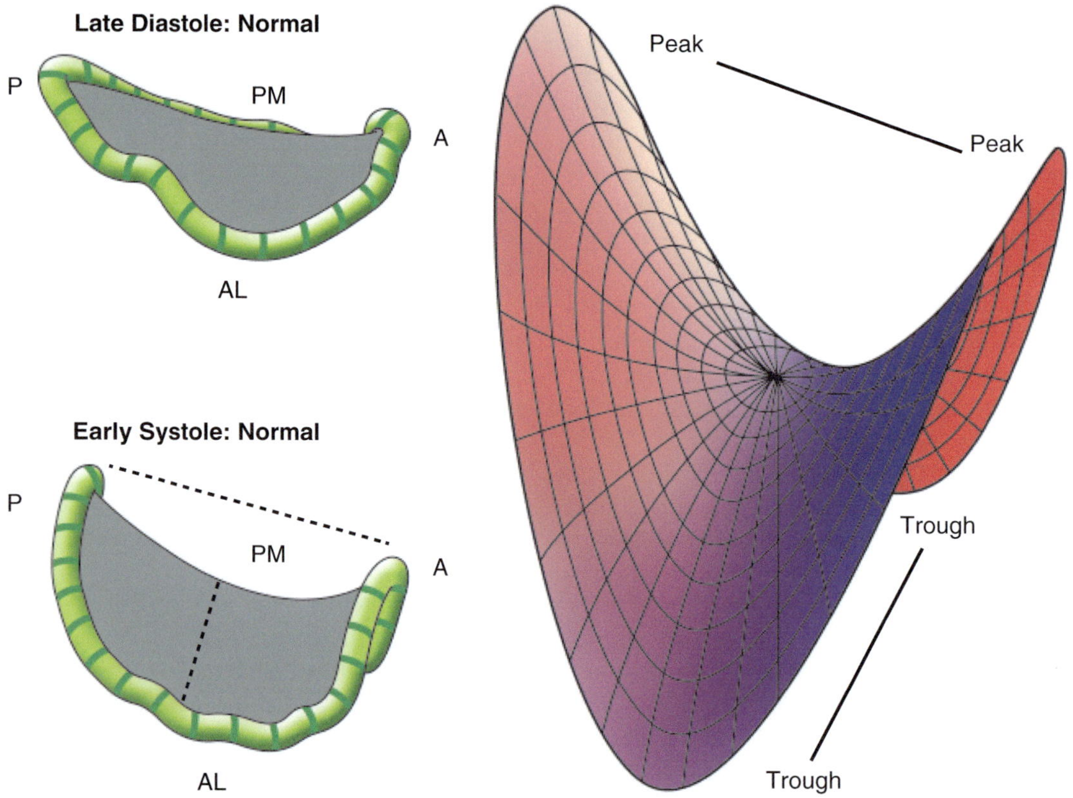

Fig. 8.4 Rendition of mitral valve annulus depicting the characteristic saddle-shaped geometry. The anterior-posterior axis (ME LAX view) encompasses the peak-to-peak distance, whereas the lateral axis (ME mitral commissural view) corresponds to the trough-to-trough distance

of the mitral valve during systole, preventing regurgitant flow into the LA.

2D Imaging of the Mitral Valve

Assessment of the mitral valve begins with two-dimensional (2D) imaging of the entire mitral apparatus using TEE (Fig. 8.5a–f) or TTE (Fig. 8.6a–d) [1–6, 8–11]. The TEE examination can be performed by starting in the ME four-chamber view and obtaining sequential multiplane images of all components of the mitral apparatus [1–3, 5, 6]. The leaflet subunits of the mitral valve can be individually viewed as a two-dimensional slice by using the available sector planes of the TEE probe at various multiplane angles (Figs. 8.3 and 8.5a–f). Detailed instructions on how to obtain the various views discussed in this chapter are described in Chap. 2. The parasternal window is a useful starting point to evaluate the components of the mitral apparatus with TTE, allowing for the development of the parasternal long-axis (PLAX) and parasternal short-axis views (PSAX) of the mitral valve [8–11] (Fig. 8.6a–d). Additional views can then be obtained through the apical window, which provides the apical four-chamber (A4C) and two-chamber views. A more detailed discussion of 2D imaging of the mitral apparatus using TTE can be found in Chap. 3. The following sections will highlight the essential 2D windows necessary to evaluate the mitral valve apparatus using TEE and TTE.

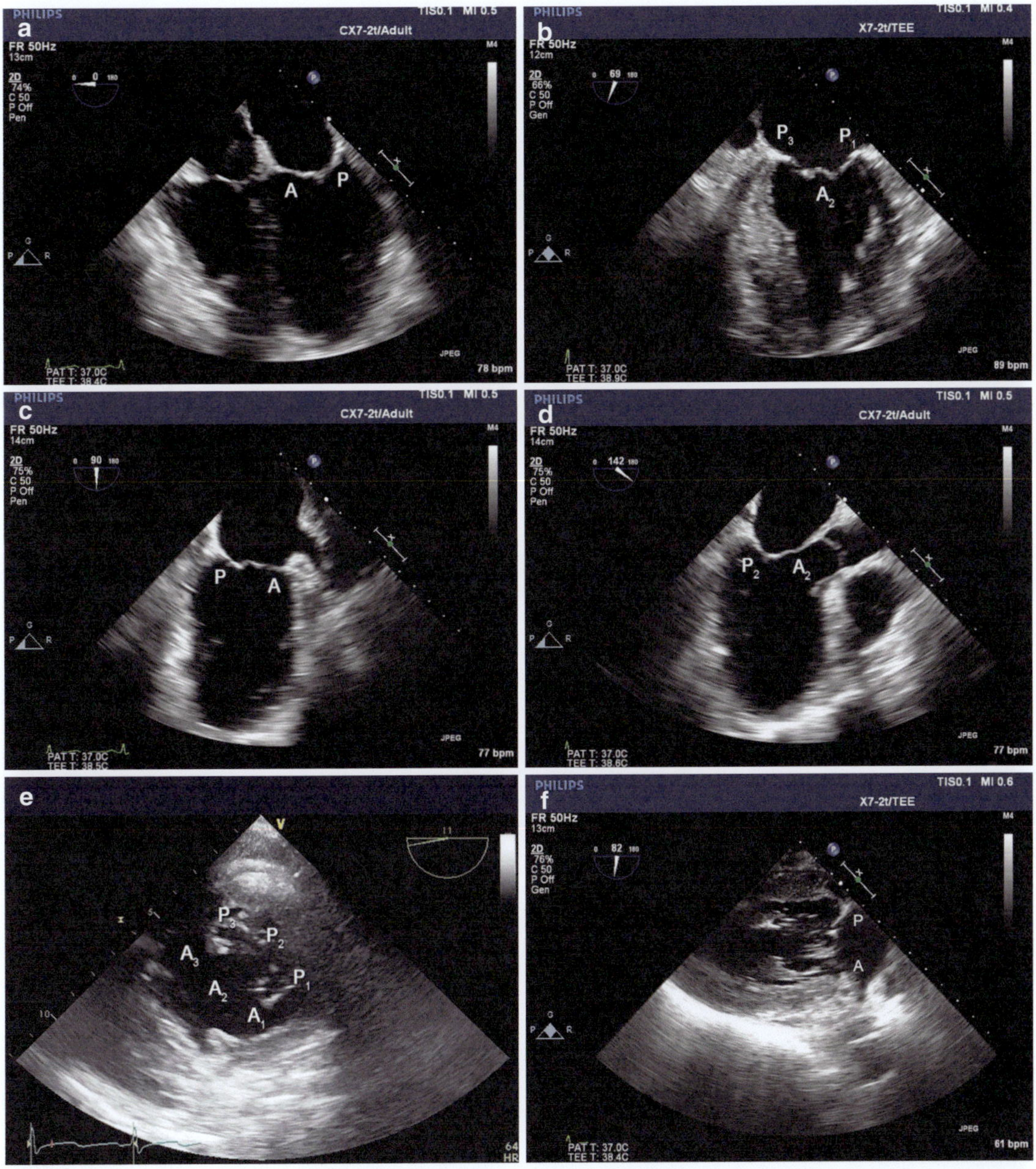

Fig. 8.5 Transesophageal echocardiography (TEE) imaging of the mitral valve apparatus. (**a**) ME four-chamber view. (**b**) ME mitral commissural view. (**c**) ME two-chamber view. (**d**) ME LAX view. (**e**) TG basal SAX view. (**f**) TG two-chamber view. *A* anterior leaflet, *P* posterior leaflet

TEE: Midesophageal Four-Chamber View (ME Four-Chamber View)

In the ME four-chamber view at 0 degrees (Figs. 8.3 and 8.5a), the anterior leaflet appears on the left side of the screen, and the posterior leaflet is on the right. The ME four-chamber view is useful for obtaining a global evaluation of mitral leaflet anatomy and motion and the adaptive changes that may occur as a result of volume stress in the upstream atrium and downstream ventricle. The ME four-chamber view is

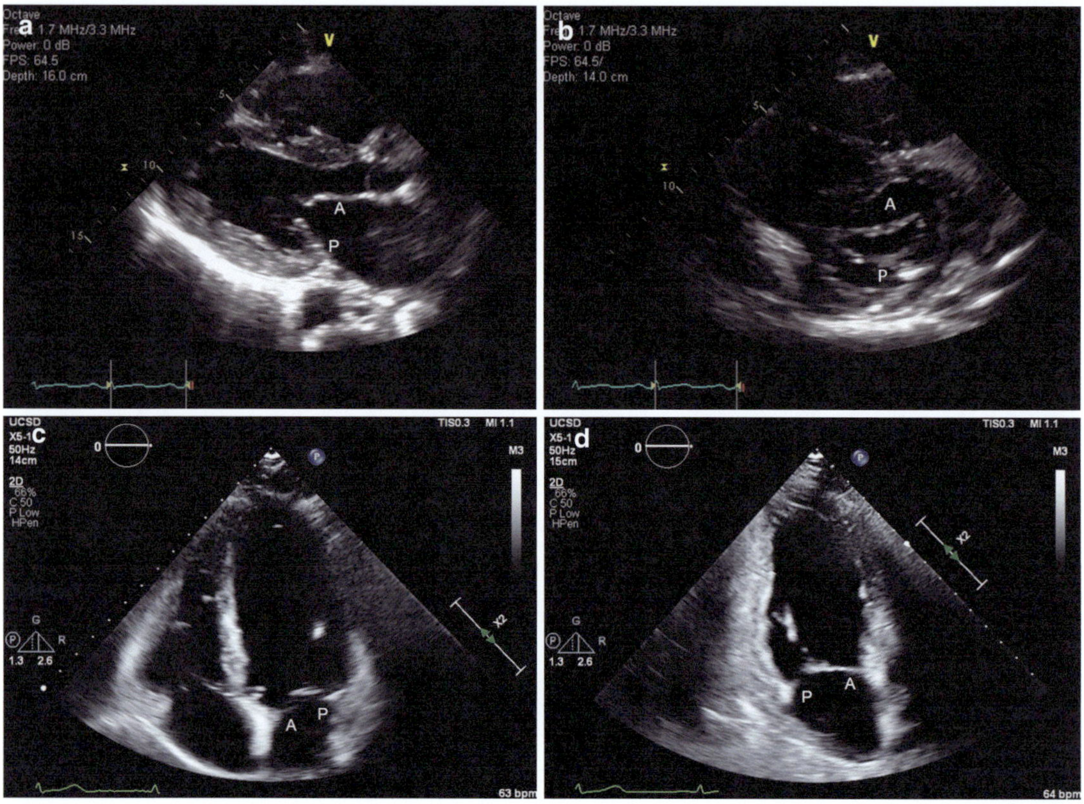

Fig. 8.6 Transthoracic echocardiography (TTE) imaging of the mitral valve apparatus. (**a**) PLAX view. (**b**) PSAX view. (**c**) A4C view. (**d**) Apical two-chamber (A2C) view. *A* anterior leaflet, *P* posterior leaflet

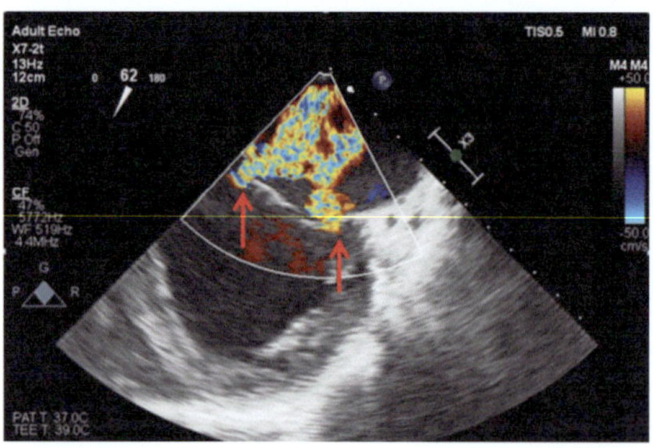

Fig. 8.7 Midesophageal mitral commissural view with color flow Doppler demonstrating two distinct jets (*red arrows*) due to a sector plane that captures only the two outer edges of the jet, omitting the central portion

also useful to evaluate the degree of mitral regurgitation (MR) using color flow Doppler [1–3, 5, 6].

TEE: ME Mitral Commissural View

The ME mitral commissural view is obtained by starting at the ME four-chamber view and rotating the multiplane angle to approximately 45–60 degrees (Figs. 8.3 and 8.5b). In this view, the middle A2 segment is flanked by the P3 scallop on the left and P1 scallop on the right of the screen [1–3, 5, 6]. The ME mitral commissural view also provides a view of both papillary muscles and their associated chordae tendineae. It is important to note that the ME mitral commissural view displays an imaging slice that traverses the semicircle-shaped coaptation line and the anterolateral and posteromedial commissures. Accordingly, color flow Doppler assessment of a regurgitant jet may appear as two distinct jets on either side of the A2 segment of the anterior leaflet, because the sector plane captures the two outer edges of the jet and omits the central portion (Fig. 8.7; Video 8.1). This often results in the incorrect echocardiographic diagnosis of two distinct jets, when in fact the image merely represents the two edges of one curved jet.

TEE: ME Two-Chamber View

The ME two-chamber view is obtained by rotating the multiplane to approximately 90 degrees (Figs. 8.3 and 8.5c). In this image plane, the anterior leaflet is located on the right and the posterior leaflet is on the left of the screen. The left atrial appendage and Coumadin ridge (a band of tissue separating the left atrial appendage and the left upper pulmonary vein (LUPV)) are often observed above and to the right of the anterior mitral leaflet. Withdrawing the probe from this position and turning slightly to the left often bring the LUPV into view, allowing for Doppler interrogations of left atrial inflow [1–3, 5, 6].

TEE: ME Long-Axis View (ME LAX View)

From the ME four-chamber view, the ME LAX view is obtained by increasing the multiplane angle to 120–150 degrees until the aortic valve and mitral valve are visualized in the same image plane (Figs. 8.3 and 8.5d) [1–3, 5, 6]. This imaging plane displays a slice of the mitral leaflets along the anterior-posterior dimension (A2-P2), perpendicular to the coaptation line. The A2 segment is displayed on the right of the screen nearest the aortic valve leaflets, and the P2 segment appears on the left side of the screen. The ME LAX view allows one to assess the anterior-posterior dimension of both the diameter of the MR jet and peak-to-peak dimensions of the mitral annulus. This imaging plane therefore offers a more accurate measurement of the width of the vena contracta, the narrowest part of a regurgitant jet at the level of the valve leaflets as measured by color flow Doppler [1–3, 5, 6].

TEE: Transgastric Basal Short-Axis View (TG Basal SAX)

The TG basal SAX view at 0 degrees (Fig. 8.5e) is obtained by either slightly withdrawing the probe or exerting anteflexion from the true transgastric (TG) midpapillary short-axis view of the LV. The imaging plane is achieved when both the anterior and posterior mitral leaflets are visualized in a short-axis "fish mouth" view. This view of the mitral valve allows for all the mitral segments to be visualized, providing a means to assess valve opening and closure qualitatively or with planimetry. The TG basal SAX view may also reveal a ruptured chordae or flail segment from this vantage. Moreover, color flow Doppler mapping of the regurgitant jet in the TG basal SAX view may reveal the origin of the coaptation defect and provide insight into the mechanism of regurgitation [1–3, 5, 6].

TEE: Transgastric Two-Chamber View (TG Two-Chamber View)

From the TG midpapillary short-axis view of the LV, rotation of the multiplane angle to ~90 degrees gives rise to the TG two-chamber view (Fig. 8.5f), which provides a perpendicular scan plane that facilitates the assessment of the subvalvular apparatus (i.e., chordae tendineae and papillary muscle-LV wall complex) [1, 2, 5, 6]. The anterolateral papillary muscle occupies a position furthest from the probe, and the posteromedial papillary muscle is displayed in the near field. This view is useful for evaluating the position and geometry of the papillary muscles, chordae tendineae, and ventricular wall complex, as well as demonstrating pathologic processes associated with these structures (e.g., papillary muscle calcification, rupture, or endocarditis).

TTE: Parasternal Long-Axis View (PLAX)

The PLAX view provides a view of the mitral valve in juxtaposition to the aortic valve, similar to the ME long-axis view with TEE (Fig. 8.6a) [8–11]. The anterior and posterior leaflets of the mitral valve are seen opening during diastole and closing with the leaflet tips overlapping at the coaptation point during systole. The identification of the anterior mitral leaflet is confirmed by observing the leaflet tip approaching or contacting the ventricular septum as it opens during diastole. The PLAX view offers an anterior-to-posterior imaging plane that corresponds to the peak-to-peak dimension of the mitral annulus. Accordingly, this imaging plane offers the echocardiographer a means to evaluate for the presence of annular dilation in the anterior and posterior dimension. The PLAX view may also prove particularly useful in identifying the presence of a prolapsing or flail leaflet segment compared to other transthoracic windows [8–11].

TTE: Parasternal Short-Axis (PSAX)

From the PLAX view, the PSAX view is obtained by rotating the transducer clockwise 90 degrees, until the indicator is directed toward the left shoulder of the patient. Careful adjustments of the probe by fanning from the superior to inferior direction may be required to properly display the mitral valve in short axis (Fig. 8.6b). Analogous to the TG basal short-axis view on TEE, the PSAX view of the mitral valve allows for the qualitative or planimetric evaluation of leaflet opening and closure. Color flow Doppler interrogation of the mitral valve in the PSAX view may also offer clues regarding the location or origin of the mitral jet from this unique vantage point from the LV [8–11].

TTE: Apical Four-Chamber View (A4C)

The TTE apical windows are obtained by placing the transducer near the point of maximal impulse on the left side of the chest, usually near the 4th–fifth intercostal space at the anterior axillary line, with the indicator directed to the left shoulder. The image is then optimized so that all four chambers are seen with the LV (near field) and LA (far field) appearing on the right side of the screen. Similarly, the right ventricle (RV) (near field) and right atrium (far field) are positioned on the left side of the screen. In the A4C view, the mitral valve apparatus is easily visualized (Fig. 8.6c) as it divides the LV and LA in this longitudinal imaging plane. In this imaging sector, the anterior leaflet can be identified by its location next to the interventricular or interatrial septum, and the posterior leaflet can be distinguished by its position next to the lateral aspect of the heart. Gross anatomical abnormalities of the mitral leaflets such as calcification or thickening can be appreciated in this view, as well as any aberrations in leaflet motion during opening or closure. The orientation of mitral flow along the path of the ultrasound wave makes the apical window usually the most accurate for Doppler measurements of mitral inflow, mitral stenosis (MS), and MR. As this imaging plane offers a longitudinal view of both the LA and LV, left atrial size can also be appreciated from the apical window. The A4C view also allows for the assessment of the pulmonary veins for measuring flow into the LA [8–11].

TTE: Apical Two-Chamber (A2C)

From the A4C view, the apical two-chamber view (Fig. 8.6d) is obtained by rotating the transducer approximately 90 degrees counterclockwise until the LA and LV are seen in a longitudinal orientation. In addition to the mitral leaflets, the left atrial appendage appears along the right side of the screen in this view. The apical two-chamber view provides another imaging plane to evaluate mitral valve leaflet motion and

Doppler interrogation of stenotic or regurgitant transmitral flow. Evidence of secondary adaptations to MR can be appreciated in this window, as the size and area of the LA and LV can be measured in the two-chamber view [8–11].

Mitral Regurgitation (Highlight Box 8.1)

Although the final common pathway of an incompetent mitral apparatus is a regurgitant jet at the level of the leaflet tips, a significant portion of MR is due to dysfunction of the valve apparatus exclusive of the leaflets themselves (e.g., LV, papillary muscles, or chordae) [5, 6, 12]. When considering the etiology or mechanism of MR, it is crucial to examine all of the associated structures above and below the leaflets in order to fully characterize the mechanism. A simplified classification scheme focusing on leaflet motion described by the cardiac surgeon Alain Carpentier may be used to identify the mechanism(s) underlying MR [1, 2, 5, 6, 8]. The Carpentier classification (see Table 8.1) centers on the evaluation of the movement of the mitral leaflets during diastole and systole, described by the following categories:

Type 1: Normal leaflet motion.
Type 2: Excessive leaflet motion.
Type 3: Restricted leaflet motion.
  3a: Restricted leaflet motion in systole and diastole.
  3b: Restricted leaflet motion in systole only.

Carpentier's classification (types 1, 2, 3a, and 3b) can yield important clues into the mechanism of MR [2, 3]. Type 1 (normal leaflet motion) consists of MR as a result of mitral valve clefts, perforations, or annular dilation [2, 5]. In type 2 (excessive leaflet motion), the excessive leaflet motion is due to leaflet prolapse or flail. In type 3a, restricted leaflet excursion during diastole and systole is often the result of a thickened or calcified leaflet secondary to rheumatic disease or a calcific process. In the type 3b subgroup, leaflet restriction occurs primarily during systole because of apical displacement of the papillary muscle or tethering of the leaflets, as can be seen with myocardial ischemia. Functional MR or MR as a result of ventricular dysfunction may also fall into the type 3b category, where the leaflets may become apically displaced and display restricted movement during coaptation [1, 2, 5, 6, 8].

Highlight Box 8.1

Mitral regurgitation	
2D	• Mitral leaflet motion (normal, excessive, restrictive) • Mitral calcification • Annular dimensions (dilated) • Left atrial enlargement, eccentric LV hypertrophy • LV wall motion abnormalities
CFD	• Qualitative assessment (jet area/LA area ratio) • Coanda effect (wall hugging jet) • Vena contracta measurement
Spectral	• Pulmonary venous Doppler (PWD) • Density of regurgitation jet profile (CWD) • PISA-based calculation of EROA

LV left ventricle, *LA* left atrium, *PWD* pulsed-wave Doppler, *CWD* continuous-wave Doppler, *PISA* proximal isovelocity surface area, *EROA* effective regurgitant orifice area

Table 8.1 Carpentier classification of mitral regurgitation

Type	Leaflet motion	Prototypical example	Surgical correction
I	Normal	Annular dilation	Annuloplasty (e.g., MV ring)
II	Excessive	P2 segment prolapse	MV repair (e.g., P2 resection, sliding annuloplasty)
IIIa	Restrictive (systolic and diastolic)	Rheumatic disease	MV replacement
IIIb	Restrictive (systolic only)	Functional/ischemic	Revascularization +/– MV repair/replacement

MR mitral regurgitation, *MV* mitral valve, *P2* middle posterior leaflet scallop

One of the main focal points of mitral valve function is the mitral annulus, which is reinforced by a network of fibroelastic tissue that serves to maintain the unique hyperbolic paraboloid (saddle-like) geometry during systole (Fig. 8.4) [8, 12–23]. Annular dilation, measured in the anterior-posterior dimension in the ME LAX or PLAX view, or distortion of the saddle-shaped geometry during systole may lead to a coaptation defect and represents an important mechanism of MR [6, 9, 19, 20]. Left atrial enlargement (e.g., due to atrial fibrillation or ventricular dysfunction) and secondary annular dilation may contribute to MR in the setting of normal leaflet anatomy and motion (Type 1). Dilation of the mitral annulus has also been implicated as a contributing mechanism in ischemic MR [24, 25].

The ventricular myocardium, anterolateral and posteromedial papillary muscles, and the network of chordae tendineae all provide the necessary foundation required for normal leaflet motion and competency (Fig. 8.1). The interpapillary distance (lateral distance) and location of the papillary muscles in relation to the ventricular wall and coaptation point plays a significant role in the overall competency of the mitral valve complex [5, 6, 22]. The major responsibility of the papillary muscle-chordae tendineae complex is to regulate leaflet movement. Excessive leaflet motion (Type 2), such as in the presence of a ruptured chord, results in leaflet prolapse and acute MR, demonstrating that the papillary muscle and chordae tendineae work together to prevent leaflet displacement into the LA.

Abnormalities in leaflet anatomy, such as those seen in degenerative diseases and endocarditis, may also result in excessive leaflet motion, a coaptation defect, and subsequent MR [2, 5, 26]. Degenerative mitral diseases (e.g., Barlow's disease and fibroelastic deficiency) comprise a range of leaflet abnormalities, characterized by chordal and leaflet thickening, mitral tissue redundancy, and excessive leaflet motion (Type 2) in the form of prolapse or flail, leading to valve incompetency (Figs. 8.8a–b and 8.9a–b; Videos 8.2, 8.3, 8.4 and 8.5) [2, 5, 26]. Infective endocarditis and the presence of bacterial vegetations on the atrial side often cause leaflet damage, leading to destruction of both the anatomy and function of the leaflets (Fig. 8.10a–b; Videos 8.6 and 8.7). Extensive damage may result in excessive leaflet motion and be classified as Type 2 MR, while healed endocarditis may have a resultant perforation in a leaflet and otherwise normal leaflet motion and be classified as Type 1.

Restriction of mitral valve leaflet motion is classified as Type 3 and may be subdivided based upon restricted movement in systole and diastole (Type 3a) or during systole only (Type 3b). Leaflet calcification and fusion, as seen in rheumatic disease (Type 3a), is an underappreciated etiology of MR where leaflet motion is impaired in both systole and diastole. In addition to marked leaflet immobility, the annulus and entire subvalvular apparatus may also deteriorate from marked calcification [2, 5, 26].

Patients with functional MR (type 3b) underscore the critical geometric relationship of the ventricular wall, papillary muscle, and chordal elements in providing a foundation for normal leaflet coaptation [4–7,]. Functional MR refers to valvular dysfunction involving the LV as the underlying cause, in the setting of normal leaflet anatomy. Most commonly, it is a result of myocardial ischemia or dilated cardiomyopathy, with distortion of the normal geometry of the ventricular myocardium, papillary muscles, and chordae network. Indeed, the proper interpapillary distance (lateral distance) and location of the papillary muscles (i.e., apical displacement) in relation to the ventricular wall and coaptation point are critical in regulating the overall competency of the mitral valve complex [4]. In the setting of myocardial ischemia, displacement of the papillary muscles toward the apex of the heart and concomitant tethering of associated chordae culminate in leaflet restriction and formation of a coaptation defect [4–7].

Grading Severity

2D Echocardiography

Prior to quantifying the severity of MR, it is prudent to examine the upstream and downstream chambers (LA and LV, respectively) for signs of

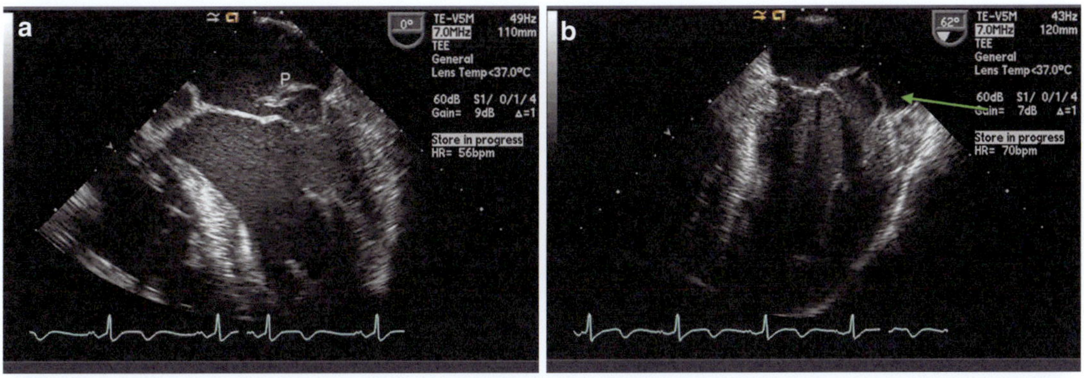

Fig. 8.8 (**a**) ME four-chamber view with a flail posterior leaflet (P). (**b**) ME mitral commissural view of the same patient with posterior leaflet prolapse of the P1–P2 segment (*green arrow*)

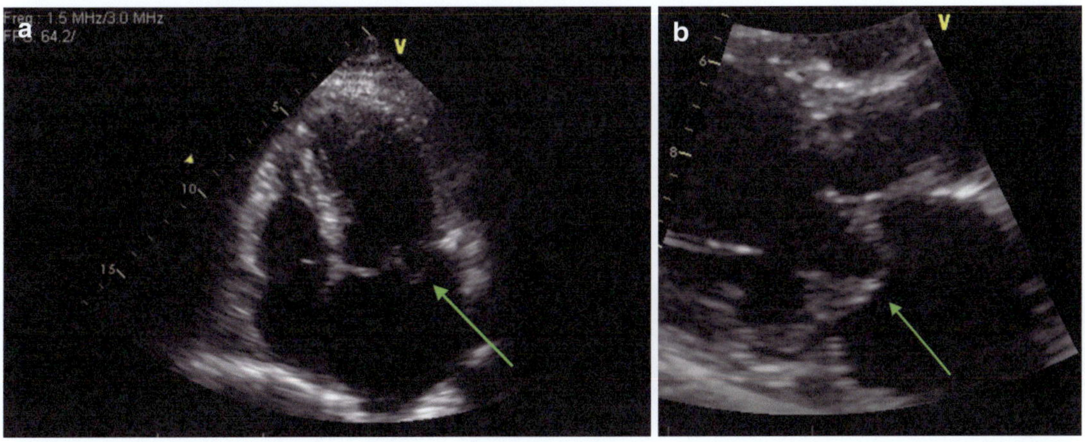

Fig. 8.9 (**a**) A4C view with posterior leaflet prolapse (*green arrow*). (**b**) PLAX view with a zoomed in perspective of the mitral valve with bileaflet prolapse (*green arrow*) during systole

adaptation to volume stress. Adaptation to chronic volume overload may lead to chamber dilation of the LA and LV, which may be appreciated on 2D imaging [5, 6, 12]. Upstream effects of left atrial volume overload and pulmonary hypertension may result in echocardiographic signs of RV dilation, tricuspid regurgitation, and interventricular septal bowing suggesting RV dysfunction. Echocardiographic signs of the downstream effects of MR may include the presence of eccentric LV hypertrophy, elevated end-diastolic volumes, and increased (presence of ventricular dysfunction) or decreased (supranormal ejection fraction in compensated chronic MR) end-systolic dimensions. After examining the adjacent heart chambers for the effects of volume overload, specific attention can then be afforded to the rest of the mitral apparatus.

Evidence of excessive leaflet motion (Type 2) is generally a result of degenerative disease of the mitral valve leading to prolapse, flail, or billowing of a leaflet segment above the annular plane [5, 6, 12, 26]. More specifically, prolapse is defined as a translation of the leaflet body above the annulus due to excess leaflet and/or chordal length during systole (Figs. 8.8a–b and 8.9a–b). The term "flail" refers to the movement of a leaflet tip above the annular plane, often because of a ruptured chordae. The presence of a ruptured chordae may often be obscured, rendering the echocardiographic distinction between prolapse and flail challenging. "Billowing" or "scallop-

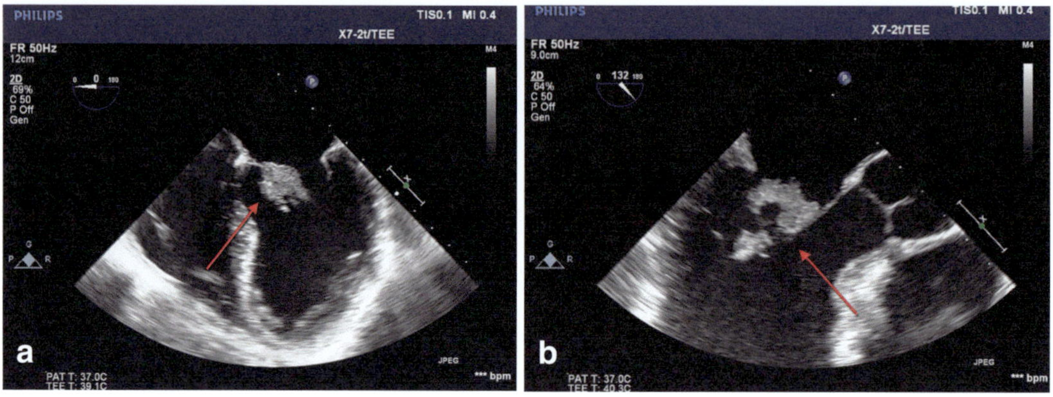

Fig. 8.10 (**a**) ME four-chamber view with anterior leaflet vegetation (*red arrow*). (**b**) ME LAX view of the same patient with an anterior leaflet vegetation (*red arrow*)

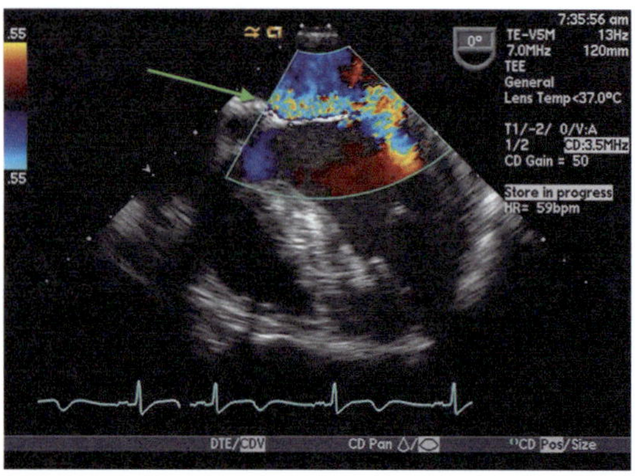

Fig. 8.11 ME four-chamber view showing posterior leaflet prolapse and corresponding jet directed away from affected leaflet (*green arrow*)

ing" is a projection of the leaflet body or segment above the annulus, with the point of coaptation remaining below the annular plane [5, 6, 26]. MR as a result of excessive motion (Type 2) of an isolated leaflet often results in an eccentric jet directed away from the diseased leaflet (Fig. 8.11; Video 8.8). Although uncommon, eccentric jets may be present in bileaflet disease if one of the leaflets is more affected than the other. Nevertheless, the appearance of an eccentric jet often signifies the presence of a structural abnormality in the mitral apparatus and warrants close examination.

Restricted leaflet motion in systole and diastole (Type 3a) is associated with rheumatic disease [27]. This differs from functional MR (Type 3b) in which restricted leaflet motion is only in systole due to leaflet tethering as a result of a dilated ventricle, papillary muscle dysfunction, or myocardial ischemia. The direction of the jet often emerges toward the affected leaflet if the restricted leaflet motion is asymmetric. In the case of symmetric bileaflet tethering, a central jet may occur [5, 6].

Color Flow Doppler

Color flow or spectral Doppler interrogation enables the echocardiographer to initially screen and map the MR jet as it flows into the LA (Fig. 8.12; Videos 8.9, 8.10, 8.11 and 8.12) [5, 6, 12, 28–30]. To optimize the image quality, it may be helpful to use the zoom function to increase the window size to the structure of interest. With a Doppler flow sector window set to capture only the LA, mapping of the MR jet can then be optimized by setting the Nyquist limit to approximately 50–60 cm/s. It is prudent to visualize any discovered MR jets in multiple views to gain a complete picture of the nature and characteristics of the regurgitant flow. In this way, jets that are difficult to visualize (i.e., eccentric jets, short duration jets) are not missed or underappreciated. It may also be helpful to make small adjustments to the probe position to maximize the quality of the image and capture the most representative jet or

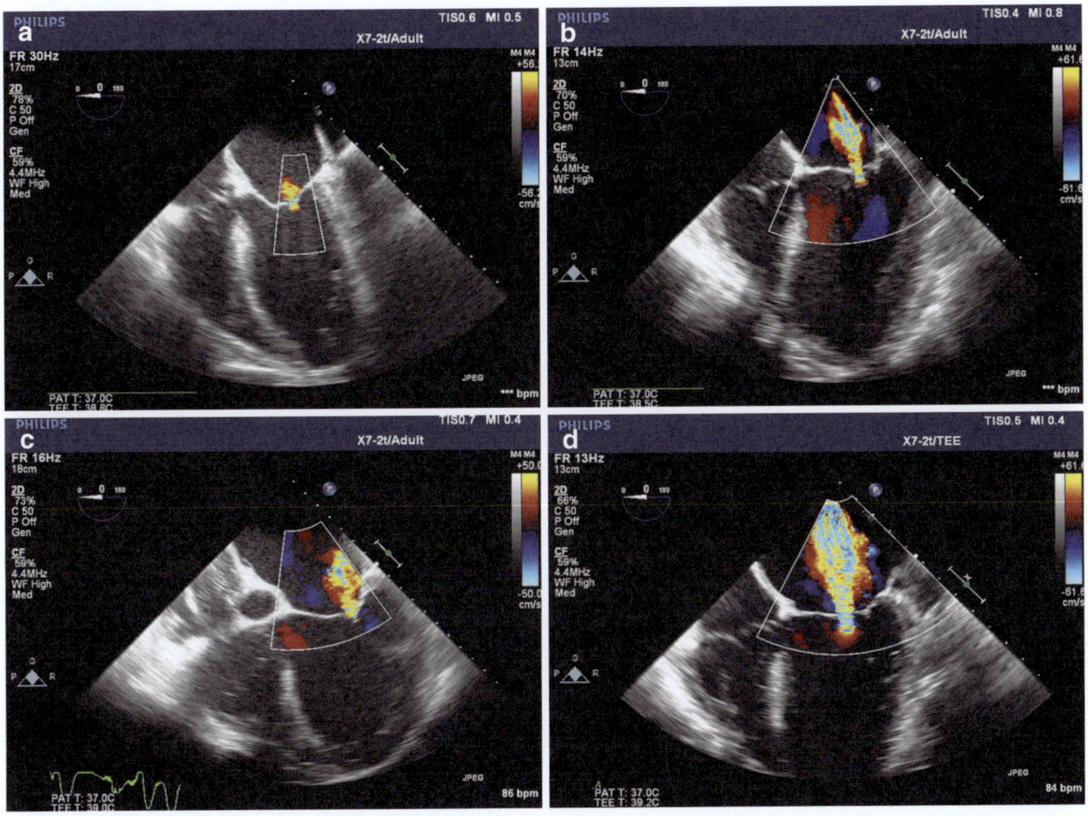

Fig. 8.12 Midesophageal four-chamber views with color flow Doppler demonstrating increasing MR severity. (**a**) Trace (1+). (**b**) Mild (2+). (**c**) Moderate (3+). (**d**) Severe (4+)

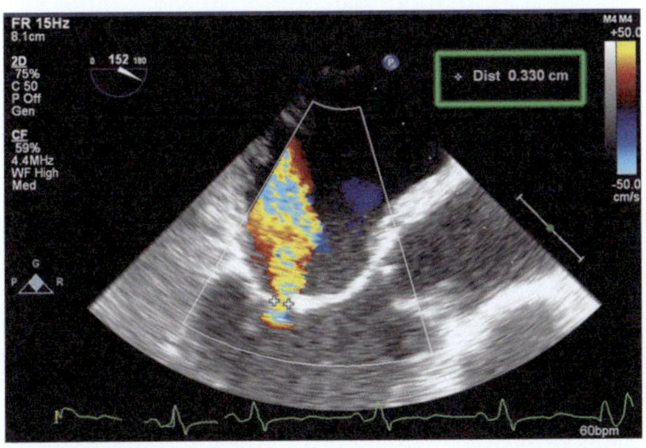

Fig. 8.13 Vena contracta measurement in the ME long-axis view. The measurement is taken at the narrowest portion, or neck, of the jet as it crosses the plane of coaptation

jets possible. For example, with TEE, this may require slight anteflexion/retroflexion or advancement/withdrawal of the probe while imaging the MR jet with color flow Doppler. Once the MR jet is fully imaged, it is important to make a qualitative assessment of the regurgitant flow focusing on the jet shape, direction, width, area, presence of eccentricity, duration, and distance traveled into the LA. Color flow Doppler examination of the MR jet is an important first step to obtaining an initial impression and grading the severity of regurgitation [5, 6, 12].

Vena Contracta

Measurement of the vena contracta is a useful method to assess the severity of MR (Fig. 8.13) [5, 6, 12, 28, 29]. The vena contracta is the narrowest part of the regurgitant jet visualized with color flow Doppler as it emerges from the regurgitant orifice at the level of the leaflet tips [5, 6, 12, 28, 29]. The ideal image captures a jet profile that consists of a proximal convergence zone (area of flow acceleration on ventricular side) and a narrow neck at the plane of the coaptation point. The vena contracta measurement is advantageous, as it is relatively independent of machine settings and loading conditions [12]. However, precise measurement of the vena contracta width can often be challenging due to difficulties in proper image acquisition and the small dimensions of the jet width. The image of the jet can be optimized by using the zoom function and setting the Nyquist limit to approximately 50–60 cm/s. The ideal acoustic window to capture the anterior-posterior dimensions (perpendicular to the coaptation point) of the regurgitant jet is the ME LAX view on TEE [1–3, 5, 6, 12] or PLAX view on TTE [8, 9]. If a jet is not visualized in the ME LAX or PLAX view, the vena contracta can also be measured in the ME four-chamber (TEE) or A4C (TTE) view, but this measurement should be interpreted with caution, as it does not measure the jet perpendicular to the coaptation point. It may be helpful to take several measurements to obtain a more precise vena contracta measurement. Vena contracta widths greater than 7 mm indicate severe MR, and a width less than 3 mm indicates mild MR (Table 8.2) [5, 6, 12, 28, 29].

Pulmonary Venous Flow Profile

Doppler interrogation of pulmonary venous flow or left atrial inflow can be used as a semi-quantitative method for grading MR severity [5, 6, 12]. Using the ME two-chamber view on TEE, the LUPV is identified by its position just above the Coumadin ridge, and flow into the LA toward the probe can be observed when applying a sample gate of color flow Doppler in this region (Fig. 8.14a). Occasionally, slight withdrawal of the probe and/or a slight leftward turn are required to optimize the image of the LUPV. With the sample volume placed approximately 1 cm into the LUPV, velocities are measured as flow moves into the LA (Fig. 8.14b). On TTE, the right upper pulmonary vein is the most convenient vein for the detection of left atrial inflow as the Doppler beam is parallel to the direction of flow in an A4C view (Fig. 8.15a–b). The velocity of blood flow into the LA during ventricular systole (atrial diastole) is typically greater than during ventricular diastole (atrial systole), yielding a systolic dominant pulmonary venous pattern (*pulm vein velocity*$_{\text{systolic}}$ > *than velocity*$_{\text{diastolic}}$; *S*/*D* > 1) [5, 6, 12].

The presence of MR may reduce the peak systolic velocity of the pulmonary venous flow as the regurgitant jet accelerates back through the LA and into the pulmonary venous bed. As the regurgitant jet flows into the pulmonary veins and meets the incoming left atrial inflow during systole, blunting ($V_{systolic} < V_{diastolic}$; $S/D < 1$), (Fig. 8.16a) or reversal (below baseline, Fig. 8.16b) of the systolic component of the pulmonary Doppler profile is observed. Systolic reversal of flow in the pulmonary venous profile is a specific but not sensitive finding of severe MR, with systolic blunting representing a more moderate degree of MR (Table 8.2) [5, 6, 12]. The poor sensitivity of the pulmonary venous flow in detecting MR is partly due to the varying degrees of left atrial compliance and the challenge of interrogating all four pulmonary veins on TEE and TTE [5, 6, 8, 9, 12].

Table 8.2 Mitral valve regurgitation Quantitative assessment

	Mild	Moderate	Severe
Vena contracta (mm)	< 3	3–7	> 7
Pulmonary venous Doppler	Normal	S-wave blunted	S-wave reversal
EROA by PISA (cm^2)	< 0.20	0.20–0.40	> 0.40

EROA effective regurgitant orifice area, *PISA* proximal isovelocity surface area

Proximal Isovelocity Surface Area (PISA)

The proximal isovelocity surface area (PISA) method is a quantitative modality for grading MR severity (Fig. 8.17a–b) [30, 31]. The PISA method is an application of the continuity equation and provides a means to calculate the effective regurgitant orifice area (EROA). In simple terms, the MR volume or flow of blood below the mitral valve is equal to the volume or flow of blood across the mitral valve. As a regurgitant jet travels toward the narrowed mitral orifice, the column of blood accel-

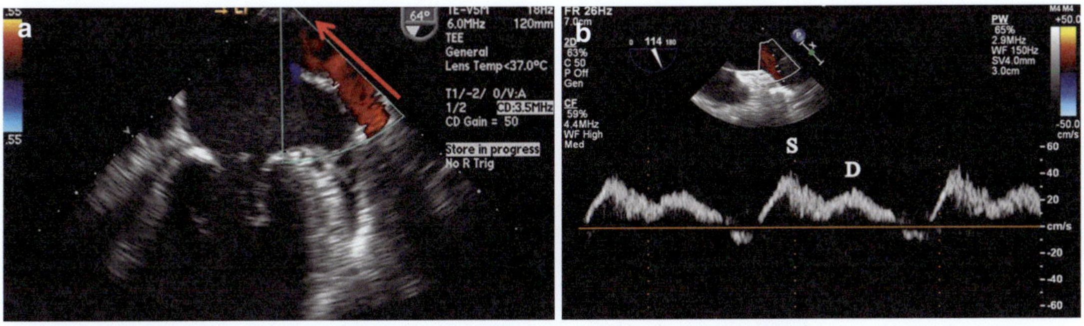

Fig. 8.14 (**a**) Upper esophageal LUPV view with color flow Doppler demonstrating LUPV flow (*red arrow*). (**b**) Pulsed-wave Doppler assessment of the right upper pulmonary veins in the upper esophageal right pulmonary vein view. In this normal spectral profile, the velocity of the systolic (S) component is greater than the diastolic (D) velocity

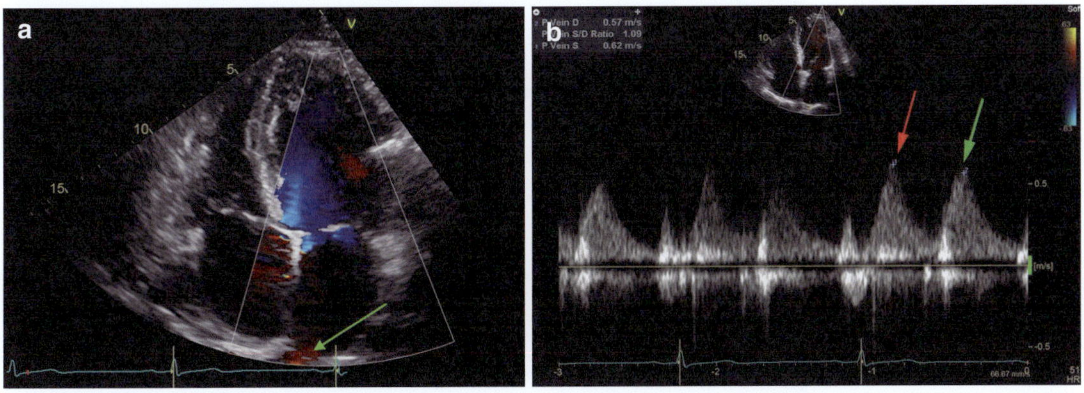

Fig. 8.15 (**a**) A4C view with color flow Doppler focused on the right upper pulmonary vein (*green arrow*). (**b**) In this normal spectral profile, the peak velocity of the systolic (S, *red arrow*) component is greater than the diastolic (D, *green arrow*) velocity

erates, and a series of concentric hemispheres are generated on the ventricular side of the mitral valve. When blood velocity increases beyond the limit of detection of the Doppler scale (Nyquist limit), the color flow map near the mitral orifice displays a high-velocity region with evidence of aliasing (blood velocities above the limit of detection appear to reverse). The flow of blood in the convergence zone (ventricular side) is equal to the product of the surface area of the first hemisphere or isovelocity shell and associated aliasing velocity (Flow = $2\pi r^2$x $V_{aliasing}$). The radius (r) of the isovelocity shell is defined by the distance from the regurgitant orifice to the border of the first aliasing velocity. The flow across the valve orifice is calculated as the product of the EROA and peak velocity of the MR jet ($V_{\mathrm{MR\ Jet}}$). For this calculation, the peak velocity of the MR jet is measured using continuous-wave Doppler interrogation parallel to the regurgitant flow.

Applying the continuity principle of equal flow on the atrial and ventricular side of the regurgitant orifice, the EROA can be calculated as follows:

$$EROA\ \mathrm{x}\ V_{\mathrm{MRjet}} = area_{\mathrm{shell}}\ \mathrm{x}\ V_{\mathrm{aliasing}}$$

$$EROA = 2\pi r^2\ \mathrm{x}\ V_{\mathrm{aliasing}} \,/\, V_{\mathrm{MRjet}}$$

where r = radius of the first isovelocity shell, V_{aliasing} = Nyquist limit, $V_{MR\mathrm{jet}}$ = peak velocity of the MR jet, and π = 3.14.

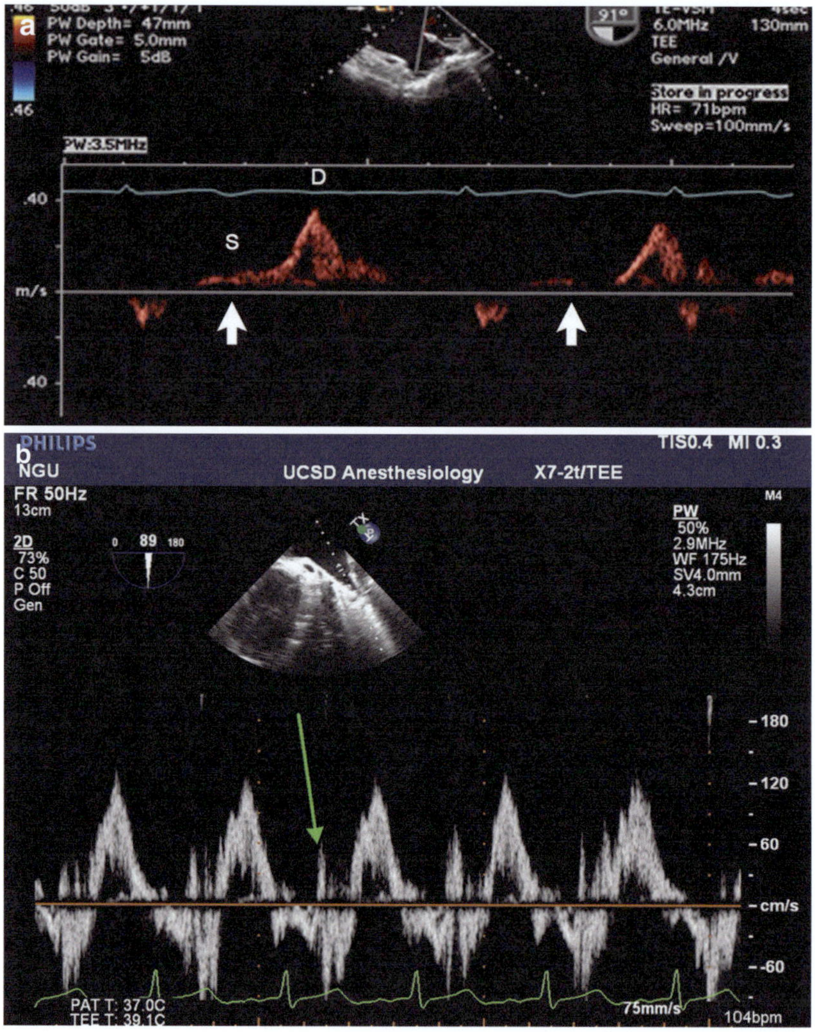

Fig. 8.16 (**a**) Pulsed-wave Doppler of the LUPV, demonstrating reduced systolic velocities (systolic blunting, *white arrows*) as a result of moderate MR. (**b**) Pulsed-wave Doppler of the pulmonary vein demonstrating reversal of systolic flow (below baseline, *green arrow*) as a result of severe MR

The PISA method allows for calculation of the EROA and represents a true quantitative measurement of MR severity. An EROA > 0.4 cm^2 corresponds to severe MR, while an EROA > 0.4 cm^2 corresponds to mild MR (Table 8.2). It is important to highlight that the PISA method has several limitations. The PISA calculation requires several steps and is based on accurate measurements of small dimensions, rendering this technique time-consuming and laborious for clinical application in the operating room or acute setting. The shape of the iso-velocity shells is also assumed to be hemispheres, when indeed they may not be. Nevertheless, the PISA method may prove useful in cases where quantitative analysis is necessary to distinguish between moderate MR from mild or severe forms [30, 31].

Hemodynamics

The MR jet is a dynamic and load-dependent valvular issue, owing to the large pressure gradient between the LV and LA during systole. The degree of MR at any point in time is sensitive to overall patient hemodynamics, with numerous studies demonstrating the dynamic nature of MR under different loading conditions. The degree of MR has been shown to alter with the reduction of preload and afterload that is often associated with induction of general anesthesia. By contrast, increasing after-

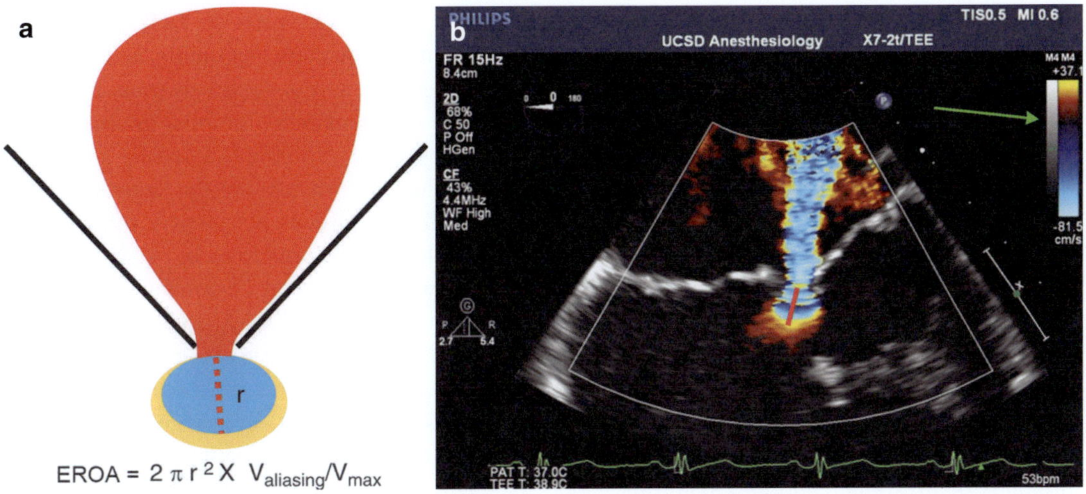

Fig. 8.17 (**a**) Calculation of the EROA of MR by PISA. (**b**) PISA radius identification (*red line*) in a ME four-chamber view. Note the shifted color flow Doppler baseline and the identified aliasing velocity (*green arrow*)

load with alpha-agonists or preload augmentation with volume administration has been shown to partially reverse the changes in MR severity under general anesthesia. The effects of general anesthesia often pose a challenge for the intraoperative echocardiographer, as the preoperative awake hemodynamics may significantly differ from that found in the operating room. It may prove useful to make note of the precise hemodynamic state of the patient at the time of intraoperative echocardiographic assessment and compare these parameters to the baseline or preoperative loading conditions [12]. Similarly, changes in physiology in the critically ill patient (e.g., sepsis) can also induce significant variation in the hemodynamic effect of MR. Changes in MR severity are important to note, as these may be reflective of new or evolving myocardial ischemia, as the aforementioned MR etiologies are intertwined with myocardial function.

Mitral Stenosis (Highlight Box 8.2)

The mitral valve assumes its largest area during diastole, as it serves as a conduit for LV filling. The normal mitral valve area is approximately 4–6 cm^2. In MS, significant elevations in the transvalvular gradient become evident as the area approaches 1.0 cm^2. Upstream from the stenotic mitral valve, a marked increase in left atrial pressure is observed, followed by chamber enlargement, stagnant blood flow, and atrial dysrhythmias. As the MS disease process progresses, marked elevations in left atrial pressure and pulmonary hypertension can precipitate right heart dysfunction. As blood converges near the narrow orifice, flow accelerates across the valve as it enters the LV. Downstream from MS, an LV with lower end-diastolic volume from restricted filling is often evident on 2D echo [27, 32].

Highlight Box 8.2

Mitral stenosis	
2D	• Mitral leaflet motion (restrictive) • Mitral annular and leaflet calcification • Left atrial enlargement. • LA spontaneous echo contrast (LAA thrombus identification • Small LV dimensions (underfilled)
CFD	• Flow acceleration on left atrial aspect • Turbulent flow entering LV
Spectral	• PHT – CWD • Mean gradient – CWD • MVA – PHT-based calculation, PISA-based calculation, planimetry

LA left atrium, *LV* left ventricle, *LAA* left atrial appendage, *PHT* pressure half-time, *CWD* continuous-wave Doppler, *MVA* mitral valve area, *PISA* proximal isovelocity surface area

2D Echocardiography

MS is typically the result of a reduction in the valve area during diastole from impaired valve opening; however, cases of functional MS may also occur due to intracardiac masses. Although rheumatic heart disease is commonly associated with mitral stenosis, nonrheumatic causes of MS have recently become more frequent in developed countries [27]. Nonrheumatic causes of MS include severe leaflet and annular calcification, congenital mitral defects like parachute deformity (in which all chordae originate from a single papillary muscle), infective endocarditis, LA thrombus or myxoma, carcinoid syndrome, and post-repair or valve replacement-associated MS [27]. The anatomic changes associated with these processes are amenable to 2D echocardiography evaluation. Besides appreciating a reduction in valve opening on 2D imaging, echocardiographic signs of calcific MS may include evidence of leaflet thickening, echogenic calcification, retraction or shortening, fusion of the commissures and leaflet immobility, as well as calcium deposition extending to the subvalvular apparatus and mitral annulus.

In the case of rheumatic MS, the characteristic doming of the anterior leaflet or formation of a "hockey stick" appearance may be appreciated in the ME four-chamber and ME LAX views on TEE (Fig. 8.18; Video 8.13) and the corresponding A4C and PLAX views on TTE. The unique pattern of calcification beginning at the leaflet tips renders this portion relatively immobile compared to the remaining mobile midportion or body. By contrast, calcific MS usually starts near the annulus and extends into the leaflets near the base, and usually does not involve the commissures or leaflet tips until later in the disease process. Two-dimensional examination of the upstream effects of MS may reveal signs of adaptation to LV inflow obstruction, including the presence of spontaneous echo contrast or early thrombus formation, LA enlargement, systolic blunting of the pulmonary venous flow, concomitant MR, dilated pulmonary arteries, RV dysfunction with paradoxical septal motion, RA enlargement with bulging of the interatrial septum, and tricuspid regurgitation. Just proximal to the stenotic mitral valve, an area of flow convergence is observed on color flow Doppler as blood accelerates into the narrow orifice. As blood crosses the plane of the valve, a population of aliasing velocities (above the Nyquist limit) emerge and are displayed as a region of turbulent flow on the color Doppler map [27].

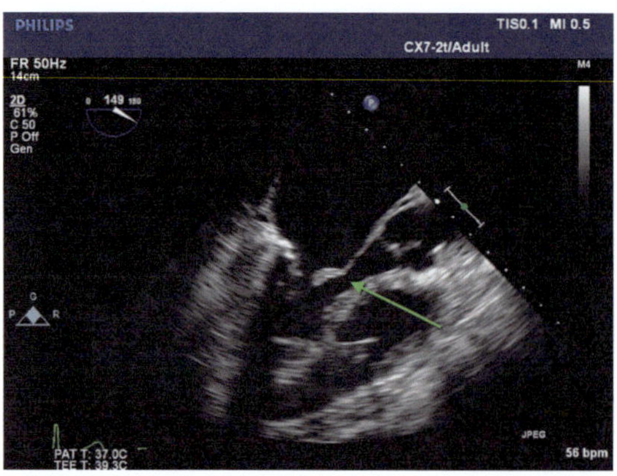

Fig. 8.18 Midesophageal long-axis view showing "hockey stick" deformity (*green arrow*) in a patient with rheumatic mitral stenosis

Quantitative Assessment of Mitral Stenosis

The following sections describe the different quantitative echocardiographic assessments of MS (Table 8.3).

Pressure Gradients

As the underlying cause of MS progresses, an increase in the LA to LV transvalvular gradient develops as flow accelerates across the narrow opening. The pressure differential (ΔP) between the LA and LV is described by the modified Bernoulli's equation or $\Delta P = 4v^2$, where v is the instantaneous peak velocity of blood across the valve and ΔP is the pressure difference or gradient. The ME four-chamber and ME LAX views on TEE [1] or the A4C view on TTE [8, 9] can

Table 8.3 Mitral valve stenosis: Quantitative assessment

Mitral Valve Stenosis: Quantitative Assessment			
	Mild	**Moderate**	**Severe**
PHT (ms)	100	200	**> 220**
Mean Gradient (mmHg)	6	6-10	**> 10**
Valve Area* (cm²)	1.6-2.0	1.0–1.5	**< 1.0**

PHT Pressure Halftime; *Valve area as determined by PHT formula, PISA calculation or Planimetry

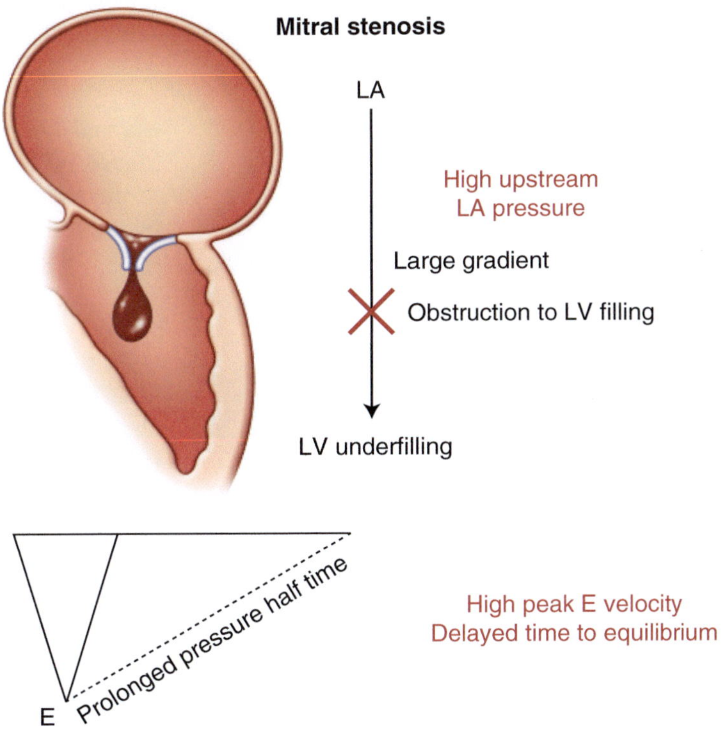

Fig. 8.19 Flow dynamics of MS resulting in an elevated peak E-wave velocity and prolonged pressure half-time downstream from the stenotic orifice

be used to measure the transvalvular gradient across the mitral valve. Using continuous-wave Doppler interrogation, the resultant transmitral inflow profile and velocity-time integral (VTI) describe the observed increase in velocities across the valve and the delayed time for the LA and LV pressures to reach equilibrium due to the stenotic orifice (Fig. 8.19). From the transmitral inflow profile, a mean gradient can be determined by tracing the area under the early filling (E-wave) and late filling (A-wave) waves in their entirety (Fig. 8.20a). The peak transvalvular gradient and velocity describe the maximal pressure differential and velocity of transvalvular blood flow, while the mean pressure gradient represents the average pressure difference of the entire column of blood moving from the LA to the LV across the stenotic orifice. The mean gradient is used in grading severity of MS [27].

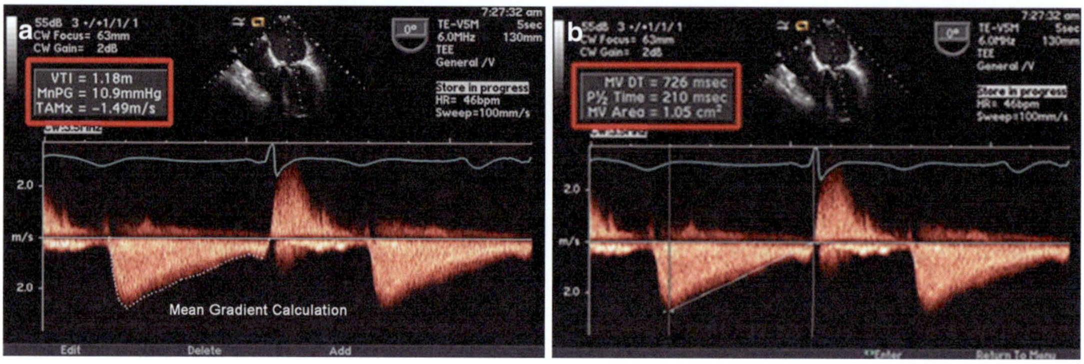

Fig. 8.20 (**a**) Continuous-wave Doppler interrogation across a stenotic mitral valve. The mean gradient of the transmitral flow profile is calculated by tracing the entire envelope, similar to a velocity-time integral. (**b**) The spectral Doppler profile is characterized by a high-velocity E-wave with a prolonged pressure half-time or deceleration time, which can be used to calculate the mitral valve area

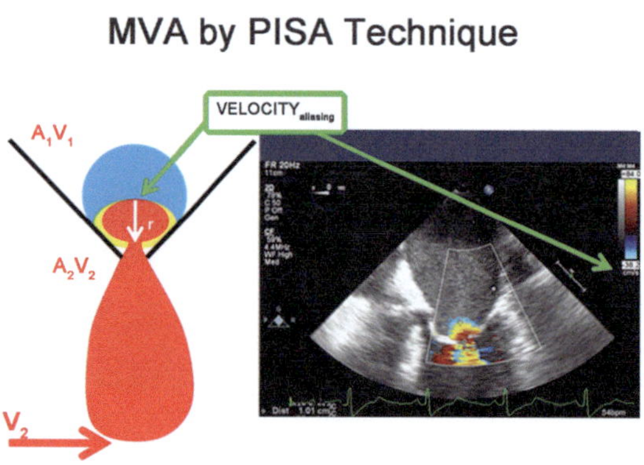

Fig. 8.21 Calculation of mitral valve area by PISA technique

Mitral Valve Area Calculations

Pressure Half-Time (PHT)

As blood moves across the stenotic mitral valve, the pressure gradient between the LA and LV begins to dissipate proportionally to the degree of stenosis. Similarly, the maximum peak instantaneous velocity of blood flow decelerates over time proportional to the severity of MS. The more severe the obstruction to flow, the longer it takes for the pressure in the LA and LV to equilibrate (Fig. 8.20b). The pressure half-time (PHT) describes the slope or rate at which the atrial and ventricular pressure differential to decrease by 50%. The more severe the stenosis, the longer it takes for the LA and LV pressures to equalize, thus a prolonged PHT. The PHT is inversely proportional to the mitral valve area (MVA) and is defined by the following equation:

$$MVA\left(\text{cm}^2\right) = 220 / PHT\left(\text{milliseconds}\right)$$

In the ME four-chamber or ME LAX view (TEE) or the A4C view (TTE), the PHT is obtained by aligning the Doppler beam parallel to the direction of flow through the MV and using continuous-wave Doppler to interrogate LV inflow. The PHT is then measured by taking the peak velocity of the E-wave (early filling) and drawing a caliper along the slope of deceleration, being careful to include the slope that encompasses the peak velocity and the baseline (point of zero velocity). The machine software will extrapolate the PHT in milliseconds and compute a mitral valve area. PHT measurements above 220 milliseconds correspond to severe MS (see Table 8.3) [6, 27].

Proximal Isovelocity Surface Area (PISA)

The PISA or flow-convergence method (Fig. 8.21) is an application of the continuity equation to measure the mitral valve area [5, 27]. As blood flow converges upon the stenotic mitral valve, a marked increase in velocity ensues, creating a series of organized hemispheres on the left atrial

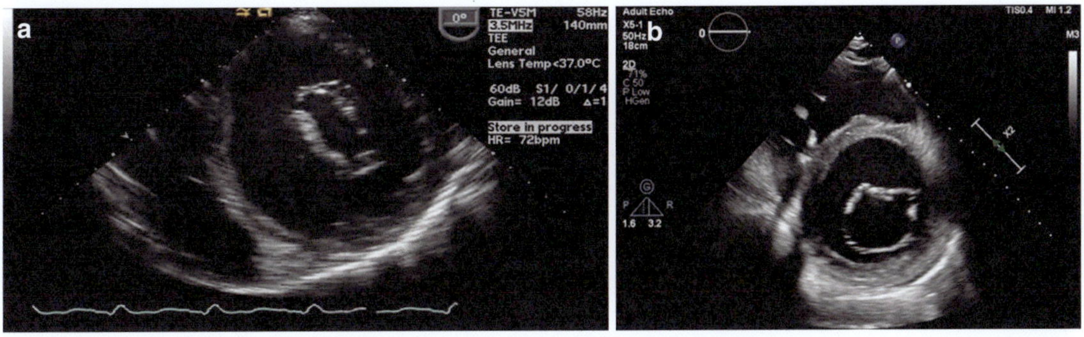

Fig. 8.22 (**a**) Transgastric basal short-axis view demonstrating the mitral valve opening. (**b**) Parasternal basal short-axis view demonstrating the mitral valve opening

side of the valve. The border between blue and red on the color flow map defines the boundary between the first isovelocity hemisphere and represents the location of the first aliasing velocity, corresponding to blood traveling faster than the limit of detection (Nyquist limit) on the color flow Doppler scale. The radius of the first isovelocity hemisphere is then carefully measured along with the angle (α) that is formed by both mitral leaflets during diastole. The product of the area of the hemisphere ($2\pi r^2$) and the aliasing velocity on the color flow Doppler scale provides the equal volumetric flow on the atrial side. The volumetric flow on the atrial side is then multiplied by the angle correction factor, $\alpha/180$ degrees, defined by the angle formed by the mitral leaflets, yielding a more accurate flow measurement. To calculate the mitral valve area, velocity of flow on the ventricular side must be measured by continuous-wave Doppler across the mitral valve. Using the ME four-chamber or ME LAX view with TEE or the view with TTE, the Doppler beam is positioned parallel to the direction of flow into the LV. The continuous-wave Doppler then produces a spectral profile that can be used to calculate the maximum velocity across the valve. Using the continuity equation where the flow of blood on the atrial side equals the flow on the ventricular side:

$$Area_{\text{hemisphere}} \text{ x } Velocity_{\text{aliasing}} = Area_{\text{mitral valve}} \text{ x } Velocity_{\text{mitral inflow}}$$

Mitral Valve Area can then be derived as follows:

$$Area_{\text{mitral valve}} = \alpha / 180^0 \text{ x } \left(Area_{\text{hemisphere}} \text{ x } Velocity_{\text{aliasing}} / Velocity_{\text{mitral inflow}} \right)$$

Planimetry

Planimetry is the direct measurement of the mitral valve area using 2D echo [1, 9, 27]. This can be achieved using the trace function from the TG basal SAX view on TEE (Fig. 8.22a) or the PSAX view on TTE (Fig. 8.22b). It is important to obtain the best image possible and utilize the freeze function on the machine to capture the valve at its maximal opening in diastole. An accurate measurement of the valve area can be maximized by advancing or withdrawing (TEE) or fanning (TTE) the probe to move the scan plane from a superior position down to the level of the smallest valve opening. If the scan plane measures the opening above the actual orifice, the mitral valve area will be overestimated.

Conclusion

Appropriate function of the mitral valve depends on the anatomy and function of all of the components of the mitral valve apparatus, including the annulus, leaflets, chordae tendineae, papillary muscles, and ventricular walls. Regurgitant or stenotic lesions can have devastating hemodynamic consequences, and recognition can help guide management. TTE or TEE can be an indispensable tool in the perioperative and acute care management of patients with mitral valve dysfunction.

Questions

1. Which of the following anatomical features distinguishes the posterior leaflet from the anterior leaflet of the mitral valve?

   a. The posterior leaflet possesses discrete scallops.
   b. The anterior leaflet possesses indentations that define the A1, A2, and A3 segments.
   c. The posterior leaflet is anchored by a rich network of fibrous tissue, rendering it more robust compared to the anterior leaflet.
   d. The anterior leaflet subtends a greater annular circumference than the posterior leaflet.

2. Which of the following echocardiographic views is generated by providing an imaging plane corresponding to the anterior to posterior dimension of the mitral annulus?

   a. Midesophageal (ME) mitral commissural view (TEE) and apical three-chamber view (TTE)
   b. ME long-axis view (TEE) and parasternal long-axis view (TTE)
   c. Apical four-chamber view (TTE) and ME four-chamber view (TEE)
   d. ME long-axis view and two-chamber view on TEE

3. Which of the following mechanism(s) may contribute to ischemic mitral regurgitation?

   a. Apical displacement of the papillary muscle-chordae tendineae complex causing leaflet restriction and failure of leaflet coaptation.
   b. Infarction of a papillary muscle and flail leaflet secondary to a ruptured chordae tendineae.
   c. Dilation and flattening of the saddle-shaped mitral annulus causing a coaptation defect.
   d. All of the above.

4. In the apical four-chamber view, which of the following statement(s) are true regarding the identification of the mitral leaflets?

   a. The posterior leaflet is located near the interatrial and interventricular septum.
   b. The posterior leaflet can be distinguished by its position next to the lateral aspect of the heart.
   c. The anterior leaflet can be identified by its close approximation to the pulmonary vein.
   d. All of the above

5. In the parasternal long-axis view, the identification of the anterior leaflet is confirmed by which of the following echocardiographic anatomical landmarks?

   a. The anterior leaflet is closest to the right ventricle and is positioned in the far field.
   b. The posterior leaflet is near the noncoronary cusp of the aortic valve.
   c. The anterior leaflet may be seen approaching or touching the interventricular septum during diastole.
   d. The anterior leaflet can be seen near the left atrial appendage.

6. According to the Carpentier classification of leaflet motion describing the mechanism of MR, which of the following is consistent with type 2 MR?

   a. Anterior wall hypokinesis and restricted leaflet movement during systole
   b. Reduced leaflet mobility due to rheumatic disease
   c. Posterior leaflet prolapse from myxomatous degeneration
   d. Perforation of the anterior leaflet from bacterial endocarditis

7. Which of the following echocardiographic findings may be observed in patients with severe MR?

   a. Spontaneous echo contrast in the left atrium
   b. Reversal of flow in the pulmonary veins evidenced by reversal of the left atrial inflow during systole
   c. Evidence of flow convergence and aliasing on the atrial side of the mitral valve using color flow Doppler
   d. Vena contracta measurement of 4.5 mm

8. Which of the following hemodynamic change(s) may contribute to a reduced degree of MR under general anesthesia?

   a. A decrease in preload from overnight fasting
   b. A reduction in heart rate from high dose narcotics
   c. A decrease in afterload from inhalational anesthetics
   d. Beta blocker administration

9. Which of the following is *least* likely to be observed in a patient with severe mitral stenosis?

   a. Thickened and calcified "echo bright" leaflets with reduced mitral opening
   b. Aliasing velocities observed on color flow mapping as blood approximates the mitral orifice
   c. Spontaneous echo contrast in the left ventricle
   d. Evidence of reduced left ventricular filling in the transgastric short-axis view

10. In a patient with severe mitral stenosis, which of the following may be observed using continuous-wave Doppler interrogation across the mitral valve during diastole?

    a. A shortened pressure half time measurement
    b. An elevated peak E velocity greater than 1 m/s
    c. A mean gradient greater than 10 mmHg
    d. A deceleration time less than 100 ms

References

1. Nicoara A, et al. Guidelines for the use of transesophageal echocardiography to assist with surgical decision-making in the operating room: a surgery-based approach: from the American Society of Echocardiography in collaboration with the Society of Cardiovascular Anesthesiologists and the Society of Thoracic Surgeons. J Am Soc Echocardiogr. 2020;33(6):692–734.
2. Cimino S, et al. Echocardiography and correction of mitral regurgitation: an unbreakable link. Cardiology. 2020;145:110–20.
3. Quader N, Rigolin VH. Two and three dimensional echocardiography for pre-operative assessment of mitral valve regurgitation. Cardiovasc Ultrasound. 2014;12:42.
4. Silverman ME, Hurst JW. The mitral complex. Interaction of the anatomy, physiology, and pathology of the mitral annulus, mitral valve leaflets, chordae tendineae, and papillary muscles. Am Heart J. 1968;76(3):399–418.
5. Sidebotham DA, et al. Intraoperative transesophageal echocardiography for surgical repair of mitral regurgitation. J Am Soc Echocardiogr. 2014;27(4):345–66.
6. Shernan SK. Perioperative transesophageal echocardiographic evaluation of the native mitral valve. Crit Care Med. 2007;35(8 Suppl):S372–83.
7. Silbiger JJ, Bazaz R. Contemporary insights into the functional anatomy of the mitral valve. Am Heart J. 2009;158(6):887–95.
8. Tan TC, et al. Standard transthoracic echocardiography and transesophageal echocardiography views of mitral pathology that every surgeon should know. Ann Cardiothorac Surg. 2015;4(5):449–60.
9. Mitchell C, et al. Guidelines for performing a comprehensive transthoracic echocardiographic examination in adults: recommendations from the American Society of Echocardiography. J Am Soc Echocardiogr. 2019;32(1):1–64.
10. Ben Zekry S, et al. Comparative accuracy of two- and three-dimensional transthoracic and transesophageal echocardiography in identifying mitral valve pathology in patients undergoing mitral valve repair: initial observations. J Am Soc Echocardiogr. 2011;24(10):1079–85.
11. Gripari P, et al. Transthoracic echocardiography in patients undergoing mitral valve repair: comparison of new transthoracic 3D techniques to 2D transoesophageal echocardiography in the localization of mitral valve prolapse. Int J Cardiovasc Imaging. 2018;34(7):1099–107.
12. Mahmood F, Matyal R. A quantitative approach to the intraoperative echocardiographic assessment of the mitral valve for repair. Anesth Analg. 2015;121(1):34–58.
13. Salgo IS, et al. Effect of annular shape on leaflet curvature in reducing mitral leaflet stress. Circulation. 2002;106(6):711–7.
14. Silbiger JJ. Anatomy, mechanics, and pathophysiology of the mitral annulus. Am Heart J. 2012;164(2):163–76.

15. Mahmood F, et al. Echocardiography derived three-dimensional printing of normal and abnormal mitral annuli. Ann Card Anaesth. 2014;17(4):279–83.
16. Padala M, et al. Saddle shape of the mitral annulus reduces systolic strains on the P2 segment of the posterior mitral leaflet. Ann Thorac Surg. 2009;88(5):1499–504.
17. Jiang L, et al. Dynamism of the mitral annulus: a spatial and temporal analysis. J Cardiothorac Vasc Anesth. 2014;28(5):1191–7.
18. Mahmood F, et al. Changes in mitral valve annular geometry after repair: saddle-shaped versus flat annuloplasty rings. Ann Thorac Surg. 2010;90(4): 1212–20.
19. Mahmood F, et al. Mitral annulus: an intraoperative echocardiographic perspective. J Cardiothorac Vasc Anesth. 2013;27(6):1355–63.
20. Mahmood F, et al. Intraoperative application of geometric three-dimensional mitral valve assessment package: a feasibility study. J Cardiothorac Vasc Anesth. 2008;22(2):292–8.
21. Owais K, et al. Three-dimensional printing of the mitral annulus using echocardiographic data: science fiction or in the operating room next door? J Cardiothorac Vasc Anesth. 2014;28(5):1393–6.19.
22. Khabbaz KR, et al. Dynamic 3-dimensional echocardiographic assessment of mitral annular geometry in patients with functional mitral regurgitation. Ann Thorac Surg. 2013;95(1):105–10.
23. Lee AP, et al. Quantitative analysis of mitral valve morphology in mitral valve prolapse with real-time 3-dimensional echocardiography: importance of annular saddle shape in the pathogenesis of mitral regurgitation. Circulation. 2013;127(7):832–41.
24. Connell JM, et al. Ischemic mitral regurgitation: mechanisms, intraoperative echocardiographic evaluation, and surgical considerations. Anesthesiol Clin. 2013;31(2):281–98.
25. Shakil O, et al. Ischemic mitral regurgitation: an intraoperative echocardiographic perspective. J Cardiothorac Vasc Anesth. 2013;27(3):573–85.
26. Shah PM. Current concepts in mitral valve prolapse--diagnosis and management. J Cardiol. 2010;56(2):125–33.
27. Wunderlich NC, Beigel R, Siegel RJ. Management of mitral stenosis using 2D and 3D echo-Doppler imaging. JACC Cardiovasc Imaging. 2013;6(11):1191–205.
28. Grayburn PA, et al. Multiplane transesophageal echocardiographic assessment of mitral regurgitation by Doppler color flow mapping of the vena contracta. Am J Cardiolo. 74(9):912–7.
29. Zoghbi WA, et al. Recommendations for evaluation of the severity of native valvular regurgitation with two-dimensional and Doppler echocardiography. J Am Soc Echocardiogr. 2003;16(7):777–802.
30. Ashikhmina E, et al. Three-dimensional versus two-dimensional echocardiographic assessment of functional mitral regurgitation proximal isovelocity surface area. Anesth Analg. 2015;120(3):534–42.
31. Lambert AS. Proximal isovelocity surface area should be routinely measured in evaluating mitral regurgitation: a core review. Anesth Analg. 2007;105(4):940–3.
32. Longo M, et al. Usefulness of transesophageal echocardiography during open heart surgery of mitral stenosis. J Cardiovasc Surg. 2000;41(3):381–5.

9 Aortic Valve

Michael Benggon

Abbreviations

2D	Two-dimensional
A5C	Apical five-chamber view
AI	Aortic insufficiency
ALAX	Apical long-axis
AR	Aortic regurgitation
AS	Aortic stenosis
AV	Aortic valve
AVA	Aortic valve area
CFD	Color flow Doppler
CSA	Cross-sectional area
CWD	Continuous-wave Doppler
LAX	Long-axis
LV	Left ventricle
LVOT	Left ventricular outflow tract
ME	Midesophageal
PHT	Pressure half time
PISA	Proximal isovelocity surface area
PLAX	Parasternal long-axis
PSAX	Parasternal short-axis
PTE	Perioperative transesophageal echocardiography
SAX	Short-axis
TEE	Transesophageal echocardiography
TG	Transgastric
TTE	Transthoracic echocardiography
VTI	Velocity-time integral

Supplementary Information The online version of this chapter (https://doi.org/10.1007/978-3-030-84349-6_9) contains supplementary material, which is available to authorized users.

M. Benggon (✉)
Department of Anesthesiology, Loma Linda University, Loma Linda, CA, USA

Introduction

The aortic valve (AV) is one of two semilunar valves in the heart; the other is the pulmonic valve. The AV allows blood that is ejected from the left ventricle to enter the systemic circulation while preventing reversal of flow back into the left ventricle during diastole. Unlike the atrioventricular (mitral and tricuspid) valves, the semilunar valves do not have associated chordae to support their form and rely on fibrous connective tissue to keep their shape. A thorough echocardiographic evaluation of the aortic valve includes assessment of the left ventricular outflow tract, aortic annulus, sinuses of Valsalva, sinotubular junction, proximal ascending aorta, and the valve leaflets (Fig. 9.1). The structure of the aortic valve is made up of three curved leaflets, or cusps, which are named by their location in relation to the coronary arteries (i.e., the left coronary cusp, right coronary cusp, and non-coronary cusp which is adjacent to the interatrial septum) (Fig. 9.2). Associated with each cusp is a sinus or concavity that forms the sinuses of Valsalva. The sinuses of Valsalva connect distally to the ascend-

T. M. Maus, C. R. Tainter (eds.), *Essential Echocardiography*,
https://doi.org/10.1007/978-3-030-84349-6_9

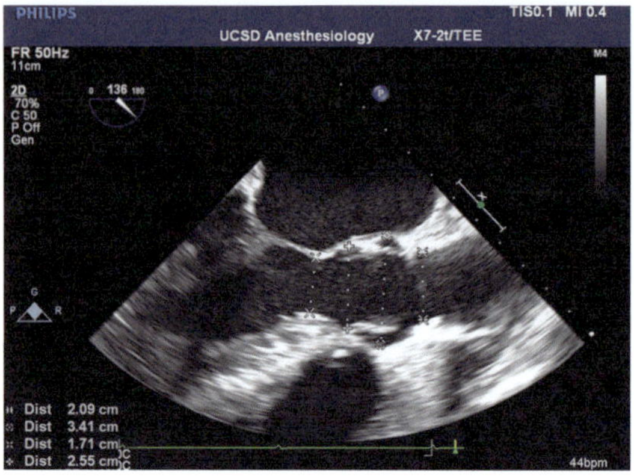

Fig. 9.1 A midesophageal long-axis view of the aortic valve. From left to right, the measured indices are the left ventricular outflow tract (LVOT), aortic annulus, sinuses of Valsalva, and the sinotubular junction

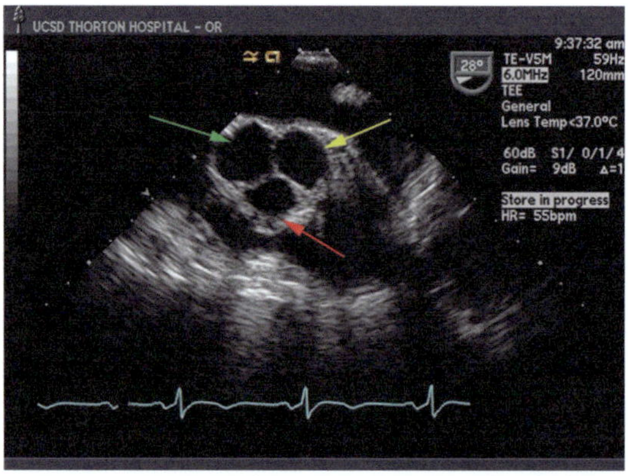

Fig. 9.2 A midesophageal aortic valve short-axis view of a normal trileaflet aortic valve. The *green arrow* indicates the non-coronary cusp (immediately adjacent to the interatrial septum, just off screen); the *red arrow* indicates the right coronary cusp (immediately adjacent to the right ventricle); the *yellow arrow* indicates the left coronary cusp

ing aorta at the sinotubular junction. The structure of these sinuses functions to allow constant blood flow to the coronary arteries while the aortic valve is open, preventing the leaflets from occluding the coronary orifices and reducing stress to the leaflets [1, 2].

The left ventricular outflow tract (LVOT) is the portion of the ventricle just proximal to the annulus of the aortic valve. It is made up of the ventricular septum and the fibrous tissue adjoining the aortic and mitral valves along the left and non-coronary aortic valve cusps and the anterior mitral valve leaflet, also known as the "intervalvular fibrosa." Dilation of these proximal or distal areas may cause structural changes to the valve that affect how the three leaflets come together or "coapt." Narrowing or stenosis will cause obstruction of blood flow.

Constant high pressure from the driving force of the left ventricle into the high-pressured systemic circulation causes cellular restructuring after birth, which makes the aortic the most durable valve. These same forces can also be detrimental in excess, causing valvular pathology over time.

Aortic Stenosis

Aortic stenosis (AS) is one of the most common cardiac pathologies in the elderly population, second only to coronary artery disease. Causes include atherosclerotic thickening of the leaflets, a congenital bicuspid aortic valve, or sequelae from rheumatic heart disease. Sclerotic thickening is the most common cause in the elderly population, while congenital bicuspid aortic valve stenosis tends to present earlier. Rheumatic heart disease, which usually presents with mitral valve involvement as well, can appear earlier or later in life, depending on when the patient was infected. Rheumatic causes of valvular disease are becoming less prevalent in developed countries. Symptoms of AS usually do not occur until the disease is severe and include exertional dyspnea, syncope, and chest pain. Once AS is symptomatic, timely replacement of the aortic valve should be performed. Delay to treatment is associated with a poor prognosis due to rapid disease progression [3].

Restriction of blood flow through the aortic valve increases afterload on the left ventricle. The left ventricle adapts by increasing its wall thickness through added muscle and fibrous tissue. This begins to affect diastolic function as the concentrically hypertrophied ventricle becomes less compliant. Ventricular relaxation during diastole decreases, further decreasing end-diastolic volumes and increasing end-diastolic pressures (see Chap. 12), resulting in cardiac congestion. Higher ejection fractions are required to maintain stroke volume and cardiac output, while compensatory neurohormonal signals such as the renin-angiotensin-aldosterone system mediate increased fluid retention [4]. Increased muscle contraction with decreased relaxation may also lead to angina from ischemia due to prolonged compression of endocardial coronary arteries. The pathology of aortic stenosis is a downward spiral that can be made acutely worse by any number of conditions (e.g., hypovolemia, tachycardia, atrial fibrillation, ischemia, and cardiac depressive agents).

Echocardiographic Evaluation (Highlight Box 9.1)

Highlight Box 9.1

Aortic stenosis	
2D	• Number of leaflets (tricuspid vs bicuspid) • Calcification (calcific vs. rheumatic) • Leaflet mobility (restriction systole +/− diastole) • Decreased systolic leaflet opening (assess severity) • Secondary changes (LAE, LVH, post-stenotic dilation)
CFD	• Flow acceleration proximal to valve • Turbulent flow distal to valve
Spectral	• Peak and mean velocities (gradients) • Aortic Valve Area (continuity equation) • Dimensionless index

LAE left atrial enlargement, *LVH* left ventricular hypertrophy

A good strategy for interrogating the aortic valve with transesophageal echocardiography (TEE) and transthoracic echocardiography (TTE) involves a three-step approach:

1. Two-dimensional (2D) inspection of the entire apparatus and associated secondary changes (i.e., ventricular hypertrophy, diastolic dysfunction, left atrial enlargement)
2. Color flow Doppler (CFD) across the valve
3. Spectral Doppler (pulsed-wave Doppler or continuous-wave Doppler (CWD)) evaluation of blood flow velocities

Basic perioperative transesophageal echocardiography (PTE)-certified practitioners should be able to evaluate the severity of a stenotic valve lesion and "if the valve lesion is considered severe, or if comprehensive quantification is required to ultimately determine the need for intervention, a consultation with an advanced PTE echocardiographer is necessary to confirm the severity and etiology of the valve pathology." Furthermore, prosthetic valves should be assessed by practitioners with advanced PTE certification [5]. Point-of-care examination should be able to identify if significant aortic stenosis or regurgitation contributes to hemodynamic instability.

Two-Dimensional Assessment

As discussed in Chap. 4, two-dimensional echocardiographic evaluation is best achieved when the structure of interest is placed perpendicular to the ultrasound beam. For TEE, visual inspection of the aortic valve is best obtained in the mid-esophageal aortic valve long- and short-axis views (ME AV LAX and ME AV SAX). Two other important TEE views, the transgastric long-axis and deep transgastric long-axis (TG LAX and deep TG LAX), should also be inspected in 2D, because their parallel orientation to the ultrasound beam provides more accurate spectral Doppler analysis. For TTE, the correlating views are the parasternal long- and short-axis views (PLAX and PSAX) and the apical five-chamber (A5C) or apical long-axis views (ALAX, also called the apical three-chamber view). Though both echo modalities are useful for AV assessment, TEE may allow more detailed visual inspection (especially when ruling out AV endocarditis [6]), because it has superior imaging quality due to the closer positioning of the transducer and lack of interference from lung tissue or ribs, etc. The goals of visual inspection include assessing leaflet motion, discerning the location and degree of calcification, and identifying any associated secondary anatomical changes. TTE benefits from closer alignment with the flow through the valve, which may provide more accurate Doppler measurements in some cases.

In all types of AS, leaflet motion tends to be restricted with decreased excursion during sys-

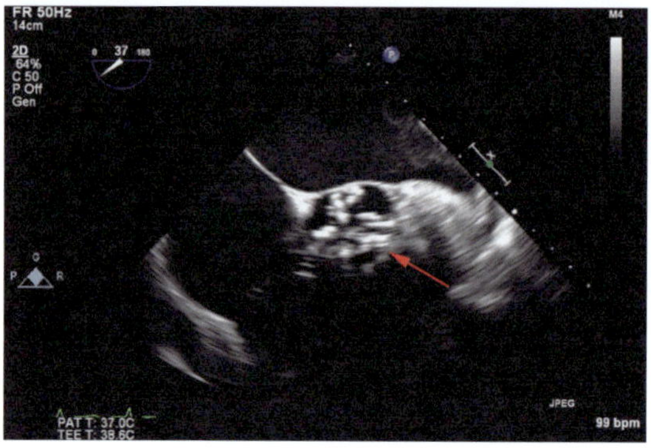

Fig. 9.3 Aortic stenosis: A ME AV SAX view of a severely calcified aortic valve (*red arrow*). Notice the clear distinction of the three leaflets ruling out congenital bicuspid disease. The patient's medical history will help distinguish between senile calcific degeneration and rheumatic disease

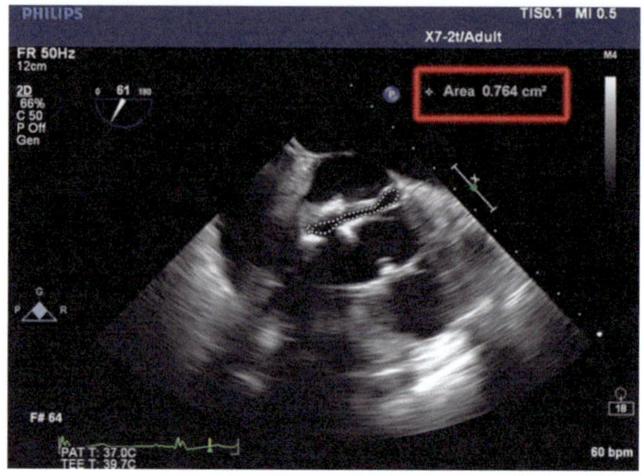

Fig. 9.5 Valve area planimetry: A ME AV SAX view of a congenital bicuspid aortic valve during mid- to late-systole. Using the trace function to outline the ejection orifice at its largest diameter gives an area of 0.764 cm^2, which constitutes severe aortic stenosis

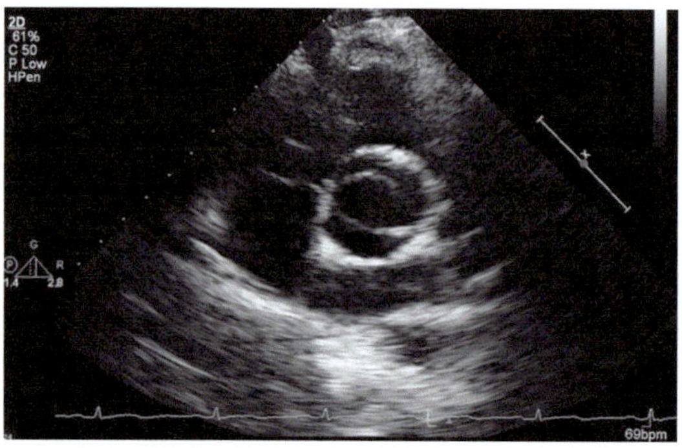

Fig. 9.4 Bicuspid aortic valve: A TTE PSAX view of a bicuspid aortic valve without stenosis

tole and potentially without appropriate coaptation during diastole. Atherosclerotic (or senile) calcific degeneration of the valve involves heavy calcification of the entire leaflet and annulus and may extend through the sinuses of Valsalva to the sinotubular junction (Fig. 9.3; Video 9.1). Congenital bicuspid valves, and especially rheumatic valves, tend to calcify along the commissures, but calcification may become so severe as to be indistinguishable from general atherosclerosis (Fig. 9.4).

Associated anatomic findings in patients with AS are secondary to the change in physiology caused by the stenosis. As mentioned above, left ventricular concentric hypertrophy develops to overcome the increase in afterload. As the disease progresses, diastolic function of the left heart will decrease, and indices for assessing diastolic function, such as E/A ratio, E' velocity, E/E' ratio, or pulmonary venous flow pattern, will begin to worsen (see Chap. 12). As the diastolic function declines, the left atrium may begin to dilate. As the disease process progresses, left heart failure with decreased ejection fraction resulting in elevated pulmonary artery pressures and even right heart dilatation and dysfunction may occur. Downstream from the valve, secondary changes include dilation of the aortic root, termed post-stenotic dilatation. Unlike laminar flow, turbulent flow exerts an outward pressure on the aortic wall and over time leads to aortic dilatation.

Using the ME AV SAX or PSAX view, the area of the aortic valve orifice can be obtained by tracing the perimeter of the leaflet tips during mid to late systole (Fig. 9.5; Video 9.2). However, this can be difficult to visualize with increasing degrees of calcification. Using CFD to identify the narrowest opening between the three leaflets during systole, and optimizing tissue echogenicity by turning down the gain, can help delineate the orifice. Aortic valve areas of 1.0–1.5 cm^2 are moderately stenosed, whereas an area less than 1.0 cm^2 is considered severe disease [7] (Table 9.1).

Two-dimensional views of the valve in the ME AV LAX or PLAX view, with or without the aid of color flow Doppler, can show the maximum distance between leaflet tips during systole (Figs. 9.6 and 9.7). A distance less than 8 mm is 97% predictive of severe disease and 100% pre-

Table 9.1 Values for grading aortic stenosis severity

	Mild	Moderate	Severe
Valve area (cm^2)	> 1.5	1.0–1.5	< 1.0
Leaflet separation distance (mm)	> 12	< 8	< 8
Mean gradient (mmHg)	< 20	20–40	> 40
Dimensionless index			< 0.25

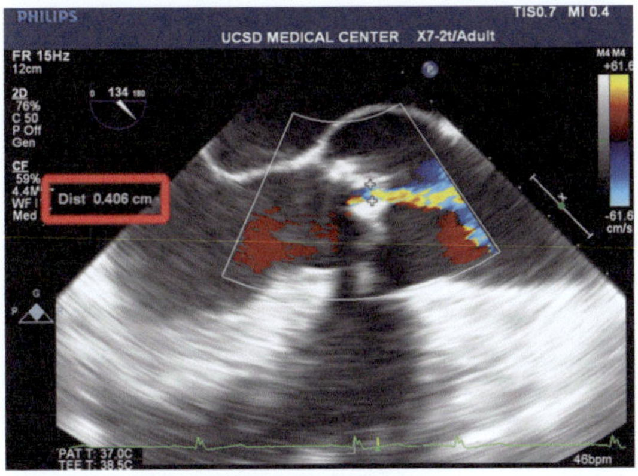

Fig. 9.6 Systolic leaflet tip distance: A ME AV LAX view of maximal leaflet tip separation during systole with the aid of CFD. This distance of 0.406 cm shows the presence of at least moderate stenosis, though likely severe

dictive of moderate or severe disease, whereas 12 mm or more is 96% predictive of mild disease or less [8]. In fact, a maximal distance of less than 8.25 mm showed a sensitivity of 89% and a specificity of 94% in diagnosing severe AS calculated by the continuity equation [9].

Color Flow Doppler

Color flow Doppler evaluation of the valve may show flow acceleration in the form of an aliasing hemisphere in the LVOT, moving toward the stenotic orifice during systole (Fig. 9.8; Videos 9.3 and 9.4). Proximal isovelocity surface area (PISA) methods may be employed; however, they are not typically utilized. Instead, recognizing the presence of flow acceleration in the LVOT on CFD should alert the echocardiographer that significant stenosis may be present. Due to the high velocity of the blood exiting the stenotic valve, CFD will show turbulent flow in the proximal aorta (Video 9.5).

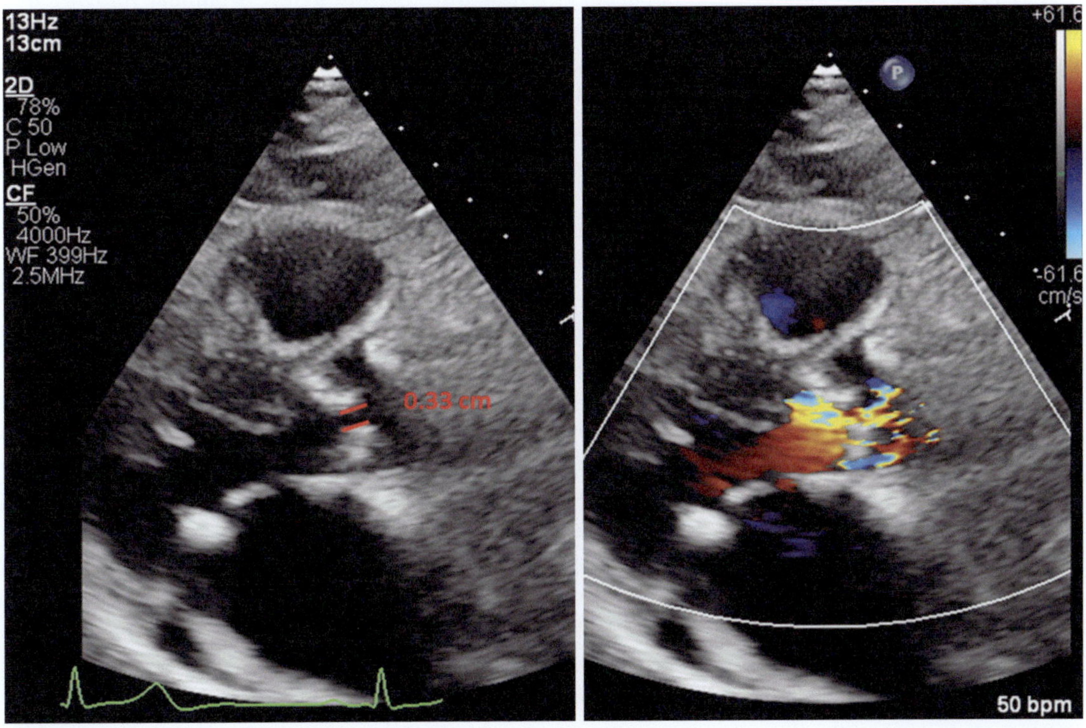

Fig. 9.7 Systolic leaflet tip distance: A PLAX view using TTE and CFD comparison to delineate maximal leaflet tip separation showing likely severe stenosis in this view

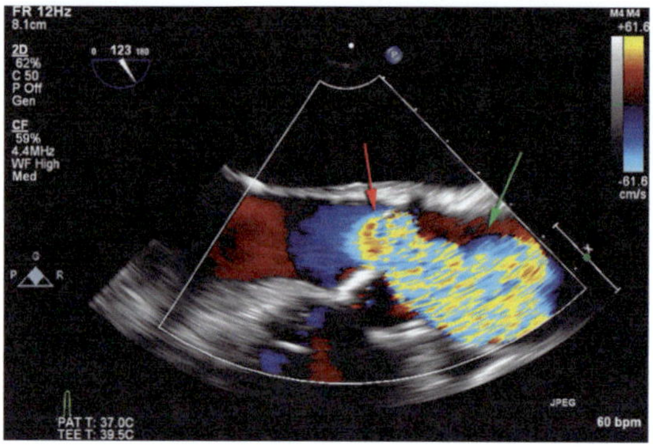

Fig. 9.8 Flow acceleration and turbulence: A ME AV LAX view of flow acceleration in the LVOT as blood flow moves into a stenotic aortic valve orifice. Note the concentric or hemispheric color pattern (*red arrow*). High-velocity flow distal to the valve causes a turbulent heterogenous color pattern indicated by the *green arrow* (versus a laminar homogenous color pattern in normal flow)

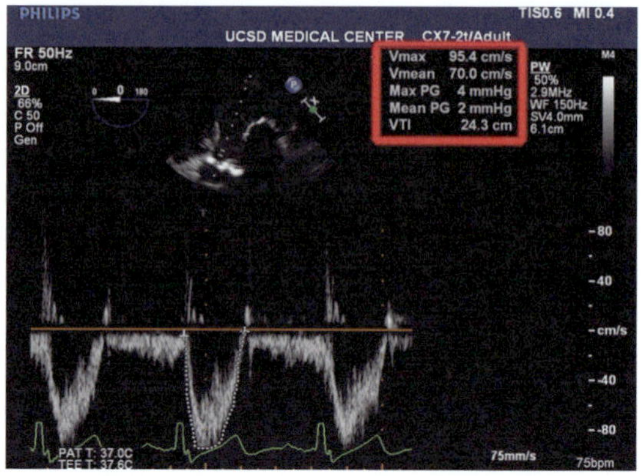

Fig. 9.9 A pulsed-wave Doppler (PWD) measurement of the LVOT 1 cm proximal to the aortic valve at the level of the sample volume (two parallel lines on the cursor). Note that the waveform occurs during systole and has a bright white outline with a black core. The wave is traced from baseline (*orange line*), and the computer calculates the velocity-time integral (VTI) from the area under the curve

Spectral Doppler

Spectral Doppler assessment of the aortic valve is best obtained in the deep TG LAX and TG LAX views with TEE, or the A5C and ALAX views with TTE, and is considered the most accurate method for quantifying aortic stenosis echocardiographically. The transgastric (TEE) and apical (TTE) views allow the Doppler line of interrogation to be parallel to the flow of blood, and therefore more accurate blood flow velocity measurements are obtained. Spectral analysis can then be utilized to estimate the valve area using the continuity equation and the pressure gradient across the valve via the modified Bernoulli equation.

The continuity equation states simply that the volume of blood in a single beat ejected through the LVOT during systole must equal the same volume ejected through the aortic valve orifice during the same single beat. Volumes of blood can be difficult to assess, but velocity of blood flow through the LVOT and aortic valve can be easily obtained using pulsed- and continuous-wave Doppler, respectively (Figs. 9.9 and 9.10a, b). In the deep TG LAX view (TEE) and A5C view (TTE), the pulsed-wave Doppler interrogation gate is placed 1 centimeter behind the aortic valve. Using the existing software on the echocardiography machine, the velocity-time integral (VTI), or the area under the curve of the systolic velocity over time, can be calculated (see Chap. 4). The tracing provides the length (cm) that a blood cell travels in one systolic beat in that given structure. The LVOT is assumed to be cylindrical in shape, and all blood flow traveling through it is laminar (moving in a similar direction at the same speed). The LVOT cross-sectional area (CSA) at the point of pulsed-wave interrogation can be calculated using the formula, $\prod r^2$. The volume of a cylinder of blood that moves uniformly through that space can be calculated by multiplying the cross-sectional area by the velocity-time integral (or cross-sectional area x length). According to the continuity equation principle of "volume in equals volume out," this cylindrical volume of blood must also pass through the aortic valve during systole. Using the deep TG LAX or the A5C view, the VTI of the aortic valve is measured using continuous-wave Doppler, and the area of the aortic valve orifice can be calculated as follows:

$$\text{LVOT volume}_{\text{systole}} = \text{AV volume}_{\text{systole}}$$

$$\text{LVOT}_{\text{CSA}} \times \text{LVOT}_{\text{VTI}} = \text{AV}_{\text{CSA}} \times \text{AV}_{\text{VTI}}$$

$$\text{AV}_{\text{CSA}} = \left(\text{LVOT}_{\text{CSA}} \times \text{LVOT}_{\text{VTI}}\right) / \text{AV}_{\text{VTI}}$$

An hourglass is a simple example of the conservation of mass principle involved. Sand

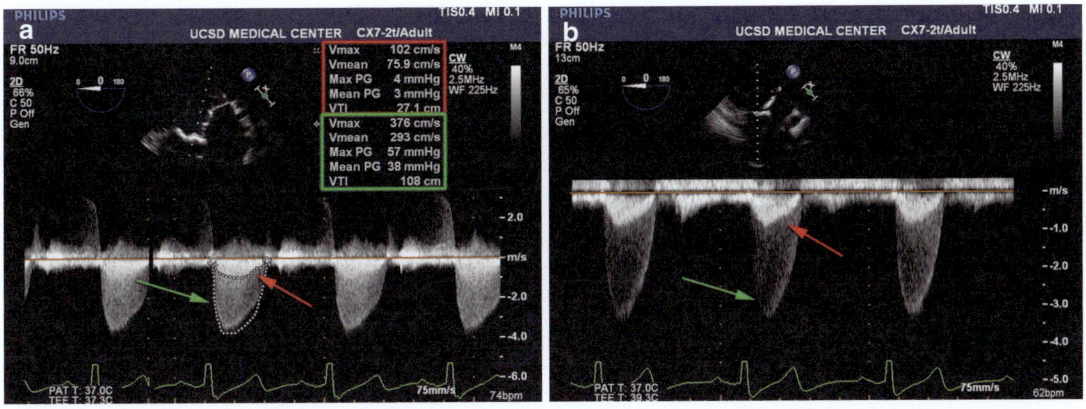

Fig. 9.10 (**a**) A continuous-wave Doppler (CWD) measurement of the aortic valve during systole. Since the valve orifice is the narrowest area along the Doppler line of interrogation, a tracing of the outer perimeter of the wave is assumed to represent the VTI at that level (*green arrow*). Note that the echocardiographer also traced a smaller waveform within the larger wave, representing the LVOT VTI (*red arrow*). This is the "double envelope" profile that can be seen with aortic stenosis, revealing a dimensionless index of 25%, indicating severe AS. (**b**) A CWD profile of a patient with aortic stenosis. The *green arrow* indicates the AV envelope, while the *red arrow* indicates the LVOT envelope

proximal to the central orifice moves in a large volume slowly, whereas sand in the narrowest part moves very quickly. However, the same volume crosses through the distal narrow portion over a fixed time period as it moves through the proximal wider area during that same time.

This technique uses VTI measurements (LVOT and AV) derived from two separate cardiac beats. While this approach to aortic valve area (AVA) is valid, it does assume that the stroke volume does not change beat to beat. This may prove false in the setting of arrhythmias (e.g., atrial fibrillation) or stroke volume changes (e.g., positive pressure ventilation). The "double envelope" technique allows the determination of LVOT and AV VTIs from a singular beat. When a CWD profile in a deep TG LAX or A5C view is obtained in a patient with aortic stenosis, the profile may display two overlapping "envelopes." Continuous-wave Doppler measures all velocities along its line of interrogation (i.e., it is "range ambiguous"). The bulk of the velocities measured are traveling slower and make up the bright inner envelope which represents the LVOT velocities. The velocities begin to accelerate to much higher speeds when traversing the stenotic aortic valve, leaving a much lighter or hollow-looking envelope (this is because blood cannot move through this narrow portion at slow speeds, and so the speed is more uniform throughout). Therefore, the lighter-shaded larger envelope represents the AV VTI (Fig. 9.10b). Obtaining both VTI measurements from a single beat removes the variability of stroke volume changes between two different beats.

One potential drawback of the continuity equation is the estimation of the LVOT area. This involves the assumption that the LVOT is circular (which may also be ellipsoid or trapezoidal), as well as the squaring of the radial measurement. Therefore, any error in the measurement of the LVOT diameter becomes significantly exaggerated, yielding potentially inaccurate AV areas. An attempt to eliminate this measurement error is the "dimensionless index," which is simply a ratio of the LVOT VTI to the AV VTI. A low ratio (less than 0.25) indicates significant velocity differences between the LVOT and AV and represents severe AS (Fig. 9.10a).

The modified Bernoulli equation eliminates negligible variables from the original formula in the clinical setting of echocardiography to come up with a simple method of determining the change of pressure across a fixed orifice based on the velocity of flow. Change is pressure (ΔP) is equal to four times the velocity of blood flow (v) squared, under physiologic conditions.

$$\Delta P = 4v^2$$

This simplified equation can easily determine the peak pressure gradient across the aortic valve using continuous-wave Doppler in a deep TG LAX (TEE) or A5C (TTE) view to determine the peak velocity. Mean pressure gradients, which evaluate the average gradient across the valve throughout systole, provide a better trend of disease severity [10]. When tracing a velocity-time profile, the ultrasound software provides peak velocity and gradient, mean velocity and gradient, as well as the VTI discussed previously. Mean aortic valve gradients of 20–40 mmHg denote moderate stenosis, whereas < 20 mmHg is mild disease [7] (see Table 9.1).

While a peak or mean gradient is less time-consuming and does provide a quick glimpse into the severity of aortic stenosis, consideration must be given in patients with a reduced stroke volume (e.g., low contractility or hypovolemia). The low stroke volume or low pressure generated from the left ventricle will be reflected in low pressure gradients, despite the presence of significant aortic stenosis, thereby underestimating the severity of AS. In this setting, the continuity equation is preferred, as the reduction in stroke volume and pressure will be reflected on both sides of the equation (the LVOT and AV).

Aortic Regurgitation (Insufficiency)

The aortic valve function involves not simply the valve leaflets themselves but also the surrounding structures of the LVOT, aortic valve annulus, sinuses of Valsalva, and the proximal ascending aorta. Defects in any of these structures may lead to aortic valve incompetency, which is referred to with the interchangeable terms aortic regurgitation (AR) or aortic insufficiency (AI) [11]. When evaluating the cause of aortic incompetency, the etiology can typically be placed into one of three groups:

1. *Aortic root dilatation:* Examples of conditions that can cause enlargement of the aortic root include connective tissue disorders (Ehlers-Danlos, Marfan, and Loeys-Dietz syndromes), ascending aortic aneurysms, aortitis, and dissections. With enlargement of the aortic root, the cusps of the valve can be pulled outward, increasing the overall diameter of the valve preventing coaptation of the leaflets. This typically produces a centrally regurgitant jet.
2. *Excessive cusp motion:* Flail leaflets that fail to coapt above the annular plane are unable to participate in valve closure and lead to incompetency. These jets tend to be eccentric in nature.
3. *Cusp integrity:* Heavy calcium deposition, fibrosis, rheumatic heart disease, bicuspid valves, and endocarditis can all cause the integrity of the valve to be compromised. The resultant regurgitant jet can be central or eccentric.

Valvular lesions that form the first two groups have the potential of valvular repair, while category three often requires valve replacement.

During evaluation of the aortic valve, care must be taken to note the current hemodynamic state of the patient (e.g., hemodynamic changes with general anesthesia). Similar to the evaluation of the mitral valve, changes in preload, afterload, and contractility can dramatically change the appearance of regurgitant aortic jets. These changes may not give a true representation of disease severity during a normal physiological state.

Echocardiographic Evaluation (Highlight Box 9.2)

Highlight Box 9.2

Aortic regurgitation	
2D	• Number of leaflets (tricuspid vs bicuspid) • Leaflet structure and mobility (calcification, prolapse, flail, perforation, malcoapt) • Surrounding pathology: Endocarditis (vegetation), aortic dissection • Measurements (LVOT, AV annulus, sinuses of valsalva, STJ) • Secondary changes (eccentric LV hypertrophy)
CFD	• Diastolic turbulent flow • Vena contracta and jet width: LVOT diameter ratio
Spectral	• Pressure half time • Deceleration slope • Diastolic flow reversal (descending thoracic aorta)

LVOT left ventricular outflow tract, *AV* aortic valve, *STJ* sinotubular junction, *LV* left ventricle

Two-Dimensional Assessment

A simple 2D evaluation will give an overall impression of the valve and supporting structural integrity, as well as to categorize the mechanism of regurgitation. Vegetations, flail leaflets, enlarged roots, heavy calcifications, valvular leaflet restrictions, or aortic dissections are among the rapidly identified pathologies apparently using 2D echocardiography. Observing a malcoaptation in two dimensions alerts the echocardiographer to AR before instituting CFD (Fig. 9.11; Video 9.6). Inspection of the valve initially in the ME AV SAX and ME AV LAX (TEE) or PSAX and PLAX (TTE) views can aid in identifying a mechanism. Measurements of the LVOT diameter, AV annulus, sinuses of Valsalva, and sinotubular junction can help ascertain the influence of an enlarged root on valvular function. Leaflet structure and mobility are key in identifying the role of calcification and restricted leaflet motion (during both systole and diastole) versus leaflet destruction and prolapse in the setting of vegetations and endocarditis. Lastly, inspection of the aortic root for aortic dissection flaps is important due to the prognostic implications of a rapid diagnosis (see Chap. 13). Therefore, while the severity of aortic regurgitation rests on CFD and spectral Doppler interrogation, 2D evaluation provides important insight into the mechanism.

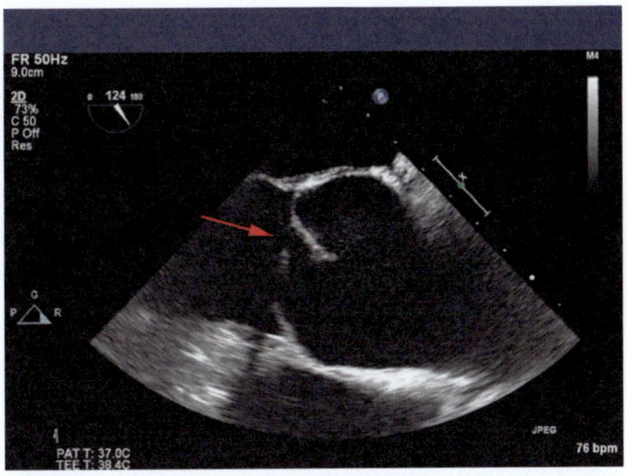

Fig. 9.11 Malcoaptation the aortic valve leaflets: A ME AV LAX view in a patient with bicuspid aortic valve disease and a dilated annulus and aortic root. The diastolic image shows a failure of coaptation (*red arrow*)

Similar to other valvular lesions, secondary anatomical changes may occur in the presence of AR, often dictated by the chronicity of the condition. Acute AR does not provide the time needed for the LV to accommodate the significant volume overload and may present with LV systolic dysfunction. Chronic AR may be associated with LV dilatation and eccentric hypertrophy to accommodate the volume overload with an enlarged stroke volume.

Color Flow Doppler

Color flow Doppler (CFD) is again useful in the short and long-axis views of the aortic valve. To identify regurgitant lesions, place the CFD box over the aortic valve, and adjust the view to show the point of leaflet coaptation (Fig. 9.12; Video 9.7). Once a lesion is identified, as with all valves, quantification of its severity into mild, moderate, or severe should be determined.

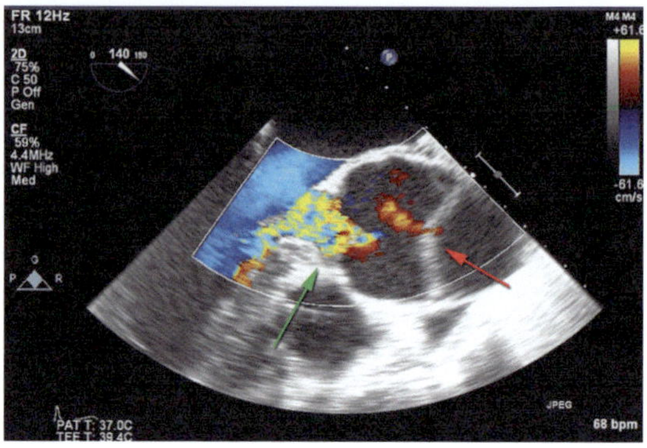

Fig. 9.12 Aortic regurgitation: A ME AV LAX view in a patient with an ascending aortic dissection and severe aortic regurgitation. The *red arrow* indicates the intimal flap (flow is seen in the intimal tear). The *green arrow* indicates the severe aortic regurgitation with flow filling the LVOT during diastole

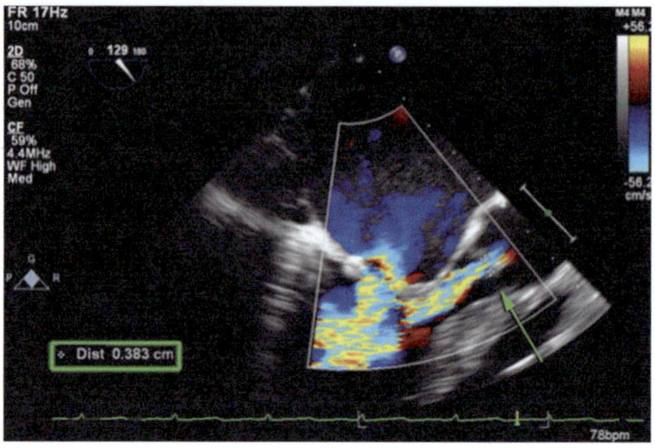

Fig. 9.13 Vena contracta: The ME AV LAX view with a color flow Doppler box over the mitral and aortic valves. Regurgitant flow can be seen entering the left ventricle. A caliper measurement (*green arrow*) is seen measuring the jet as it crosses the aortic valve showing a distance of 0.38 cm (moderate severity)

Quantification of Aortic Regurgitation

Vena Contracta

The term *vena contracta* is derived from Latin words vena = blood vessel and contracta = violated. The vena contracta "is the narrowest flow of a regurgitant jet immediately downstream from the convergence region" [12] (Fig. 9.13). Measuring a vena contracta is a simple and quick method of estimating the severity of aortic regurgitation. The probe is finely adjusted until the largest regurgitant jet across the AV plane is obtained, and then the image is acquired. The diastolic phase of the acquired image can then be examined to isolate the largest jet. The neck of the jet at its narrowest point as it crosses the aortic valve is measured. A diameter below 0.3 cm is graded as mild, 0.3–0.6 cm as moderate, and measurements above 0.6 cm considered severe regurgitation. Importantly, a vena contracta is a relatively load-independent measurement, which is a valuable characteristic to this quantitative modality.

Jet Width to LVOT Diameter

The ration of the jet width to LVOT diameter is another easily employed quantitative measure of aortic regurgitation. Similar to the measurement of a vena contracta, the regurgitant jet is optimized to find the widest regurgitant flow back through the LVOT (Video 9.8). M-mode can be combined with CFD and directed so that it images approximately 1 cm from the AV into the LVOT. The size of the jet can then be measured in relation to the width of the LVOT. A regurgitant jet that occupies between 25% and 65% of the LVOT is deemed moderate in severity. A jet size measuring less than or greater than this range is deemed mild or severe, respectively (Fig. 9.14).

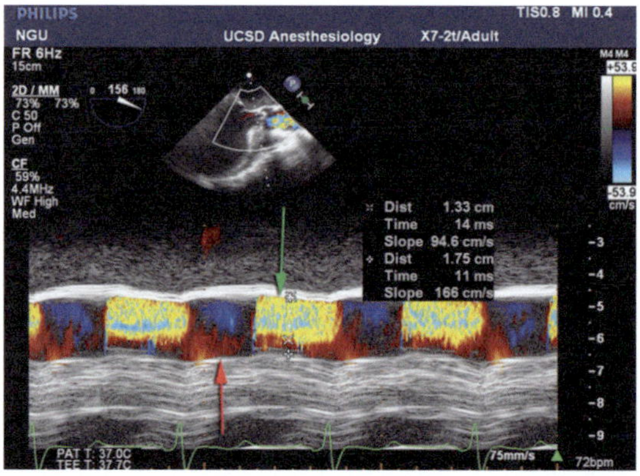

Fig. 9.14 Jet width to LVOT diameter: the M-mode cursor is placed 1 centimeter from the aortic valve into the LVOT. Note the EKG confirming the jet is in diastole (*green arrow*) as opposed to systole (*red arrow*). Measurements identify a regurgitant jet of 1.33 cm, LVOT diameter of 1.75 cm, and a ratio of jet to outflow tract of 76%, indicating severe regurgitation

Spectral Doppler

Pulsed-wave Doppler and continuous-wave Doppler can both be utilized to further quantify the severity of aortic regurgitation. These methodologies are complimentary to the CFD techniques. Like any clinical diagnosis, a collection of findings should be used to determine severity, as opposed to any one single result.

Aortic Valve Pressure Half Time

The aortic valve pressure half time (PHT), as its name suggests, is the period of time it takes for the pressure differential between the left ventricle and aorta to decrease by half. This is similar to the PHT used in mitral valve stenosis (see Chap. 8). From the deep TG LAX (TEE) or apical five-chamber or long-axis (TTE) view, a continuous-wave Doppler signal can be aligned with the jet entering the LVOT from a regurgitant lesion. The slope of the regurgitant jet from its peak velocity to the end of its decay is traced (Fig. 9.15a,b; Video 9.9). The AR PHT is then calculated by the included ultrasound software, providing a time value in milliseconds. A larger opening in the aortic valve (worse aortic regurgitation) will be noted by a more rapid equilibration of pressures between the aorta and the LVOT (faster filling). Moderate aortic regurgitation is indicated by a PHT of 200–500 ms. Values less than this are considered severe (< 200 ms), and values greater than this are mild (> 500 ms) (Table 9.2). Similarly, the slope of the deceleration line can imply the degree of AR severity. The steeper the slope, the more severe the AR, such that values greater than 3 m/s indicate severe AR, while values greater than 2 m/s indicate moderate AR.

Descending Aorta Reversal of Flow

Determining the direction of flow in the descending aorta can help confirm the severity of aortic regurgitation. In a normal patient, aortic flow in the descending thoracic aorta should be antegrade during systolic ejection, as well as during the diastolic runoff. If reversal of flow in the descending thoracic aorta during diastole is identified, aortic insufficiency is confirmed. The further from the aortic valve that the flow reversal is detected, the more severe the aortic regurgitation, such that detection of reversal in the lower descending thoracic aorta suggests severe regurgitation. However, the absence of diastolic flow reversal in the aorta does not rule out a severely regurgitant lesion. Moderate regurgitant lesions may have reversal in the proximal descending aorta, while mild regurgitant lesions typically will not have any reversal of flow within the descending aorta.

In order to make this assessment of the diastolic flow direction, a descending aortic LAX view is used with TEE, and a suprasternal notch aortic arch view (making sure to place the sam-

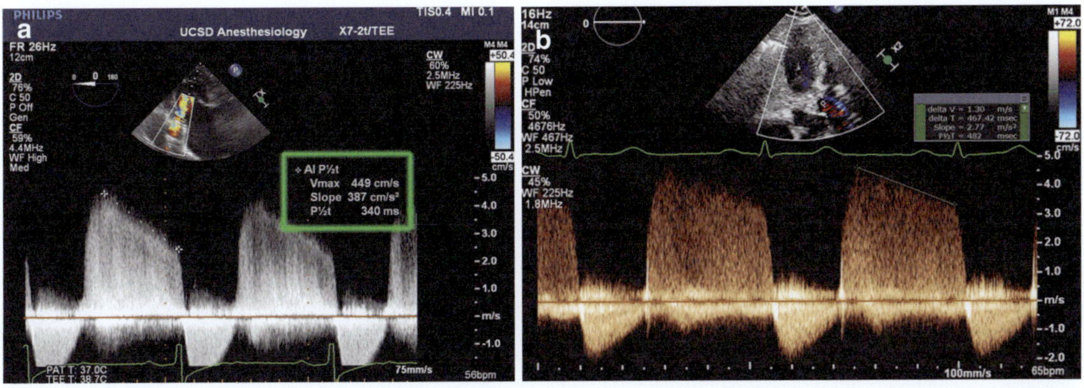

Fig. 9.15 Aortic valve PHT: (**a**) A deep TG LAX view (TEE) is obtained to align the continuous-wave Doppler beam parallel to the flow into the LVOT. The peak velocity (V_{max}) of the regurgitation is the starting point for the measurement of the jet's pressure decay. The PHT is then calculated, 340 ms (moderate aortic regurgitation). (**b**) An apical long-axis view (TTE) of AR PHT, measuring 482 ms, consistent with moderate regurgitation

Table 9.2 Values for grading aortic regurgitation severity

	Mild	Moderate	Severe
Vena contracta (cm)	< 0.3	0.3–0.6	> 0.6
Jet width/LVOT diameter ratio	< 25%	25%–65%	> 65%
PHT (ms)	> 500	200–500	< 200
Slope (m/s)		> 2	> 3

LVOT left ventricular outflow tract, *PHT* pressure half time

ple volume at least 1 centimeter distal to the left subclavian takeoff), or a subcostal long-axis view of the aorta, is used with TTE. A pulsed-wave Doppler beam is then aligned parallel to the aortic flow. A severely incompetent valve will produce holodiastolic flow reversal (Fig. 9.16a-c).

Conclusion

The aortic valve is an integral cardiac structure allowing the ejection of blood into the aorta, while maintaining a pressure gradient during diastole to provide diastolic flow into the coronary arteries and end organs, and preventing reflux of blood back in to the left ventricle. Dysfunction in the form of stenosis leads to a hindrance of systolic ejection, hypertrophy of the left ventricle, and eventual heart failure, while regurgitation may occur from multiple mechanisms and may lead to eccentric hypertrophy and congestive heart failure. Echocardiography via two-dimensional view, color flow Doppler, and spectral Doppler plays a key role in the diagnosis and management of such patients.

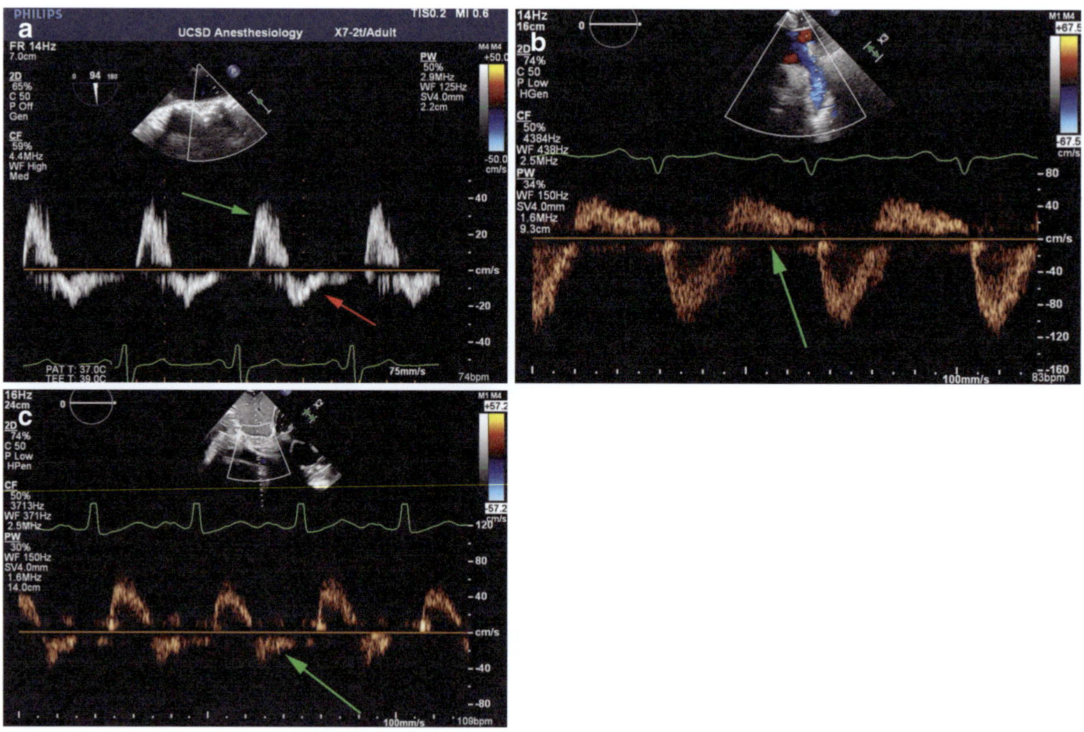

Fig. 9.16 Descending aorta reversal of flow: (**a**) A long-axis view of the descending aorta is obtained, and a pulsed-wave Doppler beam is placed within the aorta. The waveform demonstrates normal systolic forward flow (*green arrow*); however, holodiastolic flow reversal (*red arrow*) is noted, which is indicative of severe aortic regurgitation. (**b**) A suprasternal notch aortic arch view (TTE) with the pulsed-wave Doppler sample volume 1 cm distal to the left subclavian artery takeoff, showing holodiastolic flow reversal (*green arrow*). (**c**) A subcostal descending aorta long-axis view (TTE) with pulsed-wave Doppler showing diastolic flow reversal (*green arrow*)

Questions

1. Which of the following would be the most correct interpretation of the following echocardiographic image?

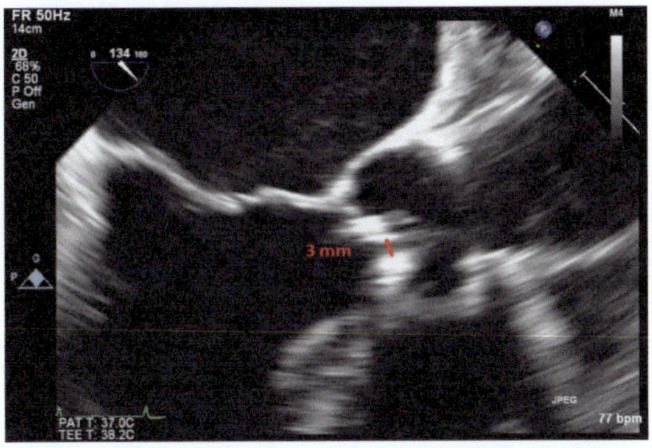

A. Measured during diastole: severe aortic insufficiency
B. Measured during systole: mild aortic insufficiency
C. Measured during diastole: severe aortic stenosis
D. Measured during systole: severe aortic stenosis

2. The spectral Doppler image shown below can be obtained from which of the following views?

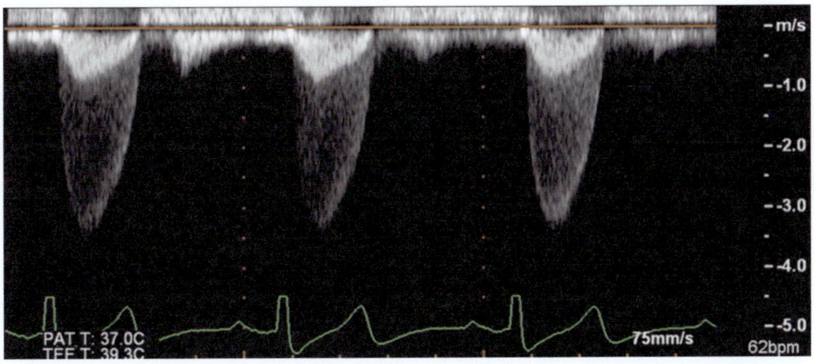

A. Apical four-chamber view
B. Deep transgastric long-axis view
C. Midesophageal long-axis view
D. Parasternal long-axis view

3. A 75-year-old man with a history of coronary artery disease and heart failure with reduced ejection fraction (25%) is evaluated for aortic stenosis with echocardiography. A peak systolic velocity through the aortic valve is measured at 2.9 m/s, with a mean pressure gradient of 30 mmHg. Which of the following is present?

A. Mild aortic stenosis
B. Moderate aortic stenosis
C. Severe aortic stenosis
D. Unable to determine

4. Which of the following is *least* likely to be associated with calcific aortic stenosis?

A. Mitral stenosis
B. Aortic aneurysm
C. Pulmonary hypertension
D. Diastolic dysfunction

5. The echocardiographic image of aortic stenosis shown below is best for determining which value?

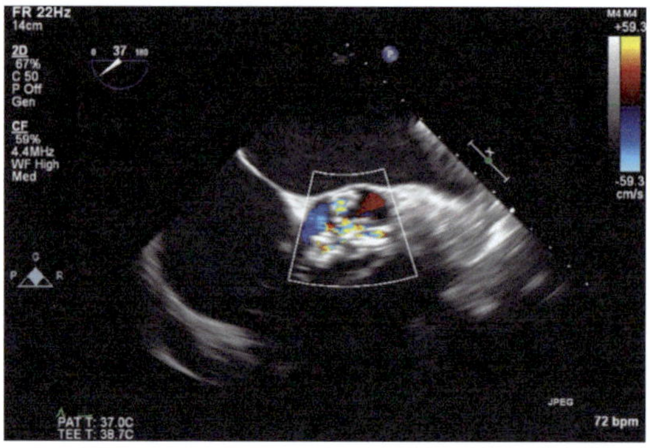

A. Planimetric valve area
B. Peak systolic velocity
C. Mean pressure gradient
D. Vena contracta

6. The following values are obtained during an echocardiographic examination: LVOT diameter 2.0 cm, LVOT VTI 32 cm, and AV VTI 100 cm. What is the approximate cross-sectional area of the aortic valve?

A. 1.0 cm^2
B. 2.0 cm2
C. 3.0 cm2
D. 4.0 cm^2

7. The echocardiographic image shown below was obtained from a midesophageal AV long-axis view using M-Mode during Color Flow Doppler. Diastole is noted between the yellow arrows. Which of the following diagnoses is apparent?

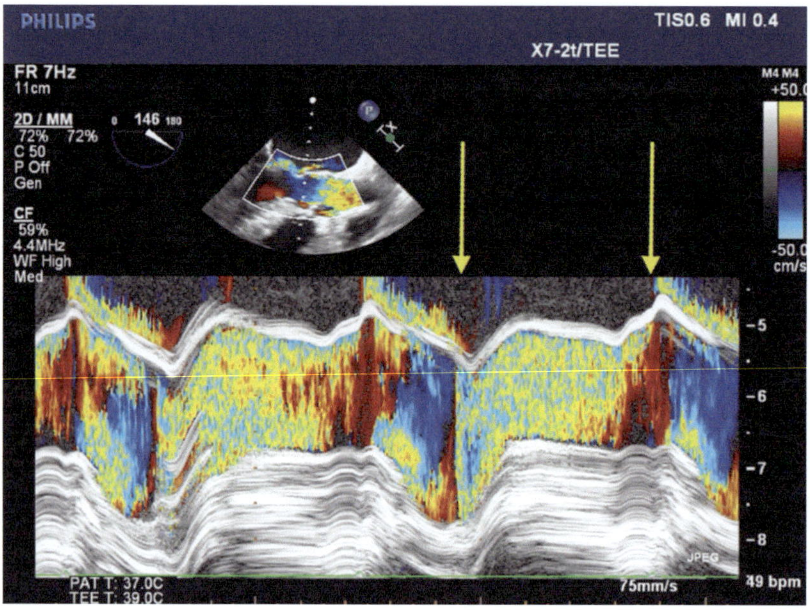

A. Mild aortic regurgitation
B. Mild aortic stenosis
C. Severe aortic regurgitation
D. Severe aortic stenosis

8. The measured diameter of a regurgitant aortic valve vena contracta in an aortic long-axis view was found to be 3.5 mm. This would indicate what degree of severity?

A. Mild
B. Moderate
C. Severe
D. Indeterminate without hemodynamic data

9. The echocardiographic image shown below was obtained from an apical three-chamber view, showing flow through the aortic valve. Which of the following can be determined from this image?

A. There is mild-moderate aortic regurgitation.
B. There is severe aortic regurgitation.
C. There is mild-moderate aortic stenosis.
D. There is severe aortic stenosis.

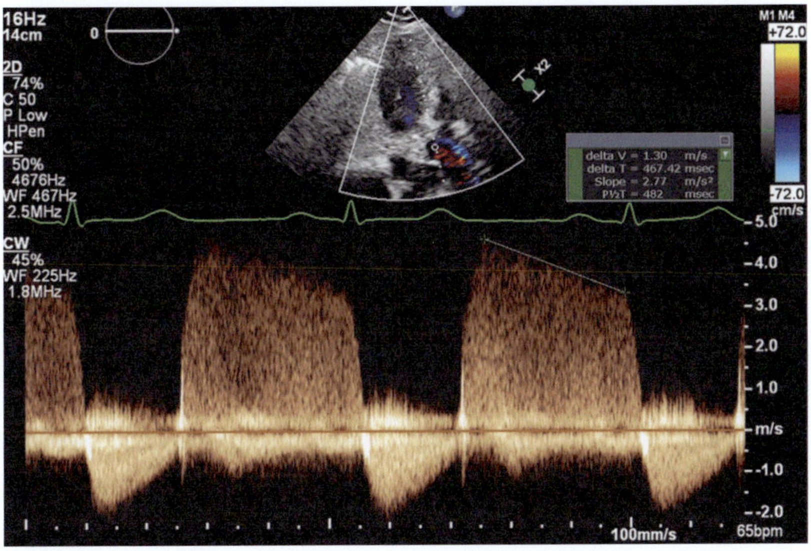

10. The pulsed-wave Doppler tracing image of the proximal descending aorta shown below indicates which of the following?

A. Mild aortic regurgitation
B. Moderate aortic regurgitation
C. Severe aortic regurgitation
D. Unable to determine

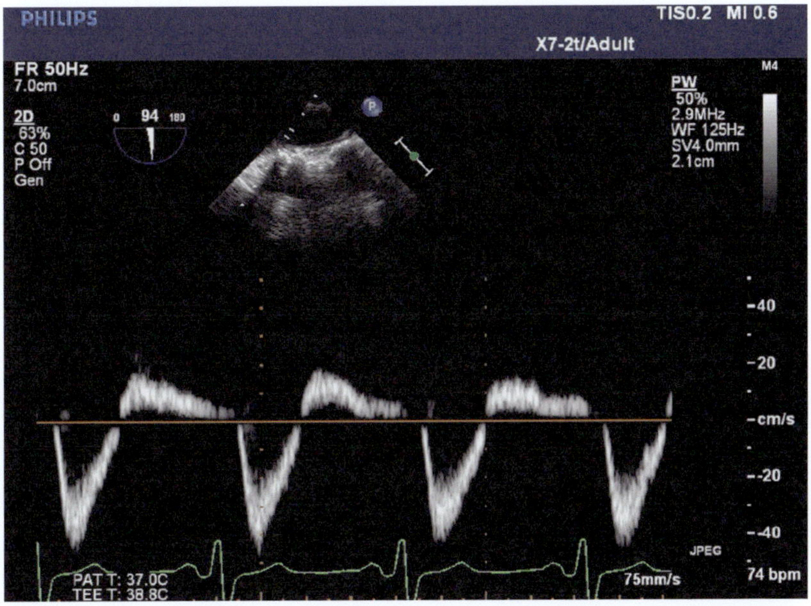

References

1. Bellhouse BJ, Bellhouse FH. Mechanism of closure of the aortic valve. Nature. 1968;217:86–7.
2. Tribouilloy CM, et al. Circulation. 2000;102:558-564.
3. Horstkotte D, Loogen F. The natural history of aortic valve stenosis. Eur Heart J. 1988;9(Suppl E): 57–64.
4. Nadir MA, Wei L, Elder D, Libianto R, Lim T, et al. Impact of renin-angiotensin system blockade therapy on outcome in aortic stenosis. J Am Coll Cardiol. 2011;58(6):570–6.
5. Reeves ST, Finley AC, Skubas NJ, Swaminathan M, Whitley WS, Glas KE, et al. Basic perioperative transesophageal echocardiography examination: a consensus statement of the American Society of Echocardiography and the Society of Cardiovascular Aneshesiologists. J Am Soc Echocardiogr. 2013;26:443–56.
6. Shively BK, Gurule FT, Roldan CA, Leggett JH, Schiller NB. Diagnostic value of transesophageal compared with transthoracic echocardiography in infective endocarditis. J Am Coll Cardiol. 1991;18(2):391–7.
7. Baumgartner H, Hung J, Bermejo J, Chambers JB, Evangelista A, Griffin BP, et al. Echocardiographic assessment of valve stenosis: EAE/ASE recommendations for clinical practice. J Am Soc Echocardiogr. 2009;22(1):1–23.
8. Godley RW, Green D, Dillon JC, Rogers EW, Feigenbaum H, Weyman AE. Reliability of two-dimensional echocardiography in assessing the severity of valvular aortic stenosis. Chest. 1981;79:657–62.
9. Jayaprakash K, Dilu VP, George R. Maximal aortic valve cusp separation and severity of aortic stenosis. J Clin Diagn Res. 2017;11(6):OC29–32.
10. Lindman B, Bonow R, Otto C. Current management of calcific aortic stenosis. Circ Res. 2013;113:223–37.
11. Bekeredijian R, Grayburn P. Valvular heart disease: aortic regurgitation. Circulation. 2005;112:125–34.
12. Lancellotti P, Tribouilloy C, et al. European association of echocardiography recommendations for the assessment of valvular regurgitation. Part 1: aortic and pulmonary regurgitation (native valve disease). Eur J Echocardiogr. 2010;11(3):223–44.

The Right Heart

10

Sophia P. Poorsattar and Dalia Banks

Abbreviations

TEE Transesophageal echocardiography
TTE Transthoracic echocardiography
RV Right ventricle
LV Left ventricle
RCA Right coronary artery
PDA Posterior descending (coronary) artery
LAD Left anterior descending (coronary) artery
AV Atrioventricular (node)
SA Sinoatrial (node)
IVS Interventricular septum
ME Midesophageal
TG Transgastric
RA Right atrium
TV Tricuspid valve
PA Pulmonary artery
RVOT Right ventricular outflow tract
SVC Superior vena cava
IVC Inferior vena cava
2D Two-dimensional
3D Three-dimensional
EF Ejection fraction
MRI Magnetic resonance imaging
PAP Pulmonary arterial pressure
PVR Pulmonary vascular resistance
PH Pulmonary hypertension
RVH Right ventricular hypertrophy
RVWT Right ventricular (free) wall thickness
TAPSE Tricuspid annular plane systolic excursion
FAC Fractional area of change
TDI Tissue Doppler Imaging
S′ Tricuspid annular velocity (systole)
IVRT Isovolumetric relaxation time
IVCT Isovolumetric contraction time
EI Eccentricity index
MPI Myocardial performance index
RVF Right ventricular failure
LVAD Left ventricular assist device

Supplementary Information The online version of this chapter (https://doi.org/10.1007/978-3-030-84349-6_10) contains supplementary material, which is available to authorized users.

S. P. Poorsattar (✉)
Department of Anesthesiology and Perioperative Medicine, University of California, Los Angeles Medical Center, Los Angeles, CA, USA
e-mail: spoorsattar@mednet.ucla.edu

D. Banks
Department of Anesthesiology, University of California San Diego Health, La Jolla, CA, USA
e-mail: dabanks@health.ucsd.edu

Introduction

The right side of the heart has historically been viewed as less important than the left side, in part because of the devastating effect of left heart dysfunction. However, recently, there has been considerable interest in understanding the function

T. M. Maus, C. R. Tainter (eds.), *Essential Echocardiography*,
https://doi.org/10.1007/978-3-030-84349-6_10

of the right ventricle (RV), as right ventricular dysfunction has been associated with increased morbidity and mortality in both perioperative and critically ill patients. Current guidelines suggest that knowledge of the echocardiographic manifestations of right heart dysfunction is essential to the perioperative and critical care echocardiographer [1]. It is easy to overlook the fact that in most cases, the right ventricle pumps the same cardiac output as the left ventricle. The main function of the RV is to enhance venous return by accommodating systemic return into a low-pressure chamber and subsequently transit blood to the left heart via the low-pressure pulmonary circuit. Recognition of right heart dysfunction due to acute pathology, such as pulmonary embolism, or chronic pathology, such as pulmonary hypertension, is key to optimal management. Transesophageal (TEE) and transthoracic (TTE) echocardiography play a significant role both in the identification and quantification of right heart dysfunction.

Right Ventricle Structure and Function

The RV forms the major portion of the anterior surface of the heart immediately behind the sternum, while the inferior border of the RV abuts the diaphragm. The right ventricle is an asymmetric crescent-shaped chamber that is wrapped around the right and antero-septal side of the left ventricle (LV). In healthy individuals, the RV cross-sectional area is roughly two-thirds the size of that of the LV. The RV is generally separated into three distinct regions, inflow, apical, and outflow, separated by a series of encircling muscular bands. The inflow portion is trabeculated and consists of the tricuspid valve, chordae tendineae, and papillary muscles. The apical portion is also a muscular portion, connecting the inflow to the smooth-surfaced outflow tract. The outflow region contains the smooth myocardial outflow tract and pulmonic valve [2, 3].

The encircling muscular bands include four individual bands; the moderator band is most important to the echocardiographer. The moderator band extends from the base of the anterior papillary muscle near the free wall to the ventricular septum. When it becomes prominent from right ventricular hypertrophy or dilation, the moderator band may be mistaken for a thrombus or intracavitary mass [4, 5]. The moderator band contains conducting fibers, and stretching or ischemia is also commonly associated with a right bundle branch pattern on EKG.

The RV wall motion is complex, characterized by a peristaltic-like motion. Contraction is sequential, beginning with the inlet portion contracting toward the apex and ending with the infundibulum. Right ventricular longitudinal shortening occurs mainly during the ejection phase of the cardiac cycle (late systole), while circumferential motion occurs mainly during the isovolumetric contraction phase (early systole) [6, 7].

The perfusion to the RV is mostly supplied by the right coronary artery (RCA), with the posterior descending artery (PDA) supplying one-third to two-thirds of the RV septum. The left anterior descending artery (LAD) may supply a portion of the apex, while branches off of the RCA, the acute marginal arteries, supply the RV free wall. Lastly, in the majority of patients, the RCA supplies perfusion to the atrioventricular (AV) node and sinoatrial (SA) nodes.

The RV provides a similar stroke volume to the LV, however, with 25% of the stroke work, due to less afterload from the low-pressure, high-compliance circuit in the pulmonary circulation [8]. As a result, the wall thickness of the RV is half that of the LV, making the RV a much more compliant chamber. The right and left ventricles share the interventricular septum (IVS) and are enclosed within the same pericardial sac. Therefore, ventricular interdependence exists. The interventricular septum (IVS) contributes to both LV and RV function, is responsible for approximately one-third of the RV stroke work under normal conditions, and is a major determinant of overall RV performance [9–11]. Normally, the IVS is shifted toward the RV free wall (concave towards the LV) during systole and diastole, contributing to RV ejection. However, this relationship is changed in conditions that lead to an increase in RV pressure or volume overload. Because the ventricles share the interventricular septum and are enclosed within the same pericardial sac, an increase in pressure or volume in the right ventricle causes the septum to shift paradoxically toward the LV, altering LV geometry and resulting in decreased LV preload and low cardiac output, a concept known as ventricular interdependence [12].

Echocardiographic Views for Evaluation of the Right Ventricle

Qualitative evaluation of the RV should allow the examiner to answer five questions, as illustrated in Table 10.1. As described in Chaps. 2 and 3, there are several views that focus on evaluation of the right heart. For most views obtained by TEE, there is generally a corresponding view with TTE that allows for the echocardiographic assessment of similar qualitative and quantitative measures. Those which are most useful for evaluation of the right heart are briefly outlined below.

TEE Views

Midesophageal (ME) Four-Chamber View

A ME view with a multiplane angle of 0–20 degrees allows for evaluation of RV chamber size, function, and anatomical variants [13, 14]. From a standard ME four-chamber view, turning the probe to the right (clockwise) allows imaging of the right atrium (RA), RV, tricuspid valve (TV), as well as the interatrial septum and IVS. This is the most commonly utilized view to assess the right heart.

Table 10.1 Outline of echocardiographic evaluation of the right heart

Echocardiographic evaluation of the RV should allow the examiner to answer the following five questions:
What is the RV Shape?
What is the RV area relative to LV area?
What is the RV free wall thickness?
How is the RV free wall motion?
What is the interventricular septal motion?

ME RV Inflow-Outflow View

Placing the right heart in the center of the imaging sector and increasing the multiplane angle to 60–90 degrees will develop the ME RV inflow-outflow view. This view demonstrates the “wrapping” nature of the RA, RV, and pulmonary artery (PA) in relation to the left heart. Assessment of the RA, TV, RV free wall, RV outflow tract (RVOT), pulmonic valve (PV), and main PA can be accomplished in this view. With an image of both the TV and PV, this view is used to help guide placement of the pulmonary artery catheter, as well as estimate RV systolic pressure.

ME Bicaval View

From the ME RV inflow-outflow view, increasing the multiplane angle to 90–110 degrees and turning the probe to the right develop the ME bicaval view. This view displays the LA, RA, and the interatrial septum. In the standard bicaval view, the superior (SVC) and inferior vena cavae (IVC), as well as right atrial appendage, are in view. Turning of the probe slightly left (counterclockwise) or increasing the multiplane angle by 10–20 degrees will bring the tricuspid valve and coronary sinus into view, which is called the ME modified bicaval tricuspid valve view [3, 13].

ME Ascending Aortic Short-Axis View

This view demonstrates the relation of the main and right PA to the ascending aorta and SVC and proves useful in identifying PA dilatation and PA thrombus (the main pulmonary artery should not be larger than the adjacent aorta), as well as confirming the position of a properly placed PA catheter.

Transgastric (TG) Midpapillary Short-Axis View

From a standard TG midpapillary short-axis view, rightward probe rotation develops an image of the crescent-shaped RV. Again, the anterolateral position of the RV in relation to the left ventricle (LV) is apparent.

TG RV Inflow View

Increasing the multiplane angle to 90 degrees from the prior view yields the TG RV inflow view. This view shows a "two-chamber" view of the right heart with a focus on the tricuspid valve and the subvalvular apparatus, as well as the right ventricular free wall.

TTE Views

Parasternal Long-Axis View

Placing the transducer at the 3rd or 4th intercostal space along the left parasternal border with the indicator directed toward the patient's right shoulder develops the parasternal long-axis view. With TEE, this view corresponds most closely with ME long-axis view; however, it is distinct in that the apex of the heart is generally not seen. At a glance, the RVOT, LV outflow tract, and left atrium (LA) should be roughly of equal width. Here, RVOT abnormalities, notably dilation, can be appreciated in relation to the other chambers in view.

Parasternal RV Inflow View

From the parasternal long-axis view, a small fan of the imaging plane anteriorly (sometimes with a small rotation counterclockwise) develops the parasternal RV inflow view. In addition to the RV and TV, this view displays the RA, SVC, and IVC and allows the echocardiographer to gain similar information to the ME bicaval or modified bicaval TV view.

Parasternal Short-Axis View (RVOT Level)

From the parasternal long-axis view, center the aortic valve in the middle of the imaging plane, and rotate the probe 90 degrees with the indicator toward the left shoulder to develop a parasternal short-axis image of the RV wrapping around the LVOT and aortic valve. This view corresponds with the inverse image of the ME RV inflow-outflow view.

Parasternal Short-Axis View (Midpapillary Level)

From the parasternal short-axis view at the RVOT level, fan the imaging plane slightly inferiorly (toward the cardiac apex) through the midpapillary level to develop a view of both ventricles in short axis. With TEE, this view corresponds with the TG short-axis midpapillary view.

Apical Four-Chamber View

Placing the transducer at the 4th or 5th intercostal space along the midclavicular line with the indicator directed toward the left flank develops the apical four-chamber view. Slight adjustments in the transducer angle and rotation to ensure the imaging plane transects the apex, tricuspid valve, and mitral valve allow full visualization of all four cardiac chambers. With TEE, this view corresponds with the inverse image of the ME four-chamber view.

Three-Dimensional Echocardiography

While this text focuses on two-dimensional (2D) echocardiography, it is important to note that three-dimensional (3D) echocardiography has gained increasing popularity for the assessment of right heart structures and function. Due to the complex geometry and contraction pattern of the RV, the application of 3D imaging has allowed perioperative echocardiographers to overcome many of the limitations and assumptions associated with assessments made in 2D and improve precision. Notably, in contrast to 2D echocardiography, 3D-generated assessments of RV volume and RV EF from both TEE and TTE have been shown to be reliable and have comparable accuracy to each other, as well as to magnetic resonance imaging (MRI) in diverse patient cohorts [15].

Physiology of the Right Heart: Adaptations to Pulmonary Hypertension

The pulmonary circulation is normally a low-pressure and low-resistance circuit, in contrast to the systemic circulation. The normal systolic, diastolic, and mean PA pressure (PAP) are 22 mmHg, 10 mmHg, and 15 mmHg, respectively. The pulmonary vascular resistance (PVR) is normally 0.9 to 1.4 Wood units (90 to 120 dynes-sec/cm^5). Pulmonary hypertension (PH) is generally defined as a mean PAP of greater than 20 mmHg or a PVR greater than 240 dynes-sec/cm^5. A mean PAP greater than 50 mmHg or a PVR greater than 600 dynes-sec/cm^5 is considered severe PH. The PVR is important, because it represents the afterload of the right ventricle (the pressure encountered during ejection) and, therefore, affects RV function and cardiac output.

Emphasis on PH classification began in 1973 at the World Health Organization conference and, since then, has undergone multiple changes as the appreciation of the disease and treatment of PH have evolved, resulting in five distinct subgroups of patients sharing specific features [14, 16, 17] [Table 10.2]. The effects on the RV in response to pulmonary hypertension are readily identified with echocardiography. The adaptations are generally categorized as RV dilation in response to volume overload (inability to properly move the volume through the pulmonary circuit) and RV hypertrophy in response to the increased afterload (inability to eject a proper stroke volume due to increased resistance). Both of these adaptations lead to RV dysfunction. Additionally, septal wall motion may become abnormal with a deviation toward the left heart, distorting the normal RV architecture, and further contributing to RV dysfunction. An echocardiographic evaluation with particular focus on the right side of the heart allows both the identification and quantification of RV dysfunction.

Table 10.2 Classification of pulmonary hypertension

Definition of pulmonary hypertension (PH)	Clinical group(s)
Precapillary: MPAP > 20 mmHg PCWP < 15 mmHg	*Group I:* Pulmonary arterial hypertension (PAH) and other subtypes of PAH *Group III:* Respiratory disease and hypoxemia *Group IV:* Chronic thromboembolic pulmonary hypertension (CTEPH) *Group V:* Miscellaneous causes
Postcapillary: MPAP > 20 mmHg PCWP > 15 mmHg	*Group II:* Left heart disease

Adapted from Simonneau, et al. [40]
MPAP Mean pulmonary artery pressure, *PCWP* Pulmonary capillary wedge pressure

Right Ventricular Enlargement

The normally thin-walled, crescent-shaped RV allows the RV to be highly compliant, accommodating a large increase in preload to maintain a normal stroke volume in the early stages of RV dysfunction. Consequently, the initial primary compensatory mechanism of RV dysfunction often is dilatation that is usually well-tolerated. With progressive dilation, the ability to maintain a normal stroke volume is lost. Qualitative visual measures are typically used to assess RV chamber size in the ME four-chamber or apical four-chamber views. RV size normally occupies two-thirds of the cross-sectional area in comparison to LV area. Additionally, the LV typically forms the cardiac apex in this view. With mild enlargement, the RV increases in size to greater than two-thirds of the LV cross-sectional area; with moderate enlargement, the cardiac apex includes both the RV and LV, and the cross-sectional areas are equal; and with severe enlargement, the RV apex dominates the cardiac apex, and the cross-sectional area of the RV exceeds that of the LV (Fig. 10.1; Video 10.1).

Additionally, two-dimensional measurements of the RV in the ME four-chamber or apical four-chamber view can be utilized to assess RV size. The RV basal dimension (the width of the TV annulus in the ME four-chamber or apical four-chamber view) ranges from 2.5 to 4.1 cm with > 4.2 cm considered to be RV dilation [18]. Longitudinal measurements from the TV annular plane to the RV apex range from 5.9 to 8.2 cm, with > 8.6 cm considered to be RV dilation [3, 18].

Right Ventricular Hypertrophy

Echocardiographic evaluation of RV wall thickness may also serve to evaluate global RV performance, because conditions of RV pressure

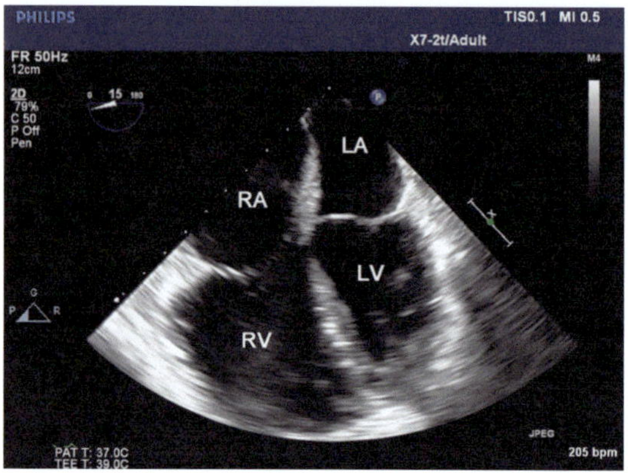

Fig. 10.1 A midesophageal four-chamber view of a patient with pulmonary hypertension and severe right ventricular (RV) enlargement. Note the size of the RV exceeds that of the left ventricle (LV) and the apex of the heart appears to be formed by the RV. *RA* right atrium, *LA* left atrium

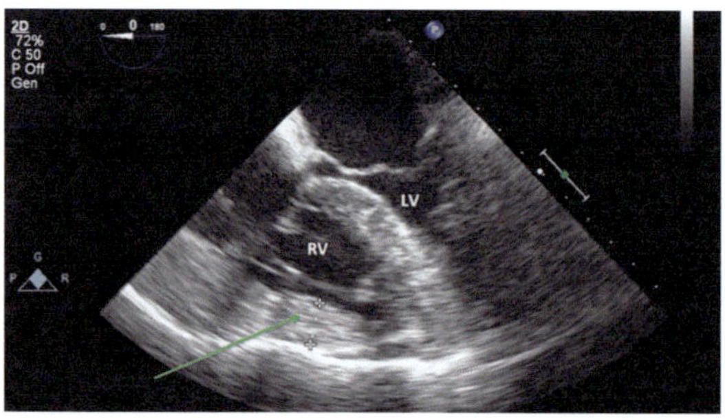

Fig. 10.2 A midesophageal four-chamber view of a patient with chronic pulmonary hypertension and resultant right ventricular hypertrophy (*green arrow*)

overload cause compensatory right ventricular hypertrophy (RVH) over time. This increase in RV myocardial mass is an effort to maintain cardiac output in the presence of increased PVR.

Echocardiographic evaluation of RV wall thickness typically assesses the lateral RV free wall. Normally, the RV is thin-walled with RV free wall thickness (RVWT) approximately half the wall thickness of the LV, measuring < 5 mm at end-diastole. RVH may be diagnosed when the RVWT is > 5 mm, while RVWT exceeding 10 mm is considered severe hypertrophy (Fig. 10.2). The best views to measure the RV free wall are the ME four-chamber or apical four-chamber, ME RV inflow-outflow or parasternal short-axis (RVOT), and TG RV inflow or parasternal RV inflow views. Measurements of RVWT occur during myocardial relaxation (diastole) and must exclude the epicardial fat layer. Additionally, the moderator band is usually more prominent in patients with RVH and is often visualized near the RV apex (Fig. 10.3; Video 10.2).

Quantitative Assessment of Right Ventricular Function (Highlight Box 10.1)

Highlight Box 10.1

Right ventricular dysfunction	
2D	• Right atrial enlargement • Right ventricular enlargement and/or hypertrophy • IAS/IVS shifted toward the left heart • Underfilled LA and LV • Decreased TAPSE (M-mode) • Decreased FAC
CFD	• Tricuspid regurgitation
Spectral	• TDI: Tricuspid annular velocity (S′) • PASP estimation • Hepatic vein confirmation of TR

IAS interatrial septum, *IVS* interventricular septum, *LA* left atrium, *LV* left ventricle, *TAPSE* tricuspid annular plane systolic excursion, *FAC* fractional area of change, *TDI* tissue Doppler imaging, *PASP* pulmonary artery systolic pressure, *TR* tricuspid regurgitation

A quantitative evaluation of RV global function is more difficult to achieve owing to its more complex shape [19, 20]. Unlike the shape of the LV, which allows some geometrical assumptions (e.g., Simpson's method of discs), the shape of the RV is complicated, as evidenced by its triangular shape in the ME four-chamber and apical four-chamber views, its "wraparound" nature in the ME RV inflow-outflow and parasternal short-axis (RVOT) views, and its crescent shape in the TG midpapillary short-axis and parasternal midpapillary short-axis views. Additionally, contraction of the RV differs from the LV's concentric and "piston-like" longitudinal contraction. The RV contracts in a peristaltic-like manner from the base toward the apex and subsequently the out-

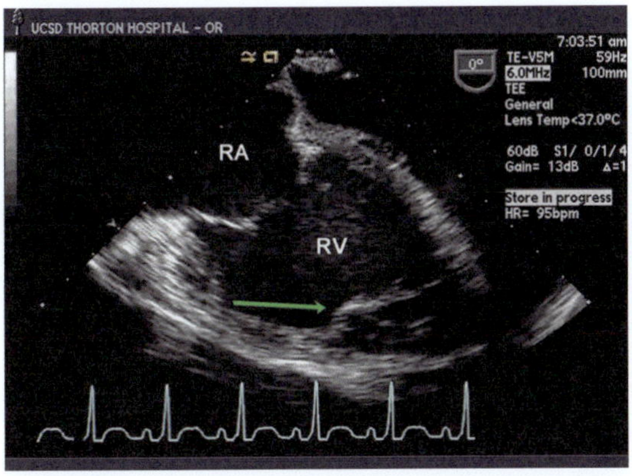

Fig. 10.3 A midesophageal four-chamber view of a patient with severe right ventricular and right atrial enlargement. A prominent moderator band (*green arrow*) is present

flow tract. The major contributor to RV ejection is the basal contraction, which therefore constitutes a basis for several methods of quantitative RV analysis. This complex shape and differing contraction have necessitated surrogate parameters to be developed and subsequently validated for RV systolic function.

Tricuspid Annular Plane Systolic Excursion

Tricuspid annular plane systolic excursion (TAPSE) measures the longitudinal movement of the tricuspid annulus toward the apex during systole. Again, the basal contraction of the RV is a large contributor to RV ejection; therefore, TAPSE is a single measurement that extrapolates and estimates global RV function. Normal TAPSE measurement is greater than 17 mm, and TAPSE values ≤17 mm are suggestive of RV systolic dysfunction [18, 19]. While often obtained as a visual estimate, measurement of TAPSE involves measuring along the RV longitudinal axis from the lateral tricuspid annulus to the apex of the RV at end-diastole and end-systole [3] (Fig. 10.4a,b). The difference in measurements constitutes the TAPSE.

TAPSE is usually acquired by TTE from an apical four-chamber view. This view allows alignment of the TV annulus to the M-mode cursor to quantify TV excursion toward the apex throughout the cardiac cycle (Fig. 10.5). While not validated for TEE, the use of a modified TG RV inflow view (deeper insertion of the probe and an increase of the multiplane angle by 10–20 degrees) can provide a less oblique angle of motion of the TV annulus to the ultrasound probe, allowing the use of M-mode echocardiography (Fig. 10.6). Some of the major limitations of TAPSE include oblique imaging of the RV (TV motion is often not aligned to the TEE ultrasound signal) and poor endocardial delineation; both can yield inaccurate measurements. Additionally, it relies on the assumption that the lateral wall of the RV is representative of the overall systolic performance of the RV, which is not valid in many disease states or after a tricuspid repair or replacement.

Right Ventricular Fractional Area Change

RV fractional area of change (FAC) is analogous to LV FAC (see Chap. 6) and serves as a surrogate measure of right ventricular ejection fraction (RV EF). Echocardiographic assessment of RV FAC is commonly performed in the ME four-chamber and apical four-chamber views and is the percentage change in ventricular area between systole and diastole, with a normal value of > 35%. While a RV FAC < 35% indicates RV dysfunction, values lower than 17% for RV FAC suggest severe RV dysfunction [18, 22]. Right ventricular FAC is obtained by tracing the RV endocardium both in systole and diastole from the annulus, along the free wall to the apex, and then back to the annulus along the interventricular septum. Care must be taken to exclude trabeculations while tracing the RV area (Fig. 10.7a,b). This measurement correlates well with RV EF by cardiac MRI [21]. Fractional area change is calculated as follows:

$$\text{FAC} = \left[\frac{\text{End-Diastolic Area} - \text{End-Systolic Area}}{\text{End-Diastolic Area}}\right] \times 100 \qquad (1)$$

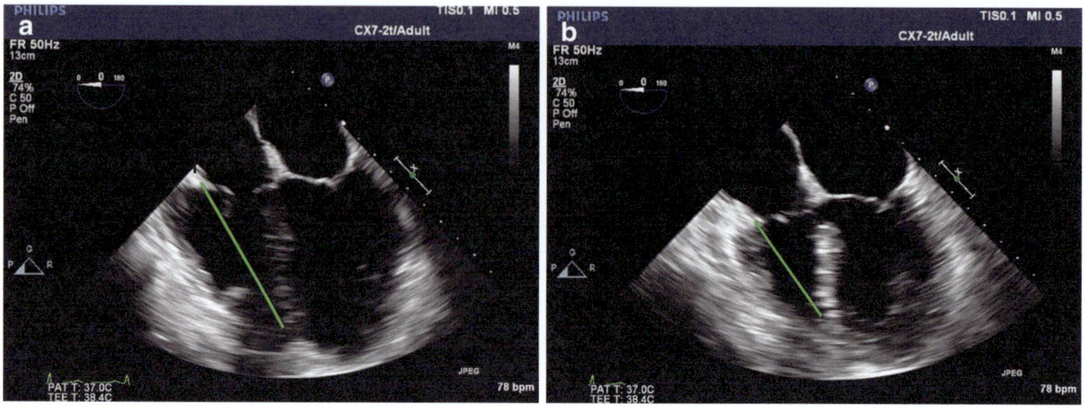

Fig. 10.4 (**a**) A midesophageal four-chamber view with a *green line* depicting measurement of the distance from the tricuspid annulus to the apex in diastole. (**b**) A systolic frame from the same patient with a *green line* depicting the distance from the tricuspid annulus to the apex. TAPSE is calculated as the difference between these two measurements

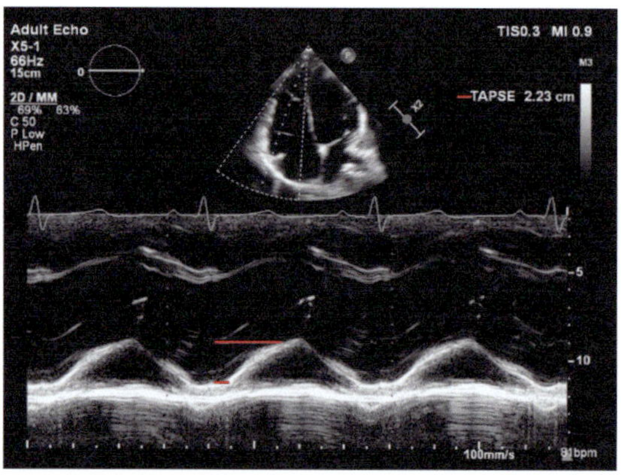

Fig. 10.5 An M-mode analysis of the lateral tricuspid annular motion in an apical four-chamber view. The *red lines* depict the distance of excursion of the lateral tricuspid annulus from the base toward the apex during systole (TAPSE)

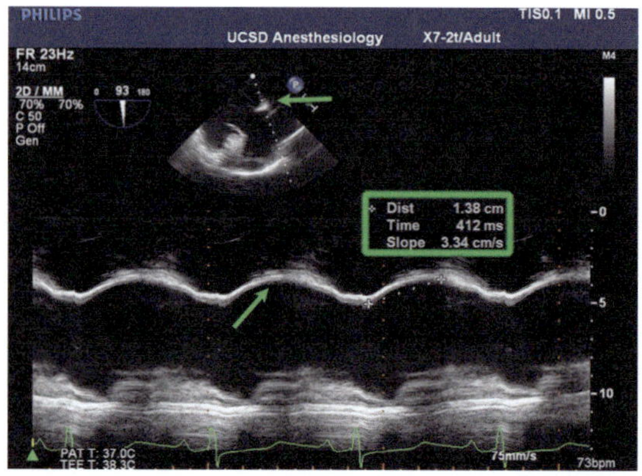

Fig. 10.6 An M-mode analysis of the lateral tricuspid annular motion in a modified transgastric right ventricular inflow view. The *green arrow* on the 2D image depicts the tricuspid annular motion on the M-mode display. TAPSE is easily measured by the movement of the annulus between diastole and systole

Tissue Doppler Imaging

Tissue Doppler imaging (TDI) is a mode of Doppler imaging that utilizes a filter to remove high-velocity, low-intensity signals (i.e., blood) and focuses on low-velocity, high-intensity signals (i.e., myocardium). Measurement of the velocity of the basal RV free wall during systole (S′) provides useful insight into RV systolic function. To obtain this measurement from either a ME four-chamber, modified TG RV inflow, or apical four-chamber view, initiate TDI and highlight the RV free wall within the imaging sector. Similar to the acquisition of the TAPSE measurement, align the cursor with RV free wall, and place the pulsed-wave Doppler sample gate at the basal RV free wall (near the lateral TV annulus) [26]. Attention to alignment of the motion of the myocardium with the ultrasound beam is key to prevent an underestimation (Fig. 10.8). The RV S′ is recorded as the highest systolic velocity. An RV S′ measurement < 9.5 cm/s is suggestive of abnormal RV function [3]. Peak systolic velocity has been demonstrated to correlate well to RV EF, as determined by cardiac MRI [20, 26]. Similar to TAPSE,

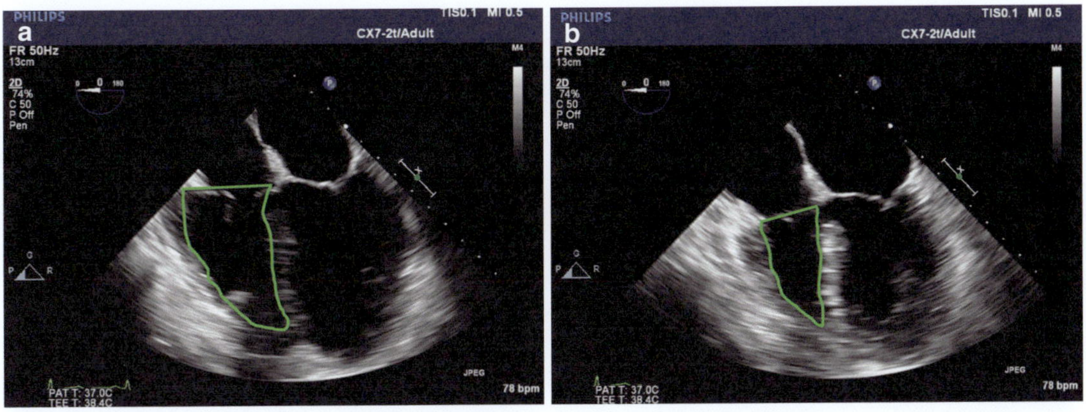

Fig. 10.7 (**a**) A midesophageal four-chamber view with a *green tracing* outlining the right ventricular area in a diastolic frame. (**b**) Systolic frame from the same patient with *a green tracing* outlining the right ventricular area. FAC is calculated as [(RV Diastolic Area – RV Systolic Area) / RV Diastolic Area] x 100

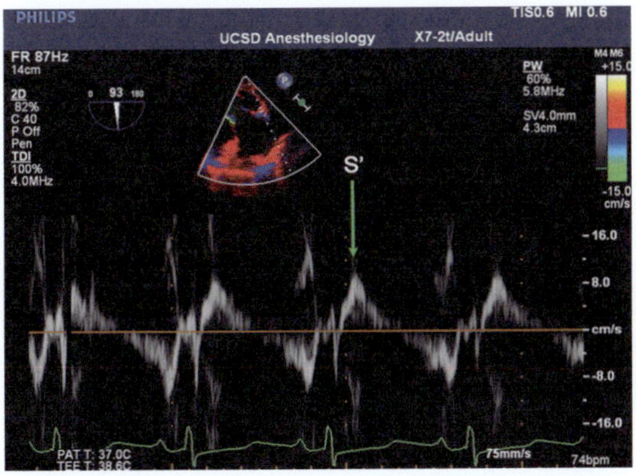

Fig. 10.8 Pulsed-wave tissue Doppler imaging (TDI) of the basal right ventricular myocardium in a modified transgastric RV inflow view. Peak tricuspid annular systolic velocity (S') is identified by the *green arrow*

this technique is limited by angle dependence of the free wall with the Doppler cursor, as well as the assumption that the basal RV free wall is representative of the overall RV systolic performance.

Right Ventricular Myocardial Performance Index

The myocardial performance index (MPI), also known as the Tei Index, is a *global estimate* of both systolic and diastolic cardiac performance of the RV during both ejection and non-ejection periods. While not routinely utilized in noncardiac surgery, MPI remains a valid method for assessing RV function. Right ventricular MPI is defined as the ratio of the total isovolumetric time (isovolumetric relaxation time (IVRT) and isovolumetric contraction time (IVCT)) divided by ejection time (ET) [23, 24].

$$\mathrm{MPI} = \left(\mathrm{IVRT} + \mathrm{IVCT}\right) / \mathrm{ET} \tag{2}$$

The index has been shown to correlate with symptoms and survival and has a prognostic value in patients with primary pulmonary hypertension [25]. Two methods may be utilized to obtain RV MPI including one based on pulsed-wave Doppler of the trans-tricuspid flow and pulmonic ejection and another based on pulsed-wave Doppler of the lateral TV annulus in TDI mode.

Evaluation of the IVS to Assess RV Function

Evaluation of RV geometry serves as a qualitative method to assess for global RV dysfunction. In the TG midpapillary short-axis or parasternal midpapillary short-axis view, the RV often appears crescent-shaped due to the higher LV pressure, causing the IVS to bulge into the lower-pressured RV. However, when RV dysfunction ensues, the compensatory RV dilation results in flattening of the septum and loss of the natural crescent shape of the RV, yielding a "D-shaped" left ventricular chamber [22] (Fig. 10.9; Video 10.3). Although RV volume overload and RV pressure overload may occur concomitantly, they may also occur separately. The timing of the septal flattening can allude to the presence of RV volume overload ver-

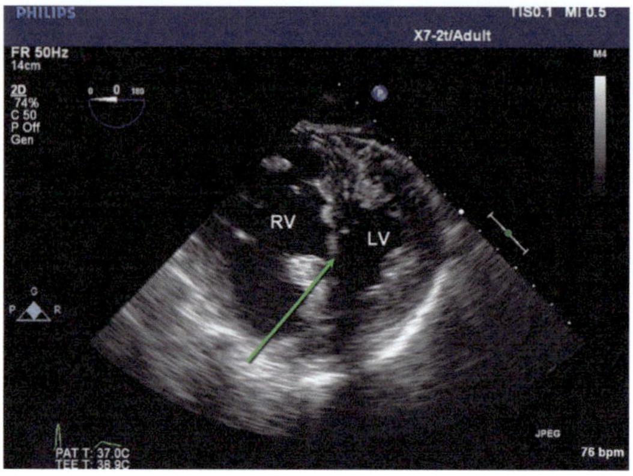

Fig. 10.9 Transgastric midpapillary short-axis view in a patient with right ventricular (RV) failure. Note the shifted interventricular septum (*green arrow*), which results in a "D-shaped" left ventricle. The presence of the shifted septum at end-diastole indicates RV volume overload, whereas at end-systole, it indicates RV pressure overload, which may occur concomitantly

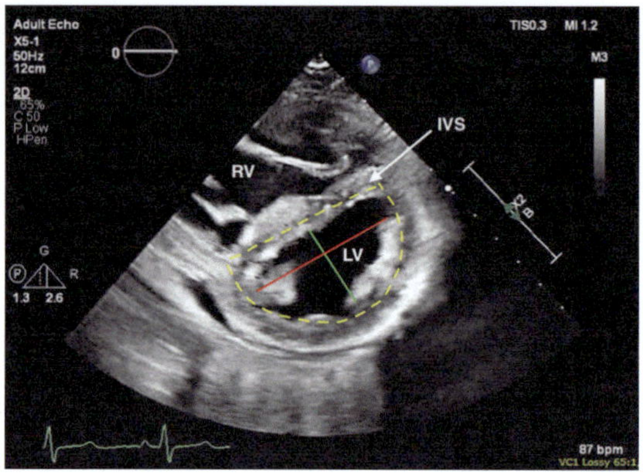

Fig. 10.10 Parasternal short-axis view in a patient with right ventricular (RV) failure. Note the shifted interventricular septum (*IVS*; *white arrow*), which results in a "D-shaped" left ventricle (*yellow dashed line*). Eccentricity index (EI) is the ratio of the LV minor axis (anterior-to-inferior; *red line*) to its perpendicular axis (septal-to-lateral; *green line*). EI value is >1 when the LV is D-shaped during end-systole in pressure overload, whereas in volume overload, it is >1 during end-diastole

sus pressure overload. With RV volume overload, the RV volume is largest at end-diastole, which corresponds to the time of peak diastolic overfilling (septal flattening at end-diastole). This is opposed to RV pressure overload, where septal flattening occurs at end-systole corresponding to when RV systolic afterload is at its peak (i.e., the time when RV pressure is the highest) [27].

The eccentricity index (EI) is an echocardiographic index for measuring the LV dimensions to differentiate RV volume overload from RV pressure overload [20]. It is the ratio of the LV minor axis (anterior-to-inferior) diameter to its perpendicular axis (septal-to-lateral) diameter using the TG midpapillary short-axis or parasternal midpapillary short-axis view. In normal individuals, the LV is round in systole and diastole, and the EI has a value of 1. The EI value is >1 when the LV is D-shaped during end-systole in pressure overload, whereas in volume overload, it is >1 during end-diastole. A high EI is an important echocardiographic predictor of mortality in pulmonary arterial hypertension (Fig. 10.10; Video 10.4).

Adaptation to Chronic Right Ventricular Overload

In chronic RV pressure overload, the RA adapts to support active atrial contribution to RV filling, leading to increased atrial distensibility, and functioning as a reservoir to support the cardiac output. These compensatory changes play an important role in maintaining cardiac output in the face of increased RV diastolic stiffness [28, 29]. Measured in the ME four-chamber or apical four-chamber view, the normal RA size upper reference limit is 5.3 cm and 4.4 cm for major (base to TV annulus) and minor (septal to lateral) axis dimensions, respectively. While the linear dimensions are easier to obtain, guidelines recommend that RA size assessment be performed by RA volume (see Chap. 11) [18]. With chronic PH, the RV dilation results in a dilated TV annulus with significant tricuspid regurgitation (TR) leading to even further RA dilatation.

Tricuspid Regurgitation

The trileaflet TV is composed of the anterior leaflet, which is the largest, the posterior leaflet, and the septal leaflet. Several echocardiographic views are used to visualize the tricuspid valve. With TEE, these include the ME four-chamber with RV focus, ME RV inflow-outflow, modified ME bicaval, TG midpapillary short-axis with RV focus, and TG long-axis views. With TTE, these views include the apical four-chamber, parasternal RV inflow, and parasternal short-axis (RVOT) views. There are several methods to assess the severity of TR; however, the most frequently used is the vena contracta measurement, with a value greater than > 0.7 cm indicating severe TR (Fig. 10.11; Video 10.5). A confirmatory method is pulsed-wave Doppler evaluation of the hepatic vein flow pattern. Evaluation of hepatic vein flow when evaluating TR is analogous to evaluating pulmonary vein flow when evaluating mitral regurgitation (see Chap. 8). Systolic hepatic flow reversal is specific to severe TR, while blunting of forward systolic flow indicates moderate TR [18] (Fig. 10.12a,b). To image the hepatic veins with TEE, perform a rightward probe rotation from the TG midpapillary short-axis view until the liver is centered. Subsequent multiplane rotation may be necessary to obtain a view of a hepatic vein with a parallel orientation to the probe. With TTE, hepatic veins can be viewed and interrogated by obtaining the subxiphoid IVC view.

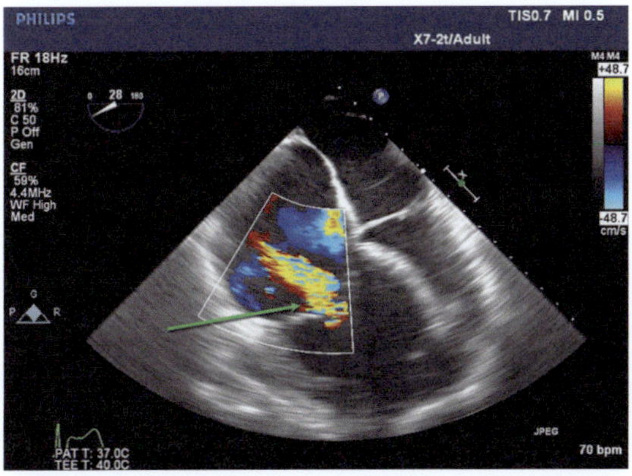

Fig. 10.11 Midesophageal four-chamber view demonstrating severe tricuspid regurgitation (*green arrow*) in a patient with a severely dilated right atrium and right ventricle

In the majority of patients who have "functional" TR, increased pulmonary and RV pressures lead to RV dilation and subsequent TV annular dilatation and leaflet tenting. The result is worsening regurgitation as the valve leaflets are unable to coapt during systole, although they are morphologically without any pathology [31]. With RV systolic failure, the diastolic pressure rises, and the IVS shifts toward the LV during diastole, subsequently raising LV diastolic pressure and further aggravating the TR [32]. Therefore, any patient with a history of PH or evidence of right heart dysfunction deserves an echocardiographic evaluation of the tricuspid valve morphology and evaluation for the causes of TR.

The presence of TR allows the opportunity to estimate the degree of PH and estimate pulmonary artery systolic pressure (PASP). As described in Chap. 4, continuous-wave Doppler measurement, combined with the simplified Bernoulli equation ($\Delta P = 4v^2$), allows measurement of the pressure gradient between the RV and the RA during systole. When added to central venous pressure (right atrial pressure), this provides an estimate of right ventricular systolic pressure, which should be equal to the PASP (assuming the absence of pulmonic stenosis). Commonly utilized views for measurement of PASP are the ME RV inflow-outflow, ME modified bicaval view, and apical four-chamber views (Fig. 10.13).

$$\text{PASP} = 4\text{x}\left(\text{TR Jet Peak Velocity}\right)^2 + \text{estimated RAP} \quad (3)$$

Pulmonary Artery

With long-standing PH, the chronically increased pressure within the PA will cause dilation beyond the normal diameter of 2.1 cm. The commonly utilized views to evaluate the main PA are the ME ascending aortic short-axis or upper-esophageal (UE) aortic arch short-axis views with TEE and the parasternal short-axis

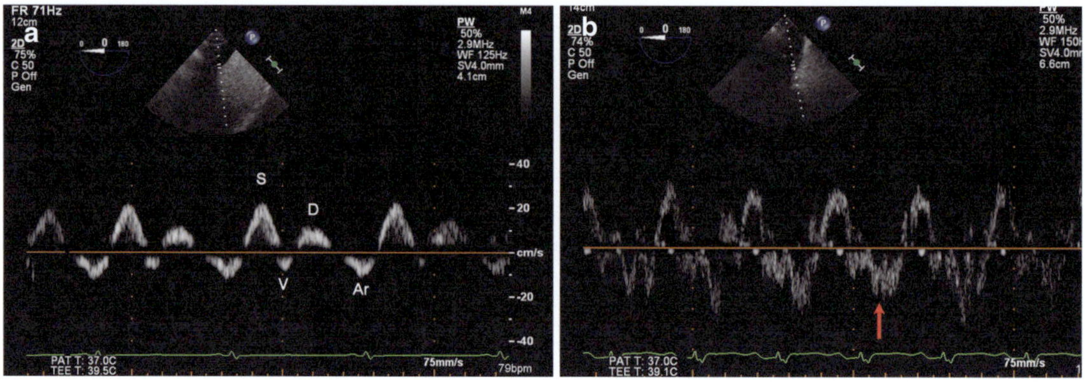

Fig. 10.12 Pulsed-wave Doppler tracing of hepatic venous flow. (**a**) The top panel demonstrates normal hepatic vein flow with positive systolic (S) and diastolic (D) waves and brief negative atrial (Ar) wave and variably present V-wave (V). (**b**) The bottom panel demonstrates systolic flow reversal (*red arrow*), confirming severe tricuspid regurgitation

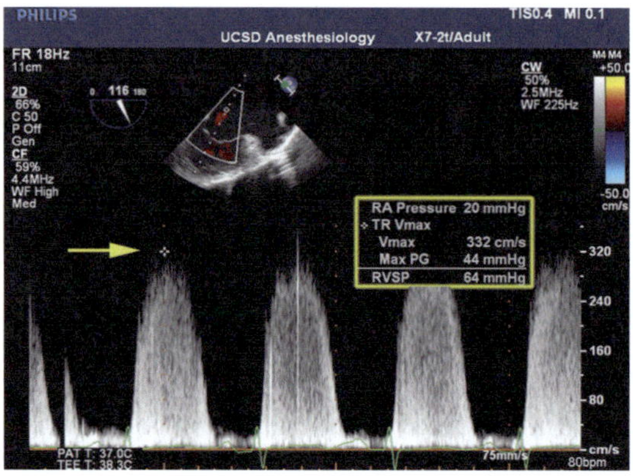

Fig. 10.13 Continuous-wave Doppler tracing of the tricuspid regurgitation jet in a midesophageal modified bicaval TV view. Applying the modified Bernoulli equation to the peak TR jet (*yellow arrow*) yields an estimation of right ventricular and pulmonary arterial systolic pressure (RA pressure is previously measured at 20 mmHg)

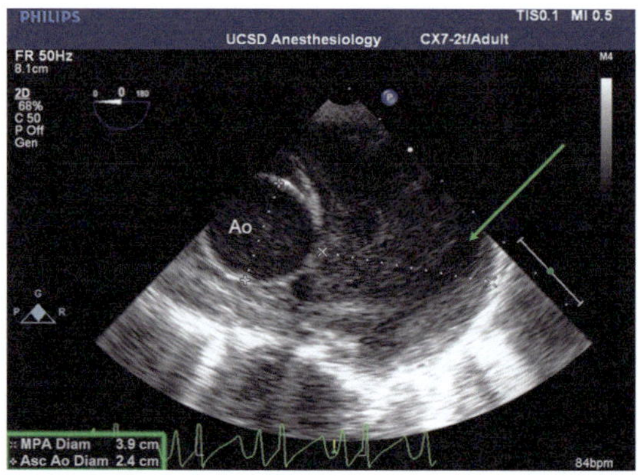

Fig. 10.14 Midesophageal ascending aortic short-axis view with slight leftward probe rotation demonstrates significant pulmonary artery dilation (*green arrow*), measuring larger than the aortic diameter. *Ao* ascending aorta

(RVOT) and parasternal short-axis (PA bifurcation) views with TTE (Fig. 10.14). A view of the main PA allows measurement of RV *cardiac output* (CO), which serves as a load-dependent index of global RV systolic function. With TEE, the right-sided stroke volume can be calculated using pulsed-wave Doppler in the ME ascending aortic short-axis or UE aortic arch short-axis views to obtain the right ventricular outflow tract (RVOT) or PA velocity-time integral (VTI) and the RVOT or PA diameter, respectively [33]. With TTE, the parasternal short-axis (RVOT) view allows the same measurements. Doppler-derived RV CO provides a method to detect right-sided CO, despite the presence of significant TR, and should be similar to the left-sided CO, in the absence of significant intracardiac shunting.

$$\text{RV CO} = \begin{bmatrix} \pi \text{ x} \left(\text{RVOT}_{\text{diameter}} / 2\right)^2 \\ \text{x VTI}_{\text{RVOT}} \end{bmatrix} \text{x HR} \quad (4)$$

Interatrial Septum

Interatrial septum position also serves as an indicator of right heart function. With RV failure, the high right-sided pressure is transmitted to the RA, leading to increasing RA pressure and shifting of the interatrial septum toward the LA. With TEE, this is usually more apparent in the ME four-chamber, ME RV inflow-outflow, or ME

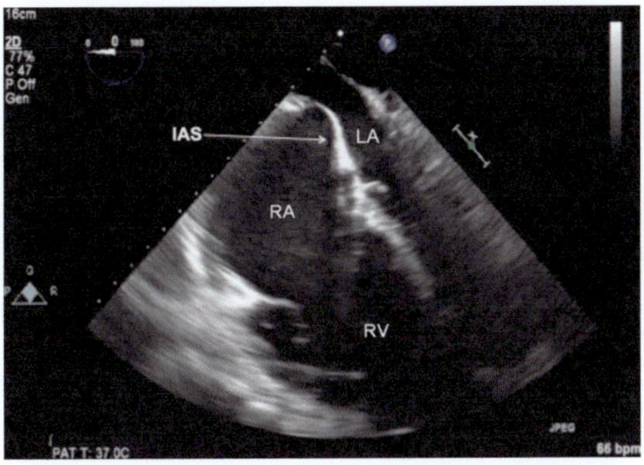

Fig. 10.15 Midesophageal four-chamber view in a patient with significant right atrial (RA) dilation and high RA pressure, noted by a shifted interatrial septum (IAS) toward the left atrium (LA). *RV* right ventricle

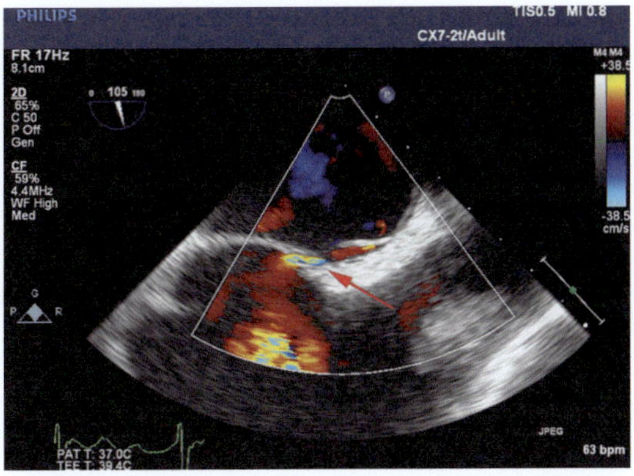

Fig. 10.16 Midesophageal bicaval view in a patient with a patent foramen ovale (*red arrow*) and right-to-left flow on color flow Doppler

bicaval views, as septal bowing toward the left atrium throughout the cardiac cycle can be appreciated (Fig. 10.15; Video 10.6). With TTE, the view of the septum can be appreciated from the apical four-chamber or parasternal short-axis (RVOT) views. In patient populations where RA pressures exceed LA pressures, there is an increased incidence of patent foramen ovale (PFO) compared to the estimated 25% of the adult population. This can lead to clinically significant right-to-left intracardiac shunting [18]. The shunting may be detected with echocardiography using color flow Doppler or agitated saline, most commonly in the ME bicaval or apical four-chamber view [30] (Fig. 10.16; Video 10.7).

Acute Pulmonary Embolism

Pulmonary embolism (PE) is a potentially fatal condition with significant morbidity and mortality when associated with hemodynamic instability [34]. An acute PE causes a sudden increase in RV afterload, resulting in RV dilation and dysfunction. The acute pressure increase also displaces the IVS, further contributing to RV failure. Both the decreased right-sided cardiac output and the septal shift lead to underfilling of the LV. Massive PE should be considered with the onset of unexplainable severe and sudden hypoxia or hypotension [35].

The most common echocardiographic findings in hemodynamically significant acute pulmonary embolism are RV dilatation and RV dysfunction, with preservation of the motility of the apex in some cases (McConnell's sign). Ninety percent of patients with a large pulmonary embolism will develop ventricular hypokinesis [36]. Other signs are dilatation of the IVC with a lack of respiratory variation, IVS flattening and paradoxical systolic motion, and PA dilatation, together with TR or pulmonary regurgitation. Patients with an acute PE will have marked prolongation of the IVCT and IVRT, resulting in an increased RV-MPI over LV-MPI, which helps differentiate chronic versus acute PH from PE. With an acute PE, there is no time for the LV to adapt, and the LV-MPI does not increase [37]. While observing an acutely dilated and dysfunctional right heart is suggestive of a PE, it is not a specific or diagnostic finding. Observation of thromboembolic material in the right heart (thrombus-in-transit), either in the RA, RV, or PA, is a diagnostic finding (Fig. 10.17; Video 10.8). However, the contrary holds true: observation of a normal-sized RA and RV with normal RV function renders the diagnosis of a hemodynamically significant PE unlikely. A thorough echocardiography exam is therefore imperative to observe the effects of acutely increased pulmonary afterload as well as to directly visualize embolized thrombi within the right heart chambers and the pulmonary arteries [37].

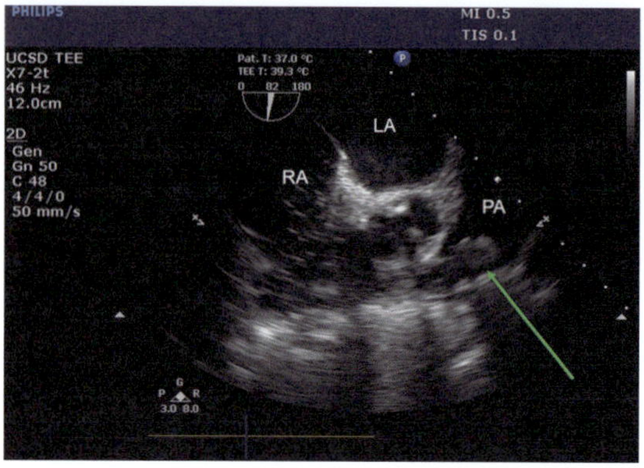

Fig. 10.17 Midesophageal RV inflow-outflow view demonstrating a thrombus-in-transit (*green arrow*) in a patient experiencing a pulmonary embolism. *RA* right atrium, *LA* left atrium, *PA* main pulmonary artery

Assessment of the Right Ventricle with Left Ventricular Assist Devices

In patients receiving left ventricular assist device (LVAD) implantation, outcomes depend on the function of the right heart and its ability to generate sufficient flow through the pulmonary vasculature to the left heart. As such, right ventricular failure (RVF) post-LVAD is associated with significantly worse morbidity and mortality. Prior to device implantation, echocardiography should be combined with clinical signs and symptoms to determine the extent of RV dysfunction in order to inform the management plan (i.e., the necessity of additional right-sided support) [38]. While no single quantitative parameter has been found to be predictive of RVF post-LVAD implantation, a purely qualitative echocardiographic assessment demonstrating more than moderate RV dysfunction is highly predictive of RVF [39]. An aggregate assessment using relevant right-sided quantitative measures, such as TR severity, RAP estimate, RV FAC, and TAPSE, may be useful in the clinical decision-making process. Post-implantation, echocardiography should be used to assess RV function in relation to volume status and LV loading and unloading and adjusting the LVAD speed. The position of the IAS and IVS and relative sizes of the RV and LV aid in this assessment. In the presence of normal loading conditions and function, both the IAS and IVS will be positioned midline. Excessive leftward deviation of the IVS, accompanied by a small LV, dilated RV, and rightward bowing IAS, suggests RVF and should prompt reductions in LVAD speed and augmentation of RV performance. Excessive rightward deviation of the IVS suggests insufficient LVAD unloading and should prompt increases in LVAD speed. The presence of both ventricles appearing small suggests hypovolemia [39].

Conclusion

Left ventricular physiology has overshadowed the study of the RV for many years. With advances in echocardiography, new opportunities have emerged for studying the important function of the RV and its effects on patient outcomes. Echocardiography is a helpful tool for the clinician who faces acutely ill patients and can help in the identification and management of right heart dysfunction, as well as identifying which patients are at highest risk of an adverse outcome related to RV failure.

Questions

1. Which of the following views is *least* helpful for assessing right ventricular function?

   A. Midesophageal right ventricular inflow-outflow view
   B. Transgastric midpapillary short-axis view
   C. Midesophageal bicaval view
   D. Apical four-chamber view

2. Which of the following suggests normal right ventricular systolic performance?

   A. Tricuspid annular plane systolic excursion (TAPSE) of 16 mm
   B. Fractional area change (FAC) of 30%
   C. Tissue Doppler S' of 10 cm/s
   D. Flattening of the interventricular septum at end-systole

3. In which clinical situation would you most expect to observe an eccentricity index (EI) > 1 during end-diastole?

    A. Atrial septal defect with a large left-to-right shunt
    B. Chronic thromboembolic pulmonary hypertension with right ventricular dilation
    C. Severe tricuspid regurgitation in a patient with infective endocarditis
    D. All of the above

4. A patient has a transduced central venous pressure of 10 mmHg and a tricuspid regurgitation peak jet velocity of 2.74 m/s. What is the estimated right ventricular systolic pressure?

    A. 20 mmHg
    B. 30 mmHg
    C. 40 mmHg
    D. 50 mmHg

5. Which of the following is true regarding the moderator band?

    A. It can be visualized in the midesophageal bicaval view.
    B. It extends from the lateral tricuspid annulus to the interventricular septum.
    C. It is easy to differentiate from thrombus or intracavitary lesion.
    D. It becomes prominent in patients with right ventricular hypertrophy.

6. Which of the following is true regarding the right ventricle?

    A. Contraction is sequential, beginning with the infundibulum contracting toward the base, and ending with the inlet portion.
    B. Its vascular supply is primarily from the circumflex coronary artery.
    C. It provides a similar stroke volume as the left ventricle.
    D. The interventricular septum contributes only to left ventricular systolic function.

7. Which of the following findings may be seen in an acute pulmonary embolism?

    A. Decreased left ventricular stroke volume
    B. Decreased contractility of the apex of the right ventricle with preserved function at the base
    C. Prolongation of the IVCT and shortening of the IVRT
    D. Decreased cardiac output with IVC collapse during inspiration

8. Which of the following is most true?

    A. The shape and function of the right ventricle is similar to the shape and function of the left ventricle.
    B. The blood supply to the right ventricle is primarily during diastole in the setting of suprasystemic pulmonary hypertension.
    C. The RVOT is not visible from the parasternal long-axis view.
    D. Trabeculations in the right ventricle are usually not visible by echo.

9. Paradoxical motion of the interventricular septum during systole is seen in which of the following?

    A. Severe acute tricuspid regurgitation due to infective endocarditis
    B. Pulmonic stenosis due to carcinoid heart syndrome
    C. Atrial septal defect with left-to-right shunt
    D. All of the above

10. What is the definition of severe RV hypertrophy?

    A. End-diastolic RV free wall thickness > 1.0 cm.
    B. End-systolic RV free wall thickness > 0.5 cm.
    C. End-systolic RV free wall thickness > 1.0 cm.
    D. End-diastolic RV free wall thickness > 0.5 cm.

References

1. Reeves ST, Finley AC, Skubas NJ, Swaminathan M, Whitley WS, Glas KE, et al. Basic perioperative transesophageal echocardiography examination: a consensus statement of the American Society of Echocardiography and the Society of Cardiovascular Anesthesiologists. J Am Soc Echocardiogr. 2013;26(5):443–56.
2. Hahn RT, Abraham T, Adams MS, et al. Guidelines for performing a comprehensive transesophageal echocardiographic examination: recommendations from the American Society of Echocardiography and the Society of Cardiovascular Anesthesiologists. J Am Soc Echocardiogr. 2013;26:921–64.
3. Rudski LG, Lai WW, Afilalo J, et al. Guidelines for the echocardiographic assessment of the right heart in adults: a report from the American Society of Echocardiography endorsed by the European Association of Echocardiography, a registered branch of the European Society of Cardiology, and the Canadian Society of Echocardiography. J Am Soc Echocardiogr. 2010;23:685–713; quiz 86-8.
4. Ho SY, Nihoyannopoulos P. Anatomy, echocardiography, and normal right ventricular dimensions. Heart. 2006;92(Suppl 1):i2–13.
5. Farb A, Burke AP, Virmani R. Anatomy and pathology of the right ventricle (including acquired tricuspid and pulmonic valve disease). Cardiol Clin. 1992;10:1–21.5.
6. Dell'Italia LJ. The right ventricle: anatomy, physiology, and clinical importance. Curr Probl Cardiol. 1991;16:653–720.
7. Jiang L, Wiegers S, Weyman A. Right ventricle. In: Weyman A, editor. Principles and practice of echocardiography. 2nd ed. Philadelphia: Lea & Febiger; 1994. p. 901–21.
8. Lee FA. Hemodynamics of the right ventricle in normal and disease states. Cardiol Clin. 1992;10:59–67.
9. Kaul S. The interventricular septum in health and disease. Am Heart J. 1986;112:568–81.
10. Lindqvist P, Morner S, Karp K, Waldenstrom A. New aspects of septal function by using 1-dimensional strain and strain rate imaging. J Am Soc Echocardiogr. 2006;19:1345–9.
11. Klima U, Guerrero JL, Vlahakes GJ. Contribution of the interventricular septum to maximal right ventricular function. Eur J Cardiothorac Surg. 1998;14:250–5.
12. Santamore WP, Dell'Italia LJ. Ventricular interdependence: significant left ventricular contributions to right ventricular systolic function. Prog Cardiovasc Dis. 1998;40:289–308.
13. Kenneth D. Horton; assessment of the right ventricle by echocardiography: a primer for cardiac sonographers. J Am Soc Echocardiogr. 2009;22:776–92.
14. Simonneau G, Hoeper MM. The revised definition of pulmonary hypertension: exploring the impact on patient management. Eur Heart J Suppl. 2019;21(Suppl K):K4–8.
15. Bartels K, Karhausen J, Sullivan B, et al. Update on perioperative right heart assessment using transesophageal echocardiography. Semin Cardiothorac Vasc Anesth. 2014;18(4):341–51.
16. Galie N, Hoeper MM, Humbert M, et al. ESC Committee for practice guidelines (CPG). Guidelines for the diagnosis and treatment of pulmonary hypertension: the task force for the diagnosis and treatment of pulmonary hypertension of the European Society of Cardiology (ESC) and the European Respiratory Society (ERS), Endorsed by the International Society of Heart and Lung Transplantation (ISHLT). Eur Heart J. 2009;30:2493–537.
17. Dadfarmay S, Berkowitz R, Kim B, et al. Differentiating pulmonary arterial and pulmonary venous hypertension and the implications for therapy. Congest Heart Fail. 2010;16:287–91.
18. Lang RM, Badano LP, Mor-Avi V, et al. Recommendations for cardiac chamber quantification by echocardiography in adults: An Update from the American Society of Echocardiography and the European Association of Cardiovascular Imaging. J Am Soc Echocardiogr. 2015;28:1–39.
19. Lindqvist P, Calcutteea A, Henein M. Echocardiography in the assessment of right heart function. Eur J Echocardiogr. 2008;9:225–34.Samad BA, Alam M, Jensen-Urstad K. Prognostic impact of right ventricular involvement as assessed by tricuspid annular motion in patients with acute myocardial infarction. Am J Cardiol 2002;90:778–81.
20. Cacciapuoti F. Echocardiographic evaluation of right heart function and pulmonary vascular bed. Int J Cardiovasc Imaging. 2009;25:689–97.
21. Perrino AC, Reeves ST. A practical approach to transesophageal echocardiography. 3rd ed. Philadelphia: Wolters Kluwer Health/Lippincott Williams & Wilkins; 2013.
22. Anavekar NS, Gerson D, Skali H, Kwong RY, Yucel EK, Solomon SD. Two-dimensional assessment of right ventricular function: an echocardiographic-MRI correlative study. Echocardiography. 2007;24:452–6.
23. Tei C, Ling LH, Hodge DO, et al. New index of combined systolic and diastolic myocardial performance: a simple and reproducible measure of cardiac function--a study in normals and dilated cardiomyopathy. J Cardiol. 1995;26:357–66.
24. Tei C, Dujardin KS, Hodge DO, et al. Doppler echocardiographic index for assessment of global right ventricular function. J Am Soc Echocardiogr. 1996;9:838–47.
25. Pavlicek M, Wahl A, Rutz T, et al. Right ventricular systolic function assessment: rank of echocardiographic methods vs. cardiac magnetic resonance imaging. Eur J Echocardiogr. 2011;12:871–80.
26. Karnati PK, et al. Myocardial performance index correlates well with right ventricular ejection fraction measured by nuclear ventriculography. Echocardiography. 2008;25:381–5.
27. Ryan T, Petrovic O, Dillon JC, et al. An echocardiographic index for separation of right ventricular

volume and pressure overload. J Am Coll Cardiol. 1985;5(4):918–27.
28. Gaynor SL, Maniar HS, Bloch JB, et al. Right atrial and ventricular adaptation to chronic right ventricular pressure overload. Circulation. 2005;112(suppl I):I-212–8.
29. Banks DA, Pretorius GV, Kerr KM, et al. Pulmonary endarterectomy: part I. pathophysiology, clinical manifestations, and diagnostic evaluation of chronic thromboebolic pulmonary hypertension. Semin Cardiothorac Vasc Anesth. 2014:Pii:1089253214536621.
30. Badano LP, Muraru D, Enriquez-Sarano M. Assessment of functional tricuspid regurgitation. Eur Heart J. 2013.
31. Antunes MJ, Barlow JB. Management of tricuspid valve regurgitation. Heart. 2007;93:271–6.
32. Mangano DT. Immediate hemodynamic and pulmonary changes following pulmonary thromboembolism. Anesthesiology. 1980;52:173.
33. Maslow A, Comunale ME, Haering JM, Watkins J. Pulsed wave Doppler measurement of cardiac output from the right ventricular outflow tract. Anesth Analg. 1996;83:466–71.
34. Kucher N, Rossi E, De Rosa M, et al. Massive pulmonary embolism. Circulation. 2006;113:577–82.
35. Mookadam F, Jiamsripong P, Goel R, et al. Critical appraisal on the utility of echocardiography in the management of acute pulmonary embolism. Cardiol Rev. 2010;18(1):29–37.
36. Hsiao SH, Lee CY, Chang SM, et al. Pulmonary embolism and right heart function: Insights from myocardial Doppler tissue imaging. J Am Soc Echocardiography. 2006;19:822–88.
37. Cohen R, Loarte P, Navarro V, et al. Echocardiographic findings in pulmonary embolism: An important guide for the management of the patient. World J Cardiovasc Dis. 2012;2:161–4.
38. Stainback R, Estep J, Agler D, et al. Echocardiography in the management of patients with left ventricular assist devices: recommendations form the American Society of Echocardiography. J Am Soc Echocardiogr. 2015;28:853–909.
39. Nicoara A, Skubas N, Ad N, et al. Guidelines for the use of transesophageal echocardiography to assist with surgical decision-making in the operating room: a surgery-based approach: from the American Society of Echocardiography in collaboration with the Society of Cardiovascular Anesthesiologists and the Society of Thoracic Surgeons. J Am Soc Echocardiogr. 2020;33(6):692–734.
40. Simonneau G, et al. Hemodynamic definitions and updated clinical classification of pulmonary hypertension. "Proceedings of the 6th World Symposium on Pulmonary Hypertension". Eur Respir J. 2019;53:1801913.

Atria

11

Quoc-Sy Nguyen and Perin Kothari

Abbreviations

A2C	Apical two-chamber
A4C	Apical four-chamber
CS	Coronary sinus
EF	Emptying fraction
IAS	Interatrial septum
IVC	Inferior vena cava
LA	Left atrium
LAA	Left atrial appendage
LAX	Long-axis
LUPV	Left upper pulmonary vein
LVEDP	Left ventricular end-diastolic pressure
ME	Midesophageal
PFO	Patent foramen ovale
PLAX	Parasternal long-axis
PV	Pulmonary vein
PWD	Pulsed-wave Doppler
RA	Right atrium
RAA	Right atrial appendage
RV	Right ventricle
SA	Sinoatrial
SAX	Short-axis
SVC	Superior vena cava
TEE	Transesophageal echocardiography
TTE	Transthoracic echocardiography

Supplementary Information The online version of this chapter (https://doi.org/10.1007/978-3-030-84349-6_11) contains supplementary material, which is available to authorized users.

Q.-S. Nguyen (✉)
Department of Anesthesiology, University of California San Diego Health, La Jolla, CA, USA
e-mail: q6nguyen@health.ucsd.edu

P. Kothari
Division of Cardiothoracic Anesthesiology, Department of Anesthesiology, Perioperative, and Pain Medicine Stanford University School of Medicine, Stanford, CA, USA

Introduction

The atrial chambers of the heart normally consist of a morphologic left and right atrium (LA and RA, respectively), separated by an interatrial septum (IAS). They are thin-walled structures that facilitate circulation by rhythmically relaxing and contracting to allow venous blood flow into the ventricles. While the overarching functions of the atria are similar, each is markedly different in structure and components. It is therefore prudent to understand the basic anatomy of each atrium to fully appreciate them in the context of echocardiography.

The Right Atrium

Anatomy

The RA is formed from the division of the primitive atria into a right side that fuses with the sinus

T. M. Maus, C. R. Tainter (eds.), *Essential Echocardiography*,
https://doi.org/10.1007/978-3-030-84349-6_11

venosus and joins at a groove called the sulcus terminalis. It receives deoxygenated blood from various sources including the superior vena cava (SVC), inferior vena cava (IVC), coronary sinus (CS), and small cardiac veins. The RA is positioned anteriorly relative to the LA. The anterior wall is comprised mainly of the right atrial appendage (RAA), which is triangular in shape and is demarcated laterally from the posterior wall by the sulcus terminalis. By surgically dissecting the RA along the sulcus terminalis and rotating the flap leftward, the internal structures can then be visualized (Fig. 11.1). The sulcus terminalis internally corresponds to the crista terminalis, which is the origin of the pectinate muscles forming the anterior wall and RAA. The crista terminalis separates the pectinate anterior wall from the smooth posterior wall, formed by the sinus venosus and the IAS.

The SVC and IVC drain into the RA laterally along the superior and inferior borders, respectively. The sinoatrial (SA) node, although not visualized, is typically located below the epicardium within the sulcus terminalis at the junction of the SVC and RA. The eustachian valve is located at the junction of the IVC and RA and is a remnant of the valve of the IVC. During fetal circulation, the eustachian valve functions to direct oxygenated blood (from the umbilical vein) through the fossa ovalis into the LA, bypassing the right heart and lungs.

The posterior wall of the RA is largely comprised of the IAS. The CS empties into the RA along the inferior aspect of the posterior wall medial to the IVC. At the opening of the CS lies the Thebesian valve (valve of the coronary sinus). At the base of the IAS near the tricuspid valve lies the AV node, which is not visualized echocardiographically.

Size

The RA can be adequately assessed via TTE and TEE, as both modalities are able to image the chamber in its entirety. Although there is less research and clinical data when compared to LA chamber quantification, TTE data from three cohorts totaling more than 2400 patients have yielded normal values for RA dimensions [1]. RA size is more gender-dependent when compared to LA size, even when indexed to body surface area (BSA) [1]. Similar to the LA, RA remodeling is not symmetric. However, the lack of standard orthogonal TTE and TEE view of the RA prevents the use of biplane imaging. Therefore, only single-plane imaging is performed for RA chamber quantification, with the recommended views being the A4C and ME 4C for TTE and TEE, respectively.

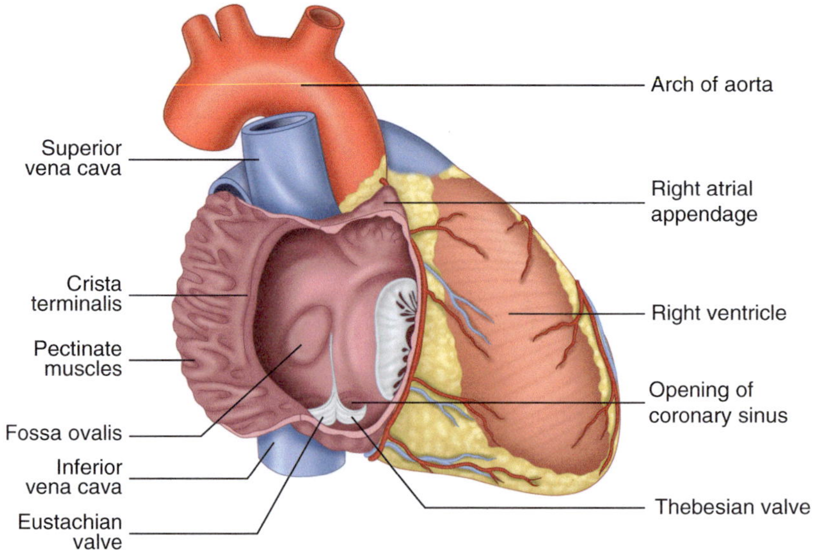

Fig. 11.1 Diagram of the heart with the right atrial free wall resected, allowing visualization of right atrial anatomy

Right atrial measurements should be performed at end-systole prior to TV opening. The three measurements for assessing RA size in order of accuracy include linear dimension, area, and volume. Normal values are shown in Table 11.1.

Linear Dimension

The linear dimensions are obtained with TTE in the A4C and TEE in the ME 4C view (Fig. 11.2a, b). The image should be optimized to maximize RA length so that it is aligned with the true long axis. Similar to the LA, the base of the RA should be at its largest size to ensure that the maximal RA short-axis area is obtained [2].

Area

Area is obtained with TTE in the A4C and TEE in the ME 4C view using planimetry to trace the endocardial border, excluding the area under the tricuspid valve (TV) annulus and RAA (Figs. 11.3 and 11.4).

Table 11.1 RA size, normal ranges, and severity by TTE

Parameter	Normal	Enlarged	Male	Female
RAd (cm/m^2) indexed by BSA Major axis			2.4 ± 0.3	2.5 ± 0.3
RAd (cm/m^2) indexed by BSA Minor axis			1.9 ± 0.3	1.9 ± 0.3
RA area (cm^2)	≤ 18	> 18		
RA volume index by BSA (ml/m^2)			25 ± 7	21 ± 6

RA right atrium, *RAd* right atrial diameter, *BSA* body surface area

Volume

Volume is obtained with TTE in the A4C and TEE in the ME 4C view. It is the recommended measurement modality for assessing RA size, as there are less geometric assumptions when compared to linear dimension and area [1]. The approaches for calculating volume are the same as for the LA and most commonly include the disc summation technique (Fig. 11.3). The disc summation technique, also known as the modified biplane or Simpson's technique, is similar to the method of left ventricular volume estimation (see Chap. 6) and estimates

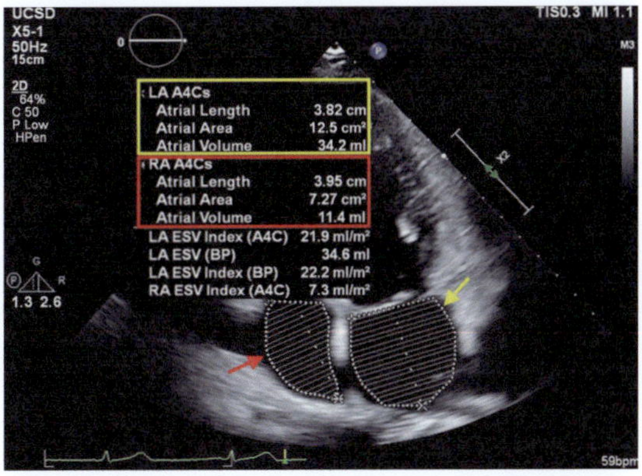

Fig. 11.3 Apical four-chamber view demonstrating a tracing of the left (*yellow arrow*) and right atria (*red arrow*). On-board software calculates atrial length, area, and volume based upon the tracing dimensions

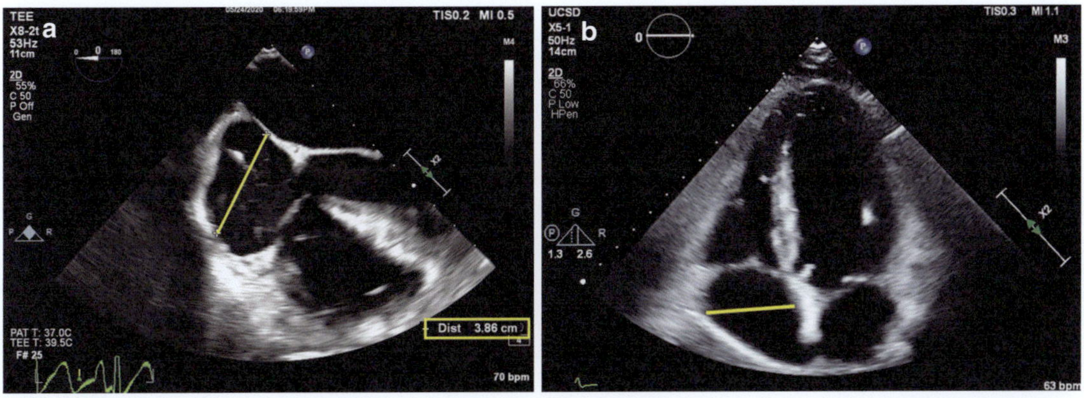

Fig. 11.2 (**a**) Midesophageal four-chamber view demonstrating linear size measurement of the right atrium (*yellow line*). (**b**) Apical four-chamber view demonstrating linear size measurement of the right atrium (*yellow line*)

right atrial volume using the diameter and height measurements to divide the RA into a stack of equal-height discs of differing diameter. The volume of each disc is calculated as $\pi r^2 \times h$ (where r is the radius of each disc and h is the height of the disc; each determined by the ultrasound machine software after tracing the RA), and the summation of the individual disc volumes results in the estimation of right atrial volume. The technique is performed with TTE in the A2C and A4C views utilizing the on-machine software and requires tracing of the RA endocardial borders, similar to the area method.

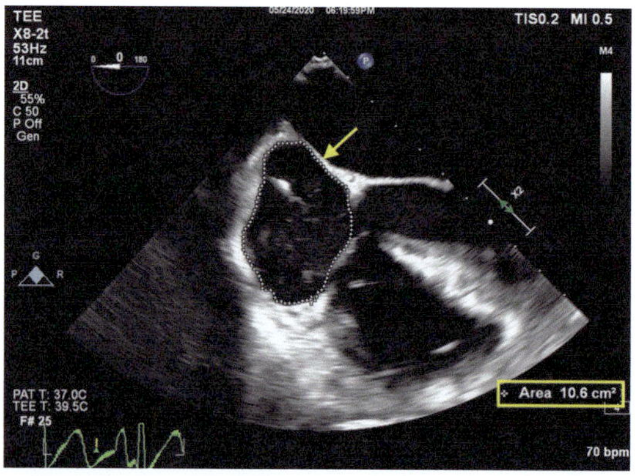

Fig. 11.4 Midesophageal four-chamber view demonstrating a tracing (*yellow arrow*) of the right atrium with resultant area calculation (*yellow box*)

The Left Atrium

Anatomy

The LA is formed from the division of the primitive atria. It receives oxygenated blood from the four pulmonary veins (PVs): left upper (LUPV), left lower (LLPV), right upper (RUPV), and right lower pulmonary veins (RLPV). The LA is positioned posterior and superior to the RA. The anterior wall of the LA is adjacent to the aortic root. The left atrial appendage (LAA) is located along the superolateral aspect of the LA, and its structure is smaller and more tubular in shape than the RAA. The LAA is bilobed in 54% and multilobed in 80% of patients [3]. The PVs enter along the posterior wall of LA. This wall is anterior and adjacent to the esophagus and thoracic aorta. The ligament of Marshall is a remnant of the oblique vein of the LA and is located on the epicardium between the LAA and LUPV. Its appearance may be confused with a

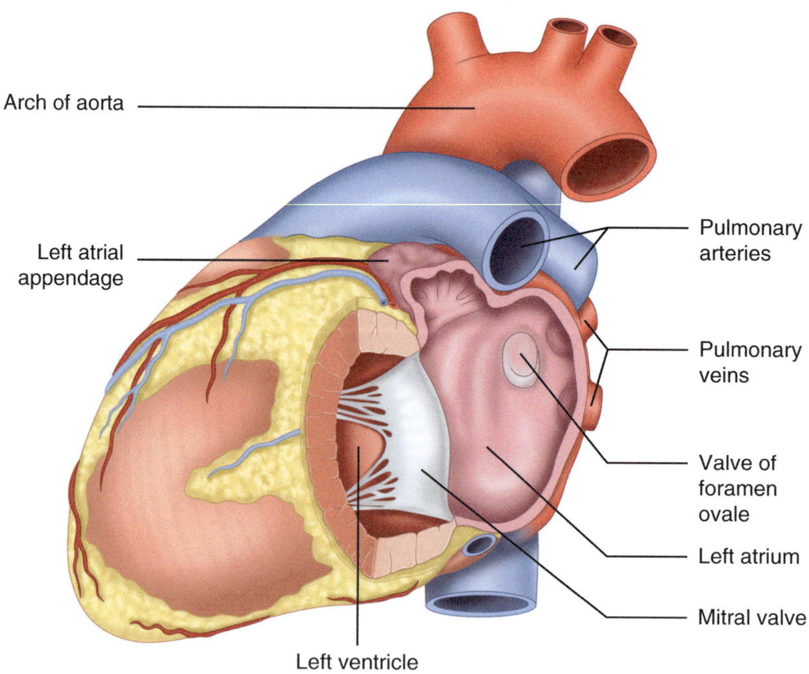

Fig. 11.5 Diagram of the heart with the left atrial free wall resected allowing visualization of left atrial anatomy

thrombus, prompting its alias, the coumadin ridge. The endocardium of the LA is smooth except for the pectinate muscles making up the LAA (Fig. 11.5). Unlike the RA, the LA does not contain a crista terminalis that demarcates the smooth and pectinate areas. The medial or septal wall of the LA contains the small crescent-shaped valve of the foramen ovale, resulting from the septum primum.

The LA functions to regulate LV filling and can be broken down into three major roles: reservoir, conduit, and pump. Each of these roles corresponds to a specific phase in the cardiac cycle and is intimately related to ventricular diastolic function. As a reservoir, the LA normally contributes roughly 40% of LV systolic volume [4]. It is affected by atrial compliance and relaxation, right ventricular (RV) systolic function, and descent of the LV base during systole. During early ventricular diastole, the LA becomes a passive conduit for PV blood flow into the LV. This normally contributes approximately 35% of LV systolic volume [4]. It is affected by atrial compliance, as well as LV relaxation and stiffness. Finally, during late ventricular diastole, the LA acts as a pump to augment ventricular filling. Active contraction of the LA normally contributes about 25% of LV systolic volume [4]. The pump function is dependent on the magnitude and timing of the intrinsic atrial contraction, in addition to being influenced by LA preload, left ventricular end-diastolic pressure (LVEDP), and LV compliance.

While the importance of LA size has been discussed extensively, there are data that LA function has an even stronger prognostic value in patients with cardiovascular disease [5]. Utilizing echocardiography, LA function can be described based on its individual roles using volumetric analysis, spectral Doppler, and tissue Doppler. Deformation analysis is a newer technique that is being increasingly studied; however it is beyond the scope of this chapter. Of note, echocardiographic evaluation of left atrial function is not routinely included in a basic perioperative echocardiography or critical care echocardiography exam.

Size

Left atrial size has a significant association with adverse cardiovascular outcomes and is a strong predictor of cardiovascular morbidity and mortality [4]. With LA enlargement, there is an increased incidence of atrial fibrillation and strokes, in addition to increased risk of mortality after myocardial infarction, and negative clinical outcomes in patients with dilated cardiomyopathy [4]. It is also an indicator of the burden and magnitude of left ventricular diastolic disease [5].

Transthoracic echocardiography is recommended for assessment of LA size, as the entirety of the atrium can be visualized. Due to the position of the TEE probe in the esophagus in close proximity to the LA, the entire LA structure cannot be visualized in a single imaging plane. This makes quantitative assessment difficult with TEE, underestimating LA area and volume when compared to TTE. While TEE is inadequate to assess area and volume, linear measurement with TEE has been correlated with TTE, though normative data is limited [6].

All TTE/TEE atrial measurements should be performed at end-systole, prior to the mitral valve opening. Care should be taken to avoid foreshortening the chamber to allow viewing of the LA at its greatest size. Once those views are obtained, the three measurements for assessing LA size include the linear dimension, area, and volume. LA parameters are shown in Table 11.2. It is important to note that while LA dimensions and

Table 11.2 LA size, normal ranges, and severity by transthoracic echocardiography

Parameter	Normal	Mild	Moderate	Severe	Male	Female
LAd AP dimension (cm)					3.0–4.0	2.7–3.8
LAd AP dimension indexed by BSA (cm/ m^2)	1.5–2.3					
LA area (cm^2)	≤20	21–30	31–40	≥41		
LA volume index by BSA (ml/m^2)	16–34	35–41	42–48	≥48		

LA left atrium, *LAd* left atrial diameter, *AP* anterior-posterior, *BSA* body surface area

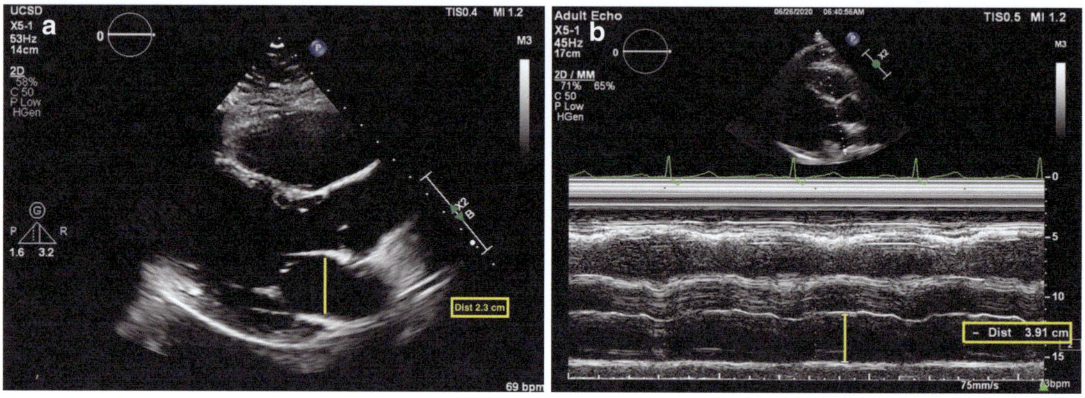

Fig. 11.6 (**a**) Parasternal long-axis view demonstrating linear size measurement of the left atrium (*yellow line*). (**b**) M-mode imaging of parasternal long-axis view demonstrating linear size measurement of left atrium (*yellow line*)

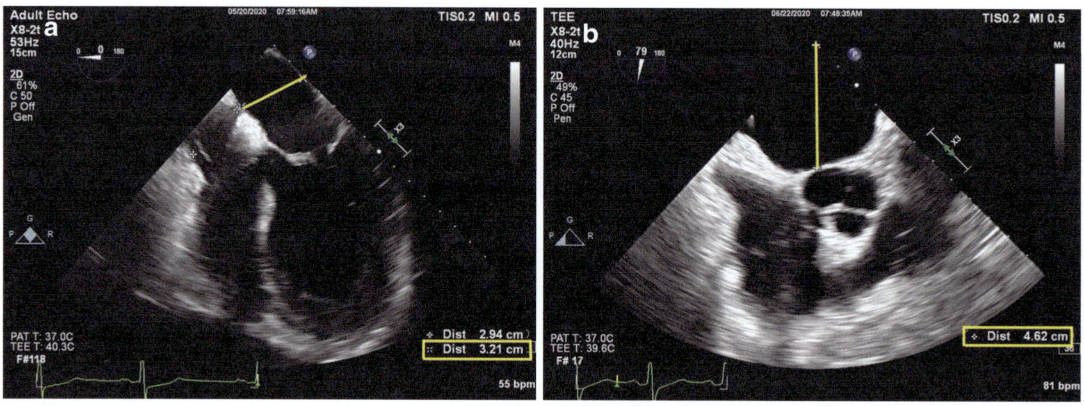

Fig. 11.7 (**a**) Linear size measurement (*yellow line*) of the left atrium in a midesophageal four-chamber view. (**b**) Midesophageal aortic valve short-axis view demonstrating linear size measurement of the left atrium (*yellow line*)

volumes are larger in men versus women, the volumes are similar when normalized to body surface area.

Linear Dimension

Linear dimension is the most widely used and reproducible measurement clinically for assessing LA size [1]. It is obtained with TTE in the parasternal long-axis (PLAX) and A4C views. In the TTE PLAX view, the anteroposterior (AP) diameter is measured at the level of the aortic sinuses (Fig. 11.6a, b). This is done using the distance function in either motion mode (M-mode) or 2D echocardiography, with the latter being the preferred method. M-mode has the advantage of having a high temporal resolution and reproducibility; however 2D imaging allows for better orientation perpendicular to the posterior wall of the LA [1]. In the TTE A4C view, measurement is made mid-atrium between the septal and lateral walls.

With TEE, linear measurement is performed on 2D imaging in the midesophageal four-chamber (ME4C), aortic valve short-axis (ME AV SAX), and aortic valve long-axis views (ME AV LAX) (Fig. 11.7a, b). Measurements made with TEE in the ME 4C view correlate with the TTE A4C view, whereas the ME AV SAX and LAX views correlate with the TTE PLAX view [6]. The assumption when using the linear dimension to quantify LA size is that the atrium enlarges equally in all directions. This is not always the case during LA remodeling; therefore linear dimension should be used in con-

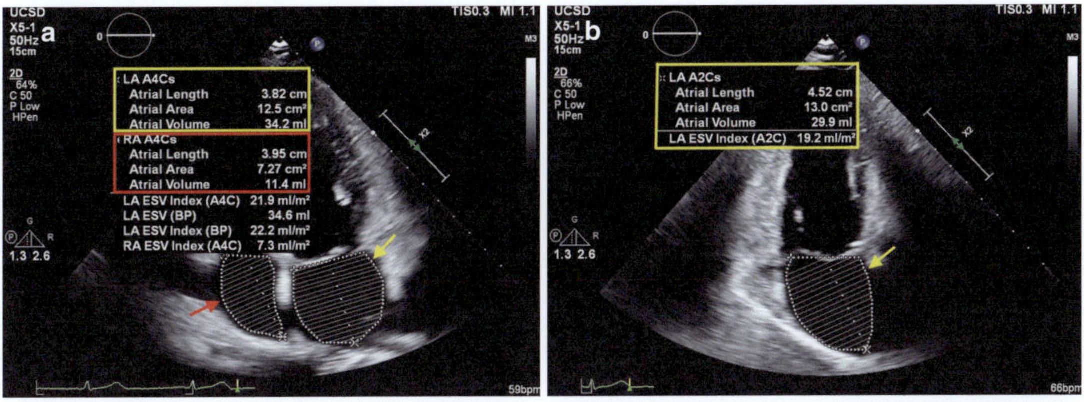

Fig. 11.8 (**a**) Apical four-chamber view demonstrating a tracing of the left (*yellow arrow*) and right atria (*red arrow*). On-board software calculates atrial length, area, and volume based upon the tracing dimensions. (**b**) Apical two-chamber view demonstrating a tracing of the left atrium (*yellow arrow*). On-board software calculates atrial length, area, and volume. Utilizing both apical four and two-chamber views allows biplane estimation of atrial volume

junction with other measurements, including area and volume.

Area

Area of the LA is obtained with TTE in the apical two-chamber (A2C) and A4C views (Fig. 11.8a, b). It should be measured in both planes if possible, as atrial dimensions may not change symmetrically. The endocardial borders should be adequately visualized, with the base of the LA at its largest size to ensure that the maximal LA short-axis area is obtained [2]. Once the view is optimized, the planimetry function can be used to trace the endocardial border of the LA. The area under the mitral valve annulus, PVs, and LAA should be excluded from this tracing. Area is a more accurate representation of true LA size when compared to linear dimension [1].

Volume

Volume is the most accurate measurement modality when compared to linear dimension and area for assessing LA size, as it theoretically accounts for changes in all directions during LA remodeling. Volume has strong prognostic value in various cardiac diseases, as well as being a stronger predictor of outcomes in cardiac patients when compared to linear dimension [1].

The disc summation technique of the LA volume estimation is utilized in a similar fashion to RA size estimation, again utilizing the diameter and height measurements to divide the LA into a stack of equal-height discs of differing diameter. The volume of each disc is calculated as $\pi r^2 \times h$ (where r is the radius of each disc and h is the height of the disc, each determined by the ultrasound machine software after tracing the LA), and the summation of the individual disc volumes results in the estimation of left atrial volume. The technique is performed with TTE in the A2C and A4C views, using the machine's software, and requires tracing of the LA endocardial borders, similar to the area method (Fig. 11.8a, b). Both planes should be obtained for better accuracy, but if that is not feasible, a single-plane technique can be utilized. While other techniques exist for LA volume estimation, the disc summation technique has fewer geometric assumptions, making it the most precise method to measure LA remodeling [1].

Volumetric analysis considers LA volume at its maximum (LA_{max}) at end-systole prior to MV opening, minimum (LA_{min}) at end-diastole with MV closing, and immediately prior to atrial systole, or the P-wave on the electrocardiogram ($LA_{pre\text{-}A}$). The total, passive, and active emptying fractions (EF) can then be calculated using the values obtained. These EFs are used to describe global LA function, as well as the relative contributions of the reservoir, conduit, and pump func-

Table 11.3 Volumetric indexes of LA function

LA function	LA volume fraction	Calculation
Global function	Total EF	$[(LA_{max} - LA_{min})/LA_{max}]$
Reservoir	Expansion index	$[(LA_{max} - LA_{min})/LA_{min}]$
Conduit	Passive EF	$[(LA_{max} - LA_{pre\text{-}A})/LA_{max}]$
Pump	Active EF	$[(LA_{pre\text{-}A} - LA_{min})/LA_{pre\text{-}A}]$

Reprinted from Hoit [7], with permission from Elsevier
LA left atrium, *EF* emptying fraction, LA_{max} maximum LA volume, LA_{min} minimum LA volume, $LA_{pre\text{-}A}$ pre-atrial systole LA volume

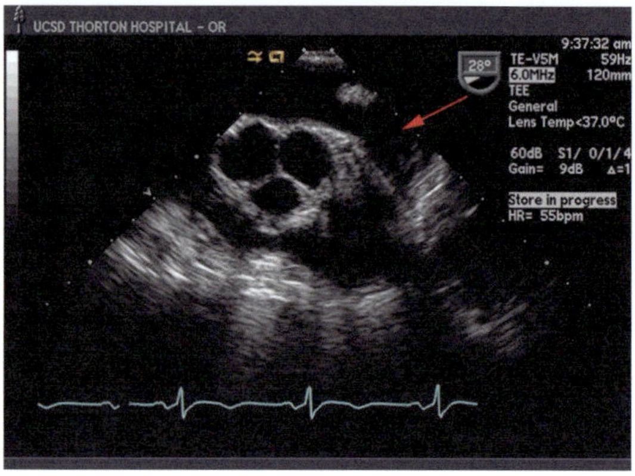

Fig. 11.9 Midesophageal aortic valve short-axis view with the left atrial appendage on the right side of the screen (*red arrow*)

tion of the LA (Table 11.3). Specifically, a total LA EF ≤ 49% has been shown to have increased risk of mortality and new-onset atrial fibrillation and atrial flutter [7]. Of important note, this method is influenced by loading conditions.

Left Atrial Appendage

TEE is the preferred modality to assess the LAA, as its more posterior position in the thoracic cavity prevents a detailed assessment by TTE. The two TEE views for optimal visualization are the ME LAA and ME AV SAX views (Fig. 11.9). If a three-dimensional ultrasound system is available, the use of the X-plane feature to obtain simultaneous orthogonal views can allow for more thorough assessment due to the often multilobed configuration of the LAA.

Echocardiographic assessment of the LAA is part of the standard exam to rule out thrombus, and TEE has a sensitivity and specificity as high as 92% and 98%, respectively [8]. Direct visualization of thrombus formation can be done via 2D and 3D echocardiography (Fig. 11.10a, b; Videos 11.1 and 11.2). It is important to note that normal cardiac structures such as the LAA pectinate muscles and coumadin ridge can be mistaken for thrombus. The observation of spontaneous echo contrast (SEC) in the LA should increase the index of suspicion of LAA thrombus and prompt a detailed examination. Spontaneous echo contrast within the LAA itself is a predictor of thromboembolic risk [3]. During conditions of low flow or blood stasis, rouleaux formation (stacking of cells) of red blood cells causes back-scattering of the ultrasound waves, creating a distinct "smoke" appearance, or spontaneous echo contrast, on imaging (Fig. 11.10a). The density of the spontaneous echo contrast is correlated with increased risk of thromboembolism [9].

Pulsed-wave Doppler (PWD) can aid the evaluation for LAA thrombus. After visualizing the LAA in the views described, place the sample volume of the PWD in the proximal 1/3 segment. In normal patients, peak emptying velocities range from 50 ± 6 cm/s to 83 ± 25 cm/s [9]. Velocities < 40 cm/s on PWD require a closer inspection, and velocities < 20 cm/s are associated with a high incidence of thromboembolism [8] (Fig. 11.11).

The Interatrial Septum

Anatomy

The IAS consists of a true and a false septa. The false septum is the interatrial groove that results from invagination of the atrium that creates a muscular rim. The true septum is formed by the septum primum and septum secundum during

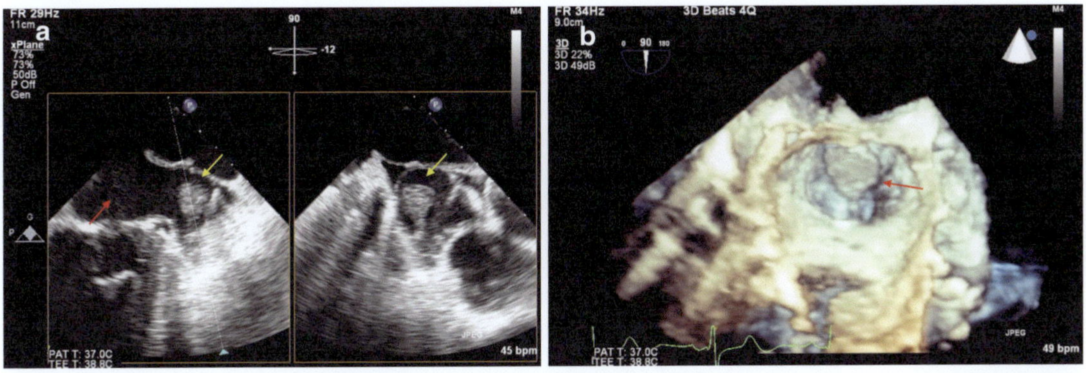

Fig. 11.10 (**a**) X-plane imaging of the midesophageal left atrial appendage view and its orthogonal image. The *red arrow* notes spontaneous echo contrast, and the *yellow arrow* notes a left atrial appendage thrombus. (**b**) Three-dimensional echocardiography of the left atrial appendage. The red *arrow* notes a left atrial appendage thrombus

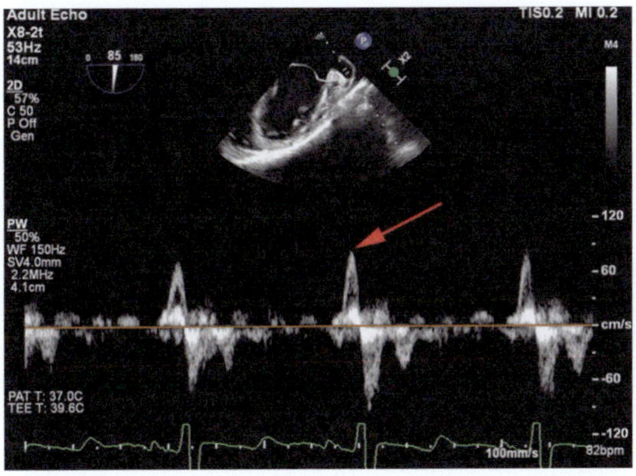

Fig. 11.11 Pulsed-wave Doppler evaluation of the left atrial appendage. The *red arrow* notes the contraction velocity of the left atrial appendage, and aids in assessing the risk of left atrial appendage thrombus formation

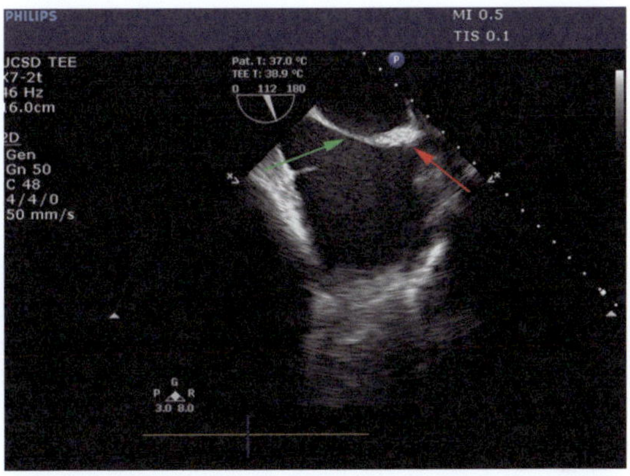

Fig. 11.12 Midesophageal bicaval view with the *red arrow* noting the muscular portion of the interatrial septum, while the *green arrow* notes the membranous portion of the interatrial septum

embryologic development. Together, the false septum leads to the muscular part of the interatrial septum, while the true septum leads to the thin, membrane-like portion of the interatrial septum seen echocardiographically (Fig. 11.12).

During septation of the left and right atria in embryologic development, the septum primum and septum secundum leave a remaining connection between the atria, termed the foramen ovale. The septum primum and secundum overlap, which acts as a one-way valve for blood flow from RA to LA and prevents flow from LA to RA. In utero, this allows oxygenated blood from the IVC to drain from the RA across the patent foramen ovale to the LA and subsequently to the systemic circulation. After birth, as LA pressure increases, the flap is functionally closed. In most patients, there is fusion of the septum primum and septum secundum with the depression formed by the septum primum on the right atrial side, called the fossa ovalis (Fig. 11.1). Up to 25% of patients may have a probe patent foramen ovale (PFO) that may be detectable with echocardiography using color flow Doppler. Reduction of the color flow Doppler scale may be needed to detect the low-velocity flow across the PFO, which typically occurs at the superior rim of the fossa ovalis. The use of a Valsalva technique and its subsequent release can aid in detection of a

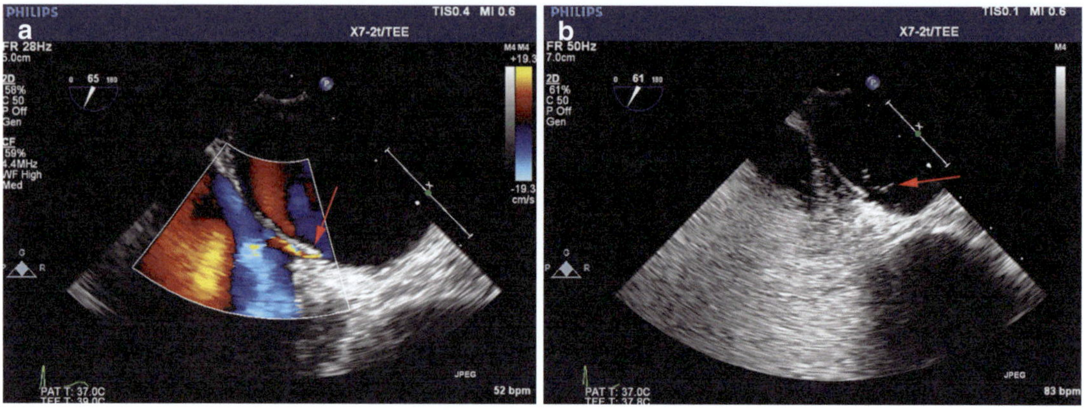

Fig. 11.13 (**a**) Modified midesophageal bicaval view of a patient with a patent foramen ovale (*red arrow*). Note the reduced color flow Doppler scale to detect the slower interatrial flow. (**b**) Modified midesophageal bicaval view with agitated saline injection in a patient with a patent foramen ovale (*red arrow*). Note the small "bubbles" crossing the interatrial septum

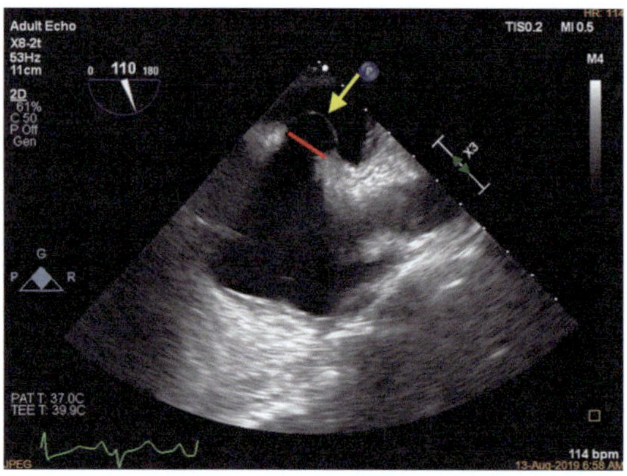

Fig. 11.14 Midesophageal bicaval view of a patient with an interatrial septal aneurysm. The *red line* indicates the neutral position of the interatrial septum, while the *yellow arrow* indicates the deviated interatrial septal aneurysm

PFO through a transient increase in right atrial pressure (above left atrial pressure) and a subsequent deviation of the IAS toward the left heart. Lastly, an agitated saline study can be utilized as contrast to detect interatrial shunting (Fig. 11.13a, b; Videos 11.3 and 11.4).

Position

The IAS can be used to estimate pressures in the LA. The septum acts like a "weathervane" that points away from the side of higher pressure toward that of lower pressure. If the septum bulges toward the LA, that indicates that the pressure in the RA is higher. If LA pressure is elevated, then the septum will bulge toward the RA. At normal physiologic pressures, the septum remains midline.

Notable variations of the IAS may be present, including interatrial septal aneurysms and lipomatous hypertrophy of the IAS. The presence of an interatrial septal aneurysm is present when the movement of the septum exceeds 1.5 cm from the midline (Fig. 11.14). Patients with an interatrial septal aneurysm have a higher prevalence of PFO and elevated risk of cryptogenic stroke. Lipomatous hypertrophy of the IAS occurs when the septum is infiltrated with fatty tissue. The fossa ovalis is typically spared, with the muscular portion of the septum appearing hypertrophied, resulting in a "dumbbell"-shaped septum (see Chap. 16). The identification of atrial septal defects is discussed in Chap. 18.

Conclusion

The atria are two thin-walled chambers that facilitate venous return and ventricular filling. Their embryological development leads to unique appearance on echocardiography with a required knowledge of anatomy and anatomic variants to prevent misdiagnosis. Recognition of chamber enlargement, spontaneous echo contrast, and LAA thrombus is essential to a complete atrial evaluation.

Questions

1. Which of the following best describes the location of the Eustachian valve?

   A. At the junction of the SVC and RA
   B. At the junction of IVC and RA
   C. At the junction of the coronary sinus and RA
   D. At the junction of the RA appendage and RA

2. Which of the following best describes the location of the coumadin ridge (ligament of Marshall)?

   A. In the right atrium near the RA appendage
   B. In the left atrium between the RUPV and RLPV
   C. In the left atrium between LA appendage and LUPV
   D. In the left atrium near the mitral valve

3. Which of the following best describes when the left atrial chamber size should be measured?

   A. At end-systole, prior to opening of the MV
   B. At end-diastole, prior to closure of TV
   C. During the P-wave
   D. During the R-wave

4. Which of the following views is *least* useful for measuring the linear dimensions of the LA?

   A. Midesophageal four-chamber view
   B. Midesophageal AV SAX view
   C. Midesophageal AV LAX view
   D. Midesophageal bicaval view

5. Which method of chamber quantification is the strongest predictor of outcomes in cardiac patients?

   A. Left atrial area
   B. Right atrial area
   C. Right atrial volume
   D. Left atrial volume

6. Which of the following is *NOT* a function of the left atrium?

   A. Reservoir
   B. Conduit
   C. Electrical current generator
   D. Pump

7. Which of the following statements about the right atrium is most correct?

   A. The RA is formed from the division of the primitive atria into a right side that fuses with the sinus venosus and joins at a groove called the sulcus terminalis.
   B. The RA is positioned posterior relative to the LA.
   C. The anterior wall is comprised mainly of the right atrial appendage (RAA), which is demarcated medially from the posterior wall by the crista terminalis.
   D. The crista terminalis is the origin of the pectinate muscles forming the posterior wall and RAA.

8. Which of the following statements is most true regarding assessment for left atrial appendage thrombus formation?

   A. Velocity measurements > 40 cm/s excludes LAA thrombus formation.
   B. The density of spontaneous echo contrast is not proportional to the risk for thromboembolism.
   C. Pulsed-wave Doppler measurement should be obtained in the middle 1/3 segment.
   D. Velocity measurements < 20 cm/s are associated with a high incidence of thrombus.

9. An interatrial septum that is displaced greater than what distance is diagnostic of an aneurysmal interatrial septum?

    A. > 0.5 cm
    B. > 1.0 cm
    C. > 1.5 cm
    D. > 2.0 cm

10. Which of the following statements is most true regarding the left atrium and interatrial septum?

    A. A LA EF $\leq$ 59% is associated with increased risk of mortality and new-onset atrial fibrillation and atrial flutter.
    B. Up to 10% of patients may have a patent foramen ovale (PFO) that may be detectable with echocardiography using color flow Doppler.
    C. A patent foramen ovale typically occurs at the posterior rim of the fossa ovalis.
    D. The minimum LA volume (LA_{min}) occurs with MV closing.

References

1. Lang RM, Badano LP, Mor-Avi V, et al. Recommendations for cardiac chamber quantification by echocardiography in adults: an update from the American Society of Echocardiography and the European Association of Cardiovascular Imaging. J Am Soc Echocardiogr. 2015;28(1):1–39.e14.
2. The American Society of Echocardiography recommendations for cardiac chamber quantification in adults: a quick reference guide from the ASE workflow and lab management task force.
3. Bansal M, Kasliwal RR. Echocardiography for left atrial appendage structure and function. Indian Heart J. 2012;64(5):469–75.
4. Ancona R, Pinto SC, Caso P, et al. Left atrium by echocardiography in clinical practice: from conventional methods to new echocardiographic techniques. ScientificWorldJournal. 2014;2014:451042.
5. Leischik R, Littwitz H, Dworrak B, et al. Echocardiographic evaluation of left atrial mechanics: function, history, novel techniques, advantages, and pitfalls. Biomed Res Int. 2015;2015:765921.
6. Hahn RT, Abraham T, Adams MS. Guidelines for performing a comprehensive transesophageal echocardiographic examination: recommendations from the American Society of Echocardiography and the Society of Cardiovascular Anesthesiologists. J Am Soc Echocardiogr. 2013;26:921–64.
7. Hoit BD. Left atrial size and function: role in prognosis. J Am Coll Cardiol. 2014;63(6):493–505.
8. Beigel R, Wunderlich NC, Ho SY, Arsanjani R. The left atrial appendage: anatomy, function, and noninvasive evaluation. J Am Coll Cardiol Img. 2014;7(12):1251–65.
9. Pathan F, Hecht H, Narula J, et al. Roles of transesophageal echocardiography and cardiac computed tomography for evaluation of left atrial thrombus and associated pathology. J Am Coll Cardiol Img. 2018;11(4):616–27.

12 Diastology

Liem Nguyen and Neal Gerstein

Abbreviations

DT	Deceleration time
IVRT	Isovolumetric relaxation time
LA	Left atrium
LV	Left ventricle
LVEDP	Left ventricular end-diastolic pressure
POI	Point of interrogation
RV	Right ventricle
TDI	Tissue Doppler imaging
TEE	Transesophageal echocardiography
TTE	Transthoracic echocardiography

Introduction

Echocardiography can be used in real time to estimate filling pressures and assess the results of hemodynamic interventions perioperatively [1, 2]. Diastology, the assessment of cardiac filling, can be performed by echocardiography using primarily pulsed-wave Doppler modalities [3]. The velocity at which blood enters a given chamber can be used to derive and estimate filling pressures. In the dynamic environment of the operating room or intensive care unit, the use of real-time echocardiography-assisted hemodynamic management may offer significant advantages when compared to the more traditional hemodynamic monitors such as the Swan-Ganz catheter [1, 2, 4–9]. Dynamic markers of left atrial (LA) and left ventricular (LV) filling by echocardiography have been shown to be a viable alternative to conventional catheter-based techniques to measure intracardiac filling pressures [1, 2]. This chapter will focus on the basics of diastolic assessment by echocardiography and highlight its potential utility in the perioperative period.

In its simplest form, the study of diastolic function by echocardiography is a means to measure the velocity at which blood flows through the heart during diastole [3]. Pulsed-wave Doppler, one of a variety of Doppler modalities, is analogous to "radar detection" as it measures the velocity of blood moving through a given chamber. A pulsed-wave Doppler signal is generated from a single transducer crystal acting as both transmitter and receiver. A short burst ultrasound wave is transmitted from the crystal toward a set sample followed by a switch to receiving and interpreting the returning echoes. Information on the velocity of blood allows the echocardiographer to derive or estimate intracardiac pressures, thus providing a means to measure the

L. Nguyen (✉)
Department of Anesthesiology, University of California San Diego Health, La Jolla, CA, USA
e-mail: liem@ucsd.edu

N. Gerstein
Department of Anesthesiology and Critical Care Medicine, University of New Mexico School of Medicine, Albuquerque, NM, USA
e-mail: NGerstein@salud.unm.edu

T. M. Maus, C. R. Tainter (eds.), *Essential Echocardiography*,
https://doi.org/10.1007/978-3-030-84349-6_12

relationship between pressure and volume in a specific chamber of the heart (e.g., LA or LV) [3, 10–13]. Beat-to-beat measurements on how the heart fills enables the anesthesiologist to optimize the determinants of stroke volume and, thus, cardiac performance. The importance of understanding diastolic filling relates to the basic of concept: *if the heart cannot fill adequately, it cannot eject adequately*.

There are two distinct properties that govern the normal filling of the heart. The first prerequisite to normal filling is an adequate drop or fall in pressure in the downstream receiving chamber (e.g., pressure drop in the LA or LV) as a result of the heart's intrinsic ability to relax (lusitropy), an energy-dependent process. The pressure drop generates the gradient necessary for adequate blood movement from one cardiac chamber to another. The second property that governs normal adequate filling is the ability for a given cardiac chamber to receive blood while simultaneously maintaining a relatively low filling pressure. The heart's pressure response to increasing volume is referred to as compliance ($\Delta V/\Delta P$). Together, the heart's ability to relax (adequate pressure drop) and remain compliant (maintain low pressure despite increased volume) are the two main properties that regulate adequate filling. It is the presence of inadequate relaxation and/or poor compliance that characterizes the onset of impaired filling. The hallmark of diastolic dysfunction is therefore a result of the inability of the heart to relax and/or remain compliant [3, 10–13].

Pulsed-wave Doppler is used to detect changes or deviations in normal blood velocity, indicating the presence of an abnormal filling process [3]. Using Doppler echocardiography, the anesthesiologist may be able to identify a shift from a normal filling state to an abnormal filling state. This data can then be used to determine how to improve and correct the filling abnormality [1, 10–13].

Phases of Diastole

There are four main phases of diastole (Fig. 12.1a): isovolumetric relaxation (IVRT), early rapid filling, diastasis, and atrial contraction [3].

1. Isovolumetric Relaxation

   The start of isovolumetric relaxation corresponds to the onset of aortic valve closure. With both the tricuspid and mitral valves closed, the chamber pressure in both ventricles decreases, creating a gradient for blood movement into the respective receiving ventricle when the atrioventricular valves are open in the next phase of diastole (early filling). IVRT is an active phase of myocardial relaxation and is energetically consuming, with the inactivation of the contractile apparatus driven by sequestration of Ca^{2+} ions into the sarcoplasmic reticulum. The pressure drop in the ventricle is the prerequisite for establishing an adequate atrial-ventricular pressure gradient for normal filling [3, 10–13].
2. Early Rapid Filling

   As the tricuspid and mitral valves open, early filling of the respective ventricle commences as blood moves into the downstream chamber. Pulsed-wave Doppler interrogation of blood flowing into the ventricle produces the characteristic E-wave (velocity of the early filling wave) on the LV or right ventricle (RV) inflow profile (Fig. 12.1a). The peak E-wave velocity is primarily dependent on the LA-LV gradient. The LA-LV gradient is a function of the large pressure drop in the LV during the IVRT phase and *not* a result of a rise in LA pressure. The deceleration time (DT) is the time it takes for atrial and ventricular pressures to equilibrate and is predicated upon the volume-pressure relationship or compliance ($\Delta V/\Delta P$) of the respective downstream receiving ventricle. Furthermore, the deceleration time is the time for the peak velocity (E-wave) of blood moving into the ventricle to reach zero, which corresponds to the time it takes for the ventricle to passively fill before the LV and LA reach equilibrium [3, 10–13].
3. Diastasis

   Diastasis, the third interval of diastole, marks the period in which the atrium and ventricle are in equilibrium with little flow moving into either chamber. This period is often truncated or shortened during higher heart rates (shorter time in diastole) and is more prolonged during lower heart rates [3, 10–13].

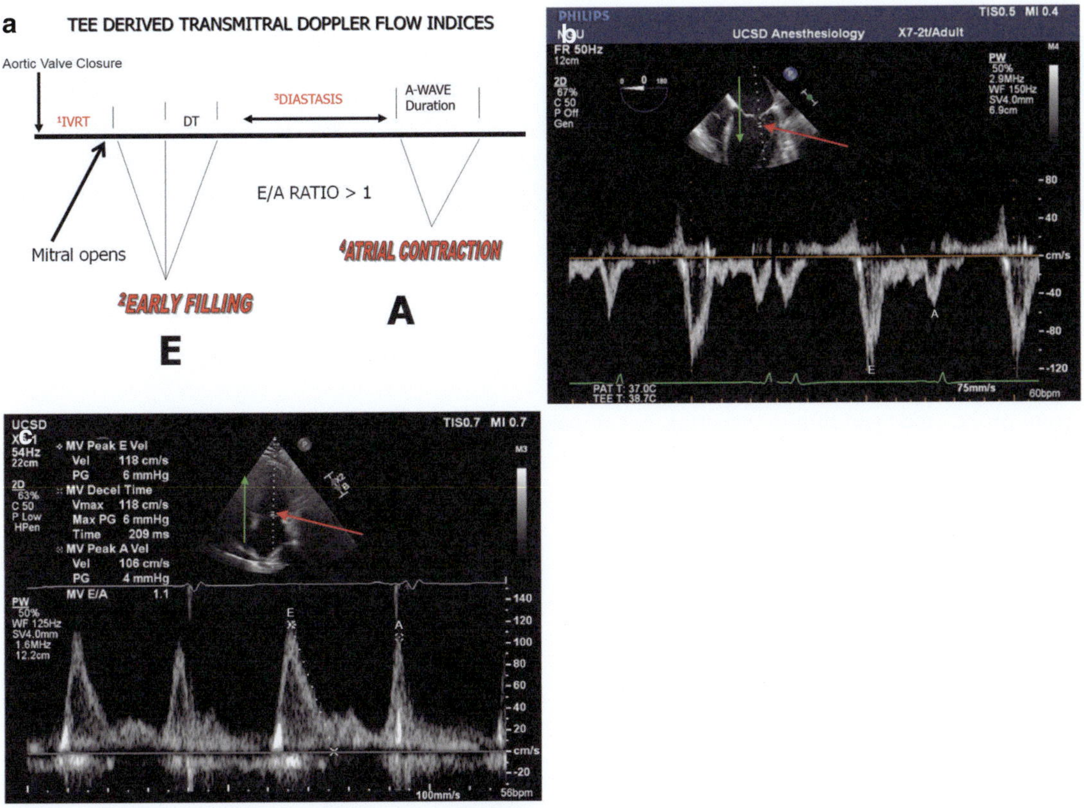

Fig. 12.1 (**a**) Diagram of a normal *TEE*-derived transmitral inflow profile encompassing the four stages of diastole (numbered with superscript). After [1]IVRT, the mitral valve opens and [2]early filling (E-wave) commences, followed by a period of pressure equalization ([3]diastasis), ending with [4]atrial contraction (A-wave). The peak E-wave velocity is proportional to the LA-LV gradient, while the deceleration time (DT) is dependent on LV compliance. (**b**) Pulsed-wave Doppler of normal *TEE*-derived transmitral inflow obtained from a ME four-chamber view. The profile is obtained by placing the point of interrogation (*red arrow*) just below the mitral leaflet tips and utilizing pulsed-wave Doppler echocardiography. Notice that the direction of flow is toward (downward) the LV indicated by the direction of the *green arrow*. (**c**) *TTE*-derived transmitral inflow obtained from an apical four-chamber view. Notice the direction of flow (upward) in the apical four-chamber view is toward the LV (*green arrow*) and the relative position of the point of interrogation (*red arrow*) of the pulsed-wave Doppler compared to TEE, giving rise to a spectral profile that is opposite in polarity. *IVRT* isovolumetric relaxation time, *DT* deceleration time, *E* early filling, *A* atrial contraction

4. Atrial Contraction

   Atrial contraction (A-wave) occurs at the latter stage of diastole and corresponds to the p-wave on the electrocardiogram. The atrial contraction or "atrial kick" mechanism transiently increases the atrial pressure and generates a "push" of blood into the receiving ventricle. The velocity of blood being "pushed" downward into the ventricle is described by the peak A-wave velocity. Diastole is finally complete when the atrioventricular valves close [3, 10–13].

Assessment of Chamber Filling: Pulsed-Wave Doppler Echocardiography

Transmitral Inflow: Measuring Flow into the Left Ventricle

The LV or transmitral inflow profile (Fig. 12.1a–c) is obtained with pulsed-wave Doppler echocardiography by setting the point of interrogation (POI) at the distal edge of the leaflet tips (ventricular side) of the mitral valve in the midesophageal four-chamber view at zero degrees [10–14] on transesophageal echocardiography (TEE, Fig. 12.1b) or apical four-chamber view on transthoracic echocardiography (TTE, Fig. 12.1c) [3]. It is important to note the relative direction of the transmitral inflow pattern when comparing TTE and TEE pulsed-wave imaging modalities (compare Fig. 12.1b, c). Though the evaluated transmitral flow is blood flow moving from the LA to the LV, the displayed spectral analysis by TTE (toward probe yielding a spectral envelope above the baseline) and TEE (away from probe and yielding a spectral envelope below the baseline) is opposite to one another. Pulsed-wave Doppler measures the velocity of blood traveling from the LA to the LV during the early filling phase of diastole. More simply, it is in part a measurement of how fast blood enters the LV. The velocity at which blood enters the LV is primarily dependent on the LA-LV gradient (Fig. 12.1a), which under normal conditions is a result of LV relaxation. As in any Doppler assessment, it is essential to align the pulsed-wave Doppler parallel to the direction of blood flow to obtain the most accurate results. The normal LV filling pattern (Fig. 12.1b, c) consists of a higher velocity E-wave (early filling), a period of diastasis (equilibrium), and a lower velocity A-wave (atrial contraction and late filling). The higher-velocity E-wave (early filling) is a consequence of the larger LA-LV gradient during the initial mitral valve opening created by LV relaxation. By contrast, during late diastole, the gradient between the LA-LV gradient is smaller due to the nearly filled LV (from the early filling phase), resulting in a lower-velocity A-wave. The end result is an E-wave velocity that is approximately 1.5 times greater than the A-wave velocity resulting in an E/A ratio of ~1.5:1.0. The DT marks the time for the peak E-velocity to reach baseline (zero velocity) and defines the time it takes for the LA and LV pressures to equilibrate. The deceleration time mathematically describes how long the early filling occurs before diastasis begins and is also a measure of LV compliance (Fig. 12.1a). A shortened deceleration time signifies a truncated filling period where the mitral valve opens and flow ceases quickly due to rapid atrial-ventricular pressure equilibration often from poor ventricular compliance. Normal deceleration times indicate that the early filling occurs over an appropriate duration signifying adequate ventricular filling and compliance [3, 10–13].

Pulmonary Venous Flow: Measuring Flow into the Left Atrium

LA inflow or pulmonary venous flow can be measured by placing the pulsed-wave Doppler point of interrogation into the left or right upper pulmonary vein utilizing a midesophageal two-chamber view on TEE (Fig. 12.2a) or apical four-chamber view on TTE (Fig. 12.2b), respectively. Using a two-chamber view on TEE, the point of interrogation is placed approximately 1 cm into the pulmonary vein near the entry point of the LA [14]. Similarly, on TTE, flow velocities into the LA can be obtained by aligning the right upper pulmonary vein in an apical four-chamber view [3]. In contrast with mitral valve inflows, as per pulsed-wave Doppler interrogation of the pulmonary veins, the direction of flow is the *same* when comparing the LA inflow profiles of TTE versus TEE (compare Fig. 12.2a, b). The resulting pulmonary vein flow velocity profile normally consists of a higher-velocity systolic wave (S-wave) and a lower-velocity diastolic wave (D-wave). The higher-velocity S-wave is a result of active LA relaxation promoting a larger gradient for forward flow from the pulmonary veins into the LA during early systole. As the mitral valve opens during early diastole, forward flow from the pulmonary veins travels down the pressure gradient into the LA and eventually into the LV, corresponding to the D-wave on the LA inflow profile. The higher-velocity S-wave is often affected by either the inability of the LA to relax adequately or an increase in LA pressure. Accordingly, a blunted or reduced S-wave velocity is often a marker of an abnormality of LA relaxation and/or compliance (Fig. 12.2c) [3, 10–14].

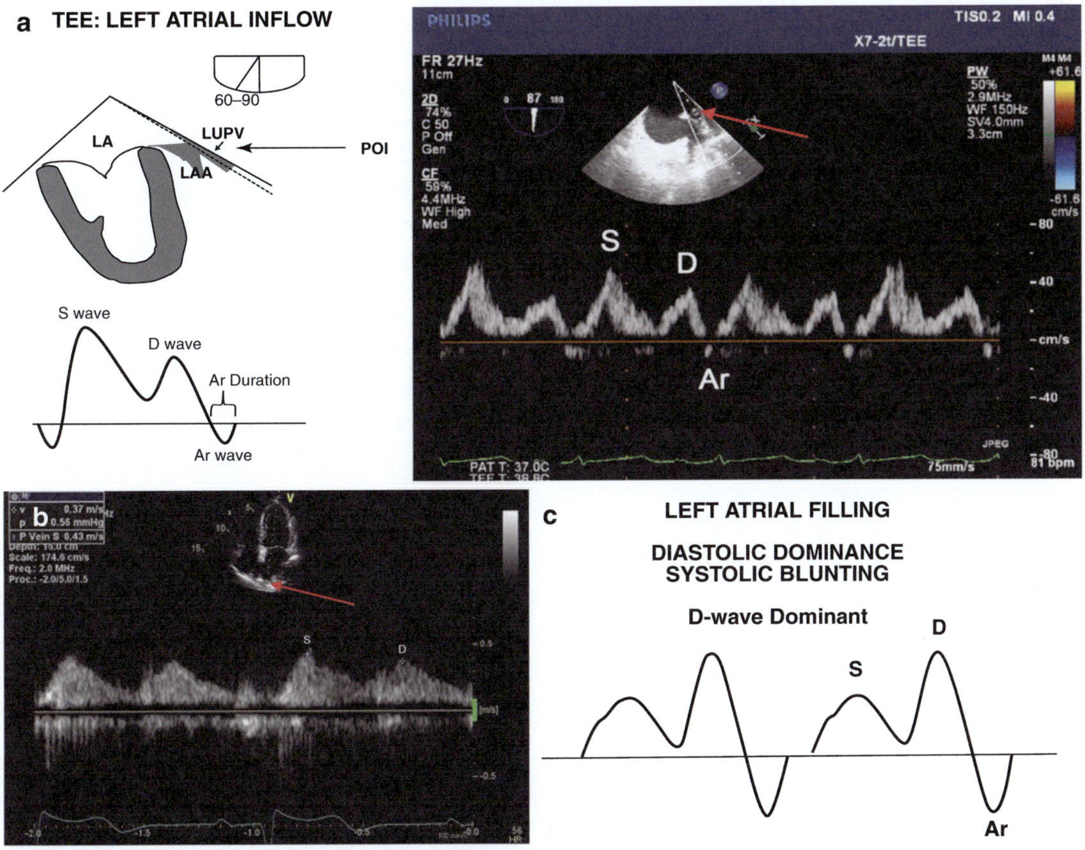

Fig. 12.2 (**a**) TEE-derived left atrial filling or pulmonary vein flow profile obtained by placing point of interrogation ~1 cm into the left upper pulmonary vein near entry of the left atrium using a ME two-chamber view. Left atrial filling or pulmonary vein flow profile consists of a higher velocity and more dominant systolic (S-wave) component and a lower-velocity diastolic (D-wave) component. (**b**) TTE-derived left atrial filling or pulmonary venous flow from using the pulsed-wave Doppler aligned with flow from the right upper pulmonary vein in an apical four-chamber view. Notice that the TTE-derived left atrial inflow spectral profile gives rise to two positive deflections (S-and D-waves) which are similar in polarity to the profile obtained on TEE. (**c**) The blunted S-wave velocity is a result of a poor left atrial relaxation and/or a rise in LA pressure. *LA* left atrium, *LAA* left atrial appendage, *LUPV* left upper pulmonary vein, *POI* point of interrogation, *S* systolic wave, *D* diastolic wave, *Ar* atrial regurgitant wave

Tissue Doppler Imaging: Measuring the Velocity of Myocardial Tissue

During the first stage of diastole, IVRT results in a net drop in LV pressure creating a pressure gradient [3]. During this period of LV relaxation, the lateral aspect of the mitral annulus and atrial myocardium moves upward (the LV is "snapping open") on TEE (Fig. 12.3a, b) [10–14] or downward on TTE (Fig. 12.3c) [3]. The movement direction and velocity of the atrial myocardium-mitral annulus can be measured using tissue Doppler imaging [3, 10–14]. Tissue Doppler imaging (TDI) is a mode of spectral Doppler that filters out blood velocities and specifically measures the movement of the myocardium exclusively. Analogous to measuring the velocity of blood moving across the mitral valve, TDI interrogation can be utilized to measure the velocity of myocardial tissue or, specifically, the translational movement of the atrial myocardium or mitral annulus during diastole [3, 14].

Employing a midesophageal four-chamber view on TEE, the TDI profile (Fig. 12.3a, b) of the lateral mitral annulus-atrial myocardium is described by two positive deflections: the first a positive signal in early diastole, carrying the designation of e` (e prime), and the second wave in late diastole with the designation of a` (a prime) [14]. Using the apical four-chamber view on TTE, the movement of the lateral mitral annulus-atrial myocardium is in the opposite direction to that compared to TEE, giving rise to two negative signals (e` and a`) directed below the baseline (Fig. 12.3b) [4]. When comparing TDI on TTE vs TEE, the direction of myocardial tissue motion during diastole is *opposite* between the two modalities (compare Fig. 13.2a, b). TTE examination of mitral annular tissue motion produces two downward deflections (e` and a`) on the spectral profile. By contrast, TEE examination of the mitral annulus yields two positive deflections (e` and a`). The onset of the e`-wave occurs just before the mitral valve opens and represents the rate of relaxation of the myocardium during the isovolumetric relaxation period (IVRT). The e`-wave velocity is therefore an index of myocardial relaxation. The TDI e`-wave velocity (normally ~10–12 cm/s) is much lower than the LV inflow E-wave velocity (~50–100 cm/s) of blood during early diastole, with a normal E/e` ratio of ≤ 8 [3]. An e`-wave velocity of less than 10 cm/s is abnormal and suggests that impaired myocardial relaxation is present. The a`-wave represents motion

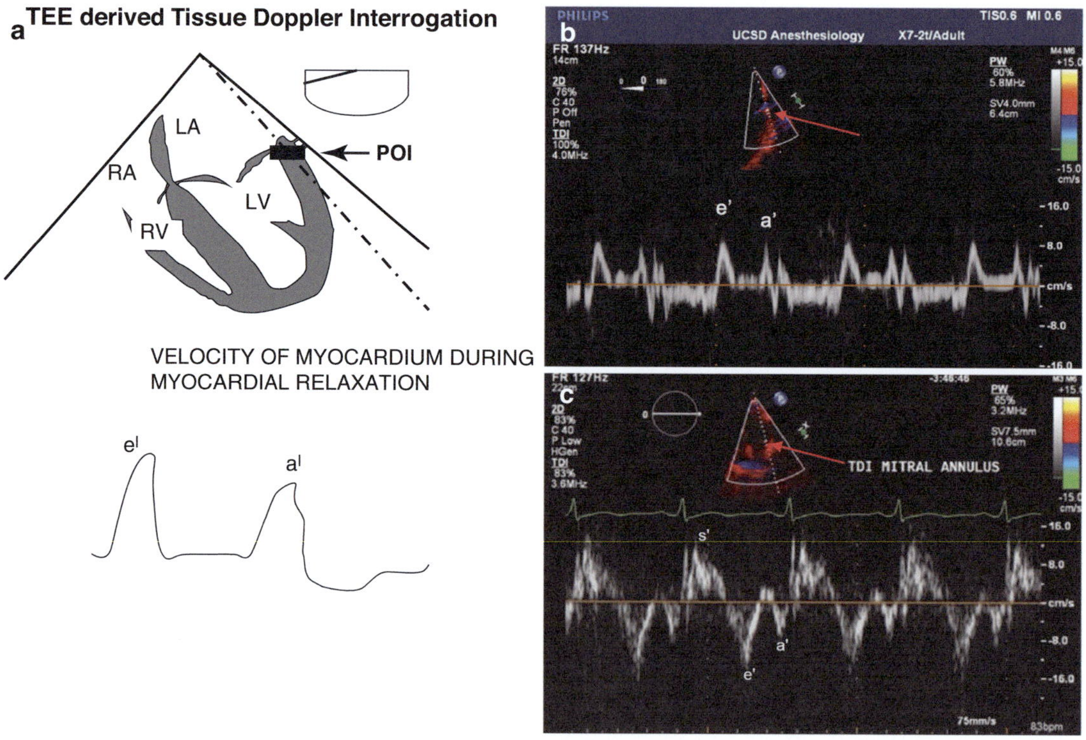

Fig. 12.3 (**a**) Tissue Doppler interrogation measuring the upward velocity of the atrial myocardium and lateral mitral annulus during diastole with TEE. The e`-wave corresponds to ascension of the atrial myocardium and lateral mitral annulus during IVRT. The a`-wave corresponds to movement of the myocardium with atrial contraction. (**b**) Tissue Doppler interrogation of the lateral aspect of the mitral annulus with TEE using a midesophageal four-chamber view. The point of interrogation (POI) is indicated by the *red arrow*. (**c**) Tissue Doppler interrogation of the lateral aspect of the mitral annulus on TTE using an apical four-chamber view. Notice that the direction of myocardial motion is in the opposite when compared to the spectral profile above obtained from TEE. The *red arrow* indicates the POI

of the atrial myocardium and lateral annulus just before atrial contraction [3, 15].

Stages of Diastolic Dysfunction: From Mild to Severe Dysfunction (Table 12.1) (Highlight Box 12.1)

Highlight Box 12.1

Diastolic dysfunction	
2D	• Left ventricular hypertrophy. • Left atrial enlargement. • Secondary right heart dysfunction from pHTN.
CFD	• Typically not utilized.
Spectral	• Assess severity: PWD: Mitral inflow. PWD: Pulmonary venous inflow. TDI: Mitral annular velocity.

pHTN pulmonary hypertension, *PWD* pulsed-wave Doppler, *TDI* tissue Doppler imaging

The term diastolic dysfunction encompasses a spectrum of abnormal filling stages of increasing severity (Fig. 12.4) [3–10–14]. On the other hand, the term diastolic heart failure describes a state of decompensation due to diastolic dysfunction as a result of redistribution of fluid into the pulmonary venous system despite a normal ejection fraction [11–13]. The first and mildest stage of diastolic dysfunction is *impaired relaxation*, characterized by the inability of the ventricle to adequately relax or decrease its pressure. The next stage on the diastolic dysfunction continuum is designated as *pseudonormalization*, which is a moderate or intermediate stage of diastolic dysfunction characterized by the combined presence of *impaired relaxation* and a compensatory elevation in LA pressure. The final and most severe stage of diastolic dysfunction is referred to as the *restrictive* form. The *restrictive* form is manifested by the presence of impaired relaxation, elevated LA pressures, and elevated LV pressures (from poor compliance) [3, 10–14].

Table 12.1 Stages of diastolic dysfunction

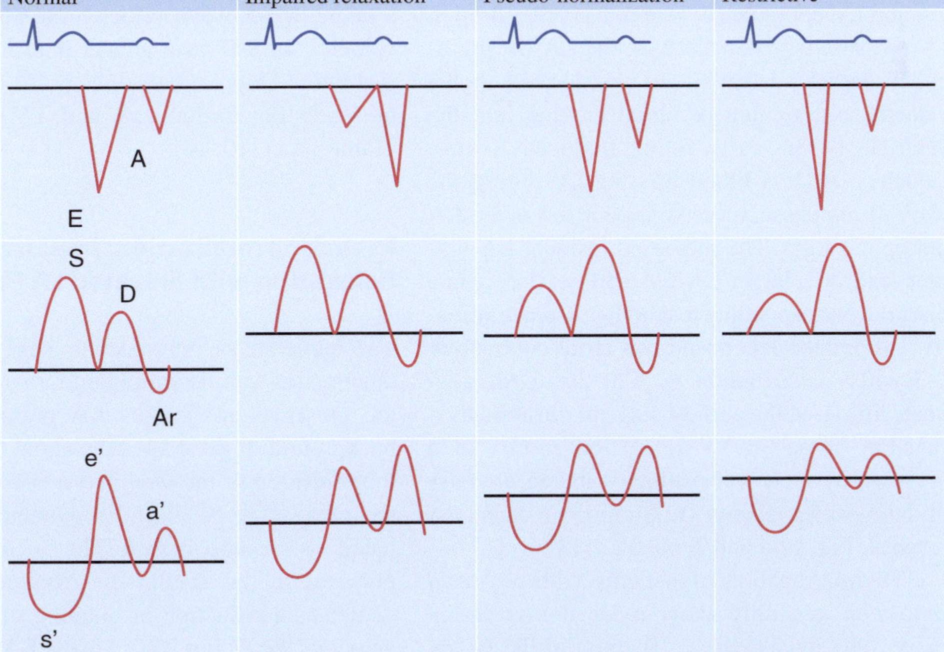

	Normal	Impaired relaxation	Pseudo-normalization	Restrictive
EKG Mitral inflow				
Pulmonary venous Doppler				
Tissue Doppler imaging				
E/e' LAP (Left Atrial Pressure)	e' > 10 Normal	E/e' < 10 Normal	E/e' = 10–14 ↑	E/e' > 14 ↑

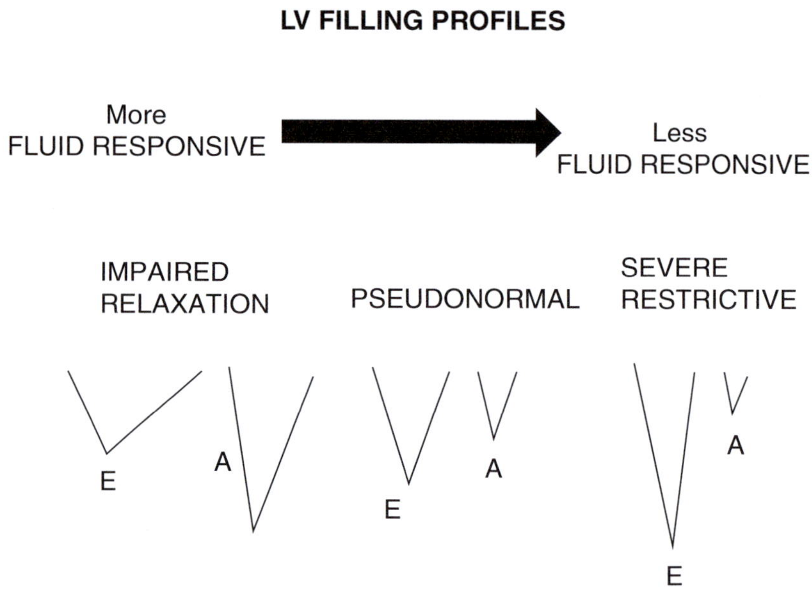

Fig. 12.4 The spectrum of diastolic dysfunction. Progression through the various stages from the left to right part of the spectrum represents an advancement from the mildest (more fluid responsive) to the most severe form (less fluid responsive) of diastolic dysfunction

Impaired Relaxation

The inability of the LV to relax marks the first stage of diastolic dysfunction and is referred to as *impaired relaxation* [3]. In this mild form of diastolic dysfunction, isolated impaired relaxation of the ventricle is present in the setting of normal LA and LV compliance. Due to a smaller drop in LV pressure (smaller $\Delta P/\Delta T$), the LA-LV gradient is decreased leading to a reduction in the velocity and amount of blood moving into the ventricle during early filling (reduced E-wave velocity). As less blood fills the LV during the early filling phase, more volume is left in the LA during diastasis. The increased residual LA volume leads to a larger LA-LV gradient during late diastole, corresponding to a higher A-wave velocity and greater dependence on atrial contraction (~30–40% contribution vs ~20–30%) for adequate filling. In the earliest stage of diastolic dysfunction, impaired LV relaxation results in a *decrease* in the E-wave velocity and an *increase* in the A-wave velocity (E/A ratio < 1 or E to A reversal, Fig. 12.4 and Table 12.1) [3].

TDI interrogation of patients with *impaired relaxation* generally show reduced myocardial tissue velocity signals (< 10 cm/s) of the lateral mitral annulus or atrial myocardium [3, 10, 15]. This corresponds with an impaired ability of the atrial myocardium-mitral annulus to move during LV relaxation. However, since the LA pressures are normal in *impaired relaxation*, the velocity of blood flowing into the LA remains normal, as evidenced by a normal left atrial inflow pattern (S-wave dominant, Fig. 12.2a, b, Table 12.1). In summary, impaired relaxation is characterized by a *decreased* E-wave velocity, *increased* A-wave velocity, an S/D ratio greater than 1, and abnormal tissue Doppler velocities (< 10 cm/s), in the presence of normal LA and LV compliance (Table 12.1) [10, 14].

Pseudonormalization: Impaired Relaxation with Elevated LA Pressure

The moderate or intermediate stage of diastolic dysfunction can be simplified by superimposing the presence of elevated LA pressures onto a background of poor LV relaxation. This defines the transition of the *impaired relaxation* stage to the next stage of diastolic dysfunction, designated as *pseudonormal*. The increase in LA pressure in the setting of impaired relaxation generates a reduction or blunting of the S-wave velocity (S < D, Fig. 12.2c) in the LA inflow (pulmonary venous flow) Doppler profile. As a result of poor LA relaxation and/or a rise in LA pressure, the pressure gradient dictating forward flow from the pulmonary veins into the LA is reduced, yielding a diastolic (D-wave) dominant profile (blunted S-wave, Fig. 12.2c) [10, 14]. The additional increase in LA pressure (larger LA-LV gradient) in the setting of impaired relaxation (E < A) produces an increase in the E-wave velocity, resulting in an apparent normalization of the E and A transmitral velocities (E > A, Table 12.1). The resulting "pseudonormal" E > A pattern and systolic blunting of the left LA profile (Fig. 12.2c) are the defining characteristics of this intermediate stage of diastolic dysfunction (Table 12.1). Furthermore, as the *pseudonormal* stage combines impaired relaxation and the presence of elevated LA pressures, TDI of the atrial myocardium and mitral annulus is abnormal (< 10 cm/s), consistent with a LV relaxation defect [3, 15]. In summary, the *pseudonormal* stage of diastolic dysfunction is an intermediate stage characterized by both impaired relaxation and elevated LA pressures. Accordingly, the distinguishing features of the *pseudonormal* stage are the presence of abnormal myocardial velocities (< 10 cm/s) and blunted S-wave velocities (diastolic dominance) on TDI and left atrial inflow, respectively (Table 12.1) [3, 10, 14].

Restrictive: Impaired Relaxation, Poor LV Compliance, and Elevated LA and LV Pressures

The progression from *pseudonormal* to the most severe or *restrictive* stage of diastolic dysfunction is marked by the addition of poor LV compliance on the background of impaired relaxation and elevated LA pressures. The *restrictive* stage features the addition of a stiff and noncompliant LV in the setting of preexisting impaired relaxation and elevated LA pressures [3, 10, 12, 14]. Marked elevations in LV pressure from poor LV compliance result in restricted LV filling and a major redistribution of volume to the LA. The large LA volume thus provides the basis for pulmonary venous congestion and symptomatic diastolic heart failure. Marked elevations in LA volume and pressure generate a much larger LA-LV gradient and faster E-wave velocity (E >> A) during early filling compared to normal (Fig. 12.4, Table 12.1). In addition, as the pressure in the LA rapidly increases, the mitral valve is forced open before the LV can adequately relax. The velocity of blood moving into the LV is very fast as the elevated LA pressure prematurely forces the mitral valve open and pushes blood downstream into the LV. However, the overall volume of LV filling is significantly diminished as the LV pressures rises abruptly (poor compliance) and rapidly equalizes with the LA, generating a very short deceleration time (time from peak E-wave velocity to zero). The end result is a small and quick "pulse" of volume that is delivered to the LV as the filling rapidly begins and ends during the early filling phase. After a period of diastasis, the elevated LV pressures are not conducive to late filling, resulting in a very small or negligible A-wave velocity during atrial contraction. In fact, when the atrium contracts during late diastole, the elevated LV filling pressures cause diastolic regurgitation into the pulmonary veins or atrial reversal (A_r, Fig. 12.2c). The most severe restricted stage of diastolic dysfunction is characterized by the unique pattern of a high velocity E-wave, low velocity A-wave (E >> A, or E/A > 2), and a shortened DT (< 150 msec) on the LV inflow or transmitral profile (Fig. 12.4, Table 12.1) [9, 10, 12, 14].

Clinical Implications of Diastolic Dysfunction: Real-Time Measurements

Pulsed-wave Doppler allows the echocardiographer to measure the velocity of blood moving between two varying cardiac structures or chambers (i.e., pulmonary vein to LA, LA to LV, etc.). This is the main clinical value of diastology. It confers the ability to evaluate how the heart fills and responds to volume in a continuous manner [4, 8, 9]. Diastology enables clinicians to identify which patients are at risk of developing elevations in chamber pressures and pulmonary venous congestion, providing the foundation to optimize hemodynamics and cardiac performance [4, 8, 9, 12, 16]. For example, in patients with impaired relaxation (i.e., E/A reversal or E/A ratio < 1) and normal LA and LV pressures, the A-wave or "atrial kick" component plays a larger role in LV filling compared to a normal profile. An increase in LA pressure with fluid therapy will therefore improve LV filling. Taken together, this early stage of diastolic dysfunction may be improved by maintaining a slow sinus rhythm, allowing more time for the LV to relax and fill, and by gentle administration of fluid to increase the LA-LV gradient [12]. Medications that may enhance LV relaxation such as milrinone, nitroglycerin, or levosimendan may also improve the relaxation abnormality and augment LV filling [12, 17–19]. On the other end of the spectrum, patients with a severe restrictive pattern with poor compliance and marked elevations in LA and LV pressures display a fixed end-diastolic volume and resultant stroke volume; hence, preload increases may not only be ineffective but may be deleterious. In cases of restrictive diastolic dysfunction, slower heart rates may actually compromise cardiac output, whereas mild elevations in the heart rate may be more beneficial [12]. Additionally, elevated LV end-diastolic pressure (LVEDP) observed in patients with a restrictive pattern may necessitate an equivalent rise in aortic pressure to optimize coronary perfusion. Judicial use of diuretics may also be warranted as marked elevations in LA and LV pressure portend a greater risk of developing congestive heart failure in the perioperative period. Patients with a restrictive pattern may therefore benefit from relatively higher heart rates, elevated aortic pressures, and avoiding further increases in LA or LV pressure [12]. The dynamic spectrum of diastolic dysfunction can be appreciated in the operating room or intensive care unit (Fig. 12.4) [1, 2, 4–10, 12, 15, 16]. A patient with a pseudonormal pattern of filling may be pushed to the right of the spectrum and progress to a restrictive form following a fluid bolus, myocardial ischemia, or acute onset valvular regurgitation. On the other hand, a patient with a restrictive pattern may improve and move to the left of the spectrum after hemodynamic optimization with diuretic therapy, careful initiation of inotropic therapy, and an increase in coronary perfusion pressure. Patients demonstrating impaired relaxation may benefit from slight increases in LA pressure and are therefore may be more fluid responsive compared to pseudonormal or restrictive patterns (Fig. 12.4). An impaired relaxation pattern may be moved to the left of the spectrum by the administration of nitroglycerin or a lusitropic agent to improve relaxation and beta-blockade medications to increase diastolic filling by maximizing early filling and atrial kick [12].

Doppler flow analysis of blood movement into the LV or LA can also be individually performed to estimate changes in filling pressures to optimize intraoperative hemodynamics as well. Using this approach, targeting a specific filling abnormality can be exploited to optimize cardiac output in real time (Fig. 12.5a, b) [8, 9, 12]. By taking serial measurements of the velocity of blood moving into the left ventricle and obtaining an LV inflow profile before and after a therapeutic intervention, the clinician can track changes in the peak E-wave velocity, A-wave velocity, or deceleration times. For example, if the deceleration time shortens after multiple fluid boluses, this suggests a right shift (Fig. 12.5a) to a less fluid-responsive state or less compliant portion of the starling curve. Similarly, flow into the LA and the pulmonary vein inflow profile can detect changes in LA pressure after fluid administration. A normal LA inflow pattern exhibiting an S-wave dominant pattern (S > D) indicates normal LA pressures. If the S-wave begins to blunt and a D-wave dominant pattern (S < D) emerges after a fluid bolus, a rise in LA pressure is the likely cause of the change in the LA inflow profile (Fig. 12.5b). A sudden increase in LA pressures signifies a shift to a less fluid-responsive state and carries a greater risk of pulmonary congestion [8, 9].

The use of intraoperative and critical care echocardiography-assisted hemodynamic management may confer additional advantages when compared to traditional static indices of chamber filling pressures [1, 2, 4–9]. One of the main advantages of echocardiography is the ability to estimate the filling pressures of the left side of the heart and com-

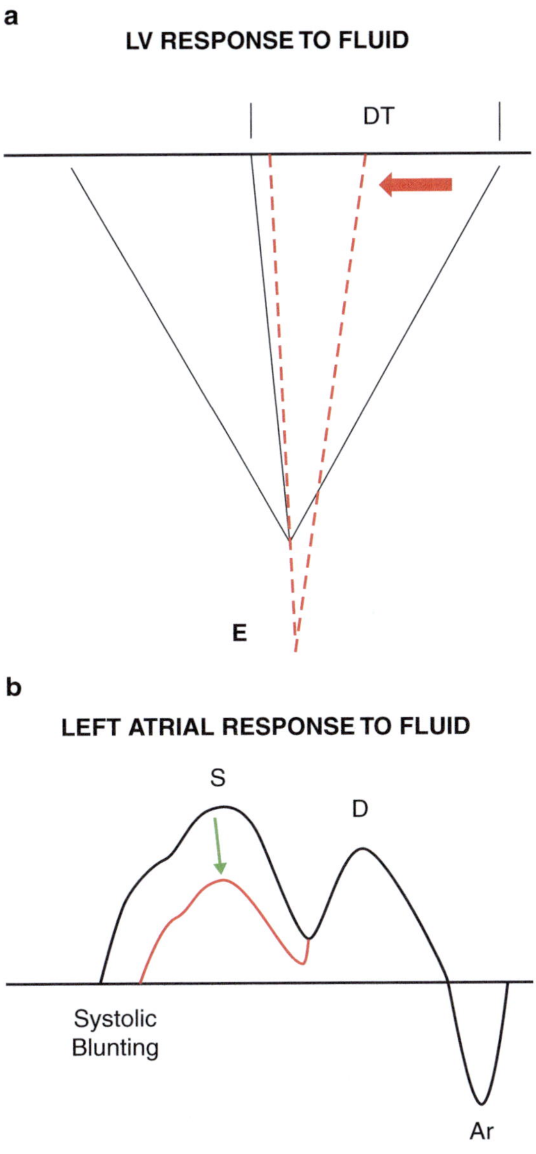

Fig. 12.5 (**a**) TEE-derived LV inflow profile at baseline (*black line*) and after a fluid challenge (*red dashed line*) demonstrating an increase in the peak E-wave velocity and shortening of the DT, corresponding to an increase in LA pressure and poor LV compliance. (**b**) TEE-derived LA inflow profile before (*black line*) and after (*red line*) a fluid challenge demonstrating systolic blunting and an increase in LA pressure. *LV* left ventricle, *DT* deceleration time, *E* early filling (*wave*), *S* systolic wave, *D* diastolic wave, *Ar* atrial regurgitant wave

bine the data with stroke volume measurements by echocardiography or by other modalities [8, 9]. The other main advantage of Doppler echocardiography is the ability to easily and repeatedly measure flow velocities and associated chamber pressures in real time. A number of reports of dynamic markers of LA and LV filling by echocardiography demonstrate their utility as viable alternatives to conventional catheter-based techniques to measure intracardiac filling pressures [5, 9]. Moreover, the use of intraoperative echocardiography-guided hemodynamic management has been shown to reduce the amount of overall fluid administration when compared to a control group [9]. The capability of performing real-time echocardiography in the operating room or intensive care unit may offer significant advantages over conventional techniques in the assessment of hemodynamics [1, 2, 4–9, 12]. At present, the ability to monitor dynamic indices of cardiac performance in real time in order to optimize hemodynamics is lacking. With continued research and broader clinical use, Doppler ultrasound has the potential to be a low cost, safe, robust, and dynamic cardiovascular monitor.

Conclusion

Evaluation of blood flow into the left atrium and left ventricle with spectral Doppler analysis allows estimation of filling pressures, providing an invaluable tool to guide hemodynamic management in real time. This assessment of diastolic function involves two main properties that govern filling in a particular chamber. The first is the ability for the chamber to relax or decrease its pressure. The second property is the ability of the chamber to maintain its compliance as filling proceeds. Cardiac chamber filling abnormalities can be detected on echocardiography, yielding a spectrum of filling patterns that characterize the various stages of diastolic dysfunction with associated clinical implications.

Questions

1. Which of the following sequences correctly describes the temporal sequence of the stages of diastole during LV filling?

A. Early filling, isovolumetric relaxation, atrial contraction, diastasis
B. Early filling, isovolumetric relaxation, diastasis, atrial contraction
C. Isovolumetric contraction, early filling, atrial contraction, diastasis
D. Isovolumetric relaxation, early filling, diastasis, atrial contraction

2. What are the two main properties that govern normal filling in the heart?

A. Compliance and elastance
B. Elastic recoil and strain rate
C. Relaxation and compliance
D. Lusitropy and inotropy

3. Which component of the pulmonary venous inflow pulsed-wave Doppler interrogation is dependent on left atrial relaxation or a decrease in left atrial pressure?

A. The early systolic (S-wave) velocity
B. The early diastolic (D-wave) velocity
C. The atrial reversal velocity (PV_{ar}) seen in late diastole
D. The velocity time integral (VTI) of the early diastolic (D-wave)

4. The velocity of blood flow across the mitral valve during the early filling period (E-wave) of diastole is primarily dependent on which of the following factors?

A. Left atrial contraction
B. A drop in LV pressure during the isovolumetric relaxation period
C. Compliance of the left ventricle
D. Diastasis

5. Patients with moderate diastolic dysfunction, characterized by a pseudonormal pattern of filling, are best described by which of the following abnormalities?

A. Elevated LA and LV pressures
B. A normal E/A ratio on LV inflow and systolic blunting of the S-wave on left atrial inflow
C. Less dependence on atrial contraction for normal filling
D. A decrease in E/e` ratio

6. Diastolic filling assessment before and after a fluid bolus demonstrates a shift from a pseudonormal pattern of filling to a restrictive pattern. Which of the following conclusions can be drawn from the "right shift" in the diastolic filling pattern?

A. The fluid bolus increased LA pressure thereby improving LV filling in the late phase of diastole.
B. The fluid bolus caused an increase in A-wave peak velocity.
C. The fluid administration increased the LVEDV and thus improved overall LV filling.
D. Elevations in LA pressure resulted in faster LV filling during early diastole (E-wave) by increasing the LA-LV gradient.

7. Which of the following indices can assist in distinguishing a normal from a pseudonormal pattern of left ventricular diastolic filling?

A. E/A ratio
B. Presence of blunting of the S-wave or a D-wave dominant left atrial inflow pattern
C. Decreased E-wave deceleration time following nitroglycerin infusion
D. A shift from a pseudonormal pattern to impaired relaxation following a fluid bolus

8. Serial Doppler assessments of pulmonary venous inflow reveal a change from a normal pattern to a new pattern characterized by blunting of the S-wave after a 500 mL IV fluid bolus. Which of the following is the most likely cause for the shift in the Doppler spectral profile?

A. Increased cardiac output
B. Reduced systemic vascular resistance and vasodilation
C. Increased left atrial pressure
D. A shift from pseudonormal to impaired relaxation

9. In a patient with a *restrictive* pattern of filling and diastolic heart failure, which of the following is most likely to contribute to pulmonary edema?

   A. Delayed LV filling due to poor LV compliance resulting in markedly elevated LA and LV pressures
   B. Atrial contraction against a high ventricular pressure, resulting in regurgitant flow into the pulmonary veins
   C. A prolonged overall LV filling period during early diastole causing a larger dependence on atrial contraction
   D. Diastolic regurgitation into the pulmonary veins due to a prolonged deceleration time and diastasis period

10. The transition from normal filling to an impaired relaxation pattern of filling is best characterized by the following.

   A. An elevation in LA pressure
   B. The inability of the LV to drop its pressure adequately
   C. Poor LV compliance
   D. Delayed mitral valve opening

References

1. Trauzeddel RF, et al. Perioperative echocardiography-guided hemodynamic therapy in high-risk patients: a practical expert approach of hemodynamically focused echocardiography. J Clin Monit Comput. 2020;35:229.
2. Ha JW. Assessing diastolic function as an important tool for clinical decision-making in critically ill patients. J Cardiovasc Imaging. 2020;28(3):165–73.
3. Nagueh SF, Smiseth OA, Appleton CP, et al. Recommendations for the evaluation of left ventricular diastolic function by echocardiography: an update from the American Society of Echocardiography and the European Association of Cardiovascular Imaging. J Am Soc Echocardiogr. 2016;29:277–314.
4. Porter TR, et al. Guidelines for the use of echocardiography as a monitor for therapeutic intervention in adults: a report from the American Society of Echocardiography. J Am Soc Echocardiogr. 2015;28(1):40–56.
5. Romero-Bermejo FJ, et al. Echocardiographic hemodynamic monitoring in the critically ill patient. Curr Cardiol Rev. 2011;7(3):146–56.
6. Ommen SR, et al. Clinical utility of Doppler echocardiography and tissue Doppler imaging in the estimation of left ventricular filling pressures: a comparative simultaneous Doppler-catheterization study. Circulation. 2000;102(15):1788–94.
7. Kanji HD, et al. Limited echocardiography-guided therapy in subacute shock is associated with change in management and improved outcomes. J Crit Care. 2014;29(5):700–5.
8. Shillcutt SK, et al. Echocardiography-based hemodynamic management of left ventricular diastolic dysfunction: a feasibility and safety study. Echocardiography. 2014;31(10):1189–98.
9. Lattik R, et al. Mitral Doppler indices are superior to two-dimensional echocardiographic and hemodynamic variables in predicting responsiveness of cardiac output to a rapid intravenous infusion of colloid. Anesth Analg. 2002;94(5):1092–9.
10. Nicoara, A. and M. Swaminathan, Diastolic dysfunction, diagnostic and perioperative management in cardiac surgery . Curr Opin Anaesthesiol. 2015;28(1): 60–6. Nicoara A, Whitener G, Swaminathan M. Perioperative diastolic dysfunction: a comprehensive approach to assessment by transesophageal echocardiography. Semin Cardiothorac Vasc Anesth. 2013;18(2):218–36.
11. Mahmood F, Matyal R. Assessment of perioperative diastolic function and dysfunction. Int Anesthesiol Clin. 2008;46(2):51–62.
12. Mahmood F, Jainandunsing J, Matyal R. A practical approach to echocardiographic assessment of perioperative diastolic dysfunction. J Cardiothorac Vasc Anesth. 2012;26(6):1115–23.
13. Matyal R, et al. Perioperative assessment of diastolic dysfunction. Anesth Analg. 2011;113(3):449–72.
14. Groban L, Dolinski SY. Transesophageal echocardiographic evaluation of diastolic function. Chest. 2005;128(5):3652–63.
15. Swaminathan M, et al. Utility of a simple algorithm to grade diastolic dysfunction and predict outcome after coronary artery bypass graft surgery. Ann Thorac Surg. 2011;91(6):1844–50.
16. Matyal R, et al. Perioperative diastolic dysfunction during vascular surgery and its association with postoperative outcome. J Vasc Surg. 2009;50(1):70–6.
17. Axelsson B, et al. Milrinone improves diastolic function in coronary artery bypass surgery as assessed by acoustic quantification and peak filling rate: a prospective randomized study. J Cardiothorac Vasc Anesth. 2010;24(2):244–9.
18. Lobato EB, Gravenstein N, Martin TD. Milrinone, not epinephrine, improves left ventricular compliance after cardiopulmonary bypass. J Cardiothorac Vasc Anesth. 2000;14(4):374–7.
19. Malik V, et al. Effect of Levosimendan on diastolic function in patients undergoing coronary artery bypass grafting: a comparative study. J Cardiovasc Pharmacol. 2015;66(2):141–7.

13 Thoracic Aorta

Sophia P. Poorsattar and Timothy M. Maus

Abbreviations

CT	Computed tomography
IABP	Intra-aortic balloon pump
MRI	Magnetic resonance imaging
TEE	Transesophageal echocardiography
TTE	Transthoracic echocardiography

Introduction

Basic perioperative transesophageal echocardiography (TEE) guidelines suggest that knowledge of echocardiographic manifestations of lesions of the great vessels is a necessary training objective. Therefore, a thorough understanding of the use of TEE in evaluating the thoracic aorta, including normal and pathologic presentations, is essential to the basic perioperative echocardiographer. This chapter will review the essential TEE and TTE views for evaluating the thoracic aorta, including potential pitfalls, and review the major aortic pathologies of aortic dissection, aortic aneurysms, aortic atheromatous disease, and thoracic aortic trauma. Evaluation of the abdominal aorta is discussed in further detail in Chap. 19.

Supplementary Information The online version of this chapter (https://doi.org/10.1007/978-3-030-84349-6_13) contains supplementary material, which is available to authorized users.

S. P. Poorsattar
Department of Anesthesiology and Perioperative Medicine, University of California, Los Angeles Medical Center, Los Angeles, CA, USA

T. M. Maus (✉)
Department of Anesthesiology, University of California San Diego Health, La Jolla, CA, USA
e-mail: tmaus@health.ucsd.edu

Echocardiographic Views of the Thoracic Aorta

The aorta is a three-layered structure, with intimal, medial, and adventitial layers, that extends from the heart immediately beyond the aortic valve through the transverse aortic arch and descends toward the lower extremity vessel branches. It is described as having five anatomical sections (Fig. 13.1):

1. *Aortic Root*, which extends from the aortic valve to the sinotubular junction (which connects the root to the ascending tubular aorta). The aortic root contains three sinuses of Valsalva, two of which contain the left and right coronary artery ostia.
2. *Tubular Ascending Aorta*, which extends from the sinotubular junction to the aortic arch.
3. *Aortic Arch*, which is the transverse portion of the aorta, with typically three great vessel branches: innominate artery, left common carotid, and left subclavian artery.

T. M. Maus, C. R. Tainter (eds.), *Essential Echocardiography*,
https://doi.org/10.1007/978-3-030-84349-6_13

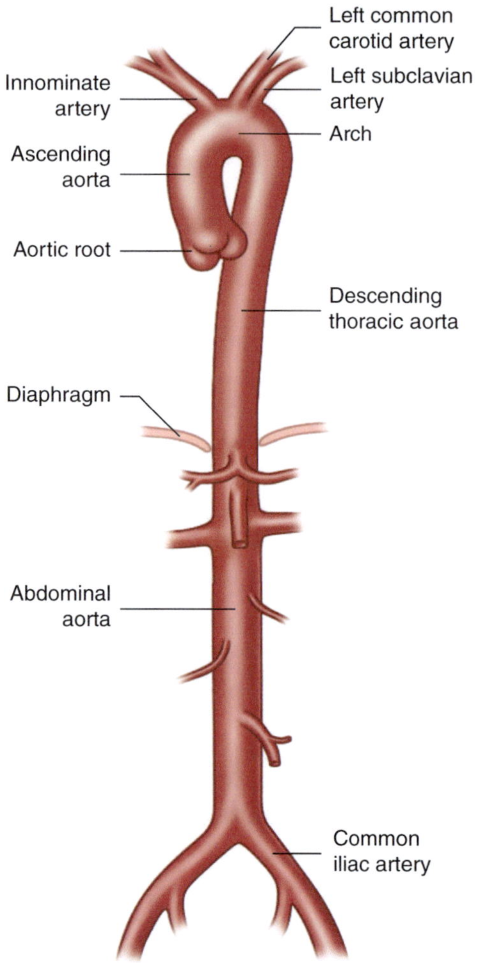

Fig. 13.1 Diagram of the entire aortic vascular system including its five anatomical components: 1. aortic root; 2. tubular ascending aorta; 3. aortic arch; 4. descending thoracic aorta; 5. abdominal aorta

4. *Descending Thoracic Aorta*, which extends from the distal edge of the left subclavian artery takeoff to the diaphragm.
5. *Abdominal Aorta*, which continues from the diaphragm to the lower extremity branch points (iliac arteries).

With TEE, the immediate proximity of the esophagus to the thoracic aorta allows excellent visualization and detection of disease states. However, limitations do exist. Because the trachea and left main bronchus are interposed between the esophagus and aorta, creating significant air-related artifact, imaging of the distal ascending aorta and proximal arch is often challenging or impossible (Fig. 13.2). Alternative echocardiographic approaches to imaging these regions include epiaortic imaging intraoperatively with an opened chest or the use of saline-filled balloons placed in the trachea. However, each of these techniques is beyond the scope of this text. While TTE also allows visualization of the aortic root, it differs from TEE in that it provides imaging windows of the distal ascending aorta and aortic arch. However, due to the distance of the probe from the aorta as it descends posteriorly in the thorax, it is less helpful than TEE for evaluating the descending thoracic aorta. As such, the combined application of both TEE and TTE allows for a complete assessment of the thoracic aorta.

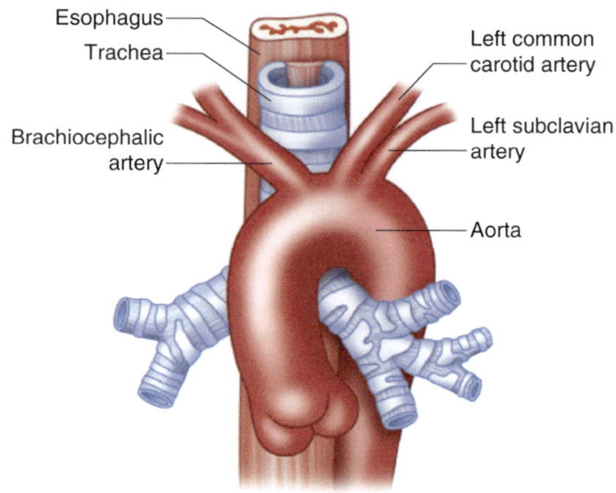

Fig. 13.2 Diagram of the distal ascending aorta, aortic arch, and proximal descending thoracic aorta, including its anterior relationship to the esophagus, with the trachea interposed. The air-filled trachea creates difficulty in TEE imaging the area is not depicted in red

TEE Views

The relationship of the esophagus to the aorta changes from cranial to caudal. The esophagus is posterior to the aorta at the cranial aspect near the arch; however, the structures twist on themselves such that the esophagus is anterior to the aorta at the gastroesophageal junction. This makes description and location of pathology dif-

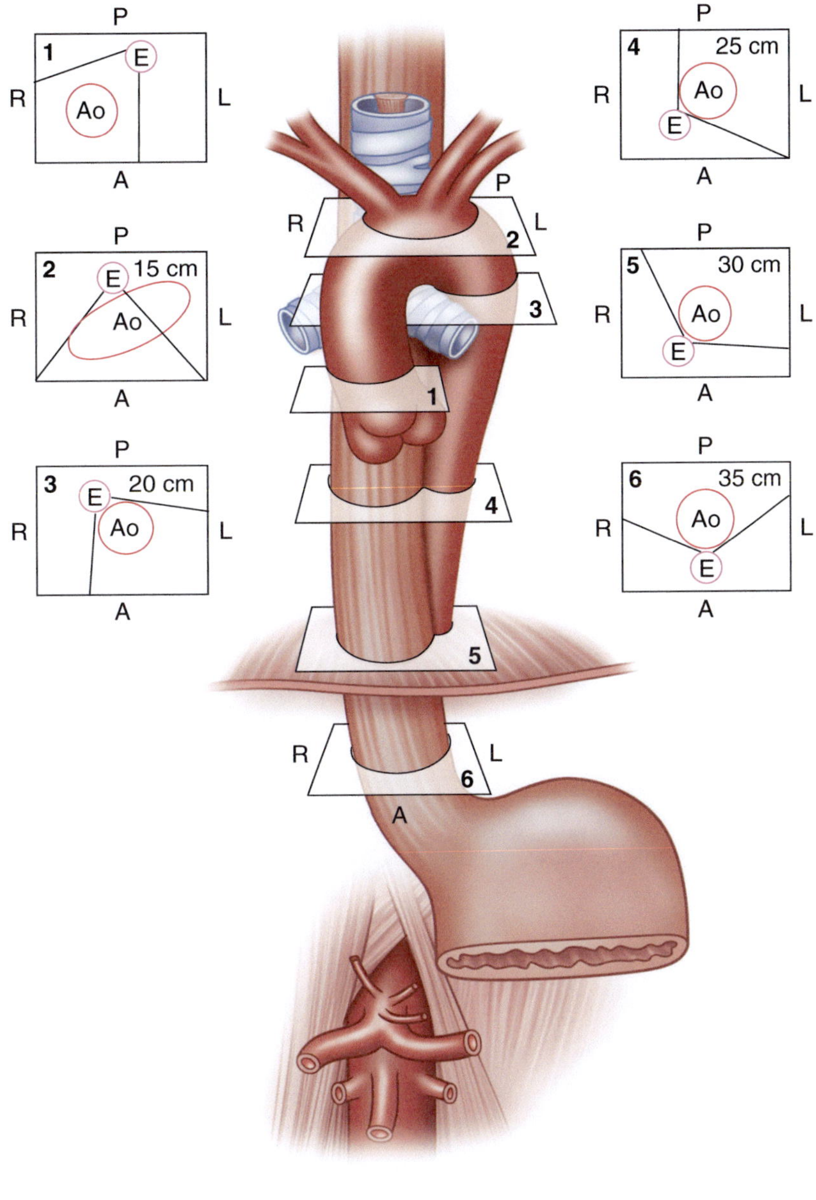

Fig. 13.3 Diagram of the thoracic aorta in relation to the esophagus. Note that when cephalad, the esophagus is positioned posterior to the aorta; however when moving caudally, the esophagus moves to an anterior position relative to the descending thoracic aorta. E esophagus

ficult because the echocardiographic imaging demonstrates a normally cylindrical shape (which appears circular in cross section) throughout the entire descending thoracic aorta (Fig. 13.3). The anterior, posterior, or lateral nature of a lesion is therefore difficult to identify. Lastly, when entering the stomach, the probe enters the intraperitoneal space *views*, while the aorta continues into the retroperitoneal space. Therefore, the probe is no longer opposing tissue near the aorta, and the abdominal aorta is not consistently imaged with TEE.

The TEE views of the aorta can largely be separated into a short- and long-axis view of each segment of the visible thoracic aorta (Table 13.1). When discussing the thoracic aorta, one must consider the aortic valve as disease of the aorta may affect the aortic valve and vice versa. The short- and long-axis views of the aortic valve provide an opportunity to evaluate the number, quality, and function of leaflets, to make appropriate measurements of left ventricular outflow tract (LVOT), aortic valve annulus, and sinotubular junction and to identify pathology such as aortic

Table 13.1 Transesophageal aortic views

Structure	Short axis	Long axis
Aortic valve	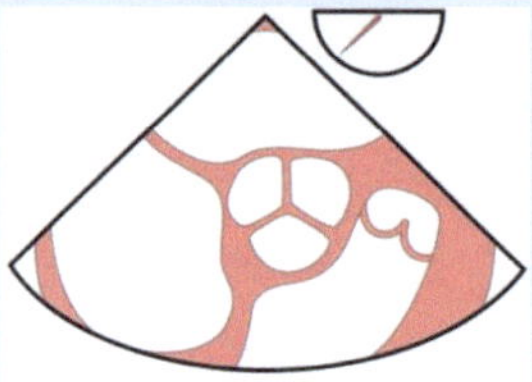 ME AV SAX	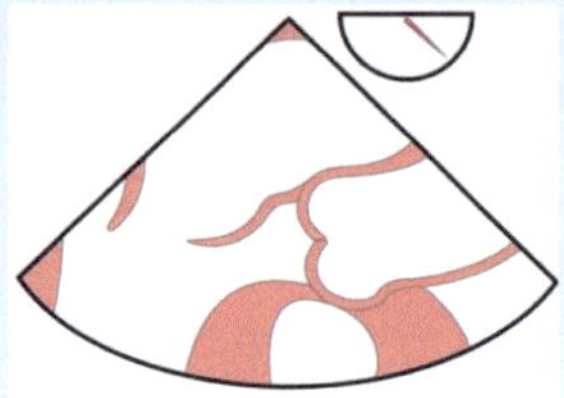 ME AV LAX
Ascending aorta	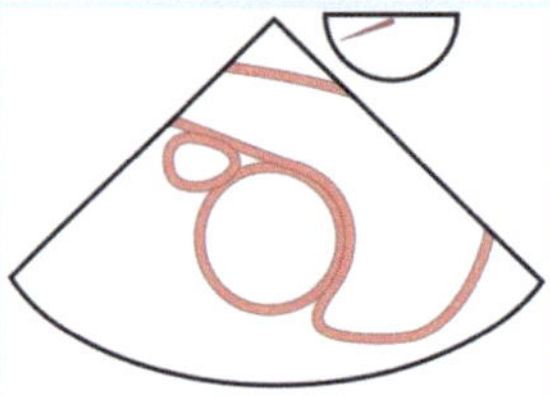 ME asc aortic SAX	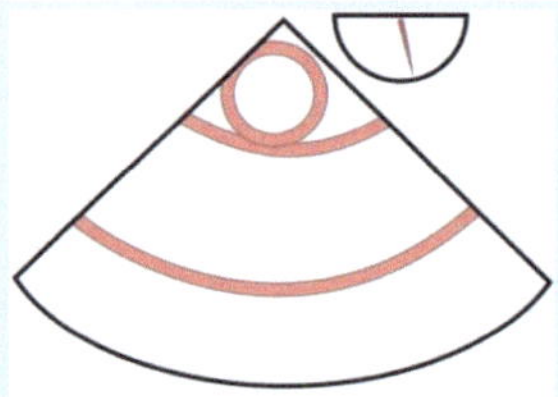 ME asc aortic LAX
Aortic arch	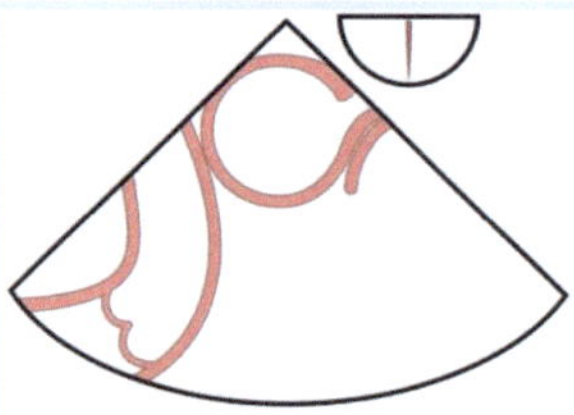 UE aortic arch SAX	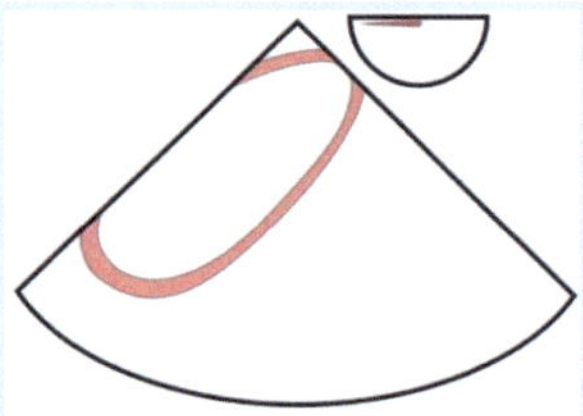 UE aortic arch LAX
Descending aorta	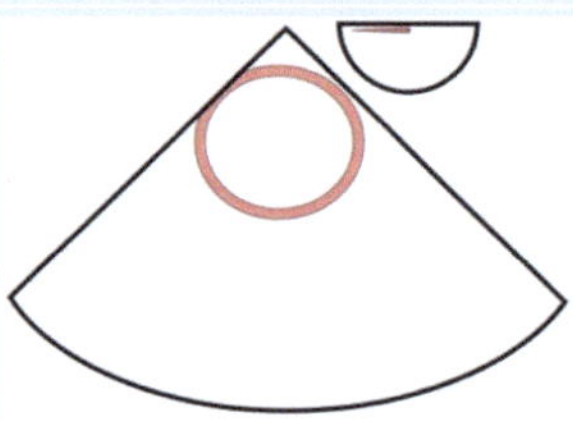 Desc aortic SAX	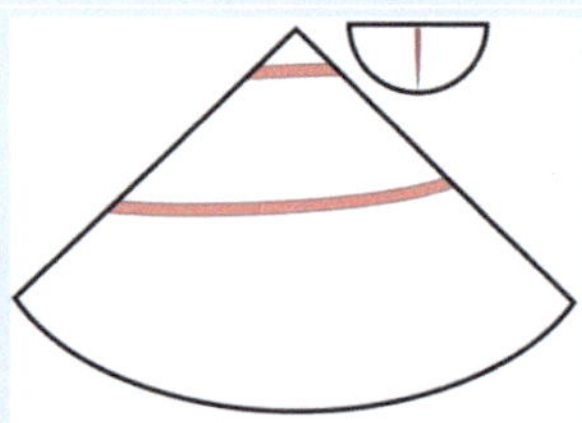 Desc aortic LAX

dissection or aneurysmal disease. The addition of color flow Doppler aids in the detection of valvular dysfunction. Withdrawing and advancing the probe at 0 and 90 degrees of multiplane allows the short- and long-axis examination, respectively, of the tubular ascending aorta. Obtaining the aortic arch views is easily achieved by rotating the TEE probe to the left until the circular descending thoracic aorta is identified and subsequently withdrawing the probe until the oval-shaped long-axis of the aortic arch is obtained. Increasing the multiplane angle to 90 degrees develops the short-axis view of the aortic arch. Of note, most commonly, the left subclavian artery takeoff is identified on the right side of the screen with the innominate vein noted *Views* distally. The left subclavian artery takeoff is an important structure for location identification in the descending aorta. As described above, determining the location of pathology in the descending aorta is difficult. Therefore, most commonly, the distance from the left subclavian artery takeoff to the pathology is used to communicate location. This technique is also utilized to properly place an intra-aortic balloon pump (IABP) within 1–2 cm distal to the left subclavian artery. Advancing the probe in both a 0- and 90-degree multiplane develops the short- and long-axis

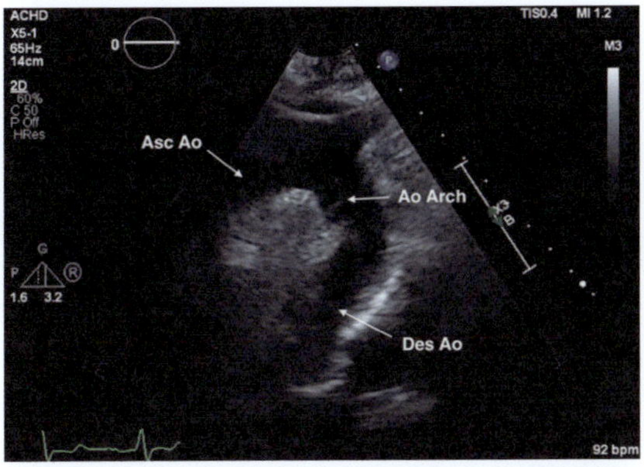

Fig. 13.4 Suprasternal view at the level of the aorta, demonstrating the distal ascending aorta (Asc Ao), aortic arch (Ao Arch), and proximal descending aorta (Des Ao). Here, the great vessels may be seen as they branch off the aortic arch

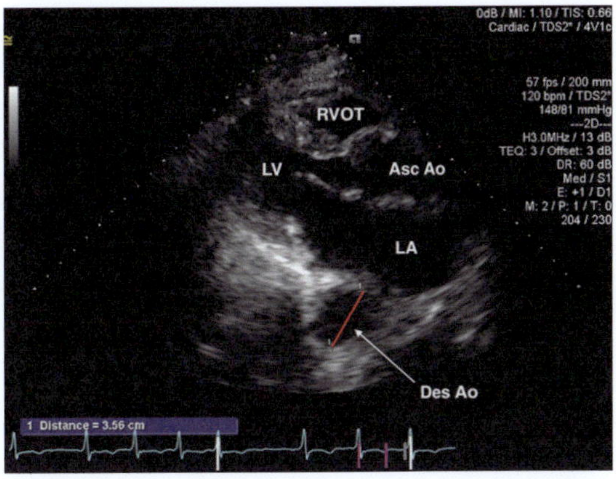

Fig. 13.5 Parasternal long-axis view with the descending aorta (Des Ao) in the fair field of the imaging sector. *RVOT* right ventricular outflow tract, *LV* left ventricle, *LA* left atrium, *Asc Ao* ascending aorta

views of the descending thoracic aorta, respectively.

TTE Views

While TEE is superior to TTE for assessment of the thoracic aorta, TTE provides the advantage of being a less-invasive, easily accessible screening modality and also allows the visualization of the TEE "blind spot" from the interposition of the trachea between the aorta and esophagus. Imaging of the aortic root and ascending aorta is best obtained through the parasternal windows, including parasternal long-axis and parasternal short-axis (right ventricular outflow tract level) views. As you follow the root to the ascending aorta, the parasternal short-axis view at the level of the pulmonary artery bifurcation allows the best assessment. From here, rotation of the probe 90 degrees or application of cross-plane imaging allows you to visualize the ascending aorta in long-axis. As you continue to follow the ascending aorta to the level of the aortic arch, the suprasternal long-axis view of the aorta provides a complete view of the aortic arch as it wraps around the right pulmonary artery. Unique to TTE, this view allows assessment of the distal ascending aorta, aortic arch with each of its three great vessels, and proximal descending aorta (Fig. 13.4). As mentioned, TTE is less helpful for evaluation of the descending aorta; however, it may be visualized in cross section in the far field of the imaging sector in the parasternal long-axis view (Fig. 13.5). Images of each of these TTE views can be found in Chap. 3.

Aortic Dissection (Highlight Box 13.1)

Highlight Box 13.1

Aortic dissection	
2D	• Large undulating mobile flap within aortic lumen • Ensure flap not due to imaging artifact • Differentiate true versus false lumen • SEC or thrombus in false lumen • Presence of pericardial or pleural effusion • Coronary artery involvement (wall motion abnormality)
CFD	• Differential flow patterns (true lumen = laminar; false lumen = sluggish) • Presence of aortic insufficiency
Spectral	• Evaluation of aortic insufficiency

Aortic dissection is typified by bleeding within the medial layer of the aorta, most commonly due to intimal tearing and separation. Propagation of bleeding within this layer separates the intima from the surrounding adventitial layer, yielding the classical dual-lumen appearance. The true lumen contains blood within the natural aortic lumen, while the false lumen is created by the force of blood ejecting through the intimal tear into the medial layer and contained by the adventitial layer.

This pathology carries a significant risk of morbidity and mortality with a 1–2% increased mortality *per hour* until definitive treatment [1]. Therefore, prompt diagnosis is of utmost concern. Patients at risk for developing an aortic dissection include those with long-standing hypertension, smoking, and connective tissue disorders [2]. Commonly-associated diseases include Marfan's syndrome, Ehlers-Danlos syndrome, bicuspid aortic valve, and coarctation of the aorta.

Two classification systems exist for classifying aortic dissections, DeBakey and Stanford [1]. The Stanford system separates any involvement of the ascending aorta into Stanford type A, which is a surgical emergency, while Stanford type B involves only the descending thoracic aorta below the left subclavian artery takeoff. Stanford type B dissections without complicating ischemia (paralysis, mesenteric ischemia, etc.) are often treated medically, while type A usually benefit from surgical treatment. The DeBakey system divides aortic dissections into three types: Type 1 involves the ascending and descending aorta, Type 2 involves the ascending aorta only, while Type 3 involves only the descending aorta below the left subclavian artery takeoff.

As mentioned above, prompt diagnosis is of paramount importance in such patients to reduce morbidity and mortality. The historical diagnostic gold standard involves angiography and the demonstration of contrast exiting the true lumen into the false lumen. The time-consuming process and increased risk of contrast-induced nephropathy have reduced this practice, being replaced by computed tomography (CT) and magnetic resonance imaging (MRI). The downside of each of these modalities is the continued need for patient transport, as well as being potentially time-consuming. While TTE may be of use as an initial screening modality, TEE also serves as an accessible portable modality while providing excellent sensitivity and specificity in the detection of aortic dissections. Shiga et al. demonstrated that TEE has a sensitivity of 98% and specificity of 95% and is comparable to CT or MRI [3]. Therefore, patients who are hemodynamically unstable and unable to be transported to an imaging suite may be evaluated by TEE in the emergency department, intensive care unit, or operating room.

The echocardiographic approach to an aortic dissection involves confirming the presence and the location of a dissection flap, as well as potentially identifying intimal tear entry/exit sites, differentiating the true versus false lumen, and identifying complicating pathologies, such as aortic insufficiency, pericardial and pleural effusions, coronary artery involvement, and ventricular dysfunction. Of note, the current basic perioperative TEE consensus statement suggests that in the setting of complex pathology such as an aortic dissection, appropriate consultation with an advanced echocardiographer or other imaging modalities is indicated [4].

Dissection Flap Identification

Identification of the intimal flap is the cornerstone of the aortic dissection diagnosis. Typically, the intimal flap is noted as a thin, undulating mobile structure that is entirely contained within the lumen of the aorta. Multiple multiplane angles should be utilized to ensure that there is a flap present, representing the separation of the true and false lumens, as occasionally artifacts can mimic a dissection flap (Figs. 13.6 and 13.7; Videos 13.1 and 13.2). With the cardiac cycle, systolic ejection into the aortic lumen causes true lumen expansion, while delayed entry of blood through the intimal tear into the false lumen causes delayed filling with sluggish or no flow. This cycling of expansion leads to the undulating mobile appearance of the intimal flap. Discussed below, the differential flow patterns may be detected with color flow Doppler to aid in identifying true versus false lumens. In addition to identifying the presence of the intimal flap, describing the location and extent of the dissection is important. Location within the ascending aorta or aortic arch denotes a surgical emergency. Dissection through adjacent structures or branches, such as the coronary arteries, great vessels, or aortic valves may also necessitate prompt surgical repair.

Echocardiography may identify not just the presence of an intimal flap but also the intimal tear site. The tear appears as an opening or communication in the intimal flap, with color flow Doppler documenting the presence of flow from the true to the false lumen (Fig. 13.8; Video 13.3). When a tear site is identified in the ascending aorta near the aortic valve, flow may be bidirectional between the true and false lumens because of pressure differentials near the aortic valve during systole and diastole. During systolic ejection, flow and pressure are higher in the true lumen with flow from true to false lumen through the tear site. During diastole, particularly with associated aortic insufficiency, the pressure is temporarily higher in the false lumen with a return of flow to the true lumen (Fig. 13.9; Video 13.4).

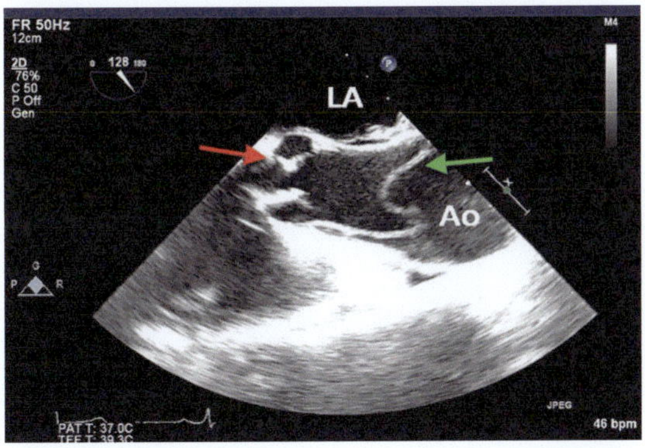

Fig. 13.6 Midesophageal aortic valve long-axis view with the probe slightly withdrawn to demonstrate more of the tubular ascending aorta. The *red arrow* points to a calcified aortic valve, while the *green arrow* indicates an undulating intimal flap within the aortic lumen. *LA* left atrium, *Ao* aorta

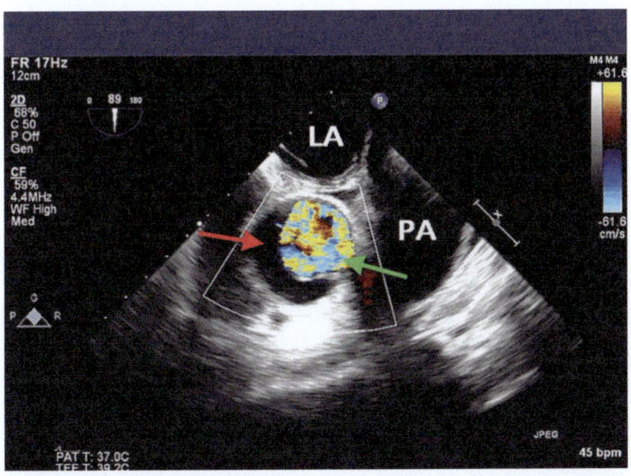

Fig. 13.7 Midesophageal view of the ascending aorta, developed by a slow withdrawal of the probe from an aortic valve short-axis view. The *green arrow* points to a true lumen with rapid early-systolic flow, while the *red arrow* indicates the false lumen with little to no flow demonstrated on color flow Doppler. *LA* left atrium, *PA* main pulmonary artery

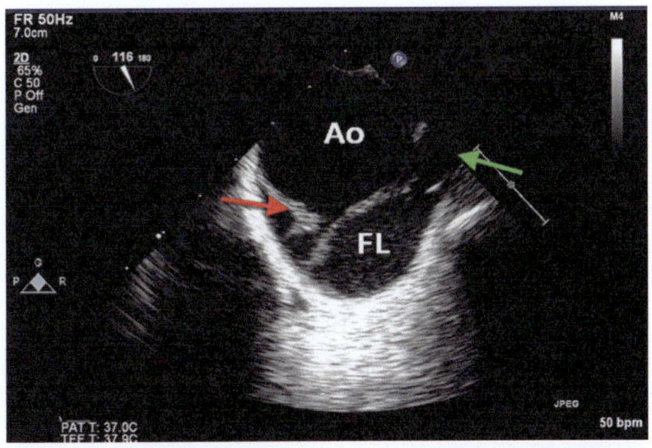

Fig. 13.8 Upper esophageal aortic arch short-axis view in a patient with an acute aortic arch dissection. The *red arrow* points to the tear site in the intimal flap. The *green arrow* indicates the left subclavian artery takeoff, which branches from the false lumen and has compromised flow. *Ao* aorta, *FL* false lumen

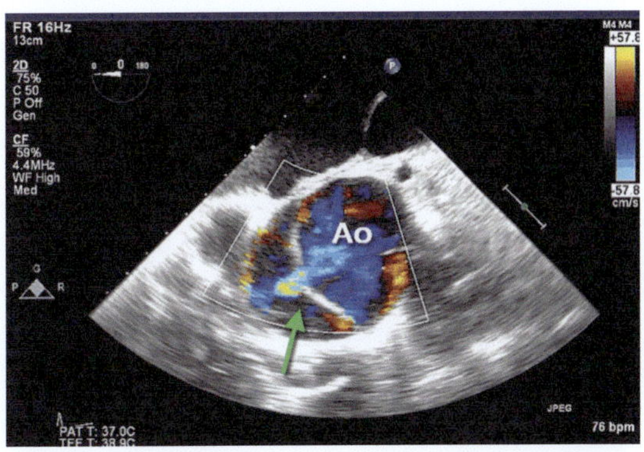

Fig. 13.9 Midesophageal ascending aortic short-axis view in a patient with an ascending aortic dissection. The *green arrow* indicates the tear site in the intimal flap with systolic flow demonstrated from the true lumen into the false lumen. *Ao* ascending aorta

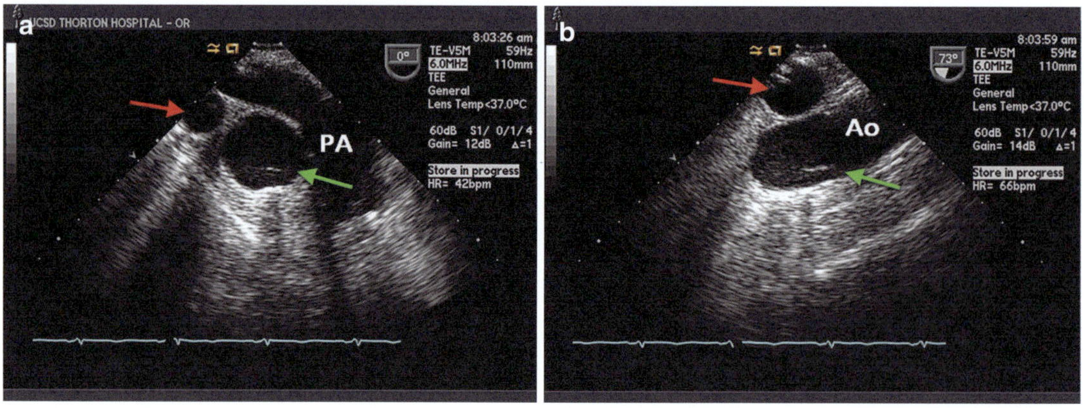

Fig. 13.10 (**a**) Midesophageal ascending aortic short-axis view, in a patient with a side lobe artifact. The *red arrow* indicates the superior vena cava. The *green arrow* indicates a side lobe artifact from a large out-of-plane specular reflector (such as a central line or pulmonary artery catheter). This linear density in the ascending aorta may be confused with an aortic dissection. (**b**) Midesophageal ascending aortic long-axis view of the same patient. The *red arrow* points to the right PA which contains a PA catheter. The *green arrow* points to a side lobe artifact which may be confused for an aortic dissection. *Ao* ascending aorta, *PA* pulmonary artery

Care must be taken to distinguish intimal flaps from imaging artifacts which, particularly in the ascending aorta, may appear as linear densities within the aortic lumen. Side lobe artifacts involve weak ultrasound beams emitted off-axis from the main imaging plane and returning from strong reflectors to the ultrasound probe. A common occurrence is a side lobe reflection from an off-plane central line or pulmonary artery catheter displayed as a linear echogenic density in the ascending aorta in the midesophageal ascending aortic short-axis view (Fig. 13.10a, b; Videos 13.5a and 13.5b). Again, it is emphasized that except in emergency situations, current consensus statement suggests that a basic echocardiographer consult an advanced echocardiographer when evaluating aortic dissections to confirm the diagnosis.

Differentiating True from False Lumens

The ability to differentiate true from false lumens serves to confirm the presence of an aortic dissection, rule out imaging artifacts, and, in the case of aortic surgery, allow the confirmation of surgical repair (lack of false lumen flow post-repair). There are several characteristics of true and false lumens that are fairly common: size, shape, systolic motion, and type or presence of flow (Table 13.2). With two-dimensional echocardiography, the true lumen is often the smaller and round-shaped lumen, while the false lumen tends to be the larger, irregularly shaped structure. The larger false lumen is often crescentic ("moon-like"), with concavity toward the true lumen. Systolic motion, as described above, involves the expansion of the true lumen with systolic ejection. Since the false lumen has delayed flow, the structure will compress during systole (Fig. 13.11a, b; Videos 13.6a and 13.6b). M-mode echocardiography may aid in identifying which structure is expanding during the systolic portion of the cardiac cycle. Lastly, color flow Doppler may be useful in differentiating if the true lumen has early-systolic laminar flow, while the false lumen has late-systolic turbulent flow. False

Table 13.2 Echocardiographic differentiation of aortic dissection true and false lumens

True lumen	False lumen
Smaller	Larger
Round	Irregular
Systolic expansion	Systolic compression
Early laminar flow	Late turbulent flow
	+/− Spontaneous contrast
	+/− Thrombus

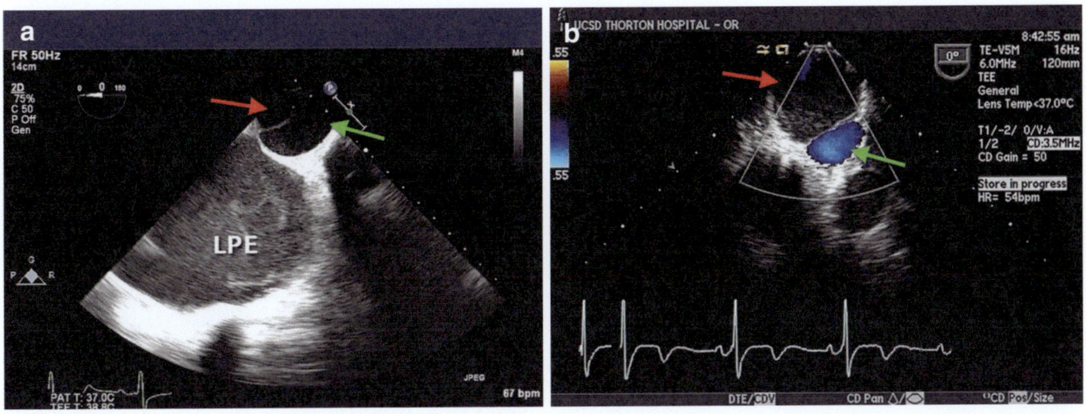

Fig. 13.11 (**a**) Descending thoracic aortic short-axis view in a patient with an aortic dissection. The *red arrow* indicates the true lumen. The *green arrow* indicates the false lumen, which contains spontaneous echo contrast. There is a large left-sided pleural effusion (LPE). (**b**) Descending thoracic aortic short-axis view with color flow Doppler in a separate patient with an aortic dissection. The *green arrow* indicates laminar flow in the true lumen and the *red arrow* indicates the false lumen with sluggish flow

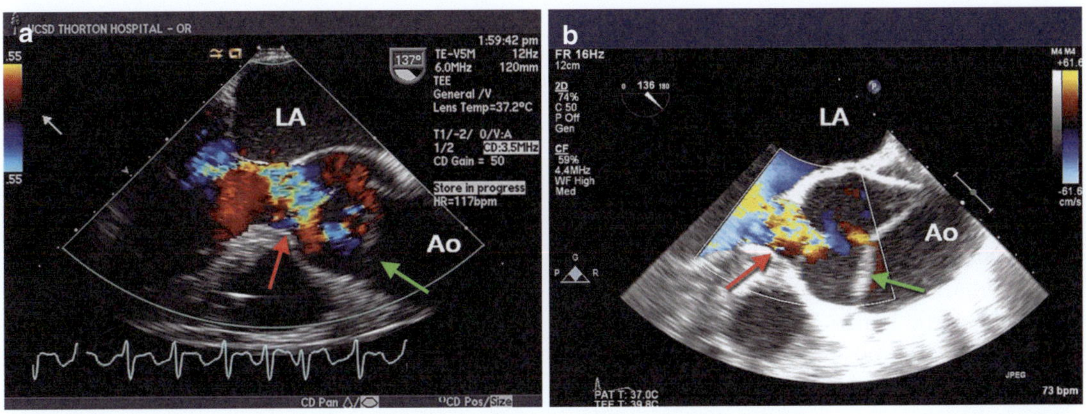

Fig. 13.12 (**a**) Midesophageal aortic valve long-axis view in a patient with an ascending aortic dissection. The *green arrow* indicates the intimal flap located near the sinotubular junction, while the red arrow indicates associated severe aortic insufficiency. (**b**) Midesophageal aortic valve long-axis view in a separate patient with an ascending aortic dissection. The *green arrow* indicates the intimal flap located near the sinotubular junction. Note the intimal tear with diastolic flow reversing back into the true lumen from the false lumen. The *red arrow* indicates associated severe aortic insufficiency. *LA* left atrium, *Ao* ascending aorta

lumens contain such sluggish flow that spontaneous echo contrast or frank thrombus may be identified.

Identifying Complicating Pathologies

The proximity of the aorta to several other anatomical structures, as well as the dependency of the branch vessels on an intact aorta, allows an aortic dissection to wreak havoc beyond just the damaged vessel itself. An advantage of echocardiography over other modalities includes its ability to evaluate surrounding structures and the effect of a dissection on those structures. As described above, the aortic valve is intimately connected to the aorta such that an aortic dissection may yield significant aortic valve dysfunction (Fig. 13.12a, b; Videos 13.7a and 13.7b). There are several mechanisms by which an ascending dissection may cause aortic insufficiency, such as the mobile flap itself impeding

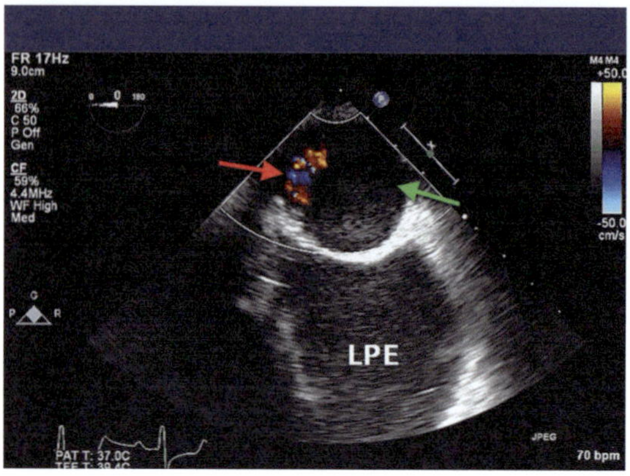

Fig. 13.13 Descending thoracic aortic short-axis view with color flow Doppler in a patient with an aortic dissection and a large left pleural effusion (LPE). The *red arrow* indicates the true lumen, while the *green arrow* indicates the false lumen

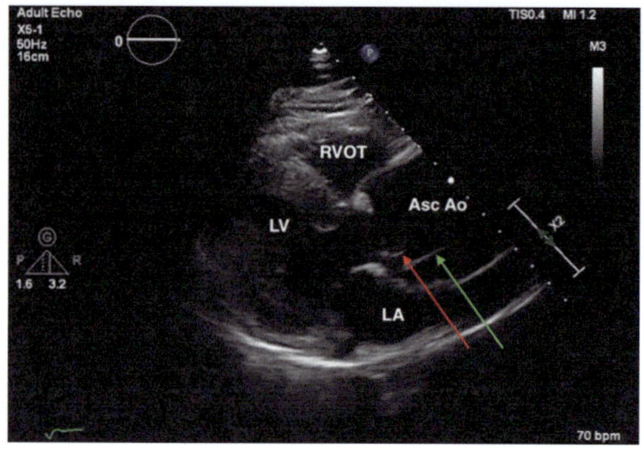

Fig. 13.14 Parasternal long-axis view in a patient with an ascending aortic dissection. The *green arrow* indicates the dissection flap extending to the aortic root with involvement of the coronary ostium. This can be distinguished from the aortic valve leaflet indicated by the *red arrow*. *RVOT* right ventricular outflow tract, *LV* left ventricle, *LA* left atrium, *Asc Ao* ascending aorta

valve closure or the large false lumen causing annular dilation or distortion and subsequent malcoaptation. A detailed evaluation of the mechanism is important in determining the need for concomitant valve replacement during aortic surgery; however this analysis is beyond the scope of this text.

In a normal state, the three layers of the aortic wall (intima, media, adventitia) contain the blood within the aortic lumen. During an aortic dissection, blood in the false lumen is now only contained by the adventitial layer, allowing a transudative process to leak into the surrounding spaces, such as the pericardial or left pleural space. An inflammatory component also appears to play a role in the development of pleural effusions [5]. Pericardial effusions are noted as an echolucent area surrounding the heart or great vessels in nearly any view, but commonly the midesophageal four-chamber or transgastric short-axis views with TEE and the apical four-chamber or parasternal short-axis (midpapillary level) with TTE. Determining tamponade physiology is discussed in the pericardium chapter (see Chap. 14). Left-sided pleural effusions are noted as an echolucent area anterior to the descending thoracic aorta in the descending aortic short-axis view (Fig. 13.13; Video 13.8). Frank rupture of the dissection into the pericardial or pleural space causes a hemorrhagic effusion, rapid accumulation of blood, and significant hemodynamic deterioration.

During evaluation of an ascending aortic dissection that is approaching the aortic root, careful evaluation should include the ostia of the main coronary arteries. The aortic root contains three sinuses of Valsalva, two of which contain coronary arteries (left and right). A proximal dissection through a coronary ostium and resultant reduction of its blood supply may result in significant myocardial ischemia or infarction (Fig. 13.14; Video 13.9). An evaluation for wall motion abnormalities should be included if coronary involvement is suspected (Fig. 13.15a, b; Videos 13.10a and 13.10b).

Lastly, aortic dissections may result in ventricular dysfunction through two major mechanisms. As previously described, acute ischemia may result in wall motion abnormalities and frank right ventricular or left ventricular dysfunction. In another fashion, acute aortic insufficiency causes abrupt volume overload to a ventricle that has not had the time to dilate and adapt to the volume overload (as in chronic aortic insufficiency). Therefore, an evaluation of biventricular function is important in the setting of ascending aortic dissections.

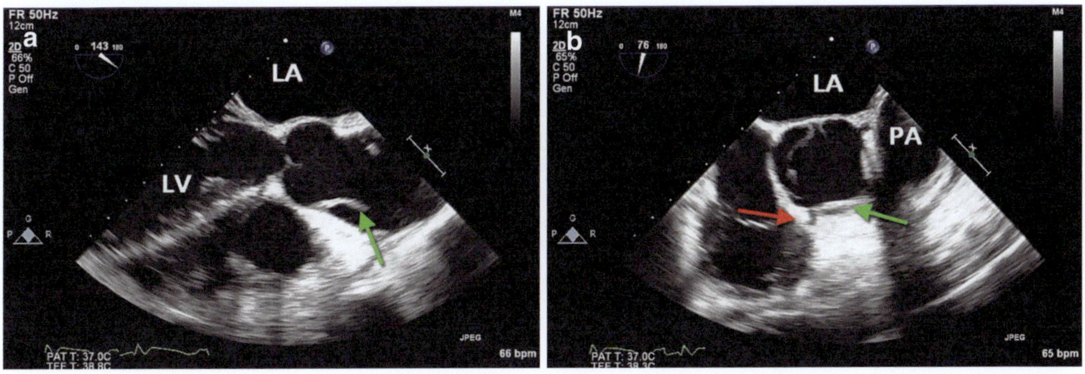

Fig. 13.15 (**a**) Midesophageal aortic valve long-axis view in a patient with an ascending aortic dissection. The *green arrow* indicates the intimal flap located near the sinotubular junction and extending into the right sinus of Valsalva. (**b**) Midesophageal aortic valve short-axis view in the same patient. The *green arrow* indicates the intimal flap located abutting the right coronary ostium (indicated by the *red arrow*). *LA* left atrium, *LV* left ventricle, *PA* pulmonary artery

Aortic Aneurysm (Highlight Box 13.2)

Highlight Box 13.2

Aortic aneurysm	
2D	• Evidence of aortic dilation (linear measurements) • Branch involvement • Aortic root involvement (aortic valve malcoaptation)
CFD	• Presence of aortic insufficiency
Spectral	• Evaluation of aortic insufficiency

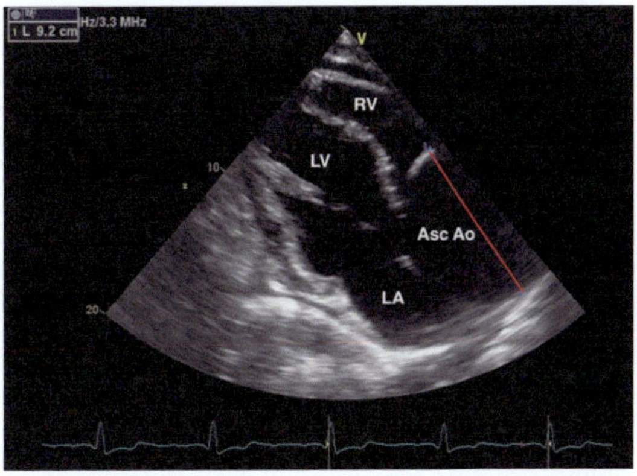

Fig. 13.16 Parasternal long-axis view in a patient with a large ascending aortic aneurysm. The *red line* indicates a dimension of 9.2 cm. *RV* right ventricle, *LV* left ventricle, *LA* left atrium, *Asc Ao* ascending aorta

Aortic dilation refers to the enlargement of the aorta beyond the upper limits of normal size. Normal adult thoracic aortic diameters are approximately 3.5–4.0 cm for the aortic root and less than 3.0 cm for the ascending and descending thoracic aorta. An aneurysm is classically described as a dilated segment of all three layers of an arterial wall with a vessel size that is beyond 150% of its normal size. Surgical repair is considered as the aorta dilates beyond 4.5–5.5 cm, taking into consideration the patients' history and risk factors [6]. Due to its noninvasive nature, TTE is often the imaging modality of choice for the screening of at-risk patients or for the serial follow-up imaging of patients with known ascending aortic aneurysms. However, as previously noted, TTE does not reliably image the descending aorta and is not used for serial assessment of this region (Fig. 13.16). Again, the close relationship of the esophagus to the aorta allows excellent TEE imaging of dilated and aneurysmal segments of the aorta. However, TEE does not carry the same potency in diagnosis of thoracic aortic aneurysm as it does in the setting of acute aortic dissection. As such, intermittent imaging by CT or MRI at longer time intervals is recommended in addition to echocardiography to allow for more accurate monitoring of the aortic diameter. In the setting of aortic aneurysms, proper surgical planning is essential to successful treatment and relies on preoperative imaging. Proper identification of tortuosity, anterior spinal arteries (including the artery of Adamkiewicz), and branch vessels may help guide management of cardiopulmonary bypass and neuroprotection strategies. Transesophageal echocardiography, however, still plays a role in the intraoperative management and in the setting of an unstable patient with an aneurysm rupture.

The echocardiographic approach to a patient with an aneurysm is similar to that of a dissection and includes determining the location and extent of disease, as well as identifying coexisting pathologies. Measurements in multiple planes may be helpful to identify the degree and extent of the aneurysm. In the setting of ascending aortic aneurysms, measurement of the aortic valve annulus and sinotubular junction may aid in assessing both the aneurysm and potential aortic valve involvement (Fig. 13.17). Care must be undertaken as proper cross-sectional measurements may be difficult in the setting of tortuosity.

Coexisting pathology with aortic aneurysm most often relates to the aorta's intimate structural relationship to the aortic valve. In the setting of aortic stenosis, the resultant post-stenotic turbulent flow in the ascending aorta leads to altered hemodynamics and an increased outward pressure. This results in post-stenotic aortic dilatation that may halt after aortic valve replacement in calcific aortic stenosis [7]. Bicuspid aortic valve disease may also progress toward aortic stenosis with attendant aortic dilatation. However, despite aortic valve replacement, aortic dilatation may continue in these patients. In addition, another group of patients with bicuspid aortic valve may present with annular dilation and aortic insufficiency without stenosis, potentially necessitating replacement of both the valve and ascending aorta (Fig. 13.18; Video 13.11). Lastly, the dilated aorta itself may have an impact on aortic valve function. As the aortic valve is crown-shaped, with attachments near the annulus at the base and the sinotubular junction at the top, dilation of the root may result in malcoaptation of the aortic valve leaflets and subsequent aortic regurgitation (Fig. 13.19; Video 13.12).

Aortic Atheroma

Transesophageal echocardiography is very sensitive to the detection of aortic atheromatous disease, and the presence of such plaque carries significant patient risk. While atheromatous disease may be detected with TTE from the suprasternal view of the aorta, it is less reliable and provides inferior visualization as compared to TEE. When atheromatous disease is noted to be

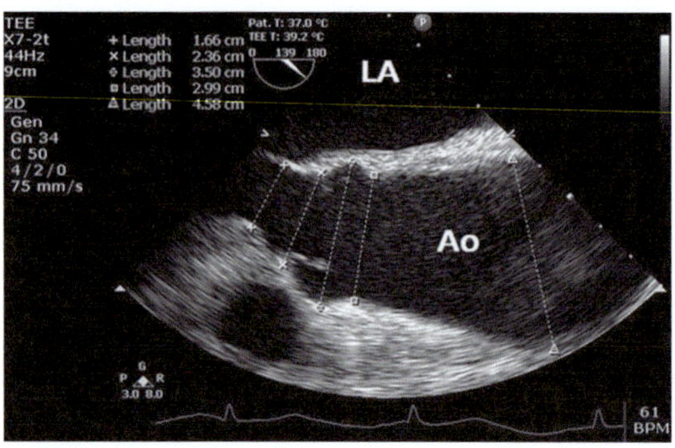

Fig. 13.17 Midesophageal aortic valve long-axis view in a patient with an ascending aortic aneurysm. Measurements of the left ventricular outflow tract, aortic annulus, sinuses of Valsalva, sinotubular junction, and ascending aorta note the presence of an ascending aortic aneurysm without significant involvement of the aortic root. *LA* left atrium, *Ao* ascending aorta

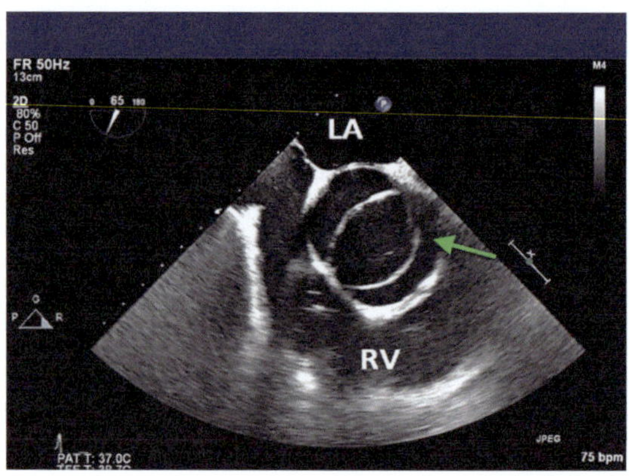

Fig. 13.18 Midesophageal aortic valve short-axis view in a patient with a bicuspid aortic valve and ascending aortic aneurysm. The *green arrow* indicates the bicuspid valve with a unified right and left coronary cusp. Note the dilated annulus. *LA* left atrium, *RV* right ventricle

greater than or equal to 4 mm in thickness, it is associated with increased risk of all vascular events, including stroke, myocardial infarction, peripheral emboli, and death [1]. The echocardiographic imaging approach includes noting severity, location, as well as mobility of the atheroma (Figs. 13.20 and 13.21a, b; Videos 13.13a and 13.13b). The grading of atheromatous disease is displayed in Table 13.3. In the setting of interventional vascular procedures, the presence of severe atheromatous disease, including plaque mobility, should be communicated to the surgical team to prevent inadvertent embolization.

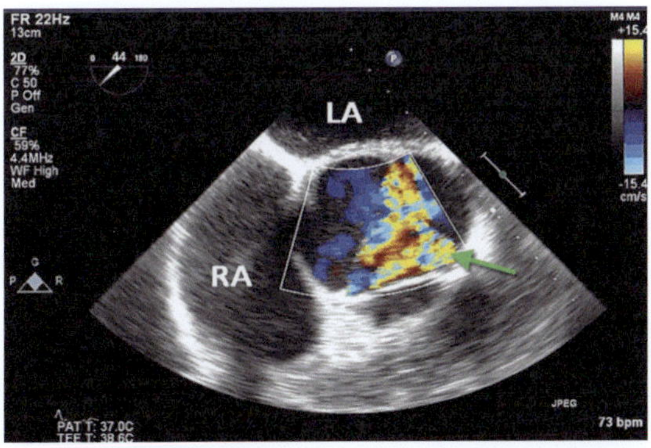

Fig. 13.19 Midesophageal aortic valve short-axis view with color flow Doppler in a patient with an ascending aortic aneurysm. The *green arrow* indicates the significant aortic insufficiency from the associated dilated annulus. *LA* left atrium, *RA* right atrium

Thoracic Aortic Trauma

The thoracic aorta has both relatively fixed and mobile portions. The junctions of these portions are often the site of injury in blunt aortic injury, mostly commonly the aortic isthmus (immedi-

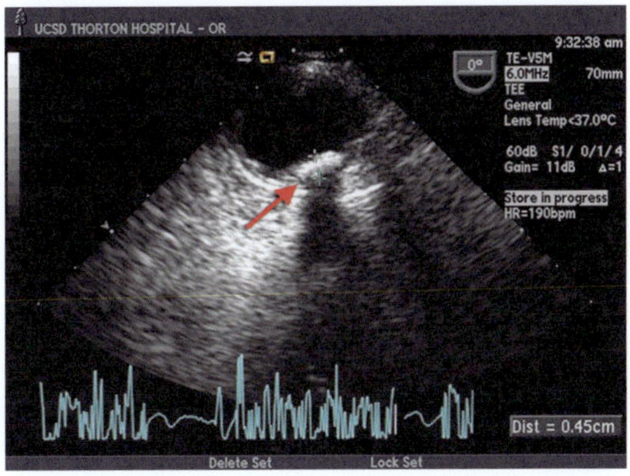

Fig. 13.20 Descending thoracic aorta short-axis view demonstrating an aortic atheroma measuring 4.5 millimeters, Grade III disease (*red arrow*)

Table 13.3 Echocardiographic grading of atheromatous disease

Grade	Description
1	Normal aorta; minimal intimal thickening
2	Extensive intimal thickening
3	Calcified aortic plaque less than 5 mm
4	Calcified aortic plaque greater than 5 mm
5	Mobile atheroma or ulcerated plaque

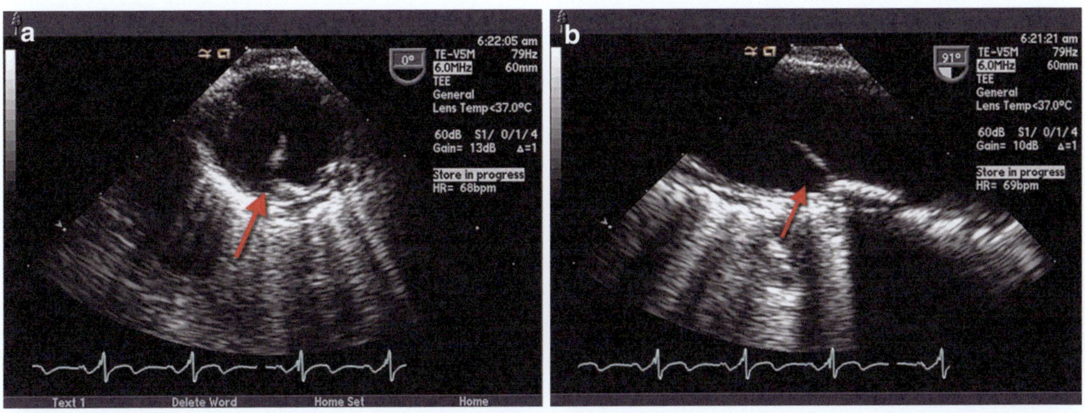

Fig. 13.21 (**a**) Descending thoracic aortic short-axis view demonstrating complex atheromatous disease. The *red arrow* indicates a large pedunculated mobile portion extending into the aortic lumen. (**b**) Descending thoracic aortic long-axis view of the same patient. The *red arrow* again points to the pedunculated mobile portion of the atheroma

ately distal to the left subclavian artery) and the ascending aorta (immediately distal to the aortic valve). The most common mechanism for this type of injury is a rapid deceleration, which transmits the sheer force between the relatively fixed and mobile portions. This usually involves damage to the aortic intima, with potential damage through the media and adventitia, including complete aortic transection [8].

Echocardiographically, aortic trauma may share characteristics of a spontaneous aortic dissection. However, on examination of a traumatic aortic injury, the medial flap tends to be thicker in appearance, the lesion is more often isolated without propagation, and there may be presence of an abnormal aortic contour, an aortic pseudoaneurysm, or a crescent-shaped intramural hematoma. A complete evaluation of the thoracic aorta in this setting should be in consultation with an advanced echocardiographer or confirmed with an alternative imaging technique.

Conclusion

Echocardiography is an excellent monitor for the diagnosis of several aortic pathologies, albeit with some limitations. Knowledge of these limitations allows this modality to be utilized in the setting of aortic dissection, aneurysm, atheroma, and trauma. The basic echocardiographer should have a sound understanding of thoracic aortic imaging with both TEE and TTE.

Questions

1. Which of the following is most true regarding distinguishing the true lumen from false lumen of an aortic dissection with echocardiography?

   (a) The false lumen has a higher systolic velocity.
   (b) The false lumen has echocardiographic evidence of stasis or thrombus.
   (c) The false lumen is often round in the short-axis view.
   (d) The true lumen has late turbulent flow in systole.

2. Which of the following is most true regarding distinguishing the true lumen from false lumen of an aortic dissection with echocardiography?

   (a) The true lumen is often crescentic in shape.
   (b) The true lumen is usually larger.
   (c) The true lumen has early laminar systolic flow on color flow Doppler.
   (d) The intimal flap moves toward the true lumen in systole.

3. Which of the following is *least* likely to be a consequence of aortic dissection?

   (a) Aortic stenosis
   (b) Myocardial infarction
   (c) Pleural effusion
   (d) Aortic insufficiency

4. Which of the following is most true regarding the use of TTE versus TEE for the identification of aortic pathology?

   (a) TTE is more sensitive and specific than TEE for the detection of aortic dissections.
   (b) The "blind spot" of the aorta with TEE imaging exists due to the interposition of the trachea between the esophagus and the aorta.
   (c) TTE is more useful than TEE for imaging of the descending aorta.
   (d) The entire thoracic aorta may be visualized by TEE imaging alone.

5. Select the correct pairing for echocardiographic grading of atheromatous disease.

   (a) Grade 2 – Minimal intimal thickening
   (b) Grade 3 – Calcified aortic plaque measuring 6 mm
   (c) Grade 4 – Calcified aortic plaque measuring 7 mm and mobile
   (d) Grade 5 – Calcified aortic plaque measuring 1 mm and mobile

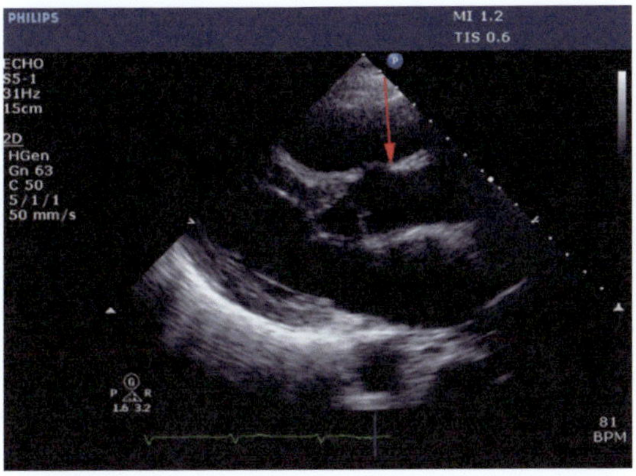

6. Which aortic section is indicated by the arrow in the figure below?

   (a) Aortic sinuses of Valsalva
   (b) Sinotubular junction
   (c) Aortic root
   (d) Tubular ascending aorta

7. A dilated segment of the aorta is considered aneurysmal when it exceeds what percent of its normal size?

   (a) 100%
   (b) 125%
   (c) 150%
   (d) 200%

8. Which of the following is most true regarding the classification systems for aortic dissections?

   (a) DeBakey Type 3 dissections are a surgical emergency.
   (b) Stanford A dissections when uncomplicated are often treated medically.
   (c) Stanford B dissections involve both the ascending and descending thoracic aorta.
   (d) DeBakey Type 2 dissections involve the ascending aorta only.

9. Which TTE view best images the "blind spot" encountered during imaging of the thoracic aorta with TEE?

   (a) Parasternal long-axis
   (b) Parasternal short-axis: pulmonary artery bifurcation level
   (c) Apical four-chamber
   (d) Suprasternal long-axis of the aorta

10. Which of the following is most true regarding the ability to distinguish artifact from a dissection flap?

   (a) Artifacts are often seen in multiple views.
   (b) Changing the angle of incidence will not affect the presence of artifacts.
   (c) A dissection flap has motion independent of the aorta.
   (d) Adjusting the imaging depth can move the artifact outside the aortic lumen.

References

1. Khalil A, Helmy T, Porembka DT. Aortic pathology: aortic trauma, debris, dissection, and aneurysm. Crit Care Med. 2007;35:S392–400.
2. Nienaber CA, Clough RE. Management of acute aortic dissection. Lancet. 2015;385:800–11.
3. Shiga T, Wajima Z, Apfel CC, Inoue T, Ohe Y. Diagnostic accuracy of transesophageal echocardiography, helical computed tomography, and magnetic resonance imaging for suspected thoracic aortic dissection: systematic review and meta-analysis. Arch Intern Med. 2006;166:1350–6.
4. Reeves ST, Finley AC, Skubas NJ, et al. Basic perioperative transesophageal echocardiography examination: a consensus statement of the American Society of Echocardiography and the Society of Cardiovascular Anesthesiologists. J Am Soc Echocardiogr. 2013;26:443–56.
5. Hata N, Tanaka K, Imaizumi T, et al. Clinical significance of pleural effusion in acute aortic dissection. Chest. 2002;121:825–30.
6. Hiratzka LF, Bakris GL, Beckman JA, et al. 2010 ACCF/AHA/AATS/ACR/ASA/SCA/SCAI/SIR/STS/SVM guidelines for the diagnosis and management of patients with thoracic aortic disease. A report

of the American College of Cardiology Foundation/ American Heart Association task force on practice guidelines, American Association for Thoracic Surgery, American College of Radiology, American Stroke Association, Society of Cardiovascular Anesthesiologists, Society for Cardiovascular Angiography and Interventions, Society of Interventional Radiology, Society of Thoracic Surgeons, and Society for Vascular Medicine. J Am Coll Cardiol. 2010;55:e27–e129.

7. Wilton E, Jahangiri M. Post-stenotic aortic dilatation. J Cardiothorac Surg. 2006;1:7.
8. Goldstein SA, Evangelista A, Abbara S, et al. Multimodality imaging of diseases of the thoracic aorta in adults: from the American Society of Echocardiography and the European Association of Cardiovascular Imaging: endorsed by the Society of Cardiovascular Computed Tomography and Society for cardiovascular magnetic resonance. J Am Soc Echocardiogr. 2015;28:119–82.

Pericardium

14

Sophia P. Poorsattar and Timothy M. Maus

Abbreviations

2D	Two-dimensional
CP	Constrictive pericarditis
RA	Right atrium
RAP	Right atrial pressure
RCM	Restrictive cardiomyopathy
TEE	Transesophageal echocardiography
TTE	Transthoracic echocardiography

Introduction

Basic perioperative transesophageal echocardiography (TEE) guidelines suggest that knowledge of the echocardiographic manifestations of the pericardium and its associated pathologies are essential to the basic perioperative echocardiographer [1]. This chapter will review the anatomy and physiology of the pericardium, essential transesophageal and transthoracic echocardiographic (TTE) views for evaluation, and major pathologies of the pericardium, including pericardial effusion, pericardial hematoma, cardiac tamponade, and constrictive pericarditis.

Anatomy and Physiology of the Pericardium

Anatomy

The pericardium is a fibrous sac surrounding the heart and proximal great vessels with an inner serous component and an outer fibrous component (Fig. 14.1a, b). The serous component is further divided into visceral and parietal layers. Each of these serosal layers is composed of a single layer of mesothelial cells and a surrounding layer of loose connective tissue. The visceral layer is an inner, thin, translucent layer, which is adherent to the epicardium. The parietal layer is an outer, thicker layer, which is adherent to the fibrous component. This outer fibrosa attaches to the sternum anteriorly and diaphragm inferiorly.

The visceral and parietal layers exist in continuity and join together at reflections points, called sinuses. The transverse sinus is created by

Supplementary Information The online version of this chapter (https://doi.org/10.1007/978-3-030-84349-6_14) contains supplementary material, which is available to authorized users.

S. P. Poorsattar (✉)
Department of Anesthesiology and Perioperative Medicine, University of California, Los Angeles Medical Center,
Los Angeles, CA, USA
e-mail: spoorsattar@mednet.ucla.edu

T. M. Maus
Department of Anesthesiology, University of California San Diego Health,
La Jolla, CA, USA

T. M. Maus, C. R. Tainter (eds.), *Essential Echocardiography*,
https://doi.org/10.1007/978-3-030-84349-6_14

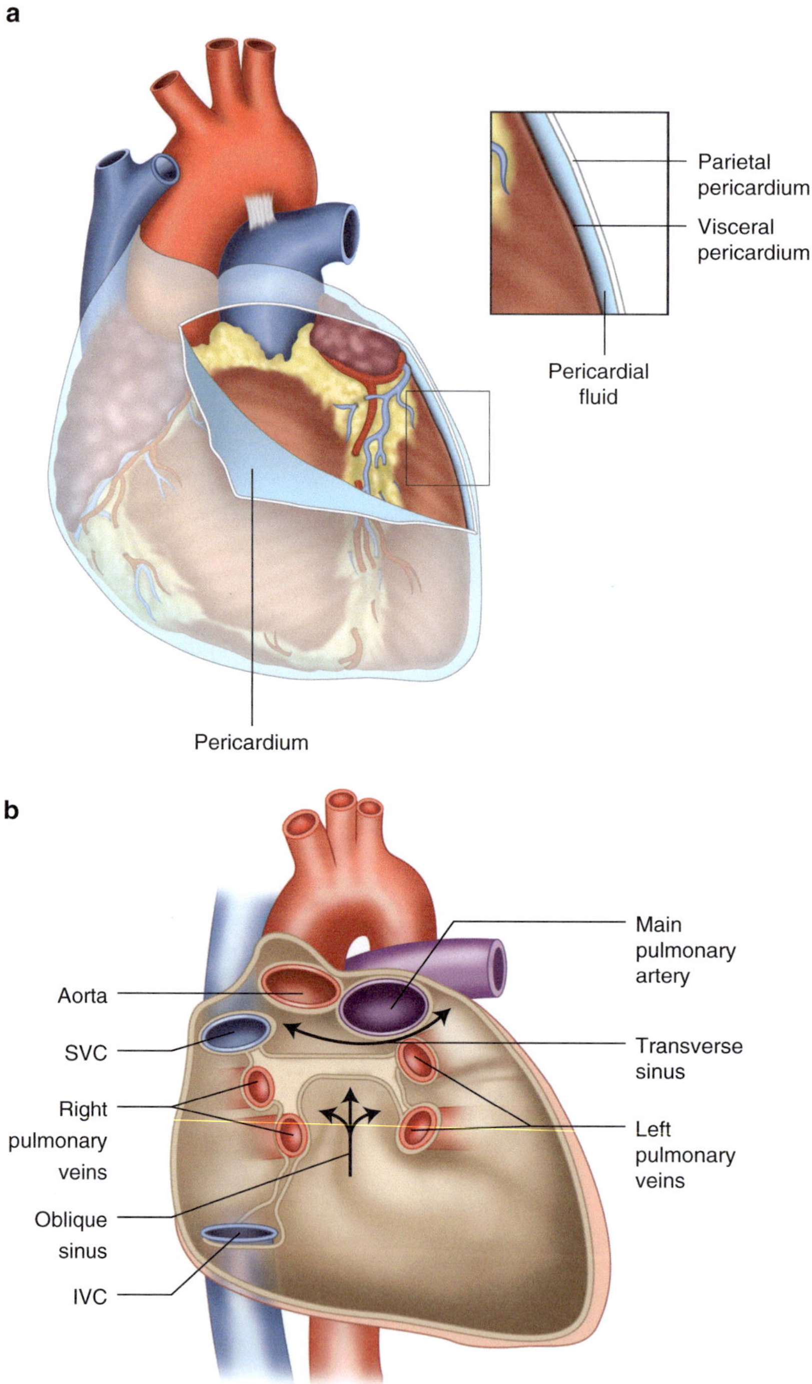

Fig. 14.1 (**a**) Anatomical drawing of the pericardium surrounding the cardiac structures. The zoomed-in portion demonstrates the parietal and visceral components of the pericardium separated by pericardial fluid. (**b**) Anatomical drawing of the pericardial space with the heart removed, demonstrating the relationship of the pericardium to the major vessels of the heart and the sinuses created at its reflection points

reflections at the base of the heart anterior to the superior vena cava and posterior to the great vessels. The oblique sinus is created by reflections posterior to the left atrium between the inferior vena cava and pulmonary veins (Fig. 14.1). The potential space created between the visceral and parietal layers is referred to as the pericardial cavity. Under normal physiologic conditions, this cavity contains between 5 and 50 mL of serous pericardial fluid.

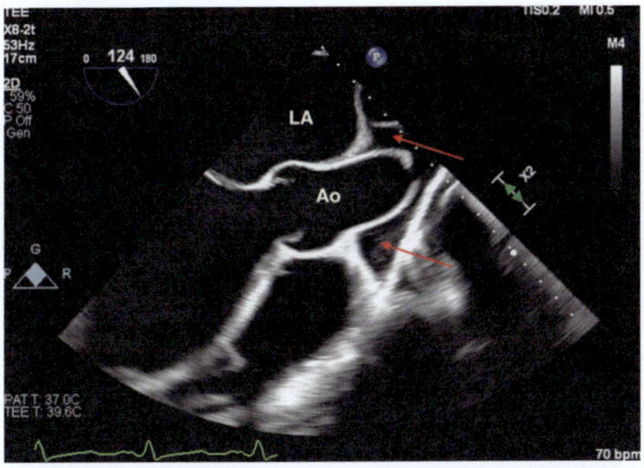

Fig. 14.2 Midesophageal long-axis view. The *red arrows* point to the transverse sinus. *LA* left atrium, *Ao* aorta

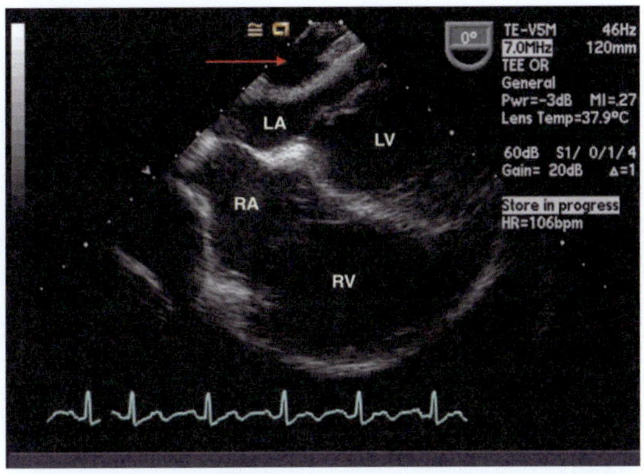

Fig. 14.4 Midesophageal four-chamber view. The *red arrow* points to the oblique sinus. *RV* right ventricle, *LV* left ventricle, *RA* right atrium, *LA* left atrium

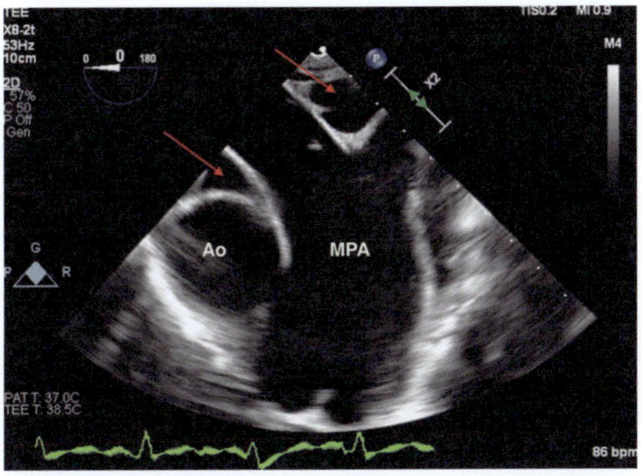

Fig. 14.3 Midesophageal ascending aorta short-axis view. The *red arrows* point to the transverse sinus. *Ao* aorta, *MPA* main pulmonary artery

Transverse Sinus

The transverse sinus is the potential space at the base of the heart anterior to the superior vena cava, superior to the atria, and posterior to the great vessels. While routinely visible when a pericardial effusion is present, the transverse sinus may be visible even when a physiologic amount of fluid is within the pericardial cavity. Fluid within the sinus can be readily appreciated as an echolucent space located between the left atrium, ascending aorta, and pulmonary artery. In the midesophageal two-chamber view, an echolucent space may be visible surrounding the left atrial appendage. In the midesophageal right ventricular inflow-outflow view, an echolucent space may be visible between the aortic valve and main pulmonary artery. In the mid-esophageal long-axis (Fig. 14.2; Video 14.1) and ascending aorta short-axis views (Fig. 14.3; Video 14.2), an echolucent space may be seen between the ascending aorta and right pulmonary artery [2]. When evaluating the sinus on echocardiography, it is important to note that hypoechoic epicardial fat may be confused with fluid accumulation or an abscess in this space.

Oblique Sinus

The oblique sinus is a thin pericardial space located posterior to the left atrium between the inferior vena cava and pulmonary veins. While the transverse sinus may be visible even with a physiologic amount of fluid, the oblique sinus is more commonly visualized when there is an abnormal fluid collection within this space. With TEE, the oblique sinus can be visualized at the level of the mid-esophagus with a collection of fluid noted posterior to the left atrium, between the left atrium and the apex of the echocardiographic window (Fig. 14.4; Video 14.3). Due to the proximity of the left atrium to the probe and the ultrasound sector width unable to visualize the entire posterior wall of the chamber, the full extent of fluid accumulation in the oblique sinus may not be appreciated with TEE [2]. Notably, post-cardiac surgery, this dependent space may accumulate blood or form a hematoma from surgical cannulation sites.

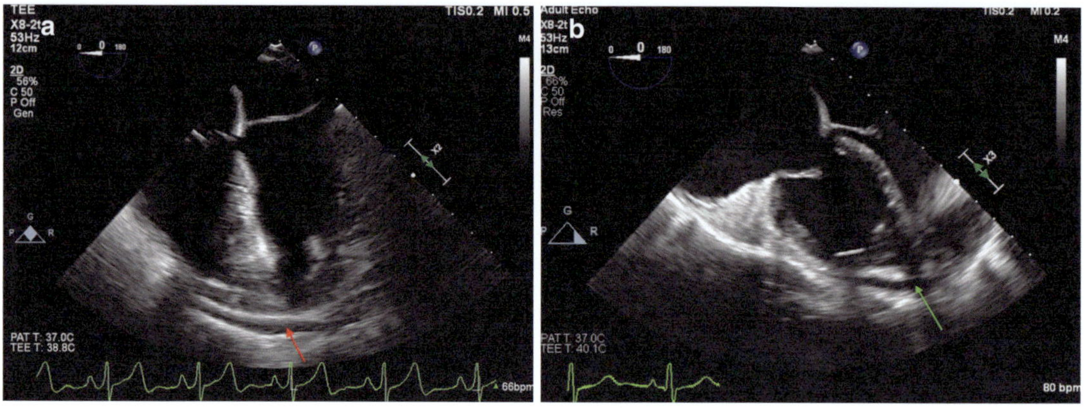

Fig. 14.5 (**a**) Midesophageal four-chamber view. The *red arrow* points to an epicardial fat pad. (**b**) Midesophageal four-chamber view with a *green arrow* pointing to a small pericardial effusion for comparison

Epicardial Fat Pad

In patients with increased visceral deposition of fat, an epicardial fat pad may be apparent in the pericardial space. Typically, this is visualized along the atrioventricular groove, the interventricular groove, or the right ventricular free wall. Epicardial fat contains coronary arteries, lymphatics, and nerve tissue. In comparison to the underlying myocardium, epicardial fat is less echogenic. Epicardial fat often has an echogenicity closer to blood, and therefore it may be difficult to distinguish from a small pericardial effusion (Fig. 14.5a, b). However, in contrast to an effusion, which is echolucent and motionless, epicardial fat is echogenic and moves in concert with the myocardium [3]. Additionally, epicardial fat has a subtle speckled appearance often lacking in effusions and is never associated with cardiac chamber collapse. In contrast to epicardial fat, which is located between the myocardium and visceral pericardium, pericardial fat may also be seen, which is adherent and external to the parietal pericardium (Fig. 14.6; Video 14.4) [4].

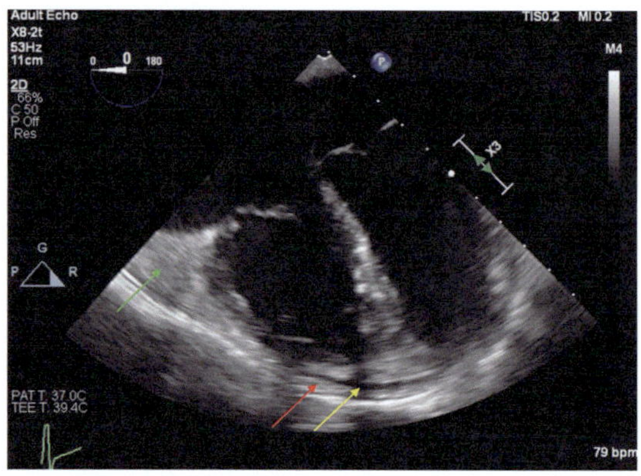

Fig. 14.6 Midesophageal four-chamber view. The *green arrow* points to epicardial fat located within the atrioventricular groove, internal to the visceral pericardium, while the *red arrow* points to pericardial fat located external to the parietal pericardium. A trace amount of pericardial fluid highlights the separation of the visceral and parietal layers (*yellow arrow*)

Function

There are several functions of the pericardium. The mesothelial cells secrete a plasma ultrafiltrate, to lubricate the heart and allow normal rotation and translation. They also hypertrophy in response to chronic fluid accumulation to allow expansion of the pericardial cavity. The thick and dense fibrosa anchors the heart within the chest and protects it from surrounding structures and infection. By encasing the heart, the pericardium serves to constrain filling of cardiac chambers, preventing overdistension and atrioventricular valvular incompetence [5].

Respirophasic Variation

Direct transmission of pressures from the intrathoracic cavity to the pericardial space alters cardiac filling during both spontaneous negative pressure breathing and mechanical positive pressure ventilation. This is termed respirophasic variation. In a patient with normal pericardium, there is no increase in transmural pressure; therefore intrathoracic and pericardial pressures are approximately equal. The true filling pressure of a cardiac chamber is determined by the transmural pressure which is the intracardiac pressure minus the pericardial pressure:

$$\text{Effective RA filling pressure} = \text{RAP} - \text{Pericardial Pressure}$$

RA right atrium, *RAP* right atrial pressure

As pericardial pressure is nearly equal to intrathoracic pressure, true RA filling pressure can be determined by:

$$\text{True RA filling pressure} = \text{RAP} - \text{Intrathoracic Pressure}$$

Therefore, negative intrathoracic pressure (spontaneous inspiration) will augment filling by increasing the true RA filling pressure, and positive intrathoracic pressure (mechanical inspiration) will reduce filling by lowering the RA filling pressure.

During spontaneous inhalation, a more negative intrathoracic pressure increases venous return to the right heart and subsequently increases right ventricular stroke volume and output. Additionally, negative intrathoracic pressure increases pulmonary venous pooling and left ventricular afterload, and in turn, there is decreased left heart filling and output. During spontaneous exhalation, a less negative intrathoracic pressure causes the opposite effect, with reduced right heart filling and output and increased left heart filling and output. During positive pressure ventilation, the opposite filling pattern is true for both inhalation and exhalation, where inspiration leads to a more positive intrathoracic pressure with reduced right heart filling and a "squeeze" of pulmonary blood into the left heart with a subsequent increase in left heart filling. These changes are reflected in the spectral Doppler patterns of the transtricuspid and transmitral inflow velocities (Fig. 14.7). Techniques for obtaining and interpreting these patterns are found in subsequent sections of this chapter and in Chap. 20.

Echocardiographic Views of the Pericardium

When visualizing the pericardium with echocardiography, the layers appear as thin, echogenic lines that surround the myocardium. Echocardiography can be used to measure the thickness of these layers, with the normal thickness being less than 2–3 mm. As mentioned, the pericardial sac normally contains a small amount of fluid interposed between these layers, which may result in a very small physiologic separation. The separate layers will be best visualized during systole as the heart contacts, with the heart and visceral pericardium sliding within and independently from the parietal pericardium. Due to the motion of the heart throughout the cardiac cycle and limitations in image quality with echocardiography, it may be difficult to distinguish between these layers. In pathologic conditions, as the layers thicken, and as fluid accumulates within the pericardial space, these anatomic features become more visible.

TEE and TTE Views

In comparison to TTE, TEE is better suited for imaging of the pericardium, as it avoids the echogenic attenuation caused by epicardial fat. When compared to computed tomography, TEE was found to be more reliable than TTE for the measurement of pericardial thickness [3].

As the pericardium encases the heart and its proximal great vessels, there are multiple basic views on two-dimensional (2D) TEE that are useful for a global assessment of the pericardium. The midesophageal four-chamber, two-chamber, long-axis, right ventricular inflow-outflow, and bicaval views allow for assessment and diagnosis of pericardial disease location, pericardial thickness, fluid collection size, and collection characteristics. Together, these views allow the echocardiographer to determine disease extent and potential suitability for procedures such as pericardiocentesis.

The midesophageal four-chamber view demonstrates the pericardium surrounding the right atrium, left atrium, right ventricular free wall in long-axis,

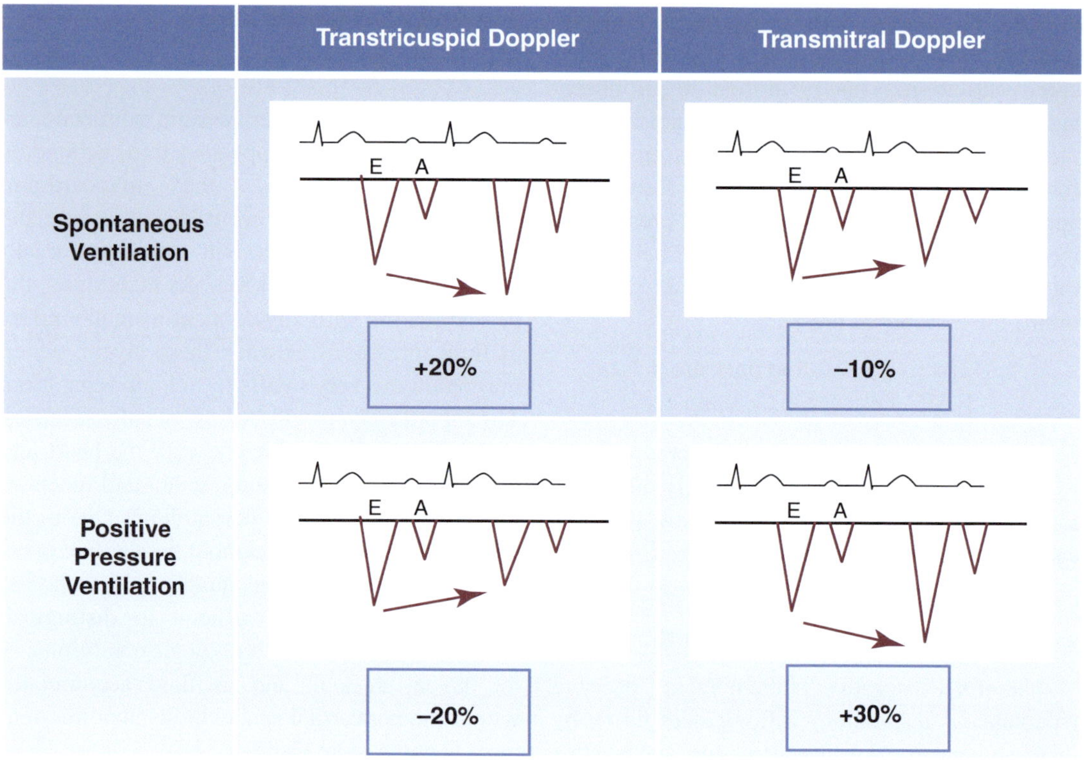

Fig. 14.7 Spectral Doppler patterns of the transtricuspid and transmitral inflow demonstrate normal respirophasic variation during inspiration for both spontaneous ventilation and positive pressure ventilation

and left ventricular anterolateral wall (see Chap. 2) and is helpful in identifying pericardial thickness, effusion, and chamber collapse in tamponade. The midesophageal two-chamber view demonstrates the pericardium surrounding the left atrium, left ventricular inferior wall, and left ventricular anterior wall. The midesophageal long-axis view demonstrates the pericardium surrounding the left atrium, ascending aorta, left ventricular inferolateral wall, and right ventricular free wall. The midesophageal right ventricular inflow-outflow view demonstrates the pericardium surrounding the right ventricular free wall in short-axis and is particularly helpful in identifying right ventricular diastolic collapse in tamponade. The midesophageal bicaval view demonstrates the pericardium surrounding the right atrium and is notably helpful in identifying right atrial collapse. At the transgastric level, the mid-papillary short-axis view also assists in evaluation of the pericardium when determining if pathology exists regionally or circumferentially [1].

Transthoracic echocardiography can provide similar information regarding the pericardium, often with very similar perspectives. When visualizing the structures identified and portions of the pericardium with TTE, the apical four-chamber view corresponds to the midesophageal four-chamber view, the parasternal long-axis view corresponds to the midesophageal long-axis view, and the parasternal short-axis view corresponds to the transgastric short-axis view (see Chap. 3).

For evaluation of inflow patterns by spectral Doppler, the chosen view will depend on optimal alignment of the Doppler cursor with the tricuspid and mitral inflows. Evaluation of tricuspid valve inflow typically occurs in a midesophageal four-chamber or modified bicaval tricuspid valve view with TEE, while an apical four-chamber view is often well-aligned for Doppler with TTE imaging. Evaluation of the mitral valve inflow, with placement of the pulsed-wave Doppler sample volume at the mitral valve leaflet tips, is in the midesophageal four-chamber with TEE, while this usually occurs in an apical four-chamber view with TTE imaging.

Indications for Echocardiography

The application of echocardiography is useful to diagnose pericardial disease, inform clinical management, and guide the success of various cardiac procedures, such as creating a pericardial window, pericardiocentesis, and pericardiectomy. As such, consensus guidelines recommend the use of echocardiography for evaluation of patients with suspected pericardial disease, including effusion, tamponade, or constrictive pericarditis, evaluation of patients with suspected bleeding into the pericardial space, and follow-up evaluation for recurrence of a pathologic pericardial process [3, 6, 7].

Pericardial Effusions (Highlight Box 14.1)

Highlight Box 14.1

Pericardial effusions	
2D	• Echolucent space between myocardium and pericardium • Semiquantification of effusion size • Circumferential vs. loculated/ regional • Presence of clot or hematoma • Systolic right atrial collapse • Diastolic right ventricular collapse
CFD	• Typically not utilized
Spectral	• Transtricuspid inflow velocities (PWD) • Transmitral inflow velocities (PWD) • Exaggeration of respirophasic variation during spontaneous ventilation

PWD pulsed-wave Doppler

Pericardial effusions occur when the amount of fluid within the pericardial space exceeds the expected physiologic amount. Echocardiography is the initial imaging modality recommended for evaluation of a suspected effusion due to its accessibility, accuracy in diagnosis, and ability to describe its physiologic effects [3]. The most important elements of the echocardiographic exam with regard to an effusion are determining the size, location, its circumferential or loculated nature, and its hemodynamic significance.

With echocardiography, pericardial effusions are often appreciated as an echolucent stripe between the visceral and parietal layers of the pericardium. A linear measurement of this stripe perpendicular to the myocardial wall at end-diastole provides a semi-quantitative estimate of the effusion volume. Effusions measuring less than 10 mm are considered small (some sources consider < 5 mm "minimal" and 5–10 mm "small"); 10–20 mm are considered moderate; and > 20 mm are considered large (Table 14.1) [8] .

Optimal imaging planes depend on the location of the effusion and whether it is circumferential (Fig. 14.8a, b) (surrounding the entire heart) or loculated (Fig. 14.9) (adjacent to a specific cardiac chamber[s]). When located anteriorly, effusions can be better appreciated in the midesophageal or parasternal long-axis views. When located posteriorly or circumferential, effusions can be better appreciated in the transgastric short-axis or parasternal short-axis views. To optimize the imaging sector, decreasing the gain setting will allow the echocardiographer to better visualize the pericardial interface, which is brightly reflective.

Pericardial Hematoma

Depending on the etiology, an effusion may be composed of differing fluid types, including transudate (serous), exudate (cells), hemopericardium (blood), or pyopericardium (pus) [3]. Distinguishing between different types of collections within the pericardial space requires experience; however, certain characteristics may aid in diagnosis. While purely transudative or exudative fluids are often visualized as an anechoic space, fibrin stranding may be evident in long-standing effusions or early clot formation, and slow swirling of spontaneous echo contrast may be evident

Table 14.1 Pericardial effusion severity and semi-quantification of volume by transverse measurement on echocardiography

	Pericardial Effusion Severity			
	Minimal	**Small**	**Moderate**	**Large**
Transverse Measurement (mm)	< 5	5 – 10	10 – 20	> 20
Approximate Volume (mL)	50 – 100	100 – 250	250 – 500	> 500

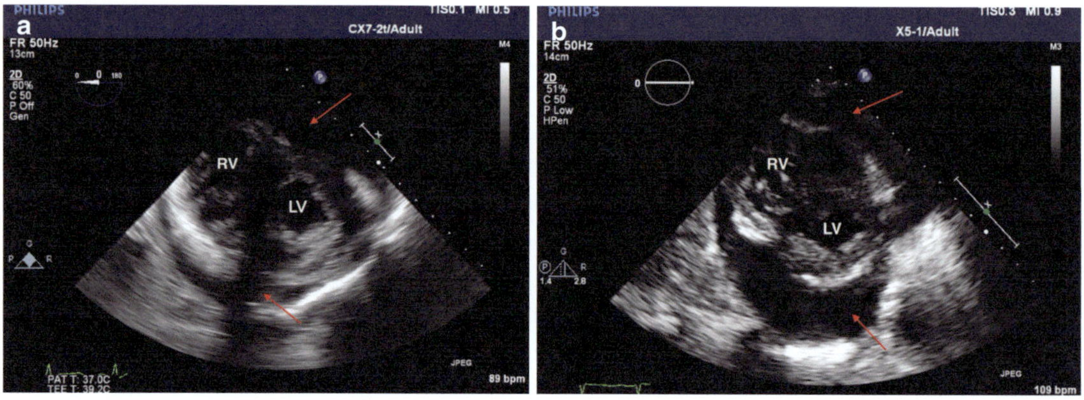

Fig. 14.8 The *red arrows* point to a circumferential pericardial effusion seen in transgastric short-axis (**a**) and parasternal short-axis views (**b**). *RV* right ventricle, *LV* left ventricle

with clumping of red blood cells (Fig. 14.10). A hemopericardium may evolve to form a thrombus, in which the collection has an echodensity approaching that of the myocardium (Fig. 14.11).

Cardiac Tamponade

The physiologic effects of a pericardial effusion depend on the size of the effusion and rate of fluid accumulation. Mesothelial cells of the serous pericardium hypertrophy to accommodate chronically expanding effusions, such that even large effusions may cause very little increase in pericardial pressure. Conversely, minimal to no hypertrophy occurs in rapidly expanding effusions (e.g., hemorrhagic), and even small effusions may cause markedly increased pericardial pressures, leading to tamponade. Accordingly, whether an effusion is large or small, once a threshold point is reached, small changes in volume will lead to large variations in pericardial pressure (Fig. 14.12) [9].

Cardiac tamponade is a clinical diagnosis and occurs when pericardial fluid accumulation impedes normal cardiac filling, which results in impaired hemodynamics. Increases in pericardial pressure are transmitted across the transmural space, and when they exceed the intracavitary pressure, collapse of the cardiac chamber occurs. The sequence of chamber collapse corresponds with the lowest intracavitary pressures (right atrium, then right ventricle) until there is equalization of the mean diastolic pressures across all chambers (equal to the pericardial pressure) and diminished cardiac output ensues. In the absence of tamponade, brief collapse

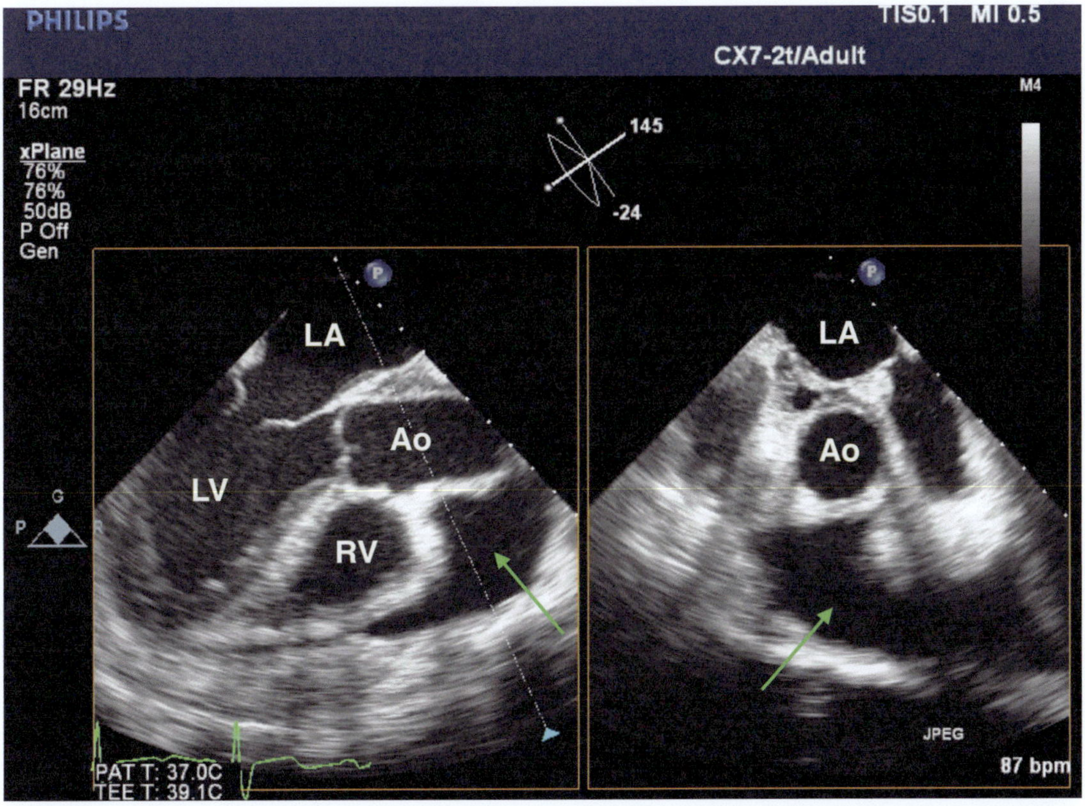

Fig. 14.9 Midesophageal long-axis view (left) with a 90-degree cross-plane image (right) at the level of the ascending aorta as indicated by the cursor. The *green arrow* points to a loculated pericardial effusion located anterior to the heart. *LA* left atrium, *Ao* aorta, *LV* left ventricle, *RV* right ventricle

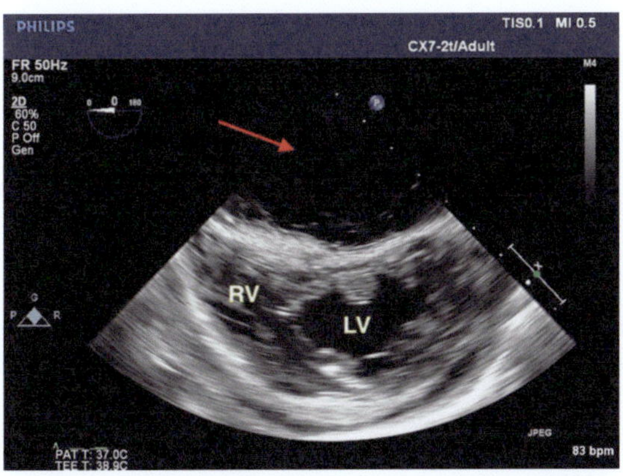

Fig. 14.10 Transgastric short-axis view. The *red arrow* points to a pericardial effusion located posterior to the left ventricle in which fibrin stranding can be seen, suggestive of early clot formation. *RV* right ventricle, *LV* left ventricle

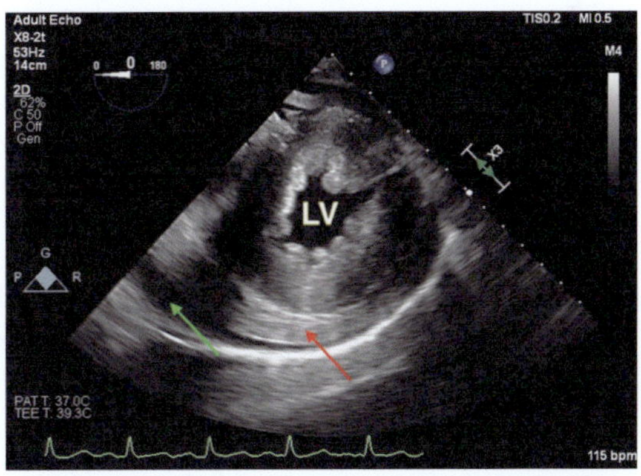

Fig. 14.11 Transgastric short-axis view. The *red arrow* points to a pericardial hematoma, while the *green arrow* points to pericardial effusion. *LV* left ventricle

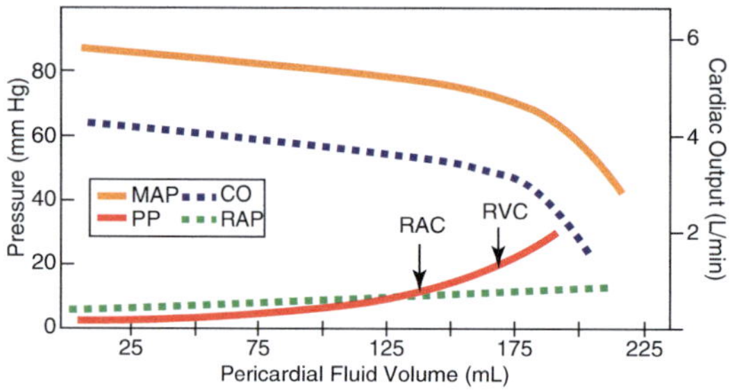

Fig. 14.12 Graphic relationship of increasing pericardial fluid volume to cardiac hemodynamics. *MAP* mean arterial pressure, *PP* pericardial pressure, *CO* cardiac output, *RAP* right atrial pressure, *RAC* right atrial collapse, *RVC* right ventricular collapse. (Reproduced with permission from Savage et al. [16])

of the right atrial free wall during diastole may occur in patients with low right atrial pressures. However, when the duration of right atrial collapse exceeds one-third of the cardiac cycle, it is 94% sensitive and 100% specific for tamponade [10]. The presence of collapse of the right ventricular free wall during diastole also suggests tamponade with the sensitivity and specificity improving as the duration of diastolic collapse increases [3]. Visualization of right atrial and right ventricular collapse is best observed from the midesophageal four-chamber and right ventricular inflow-outflow views (TEE) or the apical four-chamber view (TTE). Left atrial collapse (although rare), when present, is often visualized in conjunction with right atrial collapse. The thicker and higher-pressured left-sided structures are less likely to collapse, and when collapse is seen, it portends a bad outcome. The absence of collapse of any cardiac chamber has a negative predictive value of > 90% for tamponade [11].

During cardiac tamponade, the filling of the ventricles becomes dependent on each other, termed ventricular interdependence. As the patient spontaneously inspires, right ventricular filling is augmented. Due to higher pericardial pressure, the right ventricular filling deviates the septum toward the left, thereby impeding left ventricular filling. During expiration, the opposite occurs. Left ventricular filling increases deviating the septum toward the right and thereby impeding right ventricular filling. This phenomenon allows the spectral Doppler evaluation in spontaneous ventilating patients to help confirm the diagnosis of tamponade. As mentioned above, the variation of transtricuspid or transmitral inflow velocities is exaggerated in spontaneous negative pressure ventilation, and velocities are overall reduced in mechanical positive pressure ventilation.

The midesophageal four-chamber or apical four-chamber views allow for optimal alignment of the Doppler sample volume with the atrioventricular valves. To calculate the variation, place the pulsed-wave Doppler sample volume at the level of the atrioventricular valve leaflets, and set a sweep speed of 25–50 mm/sec to allow more beats per screen to be visualized. Using the peak E-wave velocities at expiration and inspiration, the percentage of respirophasic variation is calculated:

[Percentage of variation = 100% ×
(expiration velocity – inspiration velocity)/expiration velocity]

While patients with normal physiology demonstrate a reduction in transmitral velocities of approximately 10% during spontaneous inspiration, an exaggerated reduction of > 30% of the peak mitral E-wave velocity is suggestive of tamponade (Figs. 14.13 and 14.14; Video 14.5) [3].

Regional cardiac tamponade may also be seen, in which a loculated effusion or localized hematoma causes collapse of adjacent cardiac chambers. This is often seen in the post-cardiac surgery patient where localized bleeding collects and can compress individual cardiac chambers. This may occur near cannulation sites, such as the right atrium from venous cannulation or the left atrium from vent placement or aortic cannulation. Lastly, isolated-left heart tamponade may also occur in patients with severely elevated right-sided pressures, such as in severe pulmonary hypertension, in which an elevated pericardial pressure leads to collapse of the left atrium

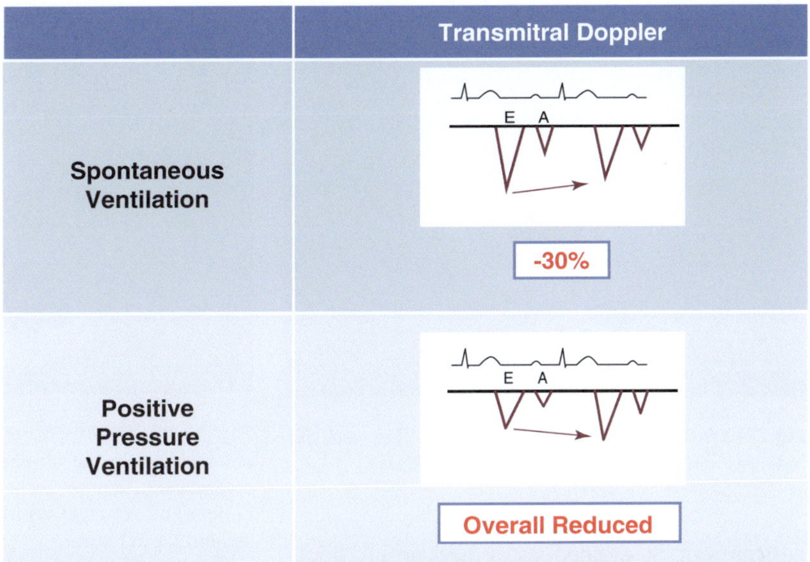

Fig. 14.13 In cardiac tamponade, spectral Doppler patterns of the transmitral inflow demonstrate exaggerated respirophasic variation during spontaneous inspiration and overall reduced inflow during positive pressure ventilation

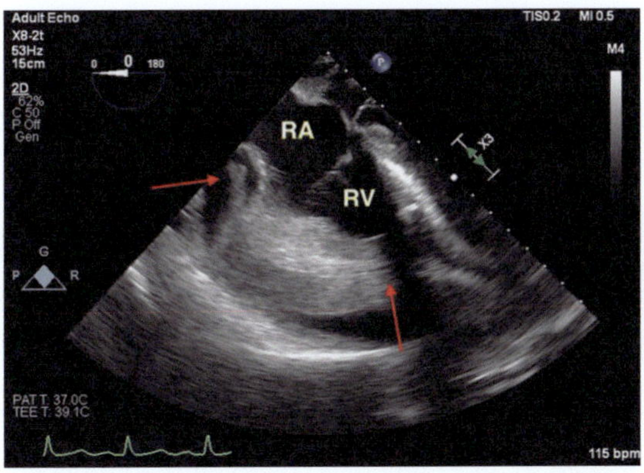

Fig. 14.14 Midesophageal four-chamber view with a right ventricular focus. The *red arrows* point to a complex pericardial effusion, with collapse of the free walls of the right atrium and right ventricle visualized. *RA* right atrium, *RV* right ventricle

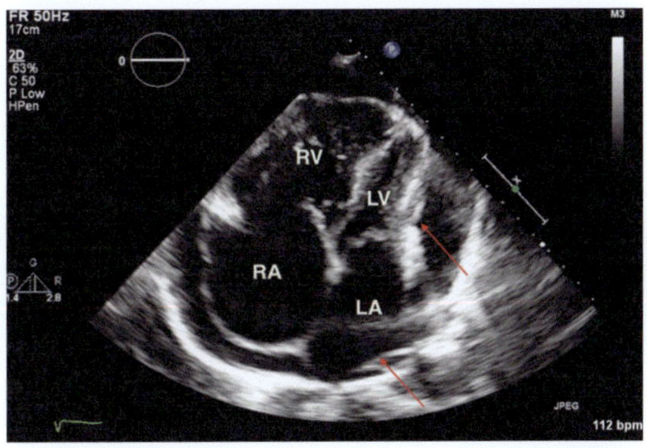

Fig. 14.15 Apical four-chamber view. A circumferential pericardial effusion can be seen with isolated collapse of the left-sided chambers (*red arrows*) in a patient with severe pulmonary hypertension. *RV* right ventricle, *LV* left ventricle, *RA* right atrium, *LA* left atrium

and/or left ventricle without collapse of the right-sided chambers (Fig. 14.15). These clinical settings require a high degree of suspicion by the echocardiographer.

Constrictive Pericarditis (Highlight Box 14.2)

Pericarditis is an inflammation of the pericardium that can be attributed to several etiologies, including immune-mediated, infectious, malignant, traumatic, uremic, and post-surgical. A normal pericardial thickness is 2–3 mm, and a thickened

Highlight Box 14.2

Constrictive pericarditis	
2D	• Thickened, highly reflective pericardium • Biatrial enlargement • Septal "bounce"
CFD	• Typically not utilized
Spectral	• Transtricuspid inflow velocities (PWD) • Transmitral inflow velocities (PWD) • Exaggeration of respirophasic variation • Restrictive diastolic profile (E much greater than A) • Normal tissue Doppler velocities

PWD pulsed-wave Doppler, *E* early diastolic mitral valve inflow velocity, *A* atrial contraction mitral valve inflow velocity

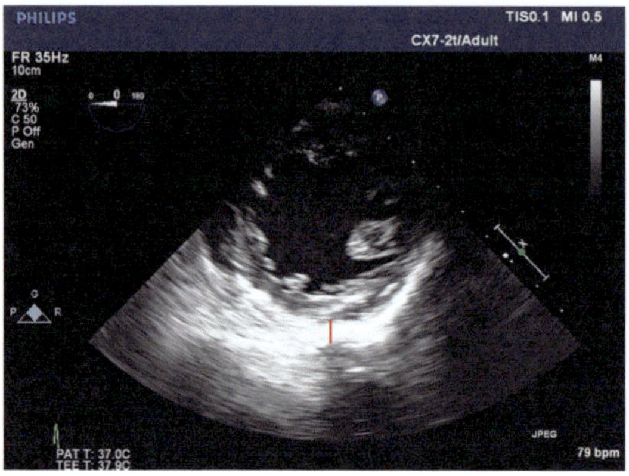

Fig. 14.16 Transgastric short-axis view. The *red line* indicates marked thickening of the pericardium

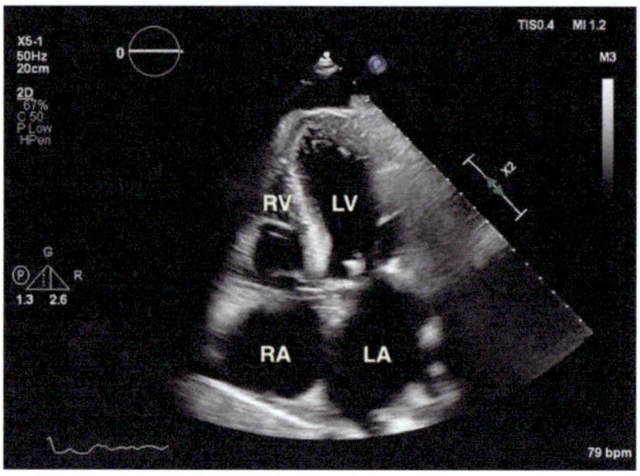

Fig. 14.17 Midesophageal four-chamber view. Biatrial enlargement in the absence of left or right ventricular enlargement can be seen in a patient with constrictive pericarditis. *RV* right ventricle, *LV* left ventricle, *RA* right atrium, *LA* left atrium

pericardium is defined as a pericardial thickness > 4 mm [3]. With echocardiography, a thickened pericardium becomes more echogenic, appearing brighter. Similar to the evaluation of pericardial effusion, multiple imaging windows should be utilized to investigate whether the thickening is localized or diffused (Fig. 14.16). Precise measurements of thickness by echocardiography are difficult, though measurements by TEE are superior to TTE [12] and comparable to those obtained by high-fidelity cardiac imaging [13].

Constrictive pericarditis (CP) is a clinical diagnosis that occurs when noncompliant pericardium leads to elevated and equalized cardiac pressures, similar to tamponade physiology. Although thickening of the pericardium may be frequently appreciated on echocardiography, it only progresses to hemodynamic compromise in 0.2–0.3% of cases [12]. As with the relationship between pericardial effusions and cardiac tamponade, a thickened pericardium may not always cause constrictive physiology, and CP may result from a pericardium with a normal thickness [14].

Several echocardiographic findings may be seen in patients with CP. As mentioned, the pericardium is often severely thickened, fibrotic, or calcified with or without pericardial adhesion (absence of detectable motion between the layers of the pericardium). Often the left and right atria are enlarged, with normal size and function of the left ventricle, in the absence of atrioventricular valvular disease (creating the "ice cream scoop on an ice cream cone" appearance) (Fig. 14.17).

Paradoxical septal motion is observed with CP, including a "septal bounce," in which early filling leads to an abrupt septal shift to the left during spontaneous inspiration followed by a second septal shift from filling by the atrial contraction. This gives the appearance of the ventricular septum having two "bouncing" movements to the left during a single cardiac cycle (Video 14.6) [15] . This septal motion is related to an exaggerated interventricular dependence, in combination with rapid early diastolic filling. Septal motion is best interrogated by TEE in the midesophageal four-chamber or transgastric mid-papillary short-axis views or by TTE with the corresponding views of apical four-chamber or parasternal short-axis views.

In addition to 2D echocardiography, spectral Doppler evaluation is useful to confirm the diagnosis of constrictive pericarditis. A restrictive filling pattern of the mitral inflow is confirmed by spectral Doppler analysis in which early diastolic filling (E-wave) is rapid and abruptly terminates as the diastolic pressure rises rapidly (see Chap. 12). The subsequent contribution from atrial contraction (A-wave) is minimal, such that the E-wave velocity exceeds the A-wave velocity by a ratio of 2:1 or greater [11] . In contrast to cardiac tamponade, in which there is primarily an exaggeration of respirophasic variation during spontaneous ventilation, with CP, there is an exaggeration of respirophasic variation during both spontaneous ventilation and positive pressure ventilation (Figs. 14.18 and 14.19).

Differentiating Constrictive Pericarditis and Restrictive Cardiomyopathy

Restrictive cardiomyopathy (RCM) is often confused with CP, since both are characterized by hemodynamic compromise related to restrictive filling patterns. However, reduced compliance in CP is due to external constraint from the abnormal pericardium, while reduced compliance in RCM is due to abnormal elastic properties intrinsic to the myocardium or intercellular matrix. On echocardiography, both pathologies result in biatrial enlargement and severe diastolic dysfunction. Findings on echocardiography that favor CP include pericardial thickening, "septal bounce," and exaggeration of respirophasic variation. The two pathologies can be differentiated by tissue Doppler imaging, as CP possesses normal tissue velocities (particularly near the septum), while RCM with its abnormal myocardium possesses reduced tissue velocities throughout the heart.

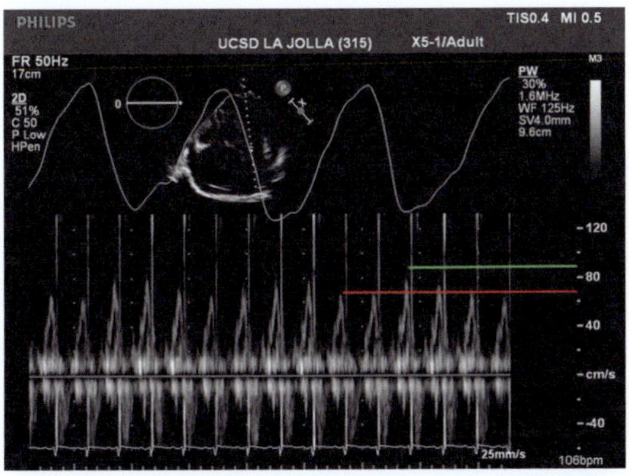

Fig. 14.18 Apical four-chamber view. Pulsed-wave Doppler of the transmitral inflow is performed during spontaneous ventilation, demonstrating the E-wave velocity decreasing by more than 25% from expiration (*green line*) to inspiration (*red line*)

Conclusion

Echocardiography is the preferred method for evaluation of the pericardium, owing to its test characteristics and ability to provide relevant physiologic data. Both transesophageal and transthoracic echocardiography can provide rapid, valuable information about the severity and sometimes the provenance, of pericardial disease, including pericardial effusion, cardiac tamponade, and constrictive pericarditis.

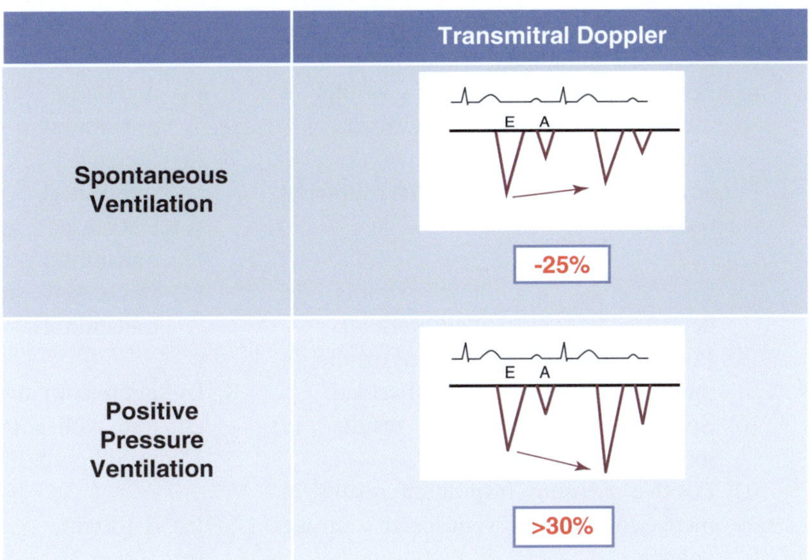

Fig. 14.19 In constrictive pericarditis, spectral Doppler patterns of the transmitral inflow demonstrate exaggerated respirophasic variation during inspiration for both spontaneous ventilation and positive pressure ventilation

Questions

1. Which of the following views does not demonstrate the transverse sinus?

   (a) Midesophageal two-chamber view
   (b) Midesophageal long-axis view
   (c) Midesophageal bicaval view
   (d) Midesophageal ascending aorta short-axis view

2. Which of the following is most true regarding differentiating epicardial fat from a pericardial effusion?

   (a) Epicardial fat is not associated with cardiac chamber collapse.
   (b) Pericardial fluid moves in concert with the myocardium.
   (c) Epicardial fat is more echogenic than myocardium.
   (d) Epicardial fat is adherent to the parietal pericardium.

3. In normal conditions, which of the following is most true?

   (a) Spontaneous inspiration results in increased filling of the left heart.
   (b) Positive pressure inspiration results in increased left ventricular stroke volume.
   (c) Spontaneous expiration results in increased pulmonary venous pooling.
   (d) Positive pressure expiration results in increased left ventricular afterload.

4. In normal conditions, which of the following is most true?

   (a) Spontaneous expiration results in decreased left ventricular afterload.
   (b) Positive pressure expiration results in increased right ventricular afterload.
   (c) Spontaneous inspiration results in increased left atrial filling.
   (d) Positive pressure inspiration results in increased right ventricular stroke volume.

5. Compared to normal respirophasic variation, what changes in atrioventricular inflow patterns do you see in constrictive pericarditis?

   (a) Exaggeration with spontaneous ventilation; exaggeration with positive pressure ventilation
   (b) Exaggeration with spontaneous ventilation; reduction with positive pressure ventilation
   (c) Reduction with spontaneous ventilation; exaggeration with positive pressure ventilation
   (d) Reduction with spontaneous ventilation; reduction with positive pressure ventilation

6. Which of the following is most true regarding cardiac tamponade?

   (a) The size of the effusion is proportional to the severity of hemodynamic effect.
   (b) Right atrial collapse indicates cardiac tamponade.
   (c) Left-sided chamber collapse is always preceded by right-sided chamber collapse.
   (d) The ventricles exhibit interdependence.

7. During cardiac tamponade, patients will exhibit which of these changes in peak E-wave velocity with spontaneous inspiration?

   (a) Increased transtricuspid; increased transmitral
   (b) Increased transtricuspid; decreased transmitral
   (c) Decreased transtricuspid; increased transmitral
   (d) Decreased transtricuspid; decreased transmitral

8. By semiquantitative assessment, a pericardial effusion with a transverse measurement of 15 mm is approximately how much volume?

   (a) < 100 mL
   (b) 100 to 250 mL

(c) 250 to 500 mL
(d) > 500 mL

9. Which of the following is not associated with constrictive pericarditis?

(a) Restrictive filling pattern
(b) Septal "bounce"
(c) Biatrial enlargement
(d) Decreased septal tissue velocity

10. Which of the following is more likely in the setting of constrictive pericarditis than tamponade?

(a) Septal "bounce"
(b) Exaggerated respirophasic variation during positive pressure ventilation
(c) Pulsus paradoxus
(d) All of the above are equally likely

References

1. Reeves ST, Finley AC, Skubas NJ, Swaminathan M, Whitley WS, Glas KE, et al. Basic perioperative transesophageal echocardiography examination: a consensus statement of the American Society of Echocardiography and the Society of Cardiovascular Anesthesiologists. J Am Soc Echocardiogr. 2013;26(5):443–56.
2. Penmasta S, Silbiger JJ. The transverse and oblique sinuses of the pericardium: anatomic and echocardiographic insights. Echocardiography. 2019;36(1):170–6.
3. Klein AL, Abbara S, Agler DA, Appleton CP, Asher CR, Hoit B, et al. American Society of Echocardiography Clinical Recommendations for multimodality cardiovascular imaging of patients with pericardial disease. J Am Soc Echocardiogr. 2013;26(9):965–1012.e15.
4. Iacobellis G, Willens HJ. Echocardiographic epicardial fat: a review of research and clinical applications. J Am Soc Echocardiogr. 2009;22(12):1311–9.
5. Savage R, Aronson S. Comprehensive textbook of perioperative transesophageal echocardiography. Philadelphia: Lippincott Williams & Wilkins; 2010.
6. Adler Y, Charron P, Imazio M, Badano L, Barón-Esquivias G, Bogaert J, et al. 2015 ESC guidelines for the diagnosis and management of pericardial diseases: the task force for the diagnosis and Management of Pericardial Diseases of the European Society of Cardiology (ESC) endorsed by: the European Association for Cardio-Thoracic Surgery (EACTS). Eur Heart J. 2015;36(42):2921–64.
7. ACCF/ASE/AHA/ASNC/HFSA/HRS/SCAI/SCCM/SCCT/SCMR 2011 appropriate use criteria for echocardiography. J Am Soc Echocardiogr. 2011;24(3):229–67.
8. Weitzman LB, Tinker WP, Kronzon I, Cohen ML, Glassman E, Spencer FC. The incidence and natural history of pericardial effusion after cardiac surgery–an echocardiographic study. Circulation. 1984;69(3):506–11.
9. Pérez-Casares A, Cesar S, Brunet-Garcia L, Sanchez-de-Toledo J. Echocardiographic evaluation of pericardial effusion and cardiac tamponade. Front Pediatr. 2017;5:79.
10. Gillam LD, Guyer DE, Gibson TC, King ME, Marshall JE, Weyman AE. Hydrodynamic compression of the right atrium: a new echocardiographic sign of cardiac tamponade. Circulation. 1983;68(2):294–301.
11. Mercé J, Sagristà-Sauleda J, Permanyer-Miralda G, Evangelista A, Soler-Soler J. Correlation between clinical and Doppler echocardiographic findings in patients with moderate and large pericardial effusion: implications for the diagnosis of cardiac tamponade. Am Heart J. 1999;138(4):759–64.
12. Ling LH, Oh JK, Tei C, Click RL, Breen JF, Seward JB, et al. Pericardial thickness measured with transesophageal echocardiography: feasibility and potential clinical usefulness. J Am Coll Cardiol. 1997;29(6):1317–23.
13. Rajiah P, Kanne JP. Computed tomography of the pericardium and pericardial disease. J Cardiovasc Comput Tomogr. 2010;4(1):3–18.
14. Talreja DR, Edwards WD, Danielson GK, Schaff HV, Tajik AJ, Tazelaar HD, et al. Constrictive pericarditis in 26 patients with histologically normal pericardial thickness. Circulation. 2003;108(15):1852–7.
15. Candell-Riera J, García del Castillo H, Permanyer-Miralda G, Soler-Soler J. Echocardiographic features of the interventricular septum in chronic constrictive pericarditis. Circulation. 1978;57(6):1154–8.
16. Savage RM, Aronson S, Shernan SK. Comprehensive textbook of perioperative transesophageal echocardiography. 2nd ed. Philadelphia: Lippincott Williams & Wilkins; 2011.

15 Perioperative Rescue Echocardiography

Byron Fergerson and Joshua Zimmerman

Abbreviations

2D	Two-dimensional
CP	Constrictive pericarditis
EF	Ejection fraction
FAC	Fractional area change
LA	Left atrium
LV	Left ventricle
LVEDA	Left ventricular end-diastolic area
LVESA	Left ventricular end-systolic area
LVOT	Left ventricular outflow tract
PA	Pulmonary artery
RA	Right atrium
RAP	Right atrial pressure
RCM	Restrictive cardiomyopathy
RV	Right ventricle
SV	Stroke volume
TEE	Transesophageal echocardiography
TTE	Transthoracic echocardiography
VTI	Velocity-time integral

Supplementary Information The online version of this chapter (https://doi.org/10.1007/978-3-030-84349-6_15) contains supplementary material, which is available to authorized users.

B. Fergerson (✉)
Department of Anesthesiology, University of California San Diego Health, La Jolla, CA, USA
e-mail: bfergerson@ucsd.edu

J. Zimmerman
Department of Anesthesiology, University of Utah, Salt Lake City, UT, USA
e-mail: Joshua.Zimmerman@hsc.utah.edu

Introduction

Echocardiography is well suited to evaluate causes of acute hemodynamic instability as it is portable and relatively noninvasive and provides information on multiple aspects of cardiovascular physiology, from contractility and valvular function to volume status and intracardiac pressures. The American Society of Echocardiography (ASE) and Society of Cardiovascular Anesthesiologists (SCA) recommend the use of transesophageal echocardiography (TEE) for acute, persistent, unexplained hypotension in the perioperative period [1]. The ASE likewise gives transthoracic echocardiography for the assessment of hemodynamic instability its highest "appropriate use score" while recognizing the value of focused cardiovascular ultrasound (FoCUS) in the emergent evaluation of unstable patients [2, 3].

A rapid, qualitative assessment of the hemodynamic state, or "eyeballing," is a cornerstone of rescue echocardiography. A detailed quantitative analysis of cardiovascular function is neither feasible nor necessary in the emergent setting. Grasping the overall hemodynamic picture, performing an intervention, and re-assessing the hemodynamics are the most practical and effective uses of echocardiography in the unstable patient. While qualitative analysis may be easier to learn, it still requires significant training and

T. M. Maus, C. R. Tainter (eds.), *Essential Echocardiography*,
https://doi.org/10.1007/978-3-030-84349-6_15

experience to avoid the "bad information is worse than none at all" situation [4].

Unfortunately, there is a paucity of data on the use of echocardiography in the setting of hemodynamic instability in the perioperative period. Markin et al. looked retrospectively at 364 rescue echocardiograms performed on cardiac and non-cardiac cases throughout the perioperative period [5]. Anesthetic management was changed in more than half of the patients with no echo-related complications. Interestingly, there was a change in surgical management in 7% of the cases as well. Griffee et al. retrospectively reviewed 37 unstable trauma patients who underwent perioperative echocardiography and demonstrated that 57% of patients were diagnosed with hypovolemia and that management changes were implemented in 49% of cases [6].

Rescue echocardiography is time-sensitive by its nature, as the etiology of hemodynamic instability must be rapidly diagnosed and acted upon. There are 28 recommended views in the most recently published comprehensive TEE exam, many of which are redundant. Redundancy is valuable in general, because it allows for visualization of structures from multiple angles. It is not, however, conducive to brevity. For this reason, a condensed examination is suggested in an emergent situation.

The "rescue TEE exam" presented in this chapter is a modification of the 11 cross-sectional views recommended by the ASE and SCA for the basic perioperative TEE exam [7]. The primary differences are the order of the views and the use of spectral Doppler to delineate between certain causes of hemodynamic instability. The rescue exam is short but covers the majority of clinically relevant pathologies. In addition, performing a consistent exam every time minimizes distraction. The views of the rescue exam are listed in Table 15.1, beginning in the mid-esophagus and ending in the stomach. Similar protocols have been studied and used effectively [5, 8, 9]. In agreement with the ASE and SCA, it is suggested to perform and store the limited exam in its entirety before focusing on segments specific to the area of interest [7]. Table 15.2 details a simple FoCUS exam that works well to evaluate the unstable patient in whom TEE is not feasible or appropriate [10].

It is important to note that rescue echocardiography is a process, not a snapshot. The cardiovascular system is complex and dynamic, potentially changing on a beat-to-beat basis. What may be considered an appropriate intervention 1 minute may not be appropriate the next. It may be difficult to discern the precise cause of a cardiovascular abnormality. In addition, it is possible that

Table 15.1 Recommended limited TEE exam

1. Midesophageal AV SAX
2. Midesophageal AV LAX
With and without CFD on the AV
Measurement of LVOT diameter
3. Midesophageal bicaval
Evaluation of SVC collapsibility
4. Midesophageal RV inflow/outflow
5. Midesophageal four-chamber
Focus first on RV then on LV
With and without CFD on the TV and MV
6. Midesophageal two-chamber
7. Midesophageal LV LAX
8. Transgastric midpapillary LV SAX
9. Deep transgastric LAX
PWD of LVOT
Calculation of stroke volume, evaluation of flow variation
10. Descending aorta SAX
11. Upper esophageal ascending aorta SAX
12. Consider additional images (including lung and abdominal) as based on the findings and clinical scenario

AV aortic valve, *SAX* short-axis, *LAX* long-axis, *CFD* color flow Doppler, *LVOT* left ventricular outflow tract, *SVC* superior vena cava, *RV* right ventricle, *LV* left ventricle, *TV* tricuspid valve, *MV* mitral valve, *PWD* pulsed-wave Doppler

Table 15.2 Recommended two-dimensional FoCUS exam views

1. Parasternal LAX
2. Parasternal midpapillary SAX
3. Apical four-chamber
4. Subcostal four-chamber
5. Subcostal IVC

LAX long-axis, *SAX* short-axis, *IVC* inferior vena cava

multiple abnormalities are present. Similar to Markin et al., a qualitative estimation – a "best guess" – of the abnormality, followed by re-evaluation after an intervention, is suggested. If parameters improve, one should continue the intervention. If they do not improve or worsen, an alternate diagnosis should be sought [5].

Some of the most common causes of hemodynamic instability will be reviewed: acute valvular and aortic pathology, tamponade, RV dysfunction, pulmonary embolism, hypovolemia, low afterload, and LV hypo- and hypercontractility.

Acute Valvular and Aortic Pathology

The echocardiographic assessments of valvular and aortic pathology (specifically dissection and traumatic rupture) are discussed elsewhere in the text and will be mentioned only briefly here (see Chaps. 8, 9, and 13). Hemodynamic instability from valvular dysfunction is most likely to occur on left-sided structures [11]. The development of acute valvular stenosis is rare and most commonly results from prosthetic valve dysfunction or thrombosis. While chronic mitral or aortic stenosis is unlikely to be the proximate cause of hemodynamic instability, their presence may make patients highly susceptible to the effects of otherwise mild hemodynamic perturbations. Acute severe regurgitation, on the other hand, is poorly tolerated and can result in hemodynamic decompensation. Endocarditis with valvular disruption or perforation is the most common cause of acute regurgitation. Other potential causes include trauma, aortic dissection, and ischemia with or without papillary muscle rupture. Evaluation of valvular regurgitation in the acute setting should be limited to a rapid, qualitative assessment, as quantitative measures may be inaccurate [11]. Color flow Doppler (CFD) is the primary modality for a visual assessment of the regurgitant jet, focusing primarily on the vena contracta. It is important to remember that the regurgitation may be a manifestation of changes in ventricular function and loading conditions induced by another cardiac abnormality.

As discussed in Chap. 13, TEE is as a reliable method to evaluate for aortic dissection [12]. The diagnosis is based on the detection of an intimal flap that divides the aorta into true and false lumens [13]. The lumens are best delineated through CFD. TEE is also valuable in assessing for the intimal tear, intramural hematomas, penetrating ulcers, and traumatic aortic injury [14].

Cardiac Tamponade (Highlight Box 15.1)

Pericardial effusions with associated tamponade physiology are particularly dangerous in the setting of general anesthesia and positive pressure ventilation. Rapid diagnosis and intervention are necessary, making echocardiography, with its portability and accuracy, the diagnostic modality of choice. Acute effusions are generally due to ischemia or trauma (blunt, penetrating, or iatrogenic) but must also be considered in the setting of inflammation, infection, malignancy, and renal or hepatic failure. Pericardial effusions are seen as hypo- or anechoic areas between the heart and the parietal layer of the pericardium (Fig. 15.1; Videos 15.1 and 15.2). A circumferential pericar-

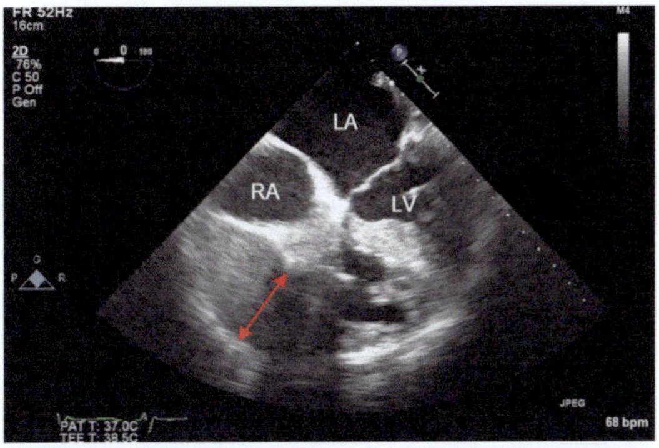

Fig. 15.1 Midesophageal four-chamber view, demonstrating an acute pericardial effusion following percutaneous transvenous lead extraction. The double-headed *red arrow* indicates the pericardial effusion. *LA* left atrium, *LV* left ventricle, *RA* right atrium

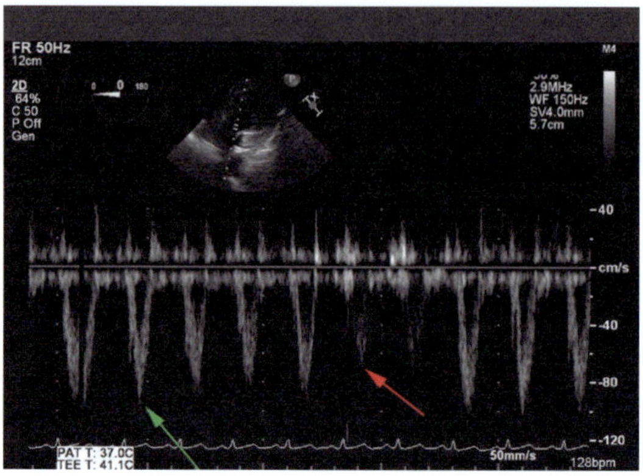

Fig. 15.2 Deep transgastric five-chamber view, with pulsed-wave Doppler placed in the left ventricular outflow tract, showing respiratory variability. The *green arrow* indicates the maximum velocity through the LVOT, while the *red arrow* indicates the minimum velocity through the LVOT during respiration

dial effusion may be identified in nearly any view as an echolucent area within the pericardium but surrounding cardiac structures; however a mid-esophageal four-chamber view (TEE) or an apical four-chamber or subcostal four-chamber view (TTE) offers the advantage of assessing for evidence of tamponade physiology. Effusions measuring less than 1 cm are considered small; 1–2 cm are considered moderate; and > 2 cm are considered large (Chap. 14, Table 14.1). Visualization of an effusion does not necessarily mean there is tamponade physiology, and the size of effusion does not correlate well with hemodynamic significance, and changes in a patient's physiology may make a previously stable effusion become hemodynamically significant. The pericardium can become quite distensible in the setting of a chronic effusion and thus may have a limited effect on intracardiac pressures and filling. However, in the case of extreme hemodynamic instability with the presence of pericardial effusion, tamponade should not be excluded. Pericardial effusions can be loculated or regional, particularly after cardiac surgery, making them difficult to locate. The localized pressure exerted on the heart in this situation can still cause cardiac tamponade.

Highlight Box 15.1

Cardiac tamponade	
2D	• Echolucent space between the heart and pericardium (may be loculated) • Effusions > 2 cm are severe, but smaller effusions may create tamponade • Chamber collapse (RA, systolic; RV, diastolic) • IVC plethora is highly sensitive, but not specific
CFD	• Typically not useful
Spectral	• > 10% respiratory variation in LVOT VTI

RA right atrium, *RV* right ventricle, *LVOT* left ventricular outflow tract, *VTI* velocity-time integral

Table 15.3 Respiratory variation in LV outflow in the setting of tamponade

	Positive pressure ventilation	
	Inspiration	Expiration
LV outflow	↑	↓

The echocardiographic diagnosis of cardiac tamponade is based on both two-dimensional and spectral Doppler findings. The normal respiratory variation in LV stroke volume (SV) seen during mechanical ventilation is exaggerated in the setting of tamponade physiology, with SV increasing on inspiration and decreasing on expiration (see below for a detailed discussion of the physiology of this variation). The variation can be detected by pulsed-wave Doppler interrogation of the left ventricular outflow tract in the deep transgastric view, using a sweep speed of 25–50 mm/sec (Fig. 15.2). Sweep speed indicates how fast the spectral Doppler refreshes on the screen (a lower speed allows the visualization of more beats per screen). A respiratory variation greater than 10% in the LV outflow tract is one of the initial echocardiographic signs of cardiac tamponade (Table 15.3) [15].

Further fluid accumulation in the pericardial space will soon cause the pericardial pressure to exceed right atrial (RA) pressure. This will be visualized as a late-diastolic collapse of the RA which will extend through at least one-third of systole (Fig. 15.3; Video 15.3). The midesophageal RV inflow/outflow and the midesophageal four-chamber are the best views to visualize this. As the pericardial pressure increases further, the RV will begin to collapse in diastole. The RV outflow tract is most likely to collapse, and thus the preferred view is the RV inflow-outflow. The thicker left-sided structures are less likely to collapse. When left-sided collapse is seen, this portends a bad outcome. Once the diagnosis is established, echocardiography can be a useful adjunct to guide needle placement during a pericardiocentesis [16]. Table 15.4 outlines the two-dimensional manifestations of tamponade.

Right Ventricular Dysfunction (Highlight Box 15.2)

Right ventricular failure (see Chap. 10) is the inability of the RV to provide adequate blood flow to the LV in the setting of a normal central venous pressure. RV failure in cardiac and non-cardiac surgeries has a very high mortality rate [17]. Potential causes of RV failure are numerous, but four common causes to consider include ischemia, acute or acute-on-chronic pulmonary hypertension, pulmonary embolism, and iatrogenic volume overload [18]. The anatomy of the RV is complex, making echocardiographic assessment challenging [19]. For this reason, we suggest performing a qualitative assessment in the emergent setting. A qualitative assessment of RV function is as good as MRI for detecting dysfunction [20]. Evaluation begins with inspection of the right-sided chambers, looking for dilation of the RV and RA. The midesophageal four-chamber, RV inflow-outflow, bicaval, and transgastric midpapillary short-axis views are helpful in evaluating the right heart with TEE. With TTE FoCUS imaging, each of the parasternal long- and short-axis, apical four-chamber, subcostal four-chamber, and inferior vena cava (IVC) long-axis views adds valuable information. Encroachment of the right heart onto the left, with right-to-left bowing of the interatrial septum

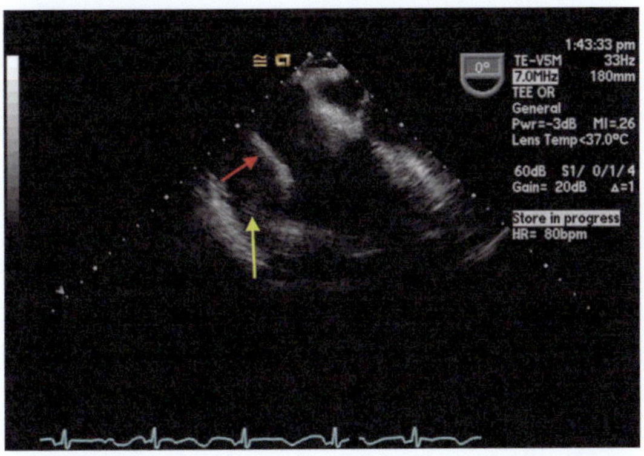

Fig. 15.3 Midesophageal four-chamber view, with right atrial collapse in the setting of a pericardial effusion, indicating tamponade physiology. The *red arrow* indicates right atrial systolic free wall collapse. The *yellow arrow* indicates the pericardial effusion

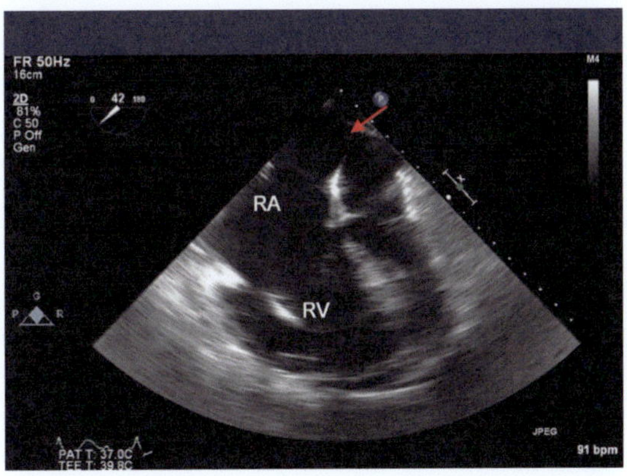

Fig. 15.4 Midesophageal four-chamber view of a patient with right heart failure. The *red arrow* indicates the atrial septal bowing due to high right atrial pressure. *RA* right atrium, *RV* right ventricle

Table 15.4 Two-dimensional manifestations of cardiac tamponade

	Systole		Diastole	
	Normal	Tamponade	Normal	Tamponade
RA	Expansion	Compression	Contraction	Contraction
RV	Contraction	Contraction	Expansion	Compression

RA right atrium, *RV* right ventricle

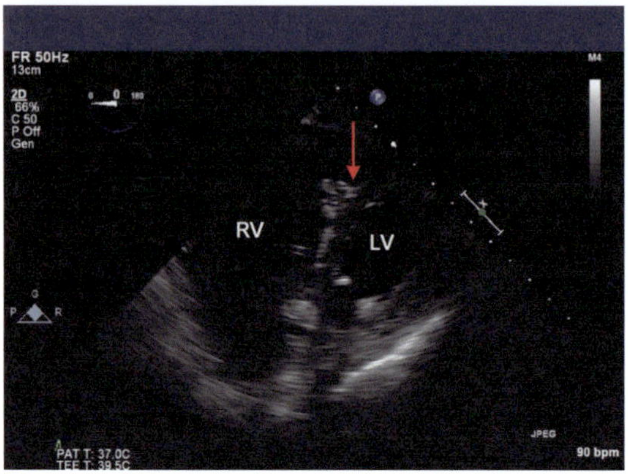

Fig. 15.5 Transgastric midpapillary short-axis view, revealing a "D-shaped" interventricular septum secondary to right ventricular failure. The *red arrow* indicates the flattened interventricular septum. *RV* right ventricle, *LV* left ventricle

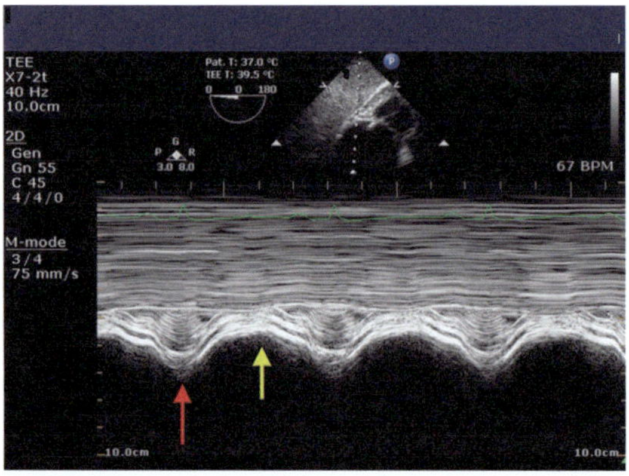

Fig. 15.6 Measurement of tricuspid annular plane systolic excursion (TAPSE), using M-mode imaging of the tricuspid annulus in the transgastric right ventricular inflow view. The *red arrow* indicates the tricuspid annulus in diastole, while the *yellow arrow* indicates the tricuspid annulus in systole. The difference in position is the TAPSE measurement

(Fig. 15.4; Videos 15.4 and 15.5) and/or a "D-shaped" left ventricle seen in the transgastric midpapillary short-axis view (Fig. 15.5; Video 15.6), indicates elevated right-sided pressures. To assess global right ventricular systolic function, one can evaluate the distance the tricuspid annulus moves toward the apex in systole (tricuspid annular systolic excursion, or TAPSE, Fig. 15.6). A reduced TAPSE (< 17 mm) suggests RV dysfunction [21]. New onset or worsening of chronic tricuspid regurgitation may indicate either RV contractile dysfunction or annular dilation. Finally, a dilated, non-collapsible IVC suggests elevated right atrial pressures and possible right-sided volume overload.

Highlight Box 15.2

Right ventricular failure	
2D	• RA and RV size (RV should be 2/3 size of LV) • Encroachment of RV into LV • "D-shaped" LV (flattened septum) • Reduced TAPSE
CFD	• New or worsened TR (dilated annulus)
Spectral	• PASP estimation

RA right atrium, *RV* right ventricle, *LV* left ventricle, *TAPSE* tricuspid annular plane systolic excursion, *TR* tricuspid regurgitation, *PASP* pulmonary arterial systolic pressure

Pulmonary Embolism (Highlight Box 15.3)

Early diagnosis and treatment can significantly reduce the mortality associated with pulmonary embolism (PE) [22]. Although echocardiography can help guide both diagnosis and management, it is not the gold standard [23, 24]. Echocardiography has a high specificity and a low sensitivity for PE (90% and 56%, respectively) [25]. Risk factors associated with PE are listed in Table 15.5.

Highlight Box 15.3

Pulmonary embolism	
2D	• Evidence of RV failure • Dilated RA and RV • Evidence of thromboembolic material in right heart (main or right PA) • McConnell's sign – Hypokinetic RV with normal RV apical function
CFD	• New or worsened TR (dilated annulus)
Spectral	• PASP estimation

RA right atrium, *RV* right ventricle, *TR* tricuspid regurgitation

Table 15.5 Risk factors associated with pulmonary embolism

Risk factor
Malignancy
Prolonged immobilization
Obesity
Tobacco use
Medications particularly
Oral contraceptives
Hormone replacement therapy
Anti-psychotics
General surgery particularly
Hip fractures
Acute spinal cord injuries
Trauma

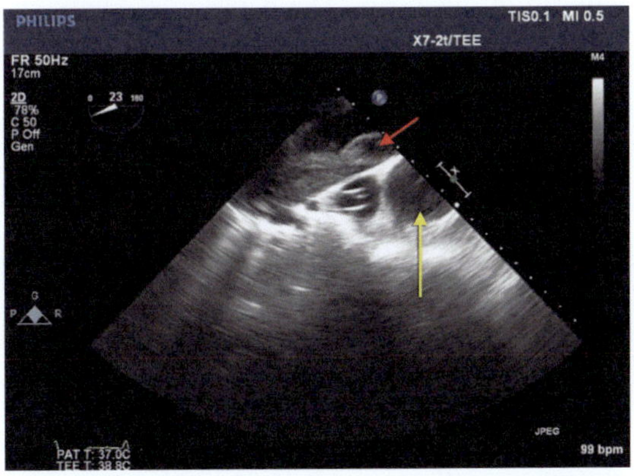

Fig. 15.7 Midesophageal ascending aortic short-axis view, with slight probe rotation to the right. There is thrombus noted in the right pulmonary artery (*red arrow*). The *yellow arrow* indicates the ascending aorta in short-axis

A thromboembolus can be found anywhere on the right side from the vena cava to the pulmonary artery (PA) and can be seen in over 80% of cases (Fig. 15.7; Video 15.7). The ideal TEE views to assess for thromboembolus include the midesophageal bicaval, RV inflow-outflow, and ascending aorta short-axis views. The main and right PAs can be seen by withdrawal of the probe into the upper esophagus, until a cross section of the ascending aorta is obtained. The left PA, on the other hand, is often obscured by the tracheobronchial tree. Thromboembolus may be apparent with TTE views which visualize the right-sided structures, particularly the RV inflow, apical four-chamber, parasternal SAX, and subcostal IVC or four-chamber views.

Although a thrombus visualized in a right-sided cardiac structure is pathognomonic of PE, right ventricular wall motion abnormalities are the most common abnormal echocardiographic findings [26]. The extent of RV dysfunction correlates with the clot burden and overall mortality [27–31]. McConnell et al. showed that a hypokinetic RV free wall and a normal or hyperdynamic apex has a sensitivity of 77% and a specificity of 94% in predicting a PE [32]. Subsequent studies, however, have found a reduced sensitivity and specificity [33]. Structural and inflammatory changes in the LV associated with a PE, as well as reduced coronary perfusion from a decrease in SV, can lead to LV dysfunction. A low LV ejection fraction is an independent predictor of mortality in the setting of acute PE [29].

Left Ventricular Dysfunction (Highlight Box 15.4)

Echocardiography is an excellent tool for the evaluation and management of LV dysfunction, particularly in the setting of myocardial ischemia. Segmental wall thickening less than 30% suggests myocardial ischemia and can manifest within seconds, making it an earlier marker of ischemia than EKG changes [34–36]. Acute ischemia is distinguished from chronic ischemia by a change in segmental wall motion from baseline by two grades (i.e., from normal to severe hypokinesis) in two or more segments (Video 15.8) [37]. Stress, inflammation, and catecholamine excess associated with acute illness can cause secondary cardiomyopathies and LV dysfunction [38]. Sepsis-induced cardiomyopathy and stress-induced cardiomyopathy, also known as takotsubo cardiomyopathy, are relatively common causes of non-ischemic LV dysfunction [38, 39].

Regardless of the etiology, the echocardiographic manifestations of LV dysfunction are similar.

Highlight Box 15.4

Left ventricular dysfunction	
2D	*Regional* • Wall motion abnormalities (thickening and excursion) *Global* • FAC or EF • LV or LA dilation • SEC *LVOT* • Movement of anterior MV leaflet during systole (SAM) • Hyperdynamic, hypovolemic LV
CFD	*Regional/global* • New or worsened MR (dilated annulus vs. papillary dysfunction) *LVOT* • New anterior MR jet from anterior MV displacement into LVOT (SAM) • Aliasing in LVOT
Spectral	*Regional/global* • Decreased SV or CO (calculated from LVOT) *LVOT* • "Dagger" shaped – Late peaking high-velocity CWD profile

FAC fractional area of change, *EF* ejection fraction, *LV* left ventricle, *LA* left atrium, *SEC* spontaneous echo contrast, *SAM* systolic anterior motion, *LVOT* left ventricular outflow tract, *MR* mitral regurgitation, *MV* mitral valve, *SV* stroke volume, *CO* cardiac output, *CWD* continuous-wave Doppler

In keeping with the concept of a qualitative echocardiographic assessment in the setting of hemodynamic instability, the SCA recommends an estimation of the LV ejection fraction when assessing who may benefit from inotropic therapy [7]. Visual estimation, or "eyeballing," has been found to be comparable to Simpson's biplane method and 3D echocardiography and requires only approximately 20 studies to become proficient [40–42]. The transgastric midpapillary short-axis (TEE) and parasternal short-axis views are the primary views used for assessing LV contractility (Fig. 15.8; Videos 15.9 and 15.10). A reduced fractional area change (FAC), which is the comparison of the LV end-diastolic area (LVEDA) and the end-systolic area (LVESA), indicates poor LV function (see Chap. 6). FAC is calculated by using the equation:

$$\text{FAC} = \left[\text{LVEDA} - \text{LVESA}\right]/\text{LVEDA}$$

Normal values are approximately the same values as those for ejection fraction (Fig. 15.9; Video 15.11) [43]. It is important to note, however, that with regional dysfunction, the midpapillary short-axis view may miss significant pathology in the basal and apical segments [44]. A brief TEE assessment of the LV in the four-chamber, two-chamber, and long-axis views looking for segmental wall motion abnormalities will aid in diagnosis. The parasternal long-axis, short-axis, and apical four-chamber views will evaluate LV function with TTE. Regardless of the modality, particular attention should be paid to the apex, as it contributes significantly to the global function of the left ventricle (Video 15.12).

Left ventricular hypercontractility resulting in dynamic left ventricular outflow tract (LVOT) obstruction may also cause hemodynamic instability and must be considered, particularly in patients whose hemodynamics worsen with inotropic support. LVOT obstruction can occur in many pathophysiologic settings (Table 15.6). LVOT obstruction results in localized increases in flow velocity during ejection due to a narrowed LVOT. This results in the anterior mitral leaflet and chordae being drawn toward the septum, causing mid- to late-systolic mitral regurgitation and LVOT obstruction [45, 46]. It is often possible to see movement of the anterior leaflet of the mitral valve toward the upper septum in the long-axis views (Fig. 15.10; Videos 15.13 and 15.14). Color flow Doppler (CFD) may show a posteriorly directed mitral regurgitant jet as well as turbulent flow in the LVOT. One author (JZ) has termed this finding the "Y-sign," and while it is neither sensitive nor specific, its appearance should lead to further investigation with spectral Doppler (Fig. 15.11, Video 15.15.) A late-peaking "dagger-shaped" spectral Doppler pattern in the LVOT is the hallmark echocardiographic finding in LVOT obstruction. Obstruction occurs late in systole because it takes time for the blood to generate

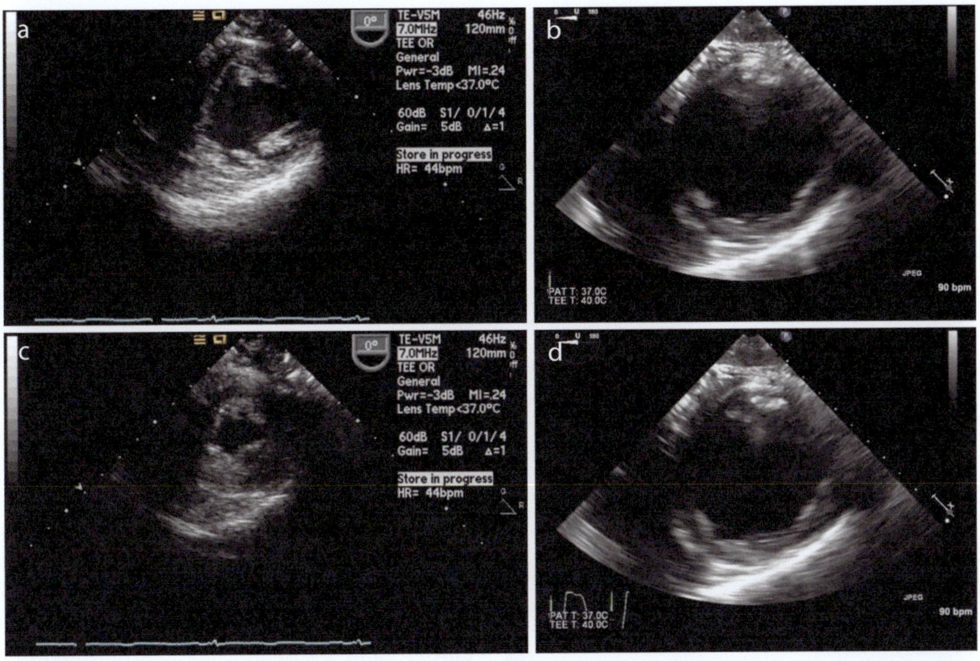

Fig. 15.8 Comparison of normal versus poor ejection fraction, using the transgastric midpapillary short-axis view. (**a**) and (**c**) are the diastolic and systolic frames, respectively, of a patient with normal systolic function. (**b**) and (**d**) are the diastolic and systolic frames, respectively, of a patient with grossly abnormal systolic function

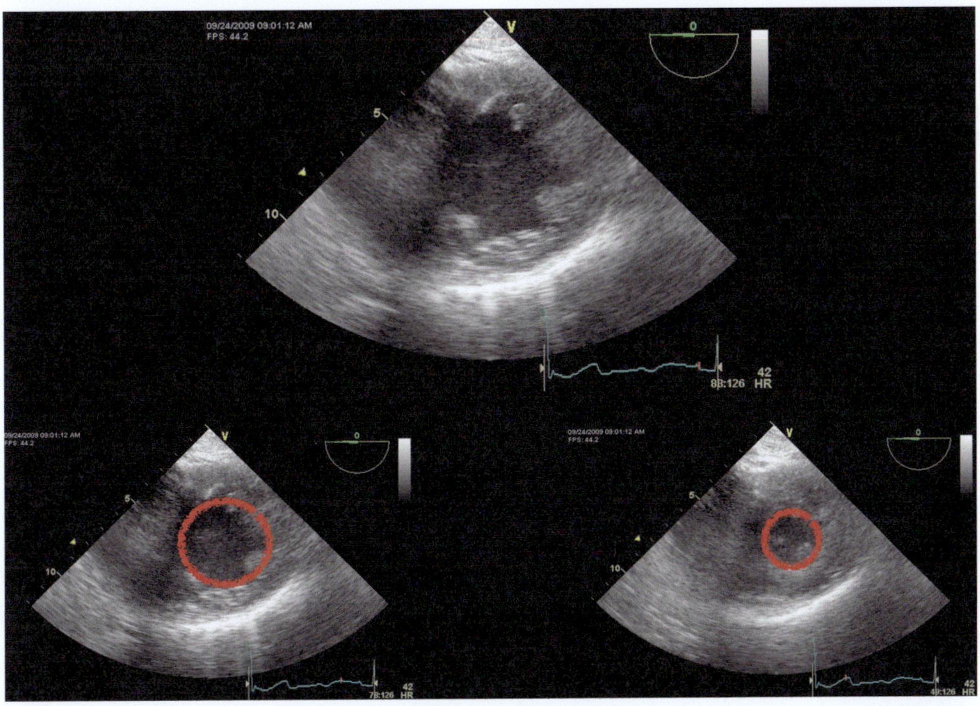

Fig. 15.9 Example of how to calculate left ventricular fractional area change. The image on the top is a transgastric short-axis view. The image on the bottom left is a rough estimate of the end-diastolic area. The image on the bottom right is a rough estimate of the end-systolic area. Fractional area change is a percentage change between the two areas

Table 15.6 Pathologies associated with left ventricular outflow tract obstruction

Hypertrophic cardiomyopathy
Hypertension
Type 1 diabetes
Myocardial ischemia
Pheochromocytoma
Takotsubo cardiomyopathy
Valvular replacements and repairs
Catecholamine administration

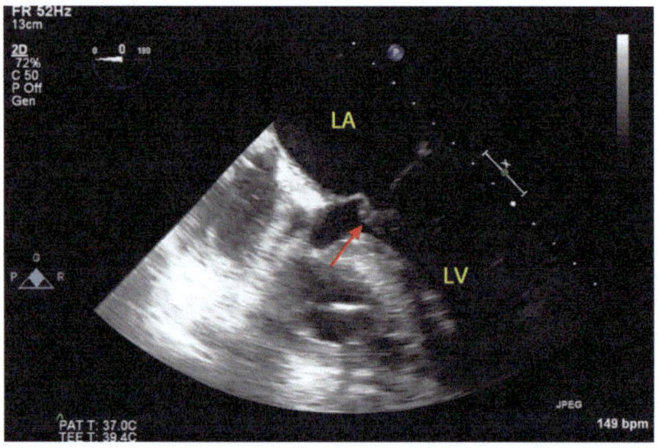

Fig. 15.10 Midesophageal four-chamber view in systole of a patient with left ventricular outflow tract obstruction. Note the anterior mitral leaflet contacting the septum (*red arrow*). *LA* left atrium, *LV* left ventricle

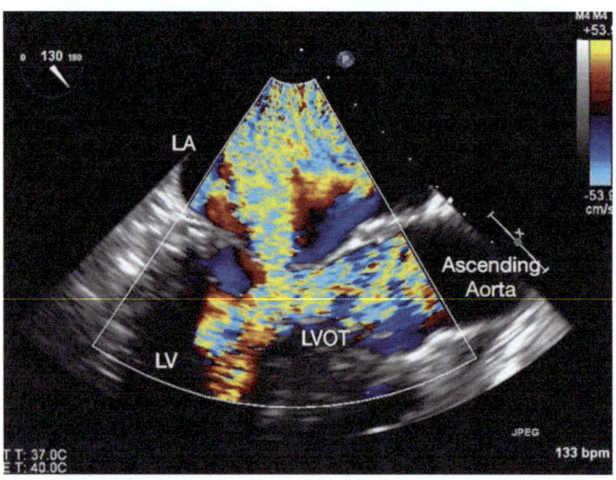

Fig. 15.11 Midesophageal aortic valve long-axis view, with color flow Doppler demonstrating the "Y-sign" of left ventricular outflow tract obstruction. Note the combination of a posteriorly directed jet of mitral regurgitation with turbulent flow in the outflow tract. *LA* left atrium, *LV* left ventricle, *LVOT* left ventricular outflow tract

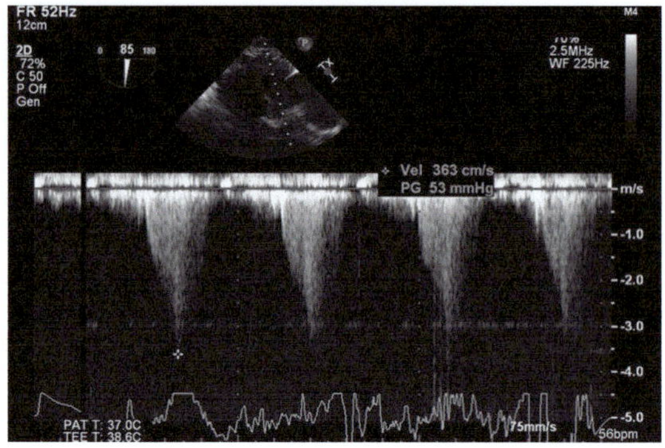

Fig. 15.12 Pulsed-wave Doppler in the left ventricular outflow tract revealing a "dagger-shaped" wave consistent with dynamic outflow obstruction

enough velocity to draw in the mitral apparatus via the Venturi effect. This dynamic property of the obstruction yields a late-peaking continuous-wave Doppler (CWD) pattern producing a "dagger" shape (Fig. 15.12). This profile is distinctly different from the fixed obstruction of aortic valve stenosis (see Chap. 9). The peak velocity of the wave will be high, consistent with an elevated pressure gradient.

Hypovolemia (Highlight Box 15.5)

The transgastric midpapillary short-axis view has been shown to be a reasonable view for estimating ventricular volume by assessments of the LV end-diastolic (LVEDA) and end-systolic (LVESA) areas [47–49]. A euvolemic patient has a "normal" LVEDA, whereas the LVEDA of a hypovolemic patient is often reduced because of decreased diastolic filling (Fig. 15.13; Videos 15.16 and 15.17). Normal value range for LVEDA is 8–14 cm^2 [50]. Several studies have confirmed the correlation between LV volume and LVEDA, although at varying strengths of correlation [51–54]. The LVESA reflects the endpoint of the LV ejection fraction (EF). A hypovolemic patient who starts off with a reduced LV diastolic volume (and thus a reduced LVEDA) will end with a reduced systolic volume (and thus reduced LVESA). A correlation between a reduced LVESA and hypovolemia has also been established [55]. Evaluation of the LVEDA and LVESA aids in qualitatively assessing volume status but often requires further evaluation to confirm.

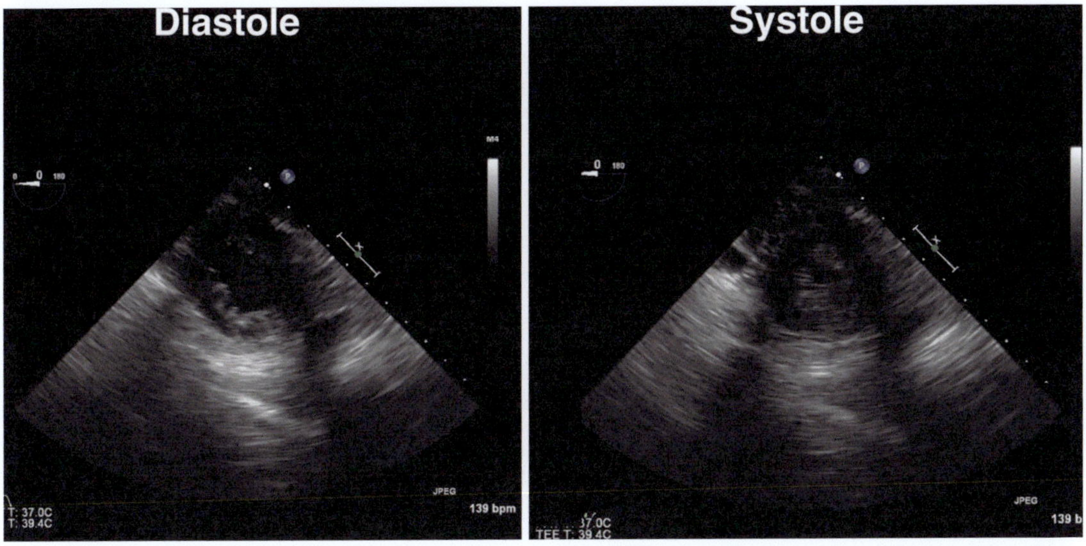

Fig. 15.13 Diastolic and systolic frames from a transgastric midpapillary short-axis view in the setting of hypovolemia. Note the small end-diastolic and end-systolic areas

Highlight Box 15.5

Hypovolemia	
2D	• Small end-diastolic area/small end-systolic area • Hyperdynamic LV
CFD	• *Typically not utilized*
Spectral	• Decreased SV or CO (calculated from LVOT) • Respiratory variation of peak LVOT velocity > 12%

LV left ventricle, *SV* stroke volume, *CO* cardiac output, *LVOT* left ventricular outflow tract

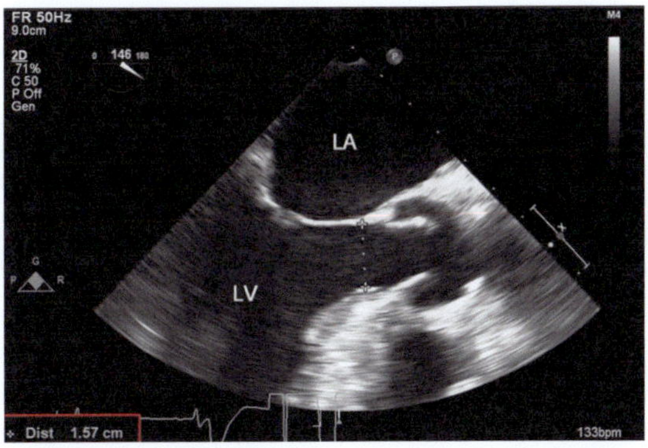

Fig. 15.14 Example of how to measure the diameter of the left ventricular outflow tract in the midesophageal long-axis view. *LA* left atrium, *LV* left ventricle

A reduced stroke volume (SV) in the setting of a normal or hyperdynamic LV strongly suggests hypovolemia as a cause of hypotension. Calculation of stroke volume assumes a cylindrical LVOT (see Chap. 4). The area of the cylinder is determined by measuring the LVOT diameter and using the following equation:

$$\text{Area} = \left(\text{LVOT diameter}\right)^2 \times 0.785$$

The LVOT diameter is usually measured in the midesophageal long-axis view within 5 mm of the aortic valve (Fig. 15.14). Small inaccuracies in measuring the diameter can introduce significant errors in the overall calculations, since the result is squared. For this reason, it is important to use the same LVOT diameter measurement for all subsequent calculations when performing serial SV measurements.

The length of the cylinder is determined by calculating the average distance a red blood cell travels in the LVOT during ejection, also called the stroke distance. Using the deep transgastric view (TEE) or apical five-chamber or long-axis (three-chamber) view (TTE), the pulsed-wave

Doppler cursor is placed in the LVOT and a systolic waveform is obtained. The waveform represents the velocities (i.e., speed and direction) of the red blood cells in the LVOT over time. The stroke distance, also called the velocity-time integral (VTI), is obtained by tracing the Doppler wave (Fig. 15.15). To better understand this concept, consider a car traveling 50 miles an hour for 2 hours. Figure 15.16 illustrates this data plotted on a graph with velocity on the Y-axis and time on the X-axis. The area of the rectangle created by these measurements yields a distance (50 mph × 2 h = 100 miles). The VTI is similar to this calculation, in that it is the area under the curve of red blood cell velocities over time. In this case, the velocities are represented by centimeters per second, the time by seconds, and the VTI by centimeters.

The overall equation for determining the SV is the following (Fig. 15.17):

$$\mathrm{SV} = (\mathrm{LVOT\ diameter})^2 \times 0.785 \times \mathrm{VTI}$$

Cardiac output (CO) can then be calculated by multiplying SV by the heart rate (HR). This method of stroke volume calculation is the recommended method for determining CO by the American Society of Echocardiography [56].

In addition to a static calculation of SV, volume status can be determined by dynamic changes in SV with respiration. Dynamic indices assess fluid responsiveness, which is the effect of

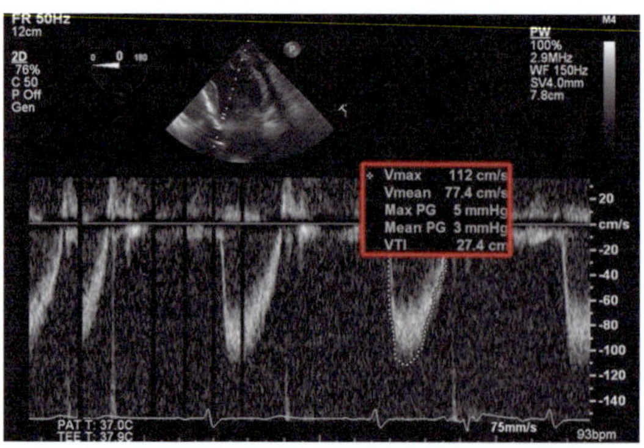

Fig. 15.15 Spectral profile from pulsed-wave Doppler placed in the left ventricular outflow tract in a deep transgastric five-chamber view. Tracing the profile provides the velocity-time integral (stroke distance)

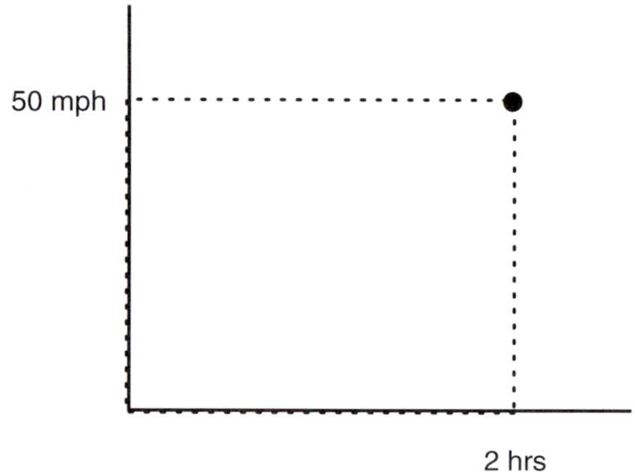

Fig. 15.16 Area under the curve for a time/velocity graph

Fig. 15.17 LVOT stroke volume calculation (Area of LVOT x Stroke Distance)

a change in preload on SV [57]. Positive pressure ventilation pushes blood out of the capillaries in the lungs into the LA and LV, augmenting LV SV. At the same time, the positive intrathoracic pressure reduces RV preload and increases RV afterload, thus reducing RV stroke volume. After several beats, the reduced RV stroke volume results in a reduced LV preload and reduced LV SV. These changes are exaggerated when the ventricles are on the steep part of the Frank-Starling curve, with the magnitude of this variation predicting fluid responsiveness. Pulsed-wave Doppler interrogation of the LVOT over time has been shown to accurately assess these changes in SV and thus predict fluid responsiveness (see Chap. 20) [58]. A lack of significant variation suggests decreased response to changes in preload (Fig. 15.18). One can use the following equation to quantitatively determine fluid responsiveness [59]:

$$\Delta V_{peak}(\%) = 100\% \times \frac{V_{max} - V_{min}}{(V_{max} + V_{min})/2}$$

V_{min} represents the minimum peak velocity in the LVOT and V_{max} the maximum peak velocity. A ΔV_{peak} of 12% or greater suggests volume responsiveness with a sensitivity of 100% and specificity of 89%. Such a calculation is often impractical in the emergent setting, and a visual estimate of the respiratory variation is often adequate.

Some patients who are found to be profoundly hypovolemic on echocardiographic evaluation have clear sources of volume loss (e.g., hemorrhage). The echocardiographer should be alert, however, to situations in which hypovolemia is an unexpected diagnosis. In these situations, the question "Where is the blood?" should be raised and additional information and imaging considered (including lung and abdominal imaging) (Table 15.7).

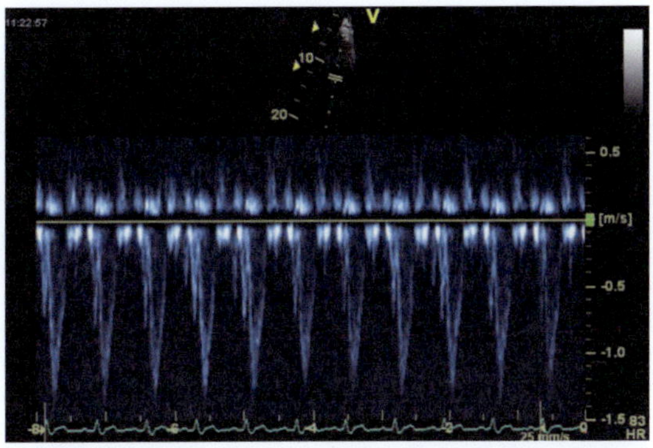

Fig. 15.18 Pulsed-wave Doppler in the left ventricular outflow tract showing minimal change in velocity with respiration

Table 15.7 Where is the blood? Considerations in unexpected hypovolemia

On the floor or in the bucket (blood loss outside the body)
Chest (pleural vs. parenchymal)
Abdomen (intraperitoneal vs. retroperitoneal)
Pelvis
Thigh
Intravascular (no true "blood loss," rather obstructive shock from pneumothorax, intra-abdominal pressure, etc.)

Low Afterload (Highlight Box 15.6)

Theoretically, the LVEDA and LVESA, typically measured in the transgastric midpapillary short-axis or parasternal short-axis view, can also help determine if the patient has a low afterload. A euvolemic patient should have a normal LVEDA, regardless of afterload. If the afterload is low, the EF should increase, which manifests as a small LVESA. Therefore, a euvolemic patient with a low afterload should have a normal LVEDA, but a reduced LVESA (Fig. 15.19; Videos 15.18 and 15.19). In contrast, a hypovolemic patient with a normal afterload should have a reduced LVEDA *and* LVESA. Table 15.8 compares LVEDAs and LVESAs in hypovolemia and low afterload. Unfortunately, a direct relationship between a low afterload and a normal LVEDA with a low LVESA has not been established, only suggested [55, 60]. A qualitative assessment of the LVEDA and LVESA can therefore only suggest hypovolemia or low afterload. Further confirmation by way of calculating the stroke volume, as described above, is often necessary. The stroke volume should be elevated in the setting of a low afterload and reduced in the setting of hypovolemia.

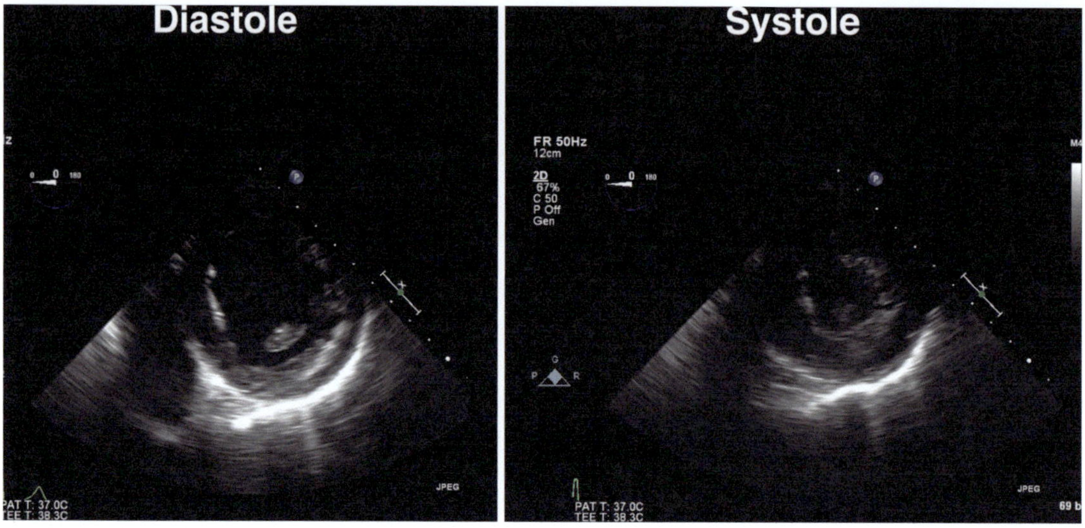

Fig. 15.19 Transgastric midpapillary short-axis view with evidence of low afterload (small end-systolic area and normal end-diastolic area)

Table 15.8 Diagnostic utility of end-diastolic area

	LVEDA	LVESA
Normal	Nl	Nl
Low afterload	Nl	Reduced
Hypovolemia	Reduced	Reduced

LVEDA left ventricular end-diastolic area, *LVESA* left ventricular end-systolic area, *Nl* normal

Highlight Box 15.6

Low afterload	
2D	• Normal end-diastolic area/small end-systolic area • Hyperdynamic LV
CFD	• *Typically not utilized*
Spectral	• Elevated SV or CO (calculated from LVOT)

LV left ventricle, *SV* stroke volume, *CO* cardiac output, *LVOT* left ventricular outflow tract

Conclusion

Echocardiography is extremely useful to the perioperative physician in assessing the cause of hemodynamic instability, aiding in both diagnosis and management. It is the diagnostic tool of choice, owing to its portability and ease of use. Not only does echocardiography help identify etiology; it also allows the practitioner to follow the effects of an intervention and make changes if necessary.

Questions

1. A 75-year-old man with a history of heart failure with a reduced ejection fraction (35%) is undergoing an exploratory laparotomy. There has been approximately 500 mL of blood loss. His blood pressure has gradually decreased through the case and is now 100/45 mmHg (mean arterial pressure 63 mmHg). Which of the following is the most appropriate next step?

   (a) Evaluate with point-of-care echocardiography
   (b) Administer 500 mL IV lactated Ringer's solution
   (c) Administer 1 unit packed red blood cells
   (d) Evaluate hemoglobin/hematocrit

2. A 35-year-old woman is in the hospital following delivery of a full-term infant by Caesarean section one day prior. She devel-

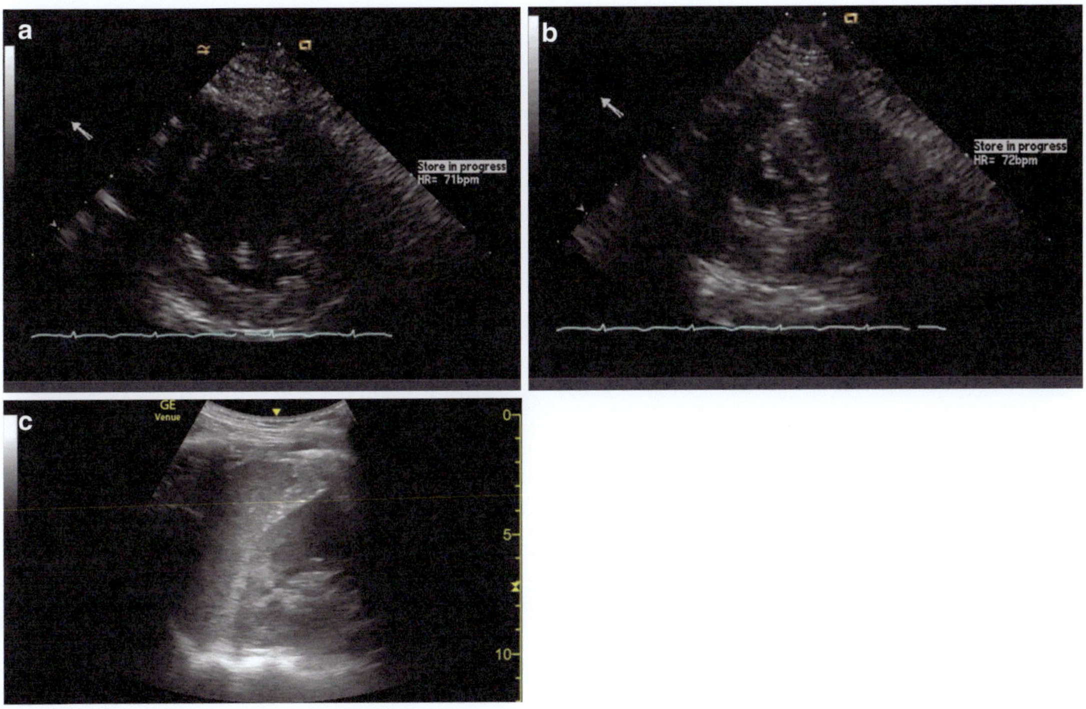

ops shortness of breath and her heart rate increases to 120 beats per minute, with a blood pressure 90/55 mmHg. Point-of-care ultrasound reveals the following images in diastole (**a**), systole (**b**), and a RUQ ultrasound image (**c**). Which of the following would be the most likely cause of the hypotension?

(a) Peripartum cardiomyopathy
(b) Acute pulmonary embolism
(c) Pelvic/intraabdominal hemorrhage
(d) Sepsis from endometritis

3. A 57-year-old man is undergoing appendectomy when he becomes acutely hypotensive. Transesophageal echocardiography reveals the following image. Which of the following is the most appropriate next step?

(a) Measure vena contracta
(b) Initiate phenylephrine infusion
(c) Measure peak velocity
(d) Initiate epinephrine infusion

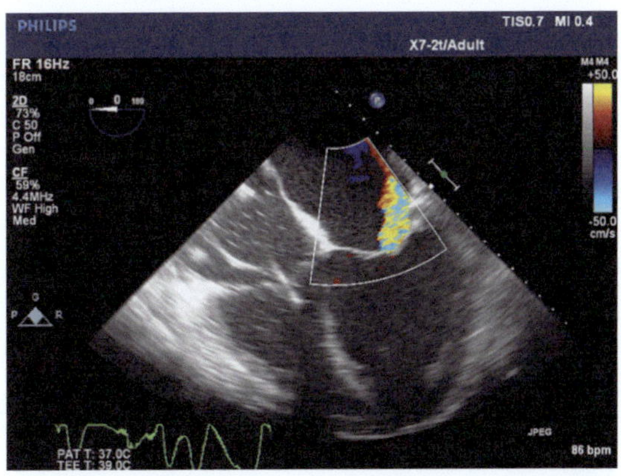

4. A 65-year-old man presents to the Emergency Department after an episode of syncope while walking. He is in moderate respiratory distress, with HR 110 BPM, BP 95/55 mmHg, RR 24, and SpO_2 90% on non-rebreather facemask. A point-of-care ultrasound examination reveals the following transthoracic image during systole. Which of the following would be the most appropriate next intervention?

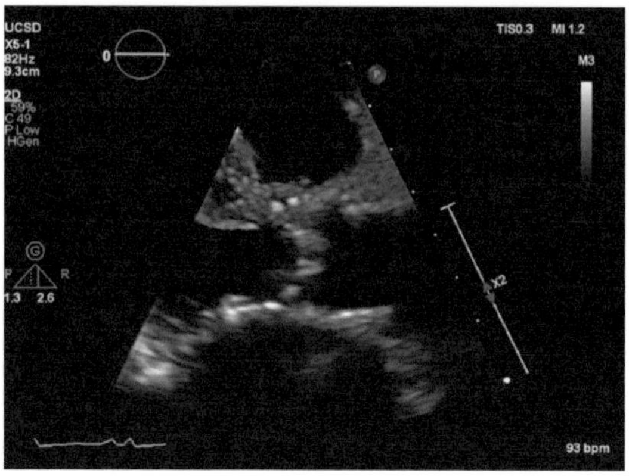

(a) Initiate epinephrine infusion
(b) Administer 500 mL IV lactated Ringer's solution
(c) Initiate norepinephrine infusion
(d) Administer 5 mg IV metoprolol

5. A 74-year-old woman is undergoing carotid endarterectomy when she becomes hypotensive. Point-of-care echocardiography reveals the following images in systole (**a**) and diastole (**b**). Which of the following is the most appropriate next step?

    (a) Administer 500 mL IV lactated Ringer's solution
    (b) Initiate epinephrine infusion
    (c) Initiate norepinephrine infusion
    (d) Decrease the imaging depth

6. A 67-year-old man is admitted to the intensive care unit for an exacerbation of chronic obstructive pulmonary disease (COPD). He was intubated prior to arrival for hypercapneic respiratory failure. His BP is 90/45 mmHg, HR 110 BPM, RR 24, and SpO_2 90% on FiO_2 1.0. Point-of-care ultrasound reveals the following image. Which of the following is the most appropriate next intervention?

    (a) Initiate heparin infusion and perform CT pulmonary angiogram
    (b) Evaluate ventilator settings
    (c) Administer 500 mL IV lactated Ringer's solution
    (d) Initiate norepinephrine infusion

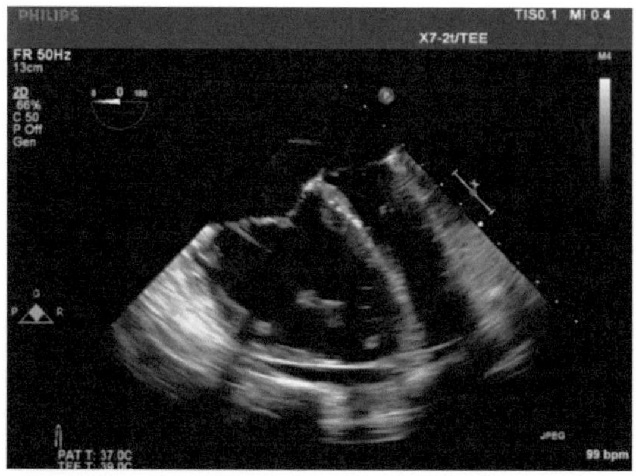

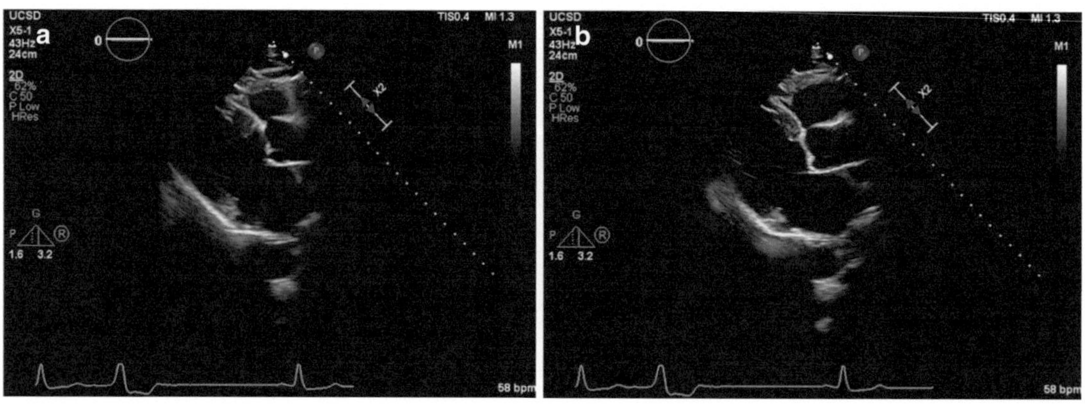

7. Which of the following can be concluded from the image provided?

    (a) Pneumothorax is not the cause of the patient's hypotension
    (b) The patient is in decompensated congestive heart failure
    (c) The patient may have a pneumothorax
    (d) The patient definitively does not have a pneumothorax

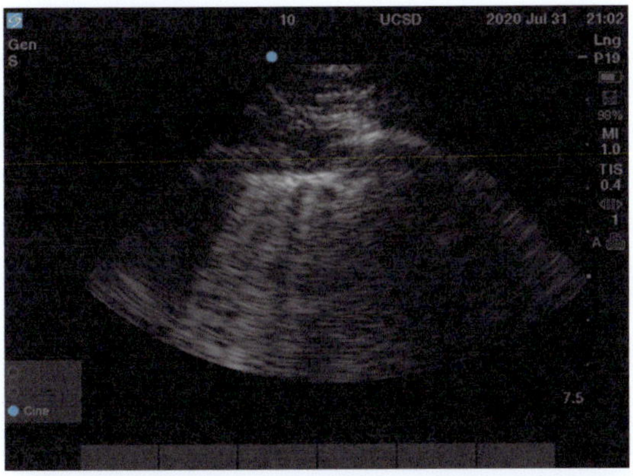

8. A 33-year-old man is recovering in the intensive care unit following a motor vehicle collision. His injuries include multiple pulmonary contusions, a grade 3 splenic laceration, and a 3 mm subdural hematoma. His temperature is 37°C, BP 95/40 mmHg, HR 120 BPM, RR 24, and SpO_2 90% on FiO_2 1.0. The following images are obtained from point-of-care echocardiography during diastole (**a**), systole (**b**), and in the abdomen (**c**). In addition to volume resuscitation, which of the following is the most appropriate next intervention?

    (a) Perform abdominal ultrasound
    (b) Perform CT abdomen and pelvis with IV contrast
    (c) Proceed to emergency exploratory laparotomy
    (d) Initiate norepinephrine infusion

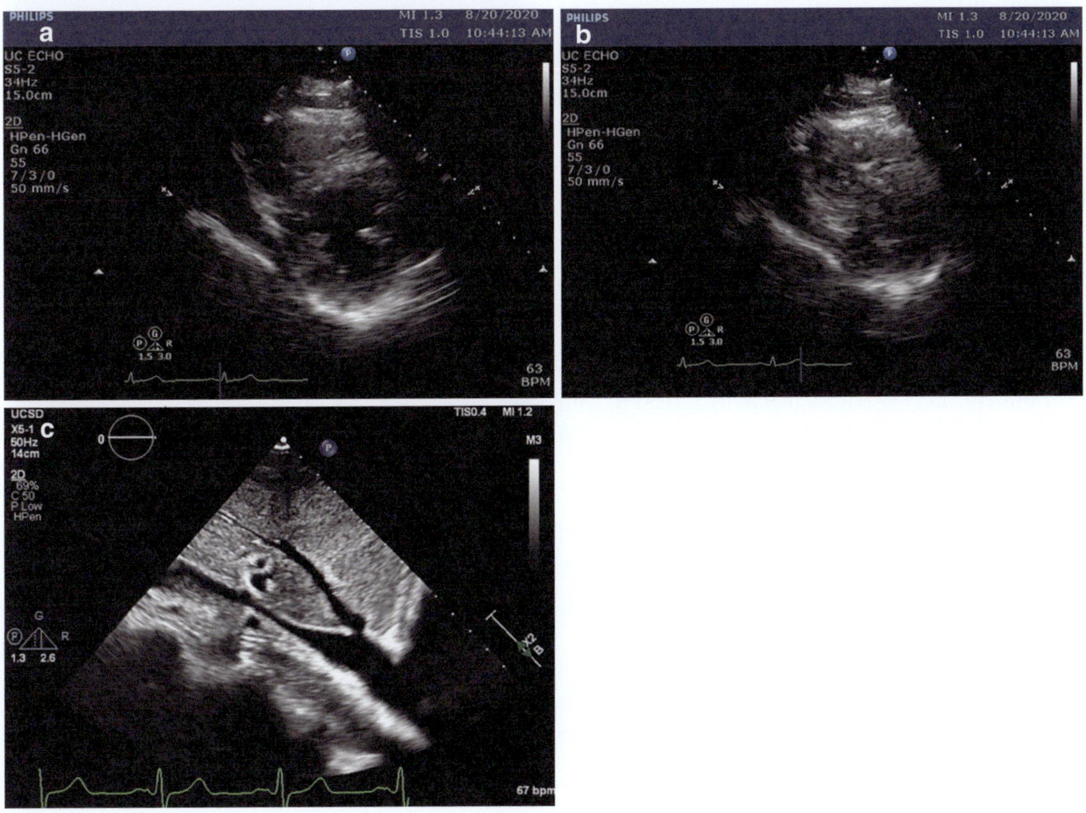

9. A 55-year-old woman is undergoing a surgical procedure for metastatic ovarian cancer. After induction of anesthesia, she becomes severely hypotensive and the following image is obtained. Which of the following is the most appropriate immediate step in management?

   (a) Evaluate mitral inflow to determine if tamponade is present
   (b) Perform pericardiocentesis to relieve tamponade
   (c) Administer 500 mL IV lactated Ringer's solution
   (d) Initiate norepinephrine infusion

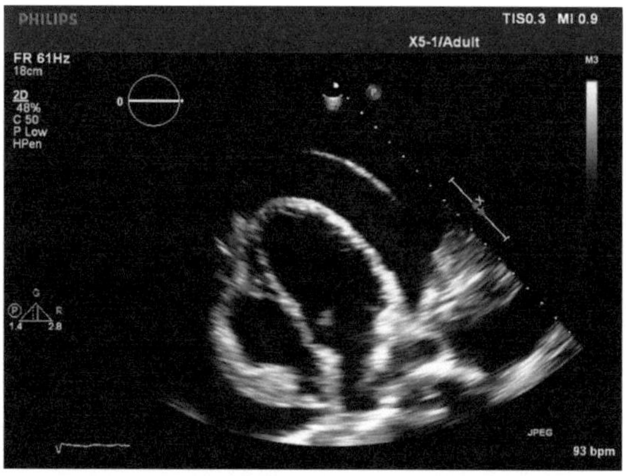

10. A 28-year-old woman is undergoing laparoscopic cholecystectomy for recurrent cholecystitis. As the surgeon insufflates the abdomen, her blood pressure suddenly decreases to 85/55 mmHg, and her HR increases to 220 bpm, with a wide complex. Which of the following is the most appropriate next step?

    (a) Perform visual estimation of LV EF and administer epinephrine if it is depressed
    (b) Evaluate LV end-diastolic area and initiate phenylephrine infusion if > 8 cm^2
    (c) Perform immediate cardioversion
    (d) Evaluate IVC diameter and administer 500 mL IV lactated Ringer's solution if < 1.5 cm

References

1. American Society of Anesthesiologists and Society of Cardiovascular Anesthesiologists Task Force on Transesophageal Echocardiography. Practice guidelines for perioperative transesophageal echocardiography. An updated report by the American Society of Anesthesiologists and the Society of Cardiovascular Anesthesiologists Task Force on transesophageal echocardiography. Anesthesiology. 2010;112(5):1084–96. https://doi.org/10.1097/ALN.0b013e3181c51e90.
2. American College of Cardiology Foundation Appropriate Use Criteria Task Force, American Society of Echocardiography, American Heart Association, et al. ACCF/ASE/AHA/ASNC/HFSA/HRS/SCAI/SCCM/SCCT/SCMR 2011 appropriate use criteria for echocardiography. A report of the American College of Cardiology Foundation Appropriate Use Criteria Task Force, American Society of Echocardiography, American Heart Association, American Society of Nuclear Cardiology, Heart Failure Society of America, Heart Rhythm Society, Society for Cardiovascular Angiography and Interventions, Society of Critical Care Medicine, Society of Cardiovascular Computed Tomography, Society for Cardiovascular Magnetic Resonance American College of Chest Physicians. J Am Soc Echocardiogr. 2011;24(3):229–67. https://doi.org/10.1016/j.echo.2010.12.008.
3. Spencer KT, Kimura BJ, Korcarz CE, Pellikka PA, Rahko PS, Siegel RJ. Focused cardiac ultrasound: recommendations from the American Society of Echocardiography. J Am Soc Echocardiogr. 2013;26(6):567–81. https://doi.org/10.1016/j.echo.2013.04.001.
4. Price S, Ilper H, Uddin S, et al. Peri-resuscitation echocardiography: training the novice practitioner. Resuscitation. 2010;81(11):1534–9. https://doi.org/10.1016/j.resuscitation.2010.07.001.
5. Markin NW, Gmelch BS, Griffee MJ, Holmberg TJ, Morgan DE, Zimmerman JM. A review of 364 perioperative rescue echocardiograms: findings of an anesthesiologist-staffed perioperative echocardiography service. J Cardiothorac Vasc Anesth. 2015;29(1):82–8. https://doi.org/10.1053/j.jvca.2014.07.004.
6. Griffee MJ, Singleton A, Zimmerman JM, Morgan DE, Nirula R. The effect of perioperative rescue transesophageal echocardiography on the management of trauma patients. A A Case Rep. 2016;6(12):387–90. https://doi.org/10.1213/XAA.0000000000000320.
7. Reeves ST, Finley AC, Skubas NJ, et al. Basic perioperative transesophageal echocardiography examination: a consensus statement of the American Society of Echocardiography and the Society of Cardiovascular Anesthesiologists. J Am Soc Echocardiogr. 2013;26(5):443–56. https://doi.org/10.1016/j.echo.2013.02.015.

8. Miller JP, Lambert AS, Shapiro WA, Russell IA, Schiller NB, Cahalan MK. The adequacy of basic intraoperative transesophageal echocardiography performed by experienced anesthesiologists. Anesth Analg. 2001;92(5):1103–10.
9. Shillcutt SK, Markin NW, Montzingo CR, Brakke TR. Use of rapid "rescue" perioperative echocardiography to improve outcomes after hemodynamic instability in noncardiac surgical patients. J Cardiothorac Vasc Anesth. 2012. https://doi.org/10.1053/j.jvca.2011.09.029.
10. Zimmerman JM, Coker BJ. The nuts and bolts of performing focused cardiovascular ultrasound (FoCUS). Anesth Analg. 2017;124(3):753–60. https://doi.org/10.1213/ANE.0000000000001861.
11. Stout KK, Verrier ED. Acute Valvular Regurgitation. Circulation. 2009;119(25):3232–41. https://doi.org/10.1161/CIRCULATIONAHA.108.782292.
12. Shiga T, Wajima Z, Apfel CC, Inoue T, Ohe Y. Diagnostic accuracy of transesophageal echocardiography, helical computed tomography, and magnetic resonance imaging for suspected thoracic aortic dissection: systematic review and meta-analysis. Arch Intern Med. 2006;166(13):1350–6. https://doi.org/10.1001/archinte.166.13.1350.
13. Evangelista A, Flachskampf FA, Erbel R, et al. Echocardiography in aortic diseases: EAE recommendations for clinical practice. Eur J Echocardiogr. 2010;11(8):645–58. https://doi.org/10.1093/ejechocard/jeq056.
14. Erbel R, Oelert H, Meyer J, et al. Effect of medical and surgical therapy on aortic dissection evaluated by transesophageal echocardiography. Implications for prognosis and therapy. The European Cooperative Study Group on Echocardiography. Circulation. 1993;87(5):1604–15.
15. Klein AL, Abbara S, Agler DA, et al. American Society of Echocardiography clinical recommendations for multimodality cardiovascular imaging of patients with pericardial disease: endorsed by the Society for Cardiovascular Magnetic Resonance and Society of Cardiovascular Computed Tomography. J Am Soc Echocardiogr. 2013;26(9):965–1012.e15. https://doi.org/10.1016/j.echo.2013.06.023.
16. Salem K, Mulji A, Lonn E. Echocardiographically guided pericardiocentesis - the gold standard for the management of pericardial effusion and cardiac tamponade. Can J Cardiol. 1999;15(11):1251–5.
17. Denault AY, Haddad F, Jacobsohn E, Deschamps A. Perioperative right ventricular dysfunction. Curr Opin Anaesthesiol. 2013;26(1):71–81. https://doi.org/10.1097/ACO.0b013e32835b8be2.
18. Zochios V. Does β2-agonist use improve survival in critically ill patients with acute respiratory distress syndrome? In: Reducing mortality in critically ill patients, vol. 353. Cham: Springer International Publishing; 2015. p. 103–9. https://doi.org/10.1007/978-3-319-17515-7_13.
19. Sheehan F, Redington A. The right ventricle: anatomy, physiology and clinical imaging. Heart. 2008;94(11):1510–5. https://doi.org/10.1136/hrt.2007.132779.
20. Drake D, Gupta R, Lloyd SG, Gupta H. Right ventricular function assessment: comparison of geometric and visual method to short-axis slice summation method. Echocardiography (Mount Kisco, NY). 2007;24(10):1013–9. https://doi.org/10.1111/j.1540-8175.2007.00510.x.
21. Lang RM, Badano LP, Mor-Avi V, et al. Recommendations for cardiac chamber quantification by echocardiography in adults: an update from the american society of echocardiography and the European association of cardiovascular imaging. J Am Soc Echocardiogr. 2015;28(1):1–39.e14. https://doi.org/10.1016/j.echo.2014.10.003.
22. Tapson VF. Acute pulmonary embolism. N Engl J Med. 2008;358(10):1037–52. https://doi.org/10.1056/NEJMra072753.
23. Konstantinides SV, Meyer G, Becattini C, et al. 2019 ESC guidelines for the diagnosis and management of acute pulmonary embolism developed in collaboration with the European Respiratory Society (ERS). Eur Heart J. 2020;41(4):543–603. https://doi.org/10.1093/eurheartj/ehz405.
24. Kurnicka K, Lichodziejewska B, Goliszek S, et al. Echocardiographic pattern of acute pulmonary embolism: analysis of 511 consecutive patients. J Am Soc Echocardiogr. 2016;29(9):907–13. https://doi.org/10.1016/j.echo.2016.05.016.
25. Miniati M, Monti S, Pratali L, et al. Value of transthoracic echocardiography in the diagnosis of pulmonary embolism: results of a prospective study in unselected patients. Am J Med. 2001;110(7):528–35. https://doi.org/10.1016/s0002-9343(01)00693-3.
26. Visnjevac O, Pourafkari L, Nader ND. Role of perioperative monitoring in diagnosis of massive intraoperative cardiopulmonary embolism. J Cardiovasc Thorac Res. 2014;6(3):141–5. https://doi.org/10.15171/jcvtr.2014.002.
27. Kjaergaard J, Schaadt BK, Lund JO, Hassager C. Quantification of right ventricular function in acute pulmonary embolism: relation to extent of pulmonary perfusion defects. Eur J Echocardiogr. 2008;9(5):641–5. https://doi.org/10.1093/ejechocard/jen033.
28. Ribeiro A, Juhlin-Dannfelt A, Brodin LA, Holmgren A, Jorfeldt L. Pulmonary embolism: relation between the degree of right ventricle overload and the extent of perfusion defects. Am Heart J. 1998;135(5 Pt 1):868–74. https://doi.org/10.1016/s0002-8703(98)70048-1.
29. Kjaergaard J, Schaadt BK, Lund JO, Hassager C. Prognostic importance of quantitative echocardiographic evaluation in patients suspected of first nonmassive pulmonary embolism. Eur J Echocardiogr. 2009;10(1):89–95. https://doi.org/10.1093/ejechocard/jen169.
30. Ribeiro A, Lindmarker P, Juhlin-Dannfelt A, Johnsson H, Jorfeldt L. Echocardiography Doppler in pulmonary embolism: right ventricular dysfunction as a predictor

of mortality rate. Am Heart J. 1997;134(3):479–87. https://doi.org/10.1016/s0002-8703(97)70085-1.
31. Sanchez O, Trinquart L, Colombet I, et al. Prognostic value of right ventricular dysfunction in patients with haemodynamically stable pulmonary embolism: a systematic review. Eur Heart J. 2008;29(12):1569–77. https://doi.org/10.1093/eurheartj/ehn208.
32. McConnell MV, Solomon SD, Rayan ME, Come PC, Goldhaber SZ, Lee RT. Regional right ventricular dysfunction detected by echocardiography in acute pulmonary embolism. AJC. 1996;78(4):469–73. https://doi.org/10.1016/s0002-9149(96)00339-6.
33. Lodato JA, Ward RP, Lang RM. Echocardiographic predictors of pulmonary embolism in patients referred for helical CT. Echocardiography. 2008;25(6):584–90. https://doi.org/10.1111/j.1540-8175.2008.00665.x.
34. Hauser AM, Gangadharan V, Ramos RG, Gordon S, Timmis GC, Dudlets P. Sequence of mechanical, electrocardiographic and clinical effects of repeated coronary artery occlusion in human beings: echocardiographic observations during coronary angioplasty. J Am Coll Cardiol. 1985;5(2):193–7. https://doi.org/10.1016/S0735-1097(85)80036-X.
35. Wohlgelernter D, Cleman M, Highman HA, et al. Regional myocardial dysfunction during coronary angioplasty: evaluation by two-dimensional echocardiography and 12 lead electrocardiography. J Am Coll Cardiol. 1986;7(6):1245–54. https://doi.org/10.1016/S0735-1097(86)80143-7.
36. Seeberger MD, Skarvan K, Buser P, et al. Dobutamine stress echocardiography to detect inducible demand ischemia in anesthetized patients with coronary artery disease. Anesthesiology. 1998;88(5):1233–9. https://doi.org/10.1097/00000542-199805000-00014.
37. Wang J, Filipovic M, Rudzitis A, et al. Transesophageal echocardiography for monitoring segmental wall motion during off-pump coronary artery bypass surgery. Anesth Analg. 2004;99(4):965–73. https://doi.org/10.1213/01.ANE.0000130614.45647.81.
38. Romero-Bermejo FJ, Ruiz-Bailen M, Gil-Cebrian J, Huertos-Ranchal MJ. Sepsis-induced cardiomyopathy. Curr Cardiol Rev. 2011;7(3):163–83. https://doi.org/10.2174/157340311798220494.
39. Chockalingam A, Mehra A, Dorairajan S, Dellsperger KC. Acute left ventricular dysfunction in the critically ill. Chest. 2010;138(1):198–207. https://doi.org/10.1378/chest.09-1996.
40. Gudmundsson P, Rydberg E, Winter R, Willenheimer R. Visually estimated left ventricular ejection fraction by echocardiography is closely correlated with formal quantitative methods. Int J Cardiol. 2005;101(2):209–12. https://doi.org/10.1016/j.ijcard.2004.03.027.
41. Shahgaldi K, Gudmundsson P, Manouras A, Brodin L-Å, Winter R. Visually estimated ejection fraction by two dimensional and triplane echocardiography is closely correlated with quantitative ejection fraction by real-time three dimensional echocardiography. Cardiovasc Ultrasound. 2009;7(1):421. https://doi.org/10.1186/1476-7120-7-41.
42. Akinboboye O, Sumner J, Gopal A, et al. Visual estimation of ejection fraction by two-dimensional echocardiography: the learning curve. Clin Cardiol. 1995;18(12):726–9. https://doi.org/10.1002/clc.4960181208.
43. Skarvan K, Lambert A, Filipovic M, Seeberger M. Reference values for left ventricular function in subjects under general anaesthesia and controlled ventilation assessed by two-dimensional transoesophageal echocardiography. Eur J Anaesthesiol. 2001;18(11):713–22. https://doi.org/10.1046/j.1365-2346.2001.00915.x.
44. Rouine-Rapp K, Ionescu P, Balea M, Foster E, Cahalan MK. Detection of intraoperative segmental wall-motion abnormalities by transesophageal echocardiography: the incremental value of additional cross sections in the transverse and longitudinal planes. Anesth Analg. 1996;83(6):1141–8. https://doi.org/10.1097/00000539-199612000-00002.
45. Sherrid MV, Gunsburg DZ, Moldenhauer S, Pearle G. Systolic anterior motion begins at low left ventricular outflow tract velocity in obstructive hypertrophic cardiomyopathy. J Am Coll Cardiol. 2000;36(4):1344–54. https://doi.org/10.1016/s0735-1097(00)00830-5.
46. Wigle ED, Rakowski H, Kimball BP, Williams WG. Hypertrophic cardiomyopathy. Clinical spectrum and treatment. Circulation. 1995;92(7):1680–92. https://doi.org/10.1161/01.cir.92.7.1680.
47. Clements FM, Harpole DH, Quill T, Jones RH, McCann RL. Estimation of left ventricular volume and ejection fraction by two-dimensional transoesophageal echocardiography: comparison of short axis imaging and simultaneous radionuclide angiography. Br J Anaesth. 1990;64(3):331–6. https://doi.org/10.1093/bja/64.3.331.
48. Ryan T, Burwash I, Lu J, et al. The agreement between ventricular volumes and ejection fraction by transesophageal echocardiography or a combined radionuclear and thermodilution technique in patients after coronary artery surgery. YJCAN. 1996;10(3):323–8. https://doi.org/10.1016/s1053-0770(96)80091-7.
49. Schmidlin D, Jenni R, Schmid ER. Transesophageal echocardiographic area and Doppler flow velocity measurements: comparison with hemodynamic changes in coronary artery bypass surgery. YJCAN. 1999;13(2):143–9. https://doi.org/10.1016/s1053-0770(99)90077-0.
50. Royse CF. Ultrasound-guided haemodynamic state assessment. Best Pract Res Clin Anaesthesiol. 2009;23(3):273–83. https://doi.org/10.1016/j.bpa.2009.02.009.
51. Cheung AT, Savino JS, Weiss SJ, Aukburg SJ, Berlin JA. Echocardiographic and hemodynamic indexes of left ventricular preload in patients with normal and abnormal ventricular function. Anesthesiology. 1994;81(2):376–87. https://doi.org/10.1097/00000542-199408000-00016.
52. Greim CA, Roewer N, Apfel C, Laux G, Schulte am Esch J. Relation of echocardiographic preload indi-

ces to stroke volume in critically ill patients with normal and low cardiac index. Intensive Care Med. 1997;23(4):411–6.
53. Swenson JD, Bull D, Stringham J. Subjective assessment of left ventricular preload using transesophageal echocardiography: corresponding pulmonary artery occlusion pressures. J Cardiothorac Vasc Anesth. 2001;15(5):580–3. https://doi.org/10.1053/jcan.2001.26535.
54. Tousignant CP, Walsh F, Mazer CD. The use of transesophageal echocardiography for preload assessment in critically ill patients. Anesth Analg. 2000;90(2):351–5.
55. Leung JM, Levine EH. Left ventricular end-systolic cavity obliteration as an estimate of intraoperative hypovolemia. Anesthesiology. 1994;81(5):1102–9. https://doi.org/10.1097/00000542-199411000-00003.
56. Quiñones MA, Otto CM, Stoddard M, Waggoner A, Zoghbi WA, Doppler Quantification Task Force of the Nomenclature and Standards Committee of the American Society of Echocardiography. Recommendations for quantification of Doppler echocardiography: a report from the Doppler quantification task force of the nomenclature and standards Committee of the American Society of Echocardiography. J Am Soc Echocardiogr. 2002;15(2):167–84. https://doi.org/10.1067/mje.2002.120202.
57. Michard F, Teboul JL. Using heart-lung interactions to assess fluid responsiveness during mechanical ventilation. Crit Care. 2000;4(5):282–9. https://doi.org/10.1186/cc710.
58. Renner J, Broch O, Gruenewald M, et al. Non-invasive prediction of fluid responsiveness in infants using pleth variability index. Anaesthesia. 2011;66(7):582–9. https://doi.org/10.1111/j.1365-2044.2011.06715.x.
59. Feissel M, Michard F, Mangin I, Ruyer O, Faller JP, Teboul JL. Respiratory changes in aortic blood velocity as an indicator of fluid responsiveness in ventilated patients with septic shock. Chest. 2001;119(3):867–73.
60. van Daele ME, Trouwborst A, van Woerkens LC, Tenbrinck R, Fraser AG, Roelandt JR. Transesophageal echocardiographic monitoring of preoperative acute hypervolemic hemodilution. Anesthesiology. 1994;81(3):602–9. https://doi.org/10.1097/00000542-199409000-00012.

Imaging Artifacts, Normal Anatomic Variants, and Common Misdiagnoses

16

Brett Cronin and Ramon Sanchez

Abbreviations

ASE	American Society of Echocardiography
AV	Aortic valve
CFD	Color flow Doppler
CT	Computed tomography
IVC	Inferior vena cava
LA	Left atrium
LAX	Long-axis
ME	Midesophageal
PWD	Pulsed-wave Doppler
RA	Right atrium
RV	Right ventricle
SAX	Short-axis
TEE	Transesophageal echocardiography
TG	Transgastric
TV	Tricuspid valve

Introduction

The ability to identify artifacts and normal anatomic variants commonly encountered during an echocardiography exam can be as important as identifying normal anatomy and function. In fact, the American Society of Echocardiography (ASE) recognizes the importance of this skill in the objectives for basic perioperative transesophageal training [1]. Lack of knowledge regarding these common anatomic structures and artifacts can result in misdiagnoses and adverse effects for patients.

The following does not represent an all-encompassing list, but rather the goal of this chapter is to describe the appearance of the artifacts and normal anatomic variants commonly encountered.

Normal Anatomic Variants/ Misdiagnoses

Epicardial and Extracardiac Fat

Echocardiographers are often asked to monitor for the development of pericardial effusions intraoperatively with TEE, and they can lead to significant hemodynamic consequences. Epicardial fat or even extracardiac fat can be confused for a pericardial effusion given its presentation as an echolucent area between the right ventricle (RV) and the pericardium or between

Supplementary Information The online version of this chapter (https://doi.org/10.1007/978-3-030-84349-6_16) contains supplementary material, which is available to authorized users.

B. Cronin (✉) · R. Sanchez
Department of Anesthesiology, University of California San Diego Health, La Jolla, CA, USA
e-mail: bcronin@health.ucsd.edu

T. M. Maus, C. R. Tainter (eds.), *Essential Echocardiography*,
https://doi.org/10.1007/978-3-030-84349-6_16

the mediastinum and chest wall, respectively (Fig. 16.1 and Video 16.1a, b). However, fat has a non-homogeneous, textured appearance that can be distinguished from a pericardial effusion by altering the gain and focus and examining the area of interest in multiple views [2].

The following echocardiography findings are normal anatomic variants that can be confused for thrombi, masses, or foreign bodies.

Eustachian Valve

The Eustachian valve is an embryologic remnant whose purpose was to shunt oxygenated blood from the right atrium (RA) to the left atrium (LA) through the foramen ovale during fetal development. The Eustachian valve can be found in adults in the midesophageal (ME) bicaval view at the junction of the inferior vena cava (IVC) and RA (Fig. 16.2 and Video 16.2) [3].

Moderator Band

Also known as septomarginal trabecula, the moderator band functions as a conduction path from the right bundle branch to the RV free wall and can become quite prominent in cases of chronic RV pressure overload (e.g., chronic pulmonary hypertension). In addition to examination in multiple views, the diagnosis of a moderator band is more likely if it moves with the cardiac cycle and the adjacent wall motion is normal (Fig. 16.3 and Video 16.3) [4].

Crista Terminalis

The crista terminalis is a smooth fibromuscular ridge located in the RA, which separates the smooth RA from the right atrial appendage (Fig. 16.4 and Video 16.4). Its appearance ranges from a ridge to pedunculated mass and can be mistaken for tumor or thrombus [3]. The superior portion of the crista terminalis also contains the

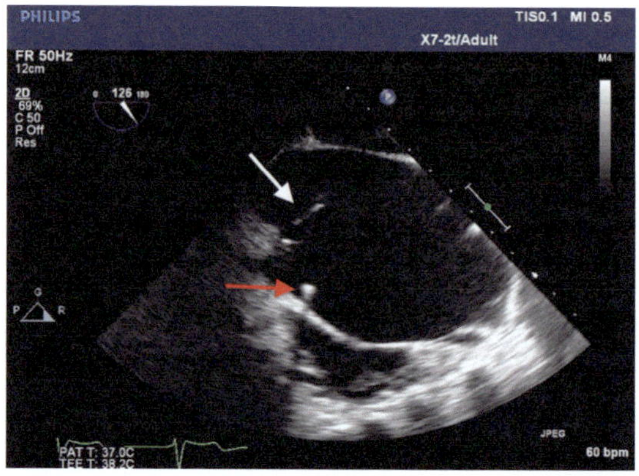

Fig. 16.2 Midesophageal bicaval view. An Eustachian valve is present at the junction of the IVC and RA (*white arrow*). A pulmonary artery catheter (*red arrow*), which is seen in cross section, is also directed toward the area of the tricuspid valve (TV)

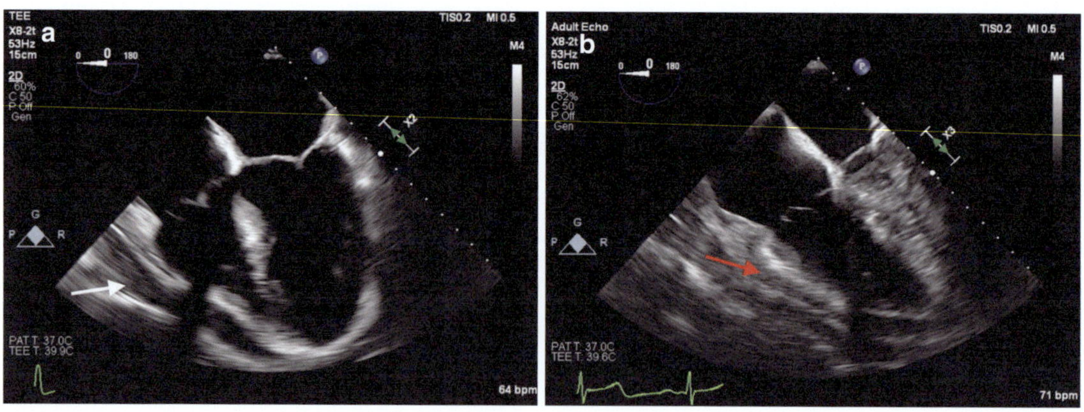

Fig. 16.1 (**a**) Midesophageal four-chamber view at end-systole. Extracardiac fat is present at seven o'clock position (*white arrow*) between the RV lateral wall and the chest wall. (**b**) ME four-chamber view with an RV focus. Epicardial fat is present between the RV lateral wall and pericardium

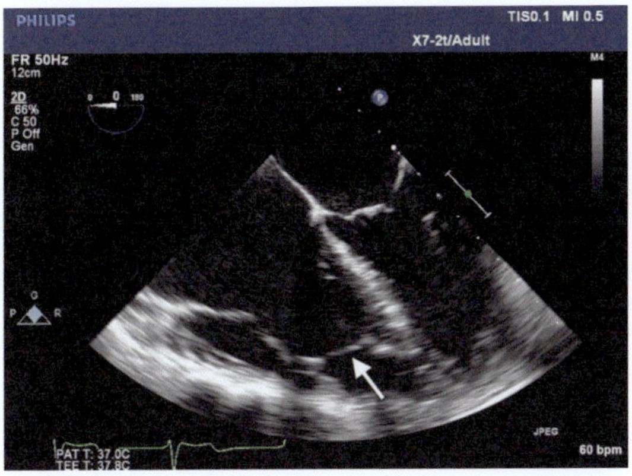

Fig. 16.3 Midesophageal four-chamber view (end-diastole). A moderator band (*white arrow*) connects the interventricular septum to the anterior papillary muscle in the distal half of the ventricle

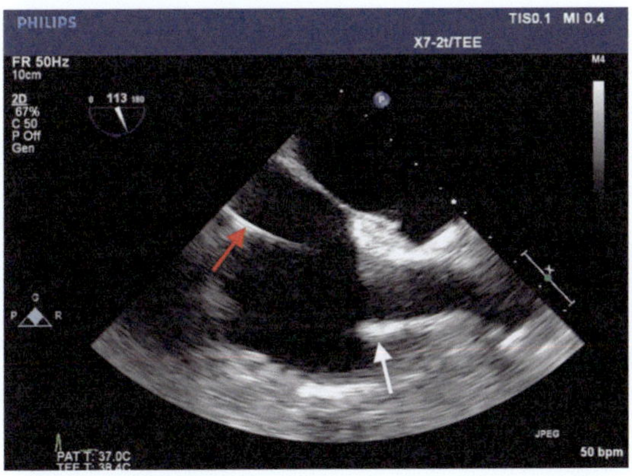

Fig. 16.4 Midesophageal bicaval view. A prominent crista terminalis (*white arrow*) is present at the superior portion of the right atrium. A pulmonary artery catheter (*red arrow*) is also visualized traversing the right atrium toward the tricuspid valve

sinoatrial node and has been implicated as the origin of atrial arrhythmias [5].

Lipomatous Hypertrophy of the Interatrial Septum

Lipomatous hypertrophy of the interatrial septum is a benign fatty infiltration of the septum that spares the fossa ovalis. This diagnosis is frequently made when the septum has a bilobed- or "dumbbell-shaped" appearance and has a thickness of > 1.5–2 cm, no other systemic explanation for the infiltration exists (e.g., amyloidosis),

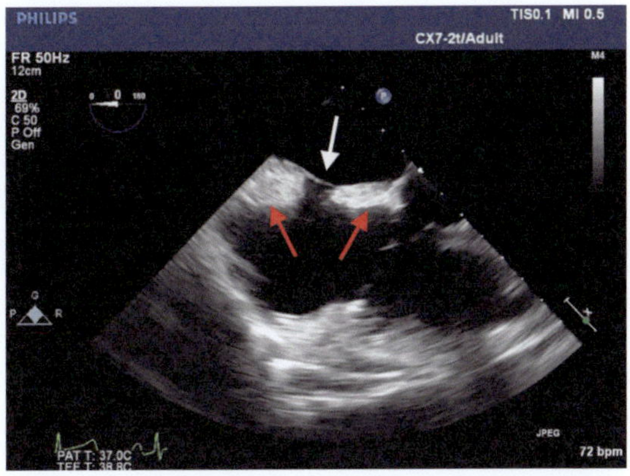

Fig. 16.5 Midesophageal four-chamber view (RV focused). Lipomatous hypertrophy of the interatrial septum is present (*red arrows*) in the near field with obvious sparing of the fossa ovalis (*white arrow*)

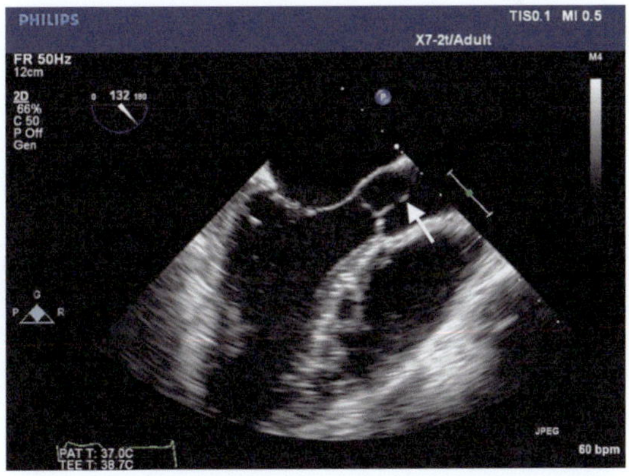

Fig. 16.6 Midesophageal long-axis view. Lambl's excrescences (*white arrow*) are present on the aortic valve extending to the level of the sinotubular junction. Please refer to the associated online video to better appreciate the classic appearance and movement of these small structures

and the fossa ovalis is spared (Fig. 16.5 and Video 16.5) [1, 6]. Additional echocardiographic evidence that makes the diagnosis more likely is heavy extracardiac fat and periaortic fat.

Lambl's Excrescences

Lambl's excrescences are typically identified on the aortic valve (AV) and originate as small thrombi on the endocardial surface at the site of valve closure (Fig. 16.6 and Video 16.6). Histologically, Lambl's excrescences are projections of fibrous tissue covered by a layer of endothelial cells [7]. While patients with Lambl's excrescences are usually asymptomatic, these small filiform (threadlike) fronds can embolize. Therefore, patients who suffer from multiple cerebrovascular accidents may be offered treatment in the form of anticoagulation or resection [8].

Fibroelastoma

Cardiac papillary fibroelastomas are benign tumors that are typically attached to the aortic side of the AV. With echocardiography fibroelastomas present as slow-growing, mobile, pedunculated masses along the line of valve closure that are more gelatinous in appearance than Lambl's excrescences (Fig. 16.7 and Video 16.7a, b) [9]. Given their predilection to thromboembolism, these masses often require surgical resection.

Nodules of Arantius

Nodules of Arantius are thickened central areas on the AV cusps (Fig. 16.8 and Video 16.8). The role of these nodules is not clear; however, it has been theorized that they have a protective role in reducing the stress on the coapting surfaces. In contrast, aortic regurgitation has been attributed to the fibrosis and hypertrophy of the nodules of Arantius in isolated patients [7].

Coumadin Ridge

The Coumadin ridge describes the normal muscular ridge located between the left upper pulmonary vein and left atrial appendage (Fig. 16.9 and Video 16.9). This structure derives its name from its frequent misdiagnosis for left atrial thrombus and subsequent prescription for anticoagulation.

Chiari Network

While a Chiari network shares its origin with the Eustachian valve, it is not simply a longer variant. A Chiari network refers to an inferiorly located, mobile, and heavily fenestrated structure in the RA (Fig. 16.10 and Video 16.10) that is associated with patent foramen ovale and atrial septal aneurysms [3].

Artifacts

The following assumptions are made when generating ultrasound images:

- Sound waves travel in straight lines to the reflector and back.
- Sound waves return to the transducer after a single reflection.
- Sound travels at exactly 1540 meters per second (m/s).

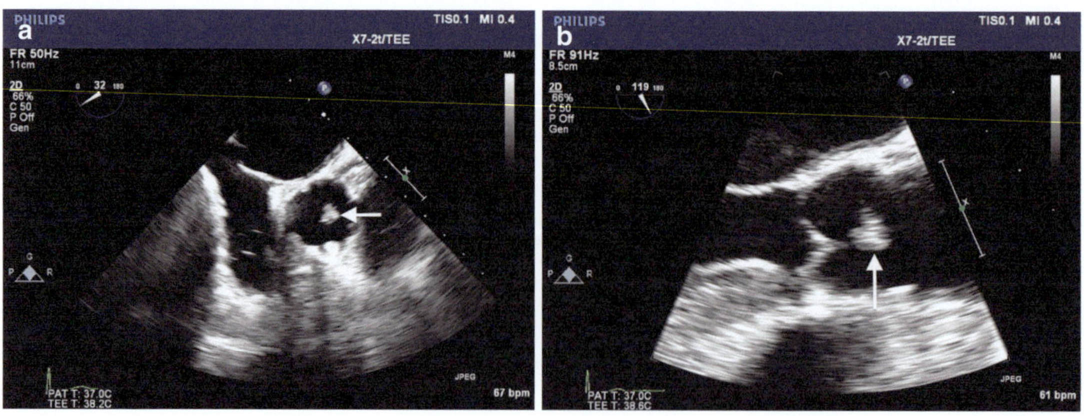

Fig. 16.7 (**a**) Midesophageal RV inflow-outflow view. A papillary fibroelastoma (*white arrow*) is visible on the aortic valve in short-axis. (**b**) Midesophageal long-axis view of the aortic valve (zoomed in). The pedunculated mass is consistent with a papillary fibroelastoma (*white arrow*) attached to the aortic valve

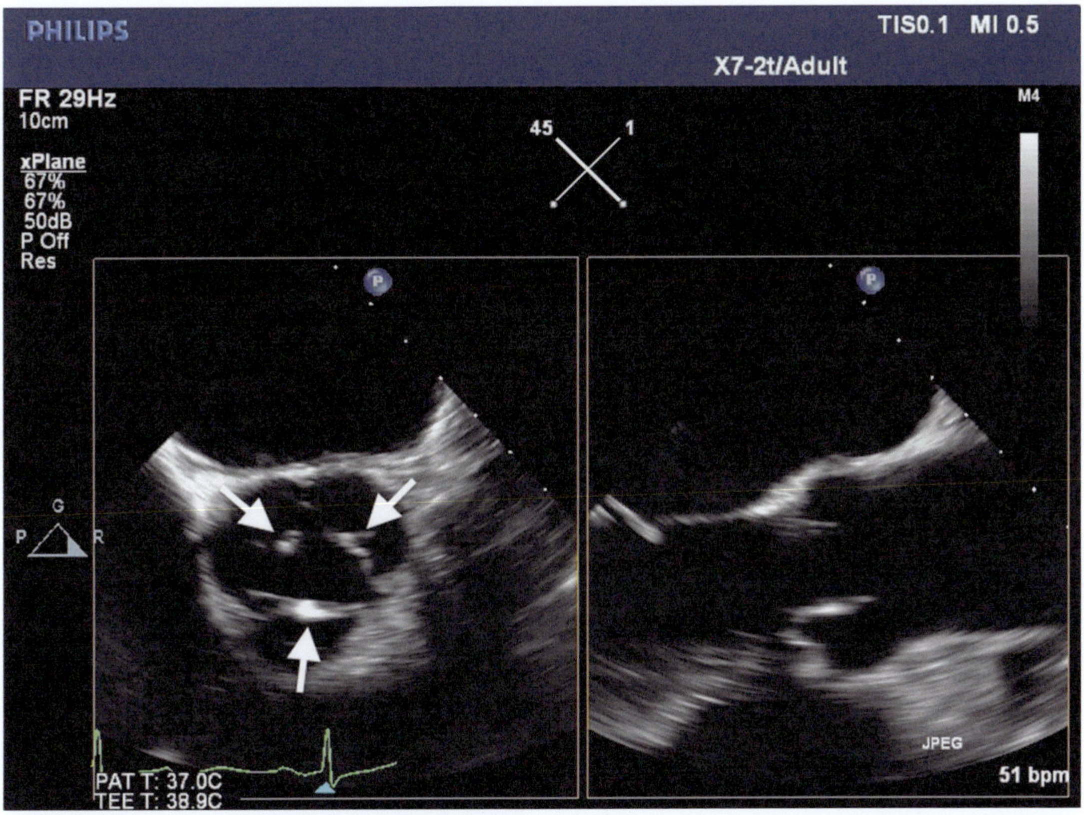

Fig. 16.8 Midesophageal aortic valve short-axis and long-axis views with X-plane (depth decreased). Nodules of Arantius (*white arrows*) are present on the center of all three AV cusps

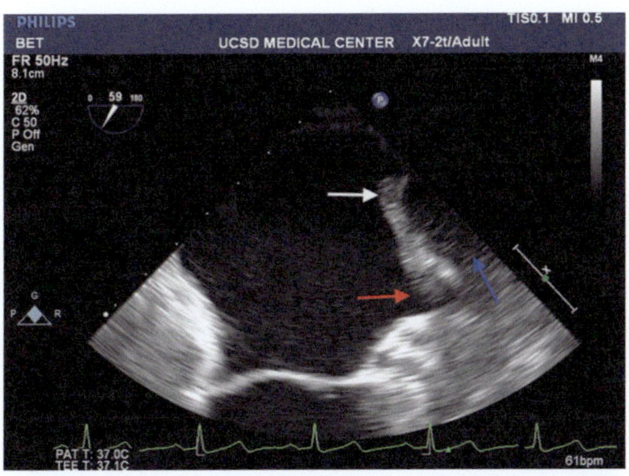

Fig. 16.9 Midesophageal mitral commissural view (depth decreased). The Coumadin ridge (*white arrow*) separates the left upper pulmonary vein (*blue arrow*) from the left atrial appendage (*red arrow*)

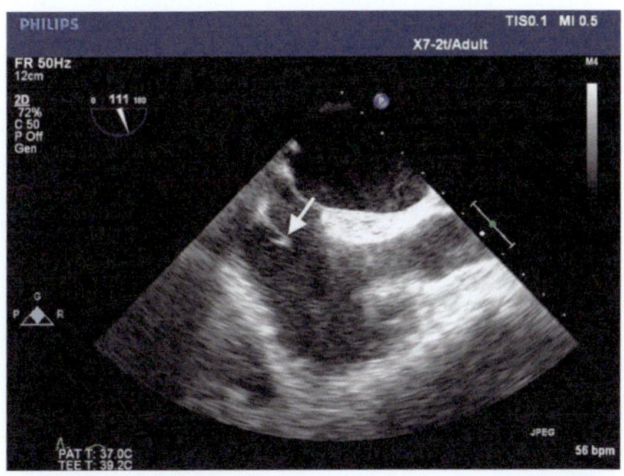

Fig. 16.10 Midesophageal bicaval view. A filamentous, mobile Chiari network (*white arrow*) is present at the junction of the IVC and RA

- Sound waves are extremely thin or pulses are small.
- Structures along the central axis of the ultrasound beam generate the images.
- Attenuation is uniform.

While these assumptions generally hold true, artifacts are generated when one or more of these assumptions are violated [10–12].

Dropout

Image generation is optimal when the object of interest is perpendicular to the ultrasound beam. Suboptimal reflections and poor image quality occur when the area of interest is parallel to the ultrasound beam or the result of anisotropy (Fig. 16.11 and Video 16.11). Alternative views, which place the area of interest perpendicular to the ultrasound beams, can be utilized to overcome imaging "dropout" in some instances.

"Railroad" Artifact

"Railroad" artifacts are an example of dropout that are generated by catheters (e.g., venous cardiopulmonary bypass cannula). Even though the cannula is three dimensional, the portions that are perpendicular to the ultrasound beam generate the strongest reflections (Fig. 16.12 and Video 16.12). These reflections produce a two-dimensional "railroad" track with a hypoechoic lumen.

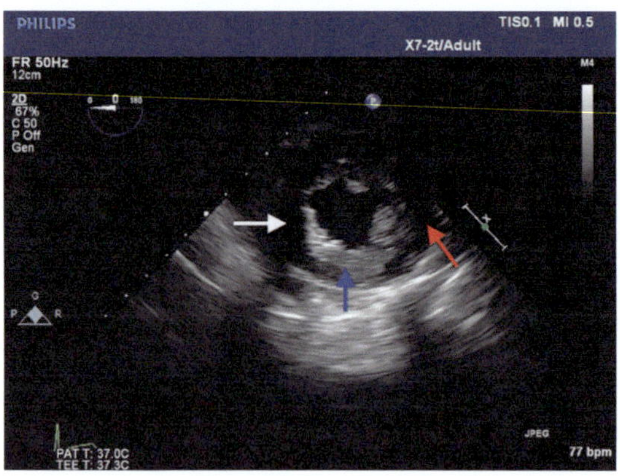

Fig. 16.11 Transgastric short-axis view. Hypo- or anechoic areas of the septal (*white arrow*) and lateral walls (*red arrow*) represent imaging dropout in the TG SAX view. Acoustic enhancement of the anterior wall is also present (*blue arrow*)

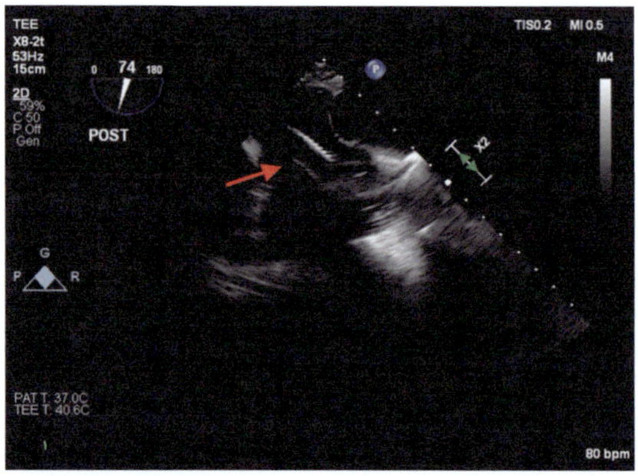

Fig. 16.12 Midesophageal modified bicaval view. A "railroad" artifact is generated by a venous cardiopulmonary bypass cannula in the RA and IVC (*red arrow*)

Acoustic Shadowing

Acoustic shadowing results from the reflection of ultrasound waves by a structure with a large acoustic impedance. The strong reflector – typically a prosthetic valve, catheter, or heavy calcification – reflects a large proportion of the ultrasound waves and thus blocks distal propagation of the ultrasound beam (Fig. 16.13 and Video 16.13). This

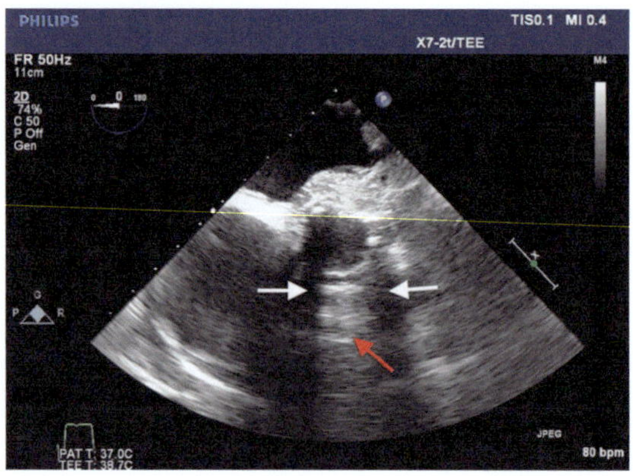

Fig. 16.13 Midesophageal AV short-axis view (modified angle of interrogation). A prosthetic AV creates a shadowing artifact (*white arrows*) which obscures visualization of the RV. In addition, a comet-tail artifact (*red arrow*), which is generated by the closely spaced annular ring and ascending aorta, is also present. Acoustic shadowing and comet-tail artifacts can both result in inadequate imaging distal to the reflecting structure(s)

results in hypoechoic areas and an inability to image the far field [11].

Acoustic Enhancement

When the assumption that attenuation is uniform throughout all tissues is violated, acoustic shadowing (see previous) or enhancement may result [12]. Acoustic enhancement is frequently encountered when a hypoechoic fluid-filled structure is located in the near field (Fig. 16.11 and Video 16.11). The lack of attenuation results in the far-field structures appearing more echogenic than the surrounding tissues.

Side Lobe

Side lobe artifacts are generated when diverging side beams, which are weaker than the central beam, encounter a strong reflector. The reflections are perceived by the ultrasound probe as being generated by the primary, central beam, and an image is incorrectly displayed (Fig. 16.14 and Video 16.14). Side lobe artifacts are typically curvilinear artifacts that maintain a constant depth along a sector arc [11].

Reverberation

A reverberation artifact is typically described as "step ladder" artifact that appears at equally spaced distances along a scan line (Fig. 16.15 and Video 16.15). The ultrasound beam bouncing back and forth between strong reflectors (e.g., calcified aorta, aerated lung tissue, or the ultrasound transducer itself) creates these artifacts. Decreasing the gain or utilizing alternative imaging planes may be helpful when this artifact is encountered [11].

Ring-Down and Comet-Tail Artifacts

Ring-down and comet-tail artifacts share a common mechanism with reverberation artifacts; however, the space between the reflectors in ring-down and comet-tail artifacts is smaller. This close proximity results in smeared or blurred artifacts [12]. Ring-down artifacts are encountered after open heart surgery due to either reflection or

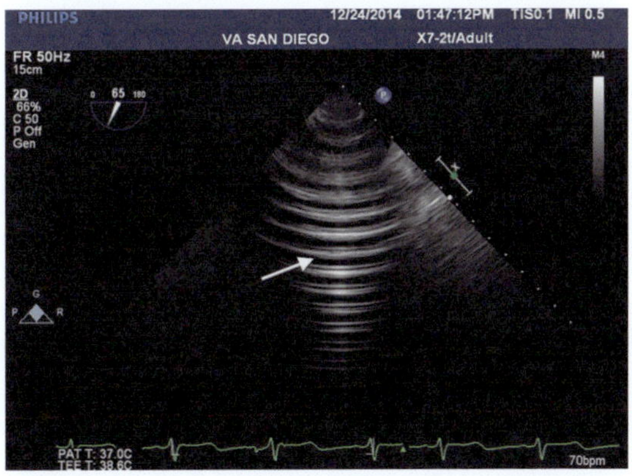

Fig. 16.15 Upper esophageal view. A reverberation artifact (*white arrow*) is generated by the tracheal rings, which is commonly encountered during probe placement

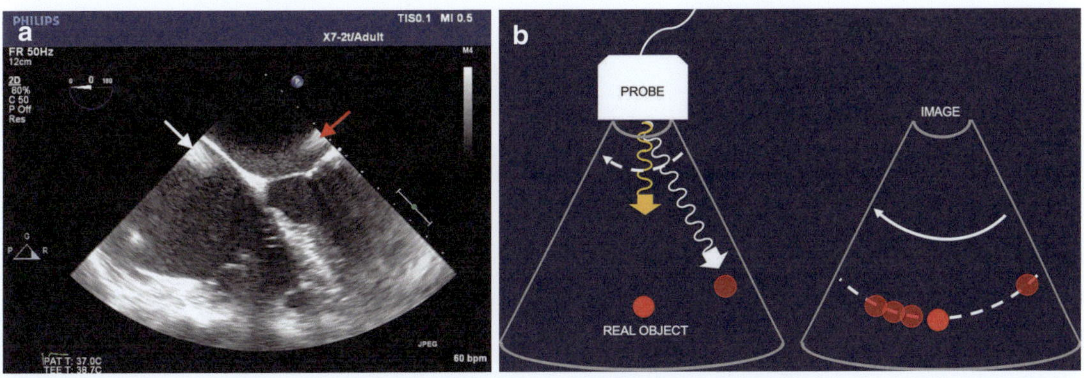

Fig. 16.14 (**a**) Midesophageal four-chamber view. Side lobes and inappropriately high gain settings result in echogenic artifacts in the RA near the interatrial septum (*white arrow*) and LA above the lateral mitral annulus (*red arrow*). (**b**) Mechanism for the generation of a side lobe artifact. The side lobe (*yellow arrow*) off the central beam (*white arrow*) encounters a strong reflector ("true object"). The resulting image displays this object in the direction of the central beam. These ghost images are repeated as the image sector is scanned radially, which produces a curvilinear or arc-like artifact

resonation of ultrasound waves by intracardiac air (Fig. 16.16 and Video 16.16). Comet-tail artifacts can be generated by two closely spaced reflectors like a prosthetic valve and the aorta (Figs. 16.13 and 16.17; Video 16.13). They are also commonly observed originating from a thickened pleural space caused by pulmonary edema, as described in Chap. 21.

Mirroring

Mirroring artifacts have a similar mechanism to reverberation artifacts. A strong reflector deflects part of the ultrasound wave which eventually returns to and is registered by the ultrasound probe. The increased transit time results in a mirror image being displayed distal to the real object (Fig. 16.18 and Video 16.17). Mirror artifacts are commonly encountered when imaging the arch of the aorta, descending aorta, or pulmonary artery catheter. A mirror image artifact of the liver above the diaphragm can also be used by the sonographer to exclude a right pleural effusion or fluid collection via abdominal ultrasound (Fig. 16.19 and Video 16.18).

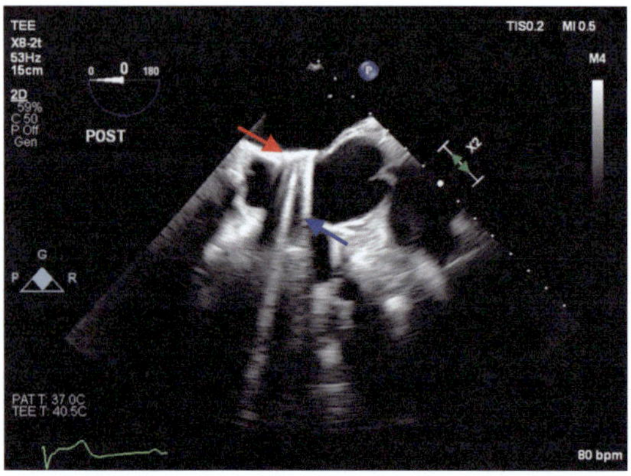

Fig. 16.16 Midesophageal modified five-chamber view. Intracardiac air (*red arrow*) is present in the LA near the interatrial septum, generating ring-down artifacts (*blue arrow*)

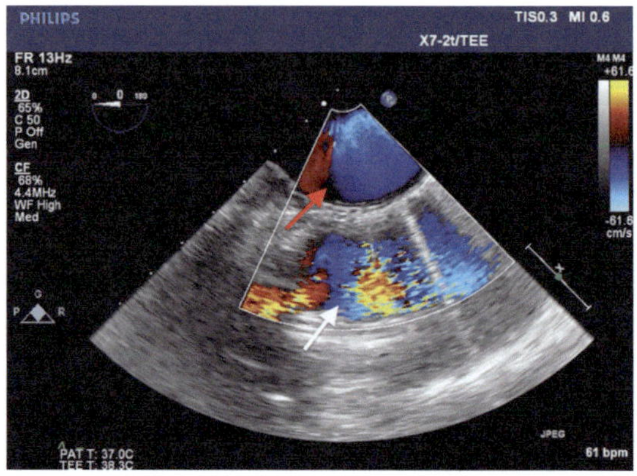

Fig. 16.18 Mirroring artifacts can occur in two-dimensional and Doppler imaging – a mirroring artifact (*white arrow*) of the aorta (*red arrow*) is displayed here with color flow Doppler

Fig. 16.17 Mechanism for the generation of a comet-tail artifact. While reflections return to the probe to produce the image at the appropriate depth (aorta) with an increasing number of reflections, the return time increases and the amplitude decreases. This results in image repetitions in the far field (aorta "B" and aorta "C") that blur together and produce a comet-tail artifact

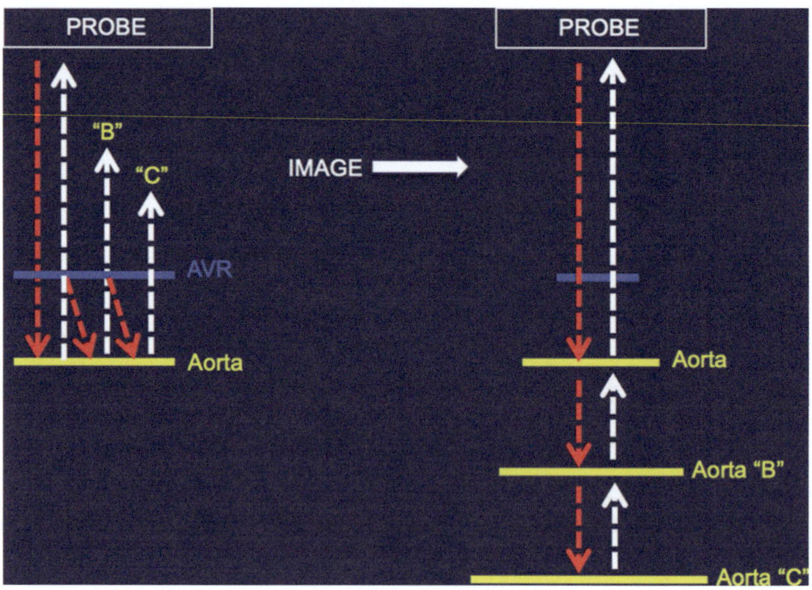

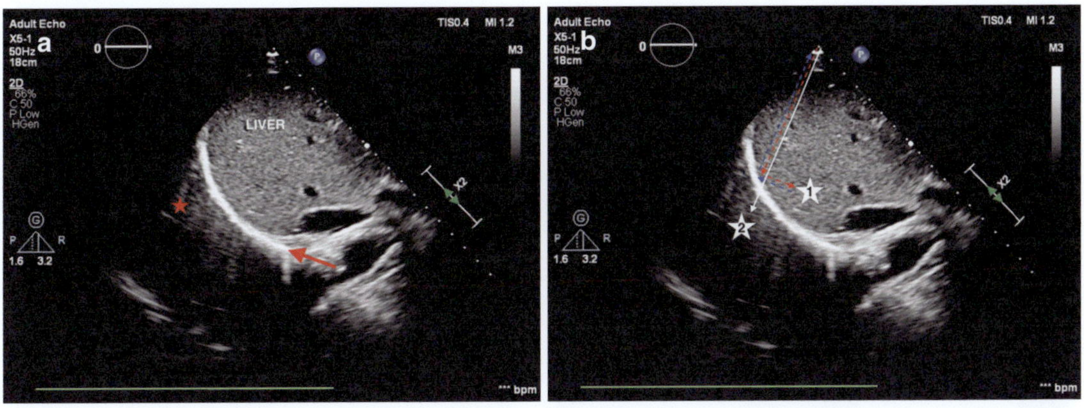

Fig. 16.19 Abdominal ultrasound – coronal image of the liver. (**a**) A mirror image of the liver (*red star*) cephalad to the diaphragm (*red arrow*). (**b**) Ultrasound waves emitted from the probe (*red dashed arrow*) reflect off a structure (*white star "1"*) after being deflected by the diaphragm. The transit time of the return waves (*blue dashed arrows*) is increased. Due to the increased transit time and the assumption that all waves travel in straight lines to the reflector and back, the mirrored structure (*white star "2"*) is produced in the far field

Spectral Doppler Mirroring

Mirroring can occur with other modalities like spectral Doppler as well. When spectral Doppler mirroring is due to cross-talk, the velocities displayed on one side of the baseline are typically denser and represent true Doppler shift. The mirrored information is less intense and in the opposite direction (Fig. 16.20). Quoted techniques to avoid generating this artifact include gain and power modifications [12].

Beam Width

A beam width artifact is directly related to lateral resolution, which refers to the ability to distinguish structures that are side by side. The ultrasound beam progressively narrows until the focal zone is reached. Distal to the focal zone, the ultrasound beam widens. Therefore, the focal zone represents the area of best lateral resolution. A beam width artifact, which is often the result of poor lateral resolution, occurs when two objects are not able to be distinguished as separate (Fig. 16.21). Instead, because of poor lateral resolution, the two objects may be displayed as one (Fig. 16.22 and Video 16.19a, b). Beam width and resulting artifacts are also important in the perpendicular plane as they relate to elevational resolution [12, 13].

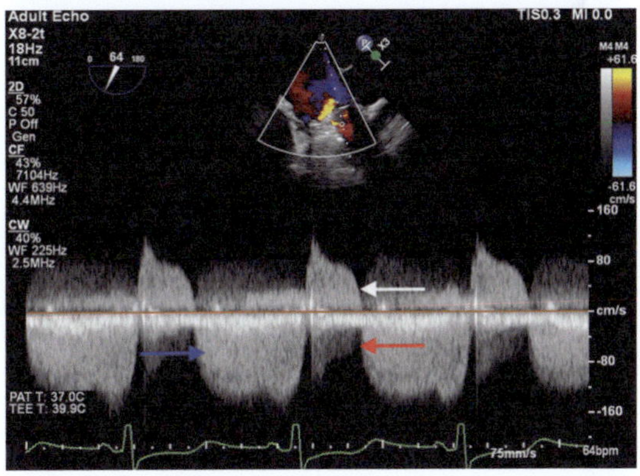

Fig. 16.20 Midesophageal RV inflow-outflow view (still image) with continuous-wave Doppler across a stenotic and regurgitant tricuspid valve. Stenosis during diastole, which is directed away from the probe and thus below the baseline (*blue arrow*), is present. During systole, there is evidence of tricuspid regurgitation (*white arrow*) and an associated spectral Doppler mirror artifact below the baseline (*red arrow*)

Aliasing Artifact

Aliasing, which can occur when utilizing both pulsed-wave Doppler (PWD) and color flow Doppler (CFD), occurs when the velocity being measured is greater than the limit of the scale. The maximum velocity measurable relates to the Nyquist limit, which is half of the pulse repetition frequency. In PWD, this results in velocities being displayed on the opposite side of the zero baseline. In CFD, this presents as rapid color changes being assigned to flow in a particular direction (i.e., from yellow to blue) and the appearance of turbulent flow (Fig. 16.23 and Video 16.20). Aliasing can frequently be addressed by changing the baseline, maximizing the velocity scale which increases the pulse repetition frequency, using a lower-frequency transducer, and decreasing the sector depth [1, 12].

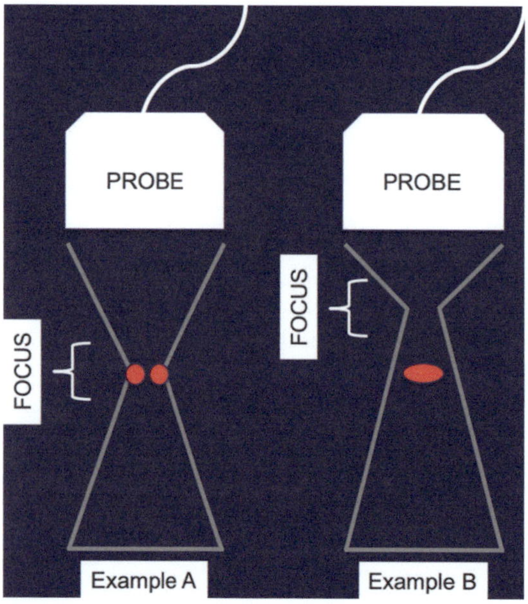

Fig. 16.21 Mechanism for the generation of a beam width artifact. In "Example A" two separate objects (*red circles*) are distinguished as two separate structures. When the focal zone is moved into the near field in "Example B," the two separate objects are located in far field. The result is a beam width artifact – the two separate structures are now indistinguishable (*red oval*)

Conclusion

In order to distinguish between anatomic variants/artifacts and pathology, the echocardiographer must utilize all information at their disposal. This includes not only a detailed knowledge of cardiac

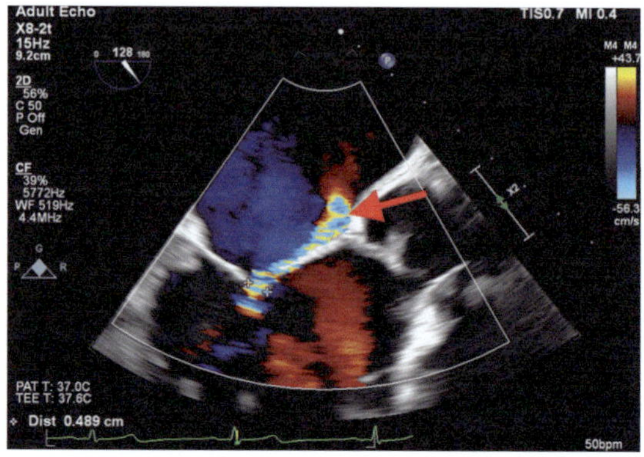

Fig. 16.23 Midesophageal long-axis view (depth reduced) with CFD. The baseline has been shifted in the direction of mitral regurgitation which results in aliasing at a lower velocity (i.e., 43.7 cm/s). When the speed of blood exceeds 43.7 cm/s, it is assigned a blue color (*red arrow*). This rapid color change is an example of CFD aliasing

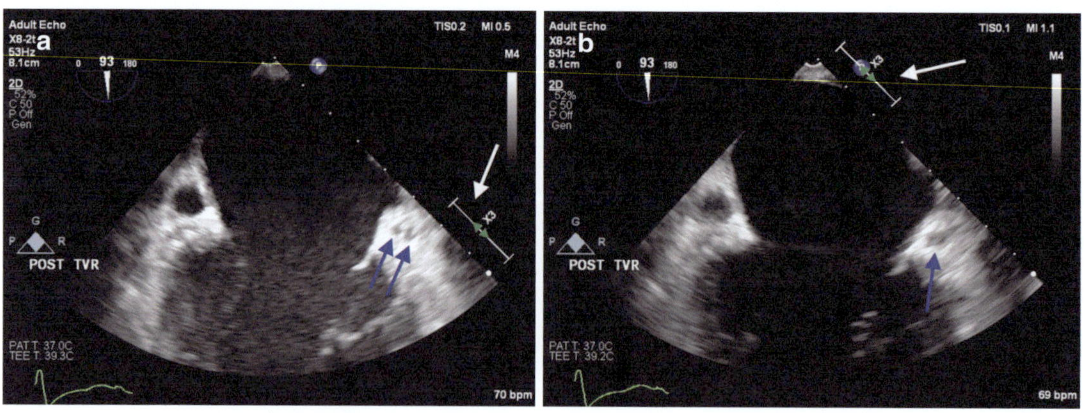

Fig. 16.22 Midesophageal two-chamber view (depth reduced). (**a**) The focal zone (*white arrow*) is positioned in the far field of the image, so the circumflex artery and great cardiac vein (*blue arrows*) are visible as two separate structures. (**b**) The focal zone (*white arrow*) is positioned in the near field, which results in a beam width artifact. The circumflex artery and great cardiac vein (*blue arrow*) no longer appear as two distinct, separate objects

anatomy but also surgical and clinical correlation (i.e., discussion with the surgeon and a full patient history) [14]. Additional evidence that a structure may be an artifact includes its adherence to the path of a scanning arc, continuance through a clearly identifiable solid structure, or disappearance in alternative views. Proper image acquisition (e.g., gain, focus, and gastric de-airing) can eliminate many artifacts or clarify an area of interest. If the diagnosis is still in question, the echocardiographer should consider utilizing echo contrast or additional imaging modalities (e.g., computed tomography, fluoroscopy) [15].

Questions

1. The "strong reflector" which generates reverberation artifacts by increasing the transit time to twice the distance from the area of interest is most commonly which of the following?

   A. Calcified aorta
   B. Pulmonary artery catheter
   C. Trachea
   D. Ultrasound probe

2. What is the speed that ultrasound travels through soft tissue?

   A. 1540 cm/s
   B. 1540 m/s
   C. 1.540 m/s
   D. 15.40 km/s

3. Which of the following artifacts is most similar to reverberation artifact?

   A. Mirroring
   B. Sidelobe artifacts
   C. Acoustic shadowing
   D. Acoustic enhancement

4. Which of the following is a pathological condition with a predilection for embolism and is an indication for surgical resection?

   A. Nodules of Arantius
   B. Lambl's excrescences
   C. Papillary fibroelastoma
   D. Chiari network

5. Which of these structures share a common embryologic origin?

   1. Crista terminalis 2. Chiari network 3. Eustachian valve 4. Coumadin ridge

   A. 1 and 2
   B. 2 and 3
   C. 2, 3, and 4
   D. 1, 2, and 3

6. Which structure is indicated by the arrow in the figure?

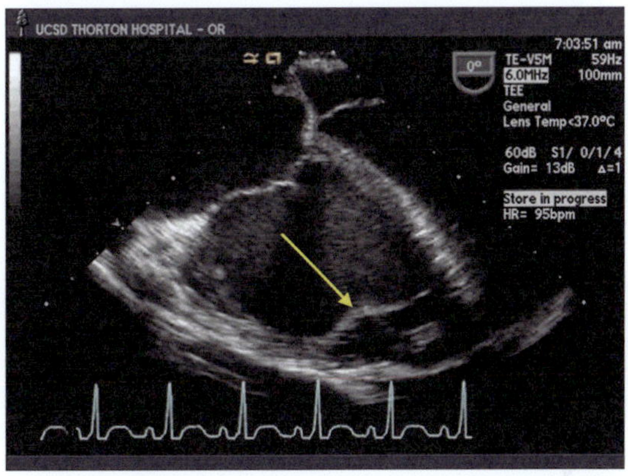

   A. Moderator band
   B. Chiari network
   C. Crista terminalis
   D. Coumadin ridge

7. Which of the following would not help to decrease aliasing artifact?

   A. Change the angle of insonation.
   B. Decreasing the Doppler scale.
   C. Using a lower frequency probe.
   D. Decreasing the sector depth.

8. The structure which separates the smooth right atrium from the right atrial appendage is the:

   A. Interatrial septum
   B. Coumadin ridge
   C. Crista terminalis
   D. Sinotubular junction

9. Often described as "dumbbell-shaped" this normal anatomical variant is often confused for a myxoma:

   A. Coumadin ridge
   B. Ebstein's anomaly
   C. Thebesian valve
   D. Lipomatous hypertrophy of the interatrial septum

10. Poor lateral resolution can result in a:

   A. Mirror artifact
   B. Beam width artifact
   C. Reverberation artifact
   D. Aliasing artifact

References

1. Reeves ST, Finley AC, Skubas NJ, Swaminathan M, Whitley WS, Glas KE, et al. Basic perioperative transesophageal echocardiography examination: a consensus statement of the American Society of Echocardiography and the Society of Cardiovascular Anesthesiologists. J Am Soc Echocardiogr. 2013;26(5):443–56.
2. Najib MQ, Ganji JL, Raizada A, Panse PM, Chaliki HP. Epicardial fat can mimic pericardial effusion on transoesophageal echocardiogram. Eur J Echocardiogr. 2011;12(10):804.
3. Tan CO, Harley I. Perioperative transesophageal echocardiographic assessment of the right heart and associated structures: a comprehensive update and technical report. J Cardiothorac Vasc Anesth. 2014;28(4):1100–21.
4. Keren A, Billingham ME, Popp RL. Echocardiographic recognition and implications of ventricular hypertrophic trabeculations and aberrant bands. Circulation. 1984;70(5):836–42.
5. George A, Parameswaran A, Nekkanti R, Lurito K, Movahed A. Normal anatomic variants on transthoracic echocardiogram. Echocardiography. 2009;26(9):1109–17.
6. Kim MJ, Jung HO. Anatomic variants mimicking pathology on echocardiography: differential diagnosis. J Cardiovasc Ultrasound. 2013;21(3):103–12.
7. Dumaswala B, Dumaswala K, Hsiung MC, Quiroz LD, Sungur A, Escanuela MG, et al. Incremental value of three-dimensional transesophageal echocardiography over two-dimensional transesophageal echocardiography in the assessment of Lambl's excrescences and nodules of Arantius on the aortic valve. Echocardiography. 2013;30(8):967–75.
8. Aziz F, Baciewicz FA Jr. Lambl's excrescences: review and recommendations. Tex Heart Inst J. 2007;34(3):366–8.
9. Hakim FA, Aryal MR, Pandit A, Pandit AA, Alegria JR, Kendall CB, et al. Papillary fibroelastoma of the pulmonary valve--a systematic review. Echocardiography. 2014;31(2):234–40.
10. Aldrich JE. Basic physics of ultrasound imaging. Crit Care Med. 2007;35(5 Suppl):S131–7.
11. Pamnani A, Skubas NJ. Imaging artifacts during transesophageal echocardiography. Anesth Analg. 2014;118(3):516–20.
12. Le HT, Hangiandreou N, Timmerman R, Rice MJ, Smith WB, Deitte L, et al. Imaging artifacts in echocardiography. Anesth Analg. 2016;122(3):633–46.
13. Bertrand PB, Levine RA, Isselbacher EM, Vandervoort PM. Fact or artifact in two-dimensional echocardiography: avoiding misdiagnosis and missed diagnosis. J Am Soc Echocardiogr. 2016;29(5):381–91.
14. Cronin B, Nguyen L, Manecke G, Pretorius V, Banks D, Maus T. Foreign body located intraoperatively using transesophageal echocardiography. J Cardiothorac Vasc Anesth. 2014;28(3):852–3.
15. Apostolidou I, Krishnan K, Keith V, Madlon-Kay R. Contrast echocardiography to differentiate artifact from left atrial thrombus. Anesth Analg. 2012;114(4):742–5.

17 Intracardiac Masses, Devices, and Foreign Bodies

Kirill Gelfenbeyn and Christine Choi

Abbreviations

CVA	Cerebrovascular accident
CVC	Central venous catheter
ECMO	Extracorporeal membranous oxygenation
IABP	Intra-aortic balloon pump
LA	Left atrium
LAA	Left atrial appendage
LV	Left ventricle
PAC	Pulmonary arterial catheter
PFO	Patent foramen ovale
RA	Right atrium
RV	Right ventricle
SVC	Superior vena cava
TEE	Transesophageal echocardiography
TTE	Transthoracic echocardiography

Supplementary Information The online version of this chapter (https://doi.org/10.1007/978-3-030-84349-6_17) contains supplementary material, which is available to authorized users.

K. Gelfenbeyn · C. Choi (✉)
Department of Anesthesiology, University of California San Diego Health, La Jolla, CA, USA
e-mail: c1choi@health.ucsd.edu

Introduction

The most commonly encountered cardiac masses are thrombi and vegetations related to endocarditis. Malignant tumors of cardiac origin are rare while secondary metastatic tumors are more common. Among primary cardiac tumors, benign tumors comprise up to 75% of cases and malignant tumors only about 25%. Intracardiac foreign bodies (e.g., intravenous catheters, atrial appendage exclusion devices, and left ventricular assist devices) are increasingly common, as more interventions become available. Intracardiac thrombi, vegetations, tumors, and foreign bodies will be discussed.

Thrombi (Highlight Box 17.1)

Highlight Box 17.1

Intracardiac thrombi	
2D	• Hyperechoic mass within cardiac chambers • Right heart: mobile, discrete, hyperechoic lesion, "thrombus-in-transit" • Right heart location: RA, RV, PA location • Left heart: less mobile, hyperechoic lesion, associated with low flow (spontaneous echo contrast) • Left heart location: LAA, LV apex

T. M. Maus, C. R. Tainter (eds.), *Essential Echocardiography*,
https://doi.org/10.1007/978-3-030-84349-6_17

Intracardiac thrombi	
CFD	Typically not useful
Spectral	• PWD of LAA – thrombi risk assessment • CWD of TR – pulmonary hypertension assessment

RA right atrium, *RV* right ventricle, *PA* pulmonary artery, *LAA* left atrial appendage, *LV* left ventricle, *PWD* pulsed-wave Doppler, *CWD* continuous-wave Doppler, *TR* tricuspid regurgitation

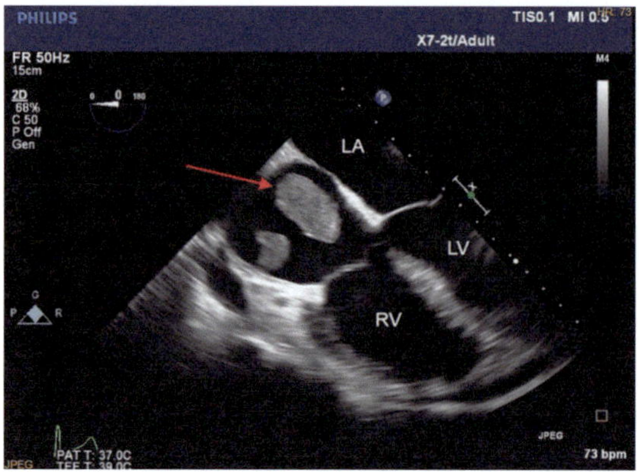

Fig. 17.1 Midesophageal four-chamber view demonstrating a homogenous right atrial thrombus (*red arrow*). *LA* left atrium, *RV* right ventricle, *LV* left ventricle

Cardiac thrombi are of particular importance, as they account for 15–40% of ischemic cerebrovascular accidents (CVA), and are associated with more severe deficits [1–3]. Thrombus formation on the left side of the heart, such as the left atrial appendage (LAA) and left ventricle, is more common compared to the right side of the heart. While left-sided thrombi are likely due to stasis of blood, right-sided thrombi are more likely from peripheral venous origin [4]. LAA thrombus is the most common cause of systemic cardioembolic event. Predisposing factors for LAA thrombus include atrial fibrillation, enlarged or bifid atrial appendage, mitral valve pathology, and poor left ventricular (LV) function. Right atrial (RA) thrombus poses its own risk and can result in pulmonary embolism or paradoxical arterial embolism via a patent foramen ovale (PFO). Predisposing factors for RA thrombus are central venous or pulmonary artery catheters and pacemaker wires. Detection of the thrombi using echocardiography will provide crucial information to determine the need for systemic anticoagulation and further treatment. Transesophageal echocardiography (TEE) is superior to transthoracic echocardiography (TTE) for detection of cardiac emboli, owing to the lack of interference from lung tissue and bone, along with the use of higher-frequency transducers yielding higher-resolution images. TEE is better-suited for imaging posterior and inferior structures of the heart due to the proximity to the esophagus. However, TTE remains a popular modality for initial assessment due to its noninvasive nature.

Intracardiac thrombus can often mimic a tumor's appearance; therefore clinical context is important. On echocardiography, thrombi typically appear as a mobile mass without a clear point of attachment (Fig. 17.1 and Video 17.1). Newly formed thrombus will be more echolucent and mobile, whereas an older thrombus will have a more hyperechoic and rounded homogenous appearance. Thrombus in the LAA is often associated with "smoke-like" appearance (spontaneous echo contrast) due to blood stasis. The left atrial appendage is best evaluated by TEE in the midesophageal two-chamber view; however scanning with various multiplane angles is essential to fully evaluate the appendage [5, 6]. Pulsed-wave Doppler velocity measurement within the LAA allows prediction of thrombogenic risk. Doppler blood flow velocity below 15 cm/s indicates a significant increase in stroke risk [7], while velocity above 40 cm/s indicates adequate blood flow within the LAA, with minimal risk of thrombosis.

Formation of ventricular thrombi is often associated with decreased ventricular function and blood stasis, typically in the setting of a large myocardial infarction, dilated cardiomyopathy, or ventricular aneurysm. Ventricular thrombi are often smooth and homogeneous in appearance (Fig. 17.2 and Video 17.2). Ventricular thrombi with more irregular borders have a higher propensity for systemic embolization. Ventricular thrombi can occasionally be visualized and assessed in the midesophageal views; however transgastric views place the LV apex closer to the transducer for imaging. It is important to evaluate thrombi from various angles to better character-

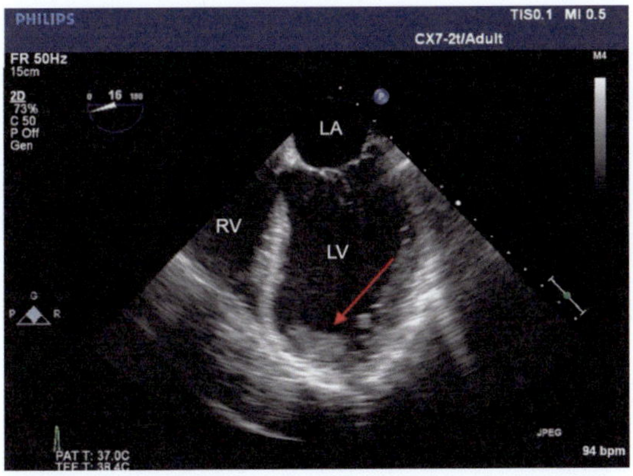

Fig. 17.2 Midesophageal four-chamber view in a patient with a large apical LV thrombus (*red arrow*). *LA* left atrium, *RV* right ventricle, *LV* left ventricle

ize them and differentiate from artifacts. It should be noted that TTE is superior to TEE for detection of left ventricular apical thrombus given the proximity of the ultrasound probe to the left ventricle [5, 6, 8].

Endocarditis (Highlight Box 17.2)

Highlight Box 17.2

Vegetations	
2D	• Hyperechoic mobile mass attached to cardiac valves • Motion independent from valvular motion • Often located atrial side of MV/TV; ventricular side of AV/PV • May be associated with foreign material: prosthetic valves, pacemaker leads
CFD	• Typically associated with valvular regurgitation • Identification of leaflet perforation
Spectral	• Assessment of valvular regurgitation

MV mitral valve, *TV* tricuspid valve, *AV* aortic valve, *PV* pulmonic valve

Endocarditis is an inflammatory disorder of the endocardium characterized by the formation of vegetations, which can be infectious or noninfectious. Vegetations are clusters of platelets, fibrin, and inflammatory cells, which may also contain microorganisms. Common risk factors are prosthetic heart valves, age-related degenerative valvular lesions, intracardiac devices, unrepaired cyanotic lesions, a history of previous endocarditis, immunosuppression, intravenous drug use, hemodialysis, and the presence of indwelling venous catheters. Gram-positive cocci are the most common causative organism.

Infective endocarditis poses significant risk to the patient; hence timely diagnosis and treatment is critical. Diagnosis is made based on the modified Duke criteria, which include three potential echocardiographic findings: presence of oscillating mobile mass, presence of abscess, or partial dehiscence of a prosthetic valve [9]. Although TTE is often utilized as an initial evaluation modality due to relative ease of exam and patient comfort, the sensitivity of the exam is limited. TEE is a superior exam and is considered the gold standard for detection and measurement of vegetations [10, 11].

Vegetations differ in presentation and appearance from thrombi and cardiac tumors. TEE allows for assessment of location, size, number, echogenicity, and mobility of vegetations to predict risk of an embolic event. Valvular vegetations resulting from infective endocarditis typically attach to the low-pressure side of the valve (i.e., the atrial side of the atrioventricular valves and ventricular side of the aortic and pulmonic valves). The typical appearance of a vegetation is an oscillating pendulum-like echogenic mass attached to the leaflet of the valve or supporting structures, with movement independent of the valve [12] (Figs. 17.3 and 17.4; Videos 17.3 and 17.4). Formation of a paravalvular abscess can occur and may appear as an echodense thickening with an echolucent cavity, typically in the annulus adjacent to the infected leaflet [13]. Destruction of the valve or distortion of the valvular or subvalvular apparatus can lead to valvular prolapse, regurgitation, flail leaflets, or perforation. Vegetations rarely result in stenosis of the valve. Perforation of the leaflet can lead to acute valvular regurgitation, resulting in significant symptomatology and acute heart failure.

Evaluation of prosthetic valve endocarditis is often more challenging, due to the presence of

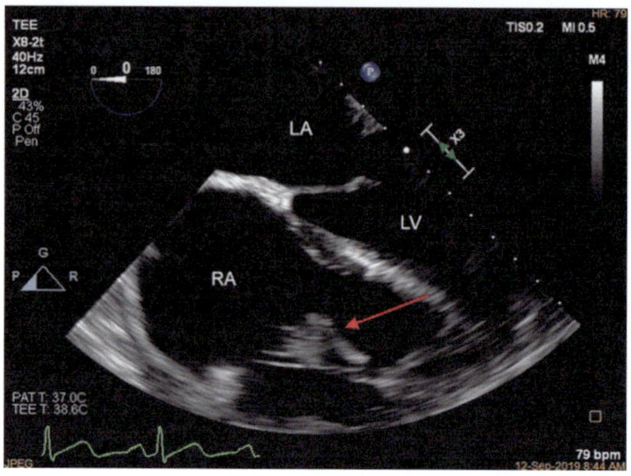

Fig. 17.3 Midesophageal four-chamber view with a large vegetation (*red arrow*) on the tricuspid valve, in a patient with endocarditis. *LA* left atrium, *RA* right atrium, *LV* left ventricle

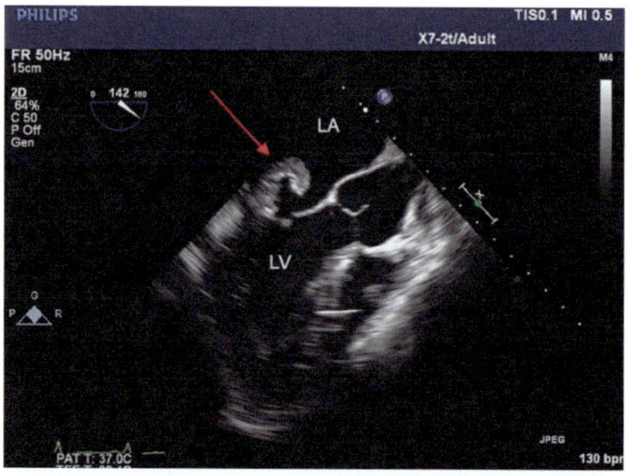

Fig. 17.4 Midesophageal long-axis view in a patient with mitral valve endocarditis and a large posterior leaflet vegetation (*red arrow*). *LA* left atrium, *LV* left ventricle

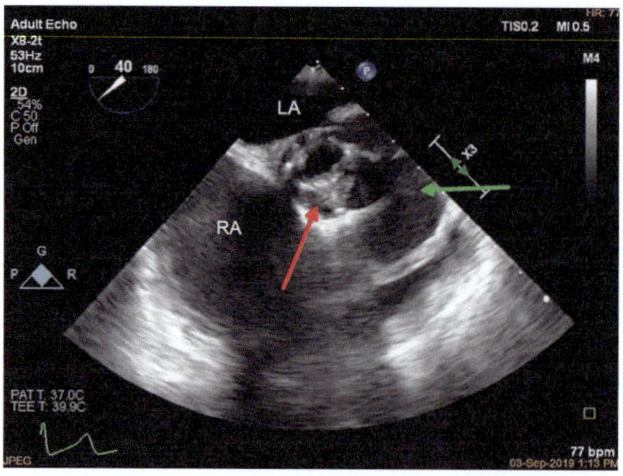

Fig. 17.5 Midesophageal AV short-axis view in a patient with bioprosthetic aortic valve endocarditis (*red arrow*) and resultant abscess (*green arrow*). *LA* left atrium, *RA* right atrium

shadowing from the prosthesis affecting the quality of the image (Fig. 17.5 and Video 17.5). The infection will likely involve an area around the ring of the prosthesis and may result in paravalvular leak, prosthesis malfunction, and dehiscence [14]. It is worth noting that endocarditis is less likely to cause stenosis of the prosthetic valve. Additionally, a negative echocardiographic exam does not completely rule out infective endocarditis [12]

In those patients with indwelling vascular catheters or implantable electronic cardiac devices (e.g., pacemaker or implantable cardiac defibrillator), bloodstream infections and formation of vegetation on the intracardiac leads or catheters may occur. Detection of vegetation is important because effective treatment will require removal of the device. On echocardiography, the vegetations will appear similar to the valvular vegetations, as a mobile echogenic mass with independent motion.

Tumors: Benign (Highlight Box 17.3)

Highlight Box 17.3

Tumors	
2D	• Variety of presentations depending on primary • Often heterogenous and irregular in shape • Most common benign – atrial myxoma with stalk from IAS • Most common malignant – sarcoma
CFD	• Associated valvular regurgitation or vessel obstruction
Spectral	• Assessment of valvular regurgitation

IAS interatrial septum

While myxomas are the most common benign cardiac tumor in adults, rhabdomyomas are the most common benign cardiac tumors in children under the age of 15 [15]. Myxomas account for about 25% of all cardiac masses and 50% of benign cardiac tumors in adults. They arise in the left atrium in 75% of cases, 20% in the right atrium, and the remaining 5% in the right or left ventricle [16, 17]. They are solitary and slowly proliferating tumors that typically attach in the fossa ovalis. They produce a variety of symptoms, including the classic triad of embolism, intracardiac obstruction, and constitutional symptoms [18]. Dyspnea on exertion and shortness of breath can occur if the mass enlarges enough to cause blockage around the mitral valve orifice. On occasion, a "tumor plop" may be auscultated as the tumor prolapses into the mitral valve orifice during diastole, mimicking mitral stenosis physiology.

With echocardiography, myxomas appear as heterogenous, irregularly shaped, grape cluster-like masses that protrude from the fossa ovalis into the atrium (Fig. 17.6 and Video 17.6). Occasionally, calcification may be seen. Color flow and spectral Doppler may be used to identify the degree of obstruction of the valvular orifice. TEE can also help with intraoperative evaluation of the mass, verification of successful removal, and ensure the absence of any other structural damage to the heart after resection. It is particularly important to evaluate for the presence of interatrial shunting if the myxoma was originally attached to the intra-atrial septum. While TTE will provide superior imaging of the myxomas involving the atria, TEE will be better in evaluating the myxoma if it involves the mitral valve.

Papillary fibroelastomas are the second most common benign cardiac tumor, accounting for about 8% of cardiac tumors [19]. They are typically a small, singular, pedunculated mass originating from valvular endocardium, attached to the valvular surface [20, 21]. They are most commonly found on the aortic side of the aortic valve or the atrial side of the mitral valve. On echocardiography, they typically appear as a small homogenous round or oval-shaped mass with well-demarcated borders. They are often attached to the valve surface with a mobile stalk, and their movement is independent of the movement of the valve involved [22] (Fig. 17.7 and Video 17.7). While these tumors are often found incidentally, surgical resection is indicated due to the potential for cerebral or coronary embolization [23].

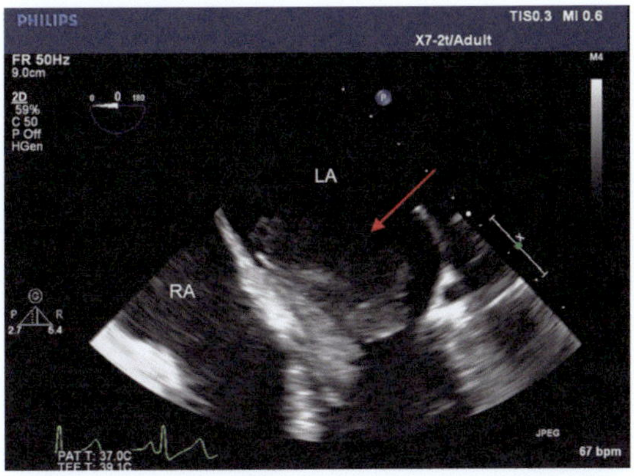

Fig. 17.6 Diastolic midesophageal four-chamber view (reduced depth) in a patient with a large left atrial myxoma (*red arrow*), attached to the interatrial septum. Note the protrusion of the left atrial myxoma into the mitral valve inlet, leading to obstruction. *LA* left atrium, *RA* right atrium

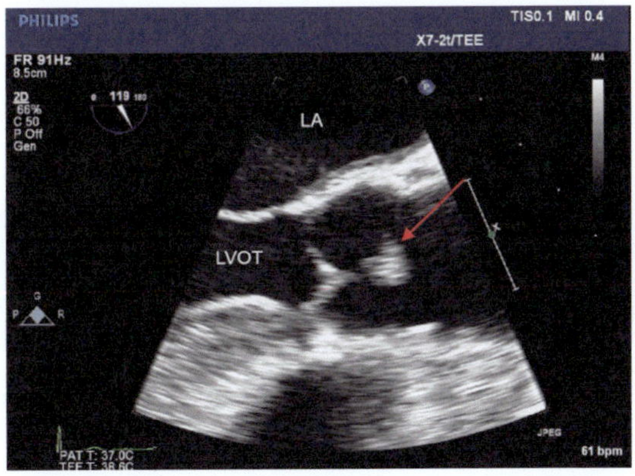

Fig. 17.7 Midesophageal AV long-axis view with a papillary fibroelastoma noted on the aortic valve (*red arrow*). *LA* left atrium, *LVOT* left ventricular outflow tract

Rhabdomyosarcoma is the most common benign cardiac tumor in infants and young children and is strongly associated with the presence of tuberous sclerosis [24]. It is most commonly found in the ventricles and can cause outflow tract obstruction of the affected ventricle. They appear on echocardiography as small, well-demarcated nodules or a pedunculated mass within the ventricle or as homogenous, hyperechoic masses when embedded within the ventricular walls [25].

Lipomas are tumors composed of adipose tissue that occur in various sizes. They appear as

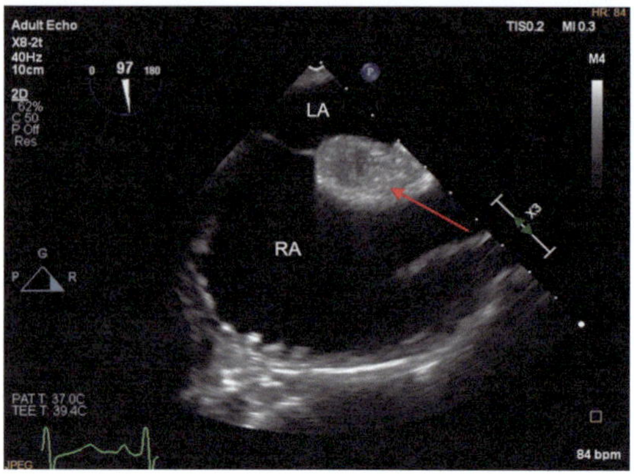

Fig. 17.8 Midesophageal bicaval view in a patient with lipomatous hypertrophy of the intra-atrial septum (*red arrow*). *LA* left atrium, *RA* right atrium

broad-based, homogenous masses that typically arise from the subendocardium [25]. They are typically asymptomatic, unless the enlargement of the mass causes compression of surrounding structures or dysrhythmias from infiltration into the conduction system of the heart. It is important to note that while lipomatous hypertrophy of the interatrial septum is not a true cardiac tumor, it can often be mistaken for one, if the degree of hypertrophy is significant. Lipomatous hypertrophy of the interatrial septum is due to infiltration of fatty adipose tissue in the proximal and distal portion of the interatrial septum, with sparing of the fossa ovalis, giving its characteristic dumbbell-shaped appearance on echocardiography (Fig. 17.8 and Video 17.8).

Some of the other rare cardiac tumors are hemangiomas and teratomas. Hemangiomas can appear as an echogenic mass speckled with echolucencies [25]. Teratomas are extremely rare in adults, and with echocardiography they can have an ill-defined cystic appearance [26]. It is important to note the potential effect of compression these masses may have on surrounding vascular or adjacent cardiac structures.

Tumors: Malignant

About 25% of primary cardiac tumors are malignant, with 95% of them being sarcomas [27]. Malignant primary cardiac tumors are more often seen on the right side of the heart, with the atrium being more common than the ventricle [28]. About 50% of all cardiac sarcomas originate in the right atrium. Secondary spread from extracardiac malignancies are more common than primary cardiac tumors, whether through metastasis or direct invasion. Uterine and renal cell carcinoma can spread along the vena cava into the right atrium.

Malignant tumors are often larger than 5 cm and tend to be invasive, involving the myocardium and endocardium. The presentation of a cardiac tumor is variable, but largely related to the location of the tumor (valvular, ventricular, or atrial). Common symptoms are heart failure, arrhythmias, and valvular dysfunction. Preferential right-sided involvement often leads to symptoms of right heart failure (e.g., peripheral edema). Rapid growth, local invasion, and hemorrhagic pericardial effusion are other signs that point to malignancy. On average, primary malignant cardiac tumors take about 16 months to diagnose from the onset of symptoms and they often carry a very poor prognosis.

Sarcomas are the most common type of primary malignant cardiac tumors, and they typically present between the third and fifth decade of life, more commonly in men [29]. Angiosarcoma is the most common subtype. It has a vascular origin and typically arises from the right atrium near the inferior vena cava. Rhabdomyosarcoma is the second most common sarcoma. Intramural infiltration at multiple sites with limited pericardial involvement is common.

With echocardiography, sarcomas often present as a large and well-delineated mass, though they may have a heterogenous appearance, with irregular echolucent areas (Fig. 17.9 and Video 17.9).

Metastatic tumors of the heart are more common than primary cardiac tumors. They commonly penetrate the muscular layer of the heart and can be of variable origin. Metastatic tumors involve the heart through direct, venous, lymphatic, or hematogenous extension. Lymphatic extension typically leads to epicardial and myocardial involvement, whereas hematogenous

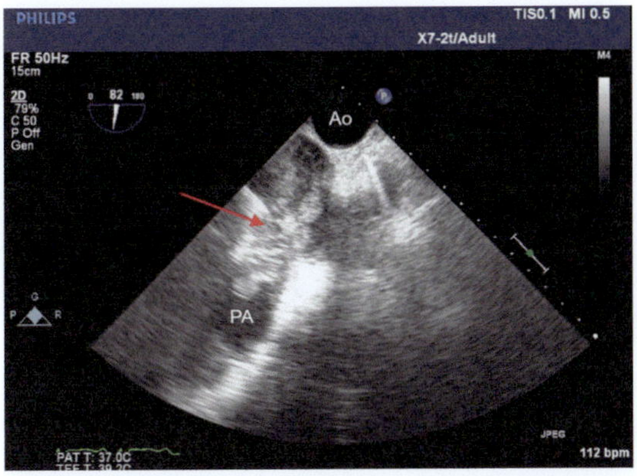

Fig. 17.9 Upper esophageal aortic arch short-axis view in a patient with a large pulmonary artery sarcoma (*red arrow*). *Ao* aortic arch, *PA* main pulmonary artery

spread leads to endocardial invasion. Pericardial involvement is not uncommon for metastatic disease.

The most common malignancies with cardiac metastasis are malignant melanomas and carcinomas of the lung and breast, followed by malignant lymphomas, and then leukemias [30]. Malignant melanoma has high propensity for hematogenous spread. More than 50% of metastatic melanoma cases involve cardiac metastasis, though most of these are not recognized antemortem. Metastasis of carcinomas of the lung and breast can result in direct invasion due to their proximity to the heart; however they spread more typically via a lymphatic route. Similar to melanoma, malignant lymphomas resulting in cardiac involvement are more often diagnosed on postmortem pathology.

Tumors with Systemic Cardiac Manifestations

Carcinoid

Carcinoid tumors are neuroendocrine tumors that can metastasize to the heart but often exert their cardiac effects through secretion of vasoactive substances. Typically, primary carcinoid tumors originate in the gastrointestinal tract and secrete serotonin and other vasoactive chemicals. These vasoactive substances typically travel via the portal venous circulation to the liver and are metabolized prior to reaching the heart. However, once the carcinoid tumor metastasizes into the liver, the vasoactive products can enter the caval circulation without being metabolized, leading to cardiac manifestations.

Classically, these vasoactive substances result in deposition of carcinoid plaques on the right-sided cardiac chambers and valves, leading to thickening and retraction of the tricuspid and pulmonic valves. The thickening results in minimal excursion during systole and diastole, and over time, the leaflets become fixed in a semi-open position, which leads to a combination of stenosis and regurgitation [31]. Left heart involvement is seen in less than 10% of carcinoid cardiac disease, [32] but can occur in the setting of bronchial carcinoid tumors and in the presence of significant intracardiac shunt. Thickening and retraction of the valves will be visible on echocardiography and may demonstrate severe tricuspid regurgitation or stenosis, pulmonic regurgitation or stenosis, and rarely left heart valvular lesions (Fig. 17.10a, b and Video 17.10a, b). The right ventricle may dilate and hypertrophy due to volume overload, and deposition of the plaque on the ventricular chamber itself can result in a restrictive cardiomyopathy [33].

Renal Cell Carcinoma

Renal cell cancer accounts for about 2–3% of all adult malignancies and is comprised of a number of subtypes, including clear cell carcinoma (75–85%), papillary renal cell carcinoma (10–15%), chromophobe renal cell carcinoma (5–10%), and oncocytomas (3–5%) [34]. Among these subtypes, variants of clear cell carcinoma are highly vascular and have a high propensity for metastasis to the right atrium and ventricle through direct invasion of the inferior vena cava, in 4–10% of cases [35]. With echocardiography, the tumor will have a hyperechoic appearance and may be visualized in the inferior vena cava or the right heart, depending on the degree of extension of

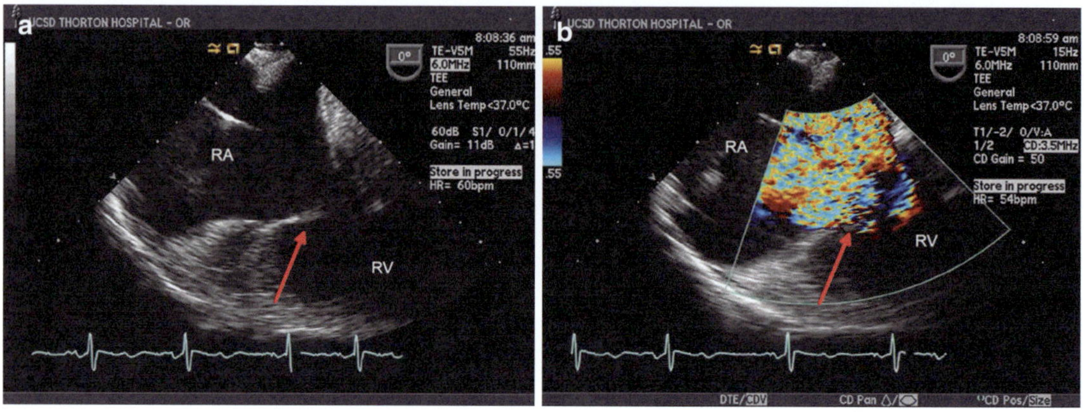

Fig. 17.10 (**a**) Midesophageal four-chamber view with an RV focus and depth reduced, in a patient with carcinoid heart disease. Note the thickened and restricted leaflet (*red arrow*). (**b**) The addition of color flow Doppler demonstrates significant tricuspid regurgitation (*red arrow*). *RA* right atrium, *RV* right ventricle

the tumor (Fig. 17.11 and Video 17.11). Intraoperatively, during resection of the renal cell carcinoma, TEE can be utilized to confirm the extension of the tumor and make real-time assessments on tumor migration and the progress of surgical resection. It can also aid in hemodynamic monitoring and evaluation of tumor embolization or compression of surrounding structures [36].

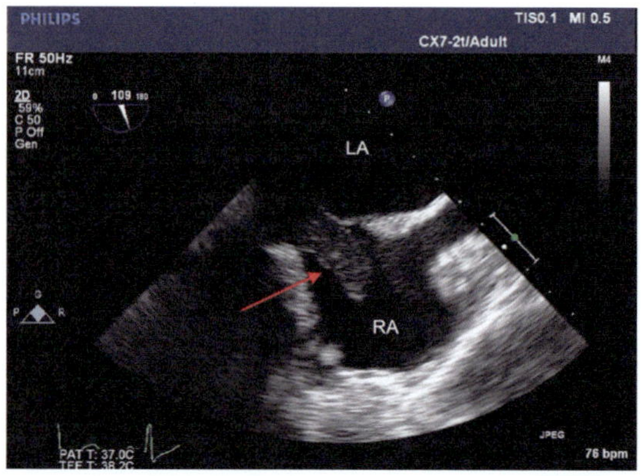

Fig. 17.11 Midesophageal bicaval view in a patient with renal cell carcinoma and subsequent IVC extension (*red arrow*). *LA* left atrium, *RA* right atrium

Foreign Bodies (Highlight Box 17.4)

Highlight Box 17.4

Foreign bodies	
2D	• Variety of presentations depending on structure and location • Hyperechoic appearance • Associated with significant artifact (shadowing, reverberation) • Echo may be utilized to guide placement or assess function
CFD	• Useful for assessing chamber occlusion (WATCHMAN device) or residual regurgitation (MitraClip) and flow (PFO occlusion device)
Spectral	• Assessment of valvular regurgitation

During echocardiographic examination of the heart, it is important to be familiar with intracardiac devices, catheters, and foreign bodies that may be present. In certain situations, it will be important to evaluate the location and function of a particular device or catheter, while in other instances, these devices can make evaluation of cardiac function more difficult due to the presence of artifacts and shadowing.

Intravascular Catheters

Central venous catheters (CVCs) and pulmonary arterial catheters (PACs) are frequently placed in the operative and acute care settings, and potential complications include vascular injury, cardiac arrhythmias, pneumothorax, hemothorax, and incorrect location. Echocardiography can be used to localize catheters and help with evaluation of frequently encountered complications. CVCs will have a hyperechoic appearance on echocardiography and should terminate in the lower portion of the superior vena cava (SVC), above the junction with the right atrium [37]. The catheter tip should be parallel with the SVC, and free floating; otherwise pressure on the vascular wall can cause erosion and lead to devastating complications. CVCs should not enter the heart per FDA recommendations [38], because catheters floating in the right atrium can trigger arrhythmias and give incorrect central venous pressure readings.

Pulmonary artery catheters are less frequently utilized today; however they may be necessary in the patients undergoing complex cardiovascular procedures. Traditionally, placement of the PAC has been guided by the pressure waveform; however, the exact location of the tip can be difficult to elucidate using this technique. Placement of PACs under TEE visualization is a useful technique and allows for visualization of the catheter tip as it enters into the main pulmonary artery (see Chap. 23), preventing excessive catheter advancement, which could result in devastating complications such as PA rupture [39]. The balloon for the PAC will appear to have a hyperechoic shell with a hypoechoic center and will typically bounce around in the cardiac chambers during insertion. The PAC itself will also have a thin, hyperechoic appearance and can be seen freely moving with each heartbeat. PACs will be most easily visualized in the midesophageal four-chamber, RV inflow-outflow, and ascending aorta short-axis views (TEE) or with the parasternal RV inflow or parasternal short-axis views (TTE) (Figs. 17.12 and 17.13; Videos 17.12 and 17.13).

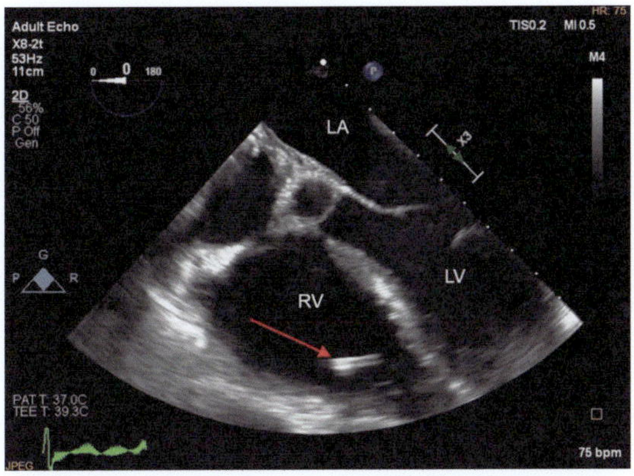

Fig. 17.12 Midesophageal four-chamber view in a patient with a pulmonary artery catheter in place (*red arrow*). *LA* left atrium, *RV* right ventricle, *LV* left ventricle

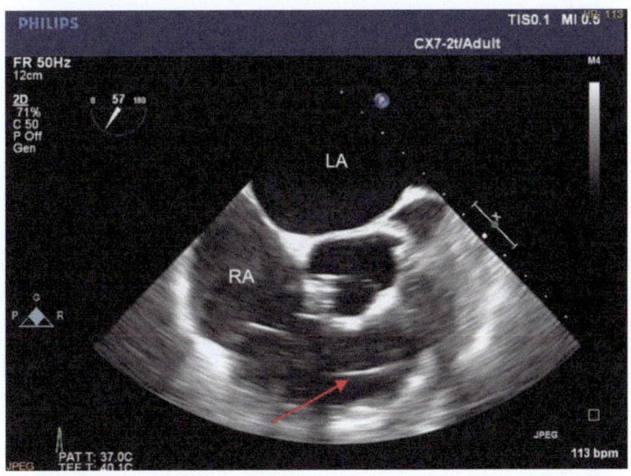

Fig. 17.13 Midesophageal RV inflow-outflow view in a patient with a pulmonary artery catheter in place (*red arrow*). *LA* left atrium, *RA* right atrium

Prosthetic Valves

Echocardiography is an excellent and important tool for the evaluation of prosthetic valves. Although there is a large variety of prosthetic valves, broadly they can be divided into two major categories based on their composition: mechanical and biological. Typically, mechanical valves will have an outer ring, which is sewn in with an occlusive valve, (ball-in-cage, tilting disk, or bileaflet valve). Biological valves can be made of various materials such as bovine, porcine, or human cadaveric tissue or a combination of synthetic and natural materials. Although any native valve can be replaced or repaired, the most common prostheses encountered are in the aortic and mitral valve positions.

Echocardiographic evaluation of the prosthesis is similar to that of native valves in principle; however, it is more challenging due to imaging artifacts. The evaluation should generally begin

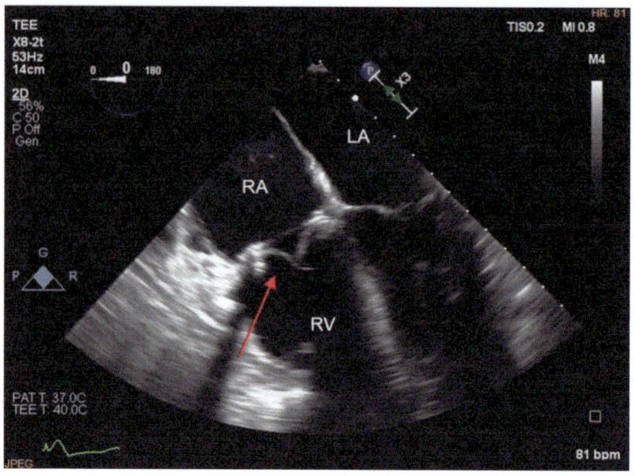

Fig. 17.14 Midesophageal four-chamber view in a patient after bioprosthetic tricuspid valve replacement. *LA* left atrium, *RA* right atrium, *RV* right ventricle

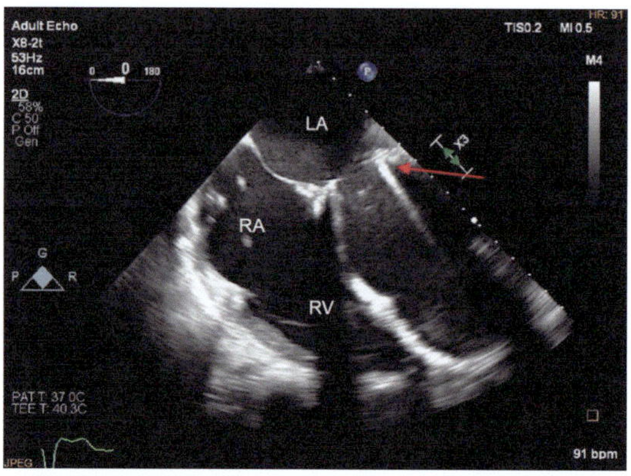

Fig. 17.15 Midesophageal four-chamber view in a patient after mechanical mitral valve replacement. *LA* left atrium, *RA* right atrium, *RV* right ventricle

with TTE, due to relative ease and noninvasive nature of the exam. However, the TTE exam can often be limited by the body habitus of the patient, small acoustic windows, and shadowing from the prosthesis. The TEE exam will allow for much higher resolution and provide additional views to better evaluate motion and flow across the valve (Figs. 17.14 and 17.15; Videos 17.14 and 17.15). Attention should be placed on determining the type of valve, evaluating mobility of the leaflets, checking the integrity of the ring position and paravalvular leaks, and detecting any calcifications or structural abnormalities [40]. Some of the more frequent complications of prosthetic valves include structural valve deterioration, valve thrombosis, embolism, endocarditis, valve stenosis, and regurgitation. Biological valves should have thin leaflets resembling that of native valves and must be inspected for tears, thickening, or calcifications.

Cardiovascular Implantable Electronic Devices

It is estimated that up to one million cardiac devices are implanted annually worldwide [41]. Therefore, it is important to be familiar with the appearance and common locations of these devices that may be encountered during TTE or TEE exam. Typical devices are permanent pacemakers, cardiac resynchronization devices, and implantable cardiac defibrillators. Newer leadless pacemakers are available; however the majority of devices encountered will be classic devices with intravascular cardiac leads. Over time, complications may arise with intracardiac leads, such as lead malfunction, dislodgment, breakage, and the rare but well-known complication of vegetation and thrombus formation. On echocardiography, leads will appear hyperechoic. A mobile, echodense structure on ® the leads should raise suspicion for vegetations or thrombi.

MitraClip™

One of the newer, but well-established techniques to improve functional mitral valve regurgitation is placement of a MitraClip™ device (Abbott, Abbott Park, Illinois). This percutaneous technique is used for patients with significant symptomatic mitral valve regurgitation, who are not surgical candidates due to high perioperative mortality risk. TTE is an important initial step in assessing and quantifying the severity of the mitral valve disease [42]. TEE is the principal imaging modality used for qualitative assessment of the regurgitation and guidance during the procedure [43]. The procedure relies on a transseptal puncture technique, followed by the advancement of the device into the LV just past the mitral valve, and then deployment of the device over incompetent cusps, effectively bringing the leaflets together and reducing the regurgitant jet. Once in the correct position, the device will be visualized as a hyperechoic object that holds the anterior and posterior mitral valve leaflets together. Color flow Doppler will show any residual regurgitation as regurgitant jets on either side of the MitraClip (Fig. 17.16 and Video 17.16). Continuous-wave Doppler can be still be utilized post-procedure to measure pressure gradients across the valve.

Atrial Appendage Occlusion Devices

Atrial fibrillation is the most common sustained arrhythmia in the United States, affecting millions [44]. The most feared complication of this disease is embolic stroke, with the frequent source being intracardiac clot formation due to relative blood stasis in the left atrial appendage (LAA). While pharmacological anticoagulation has been the mainstay for many years, the risk of bleeding complications has led to alternative strategies to reduce the risk of clot formation. Percutaneous left atrial appendage closure devices have been developed, including the WATCHMAN (Boston Scientific, Marlborough, Massachusetts) and the Amplatzer Amulet (Abbott, Abbott Park, Illinois).

TEE is essential in placement of these devices, because TTE only provides limited echocardiographic windows for LAA evaluation. Initially, echocardiography is used to identify the size and depth of the LAA and assess for any contraindications to placement of the device (e.g., LAA thrombus, PFO, ASD, or mitral valve regurgitation). The device is then advanced, and deployment is monitored and guided by the echocardiography. Real-time TEE allows for precise evaluation of its position, as well as rapid detection of any major complication, such as perforation and formation of cardiac tamponade [45]. Once placed, the device will be visualized as a hyperechoic parachute-like structure nestled into the LAA (Fig. 17.17 and Video 17.17).

PFO Closure Devices

A patent foramen ovale (PFO) is the most common congenital cardiac abnormality and estimated to be present in about 25% of the adult population. PFO is the result of incomplete fusion

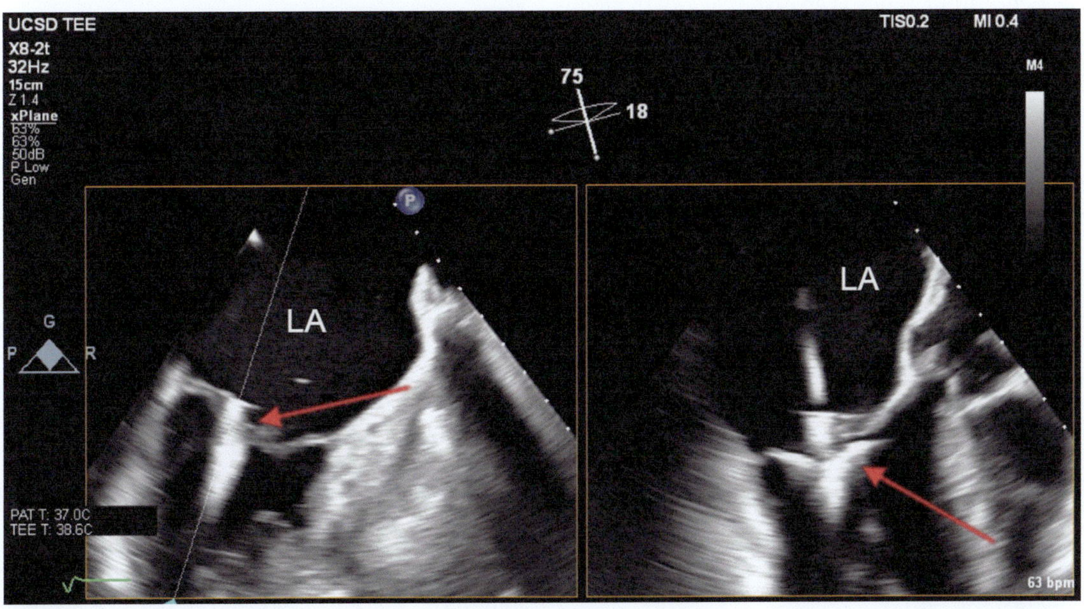

Fig. 17.16 X-plane imaging simultaneous ME mitral commissural view (left) and ME long-axis view (right) during MitraClip (*red arrow*) placement. *LA* left atrium

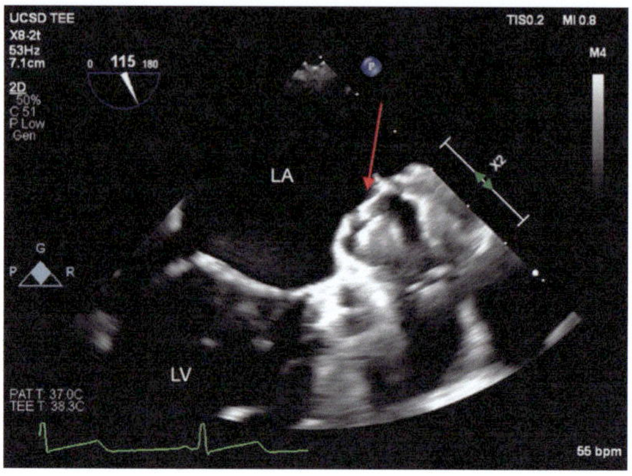

Fig. 17.17 ME left atrial appendage view in a patient after WATCHMAN device (*red arrow*) placement. *LA* left atrium, *LV* left ventricle

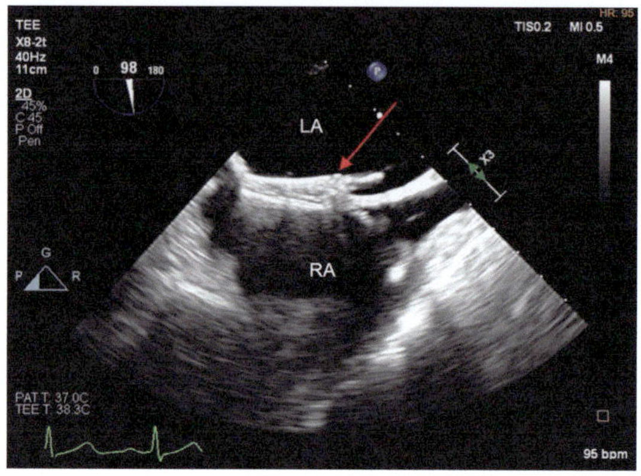

Fig. 17.18 Midesophageal bicaval view in a patient after placement of a PFO closure device (*red arrow*). *LA* left atrium, *RA* right atrium

between the septum primum and secundum, maintaining a patent "one-way valve" between the right and left atria, rather than a missing area of tissue. Although PFOs have been linked to a variety of conditions, such as migraines and decompression sickness, perhaps the most important consequence is the potential for paradoxical embolism [46]. This occurs when venous emboli cross from the RA to the LA via the PFO, bypassing the pulmonary circulation, which can result in stroke or coronary artery occlusion.

Echocardiography is an essential tool in identifying PFO, often initially using TTE, followed by a confirmatory TEE. The diagnosis is made by either color flow Doppler or by visualizing peripherally injected agitated saline bubbles cross the intra-atrial septum. The detection is improved by release of a Valsalva maneuver preceding the injection to increase right atrial pressure relative to left atrial pressure. With appropriate anatomy, PFO closure is performed via a percutaneous technique with an occlusive device. Although a variety of these devices exist, the most commonly used devices are of a double-disc design, with a small stem in between [47]. Closure is typically performed in a cardiac catheterization laboratory under visualization with fluoroscopy; however TEE has been shown to be an effective and safe modality in sparing patients from radiation and contrast use [48].

A catheter is introduced across the PFO, followed by sizing and deployment of the appropriate device. Complete closure will take several months and depends on the endothelialization of the device. Echocardiography should be performed within 6 months to confirm closure (Figs. 17.18 and 17.19; Videos 17.18 and 17.19).

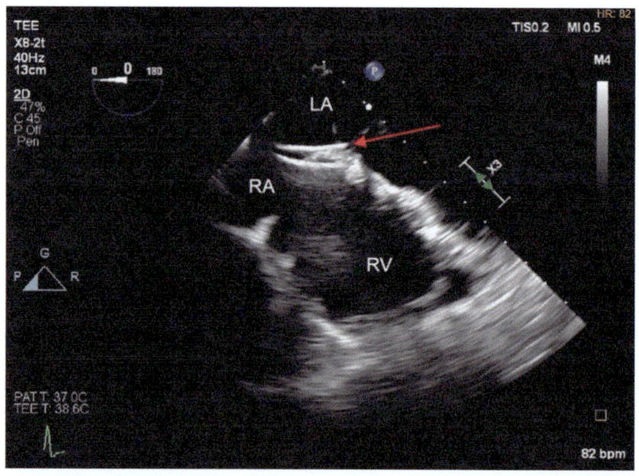

Fig. 17.19 Midesophageal four-chamber view in a patient after placement of a PFO closure device (*red arrow*). *LA* left atrium, *RA* right atrium, *RV* right ventricle

Mechanical Circulatory Support

In the last decade, there has been a substantial increase in use of mechanical circulatory devices. These devices can be implanted for short- or long-term therapy. Short-term devices include extracorporeal membranous oxygenation (ECMO), intra-aortic balloon pump (IABP),

TandemHeart® (LivaNova, PLC, London, United Kingdom), and Impella® (Abiomed, Danvers, Massachusetts). There are two major types of ECMO therapy available. Veno-venous ECMO (VV ECMO) therapy is typically utilized to support respiratory failure in patients with preserved cardiac function, and veno-arterial ECMO (VA ECMO), which gives the ability to support both cardiac and respiratory functions and, in many aspects, resembles the cardio-pulmonary bypass machine utilized in the operating room.

One configuration of VV ECMO allows for cannulation through a single site with a dual-lumen catheter (e.g., Avalon Elite® [Getinge, Goteborg, Sweden], or Protek Duo® [LivaNova, PLC, London, United Kingdom]). The Avalon Elite® catheter that has multiple drainage orifices in the superior and inferior vena cava and a return orifice directed across the tricuspid valve is commonly used. Echocardiography, particularly TEE, plays an important role in placement of such catheters. The catheter wall will have a bright lucent appearance with a dark central core (Fig. 17.20 and Video 17.20). CFD can be used to visualize flow patterns from the cannula directed toward the tricuspid valve. The ability to visualize the catheter entry will reduce risks of structural damage which is of concern due to the size the catheter. Echocardiography will ensure correct position during initial placement and may be frequently needed for catheter readjustment due to movement [49]. Similarly, echocardiographic guidance may help insertion of the Protek Duo® catheter, in a fashion similar to insertion of a PAC.

If the dysfunction is limited to the left ventricle, without respiratory involvement then a temporary left ventricular assist device such as an Impella (Abiomed, Danvers, Massachusetts) or TandemHeart® (LivaNova, PLC, London, United Kingdom) can be utilized. The Impella CP® device uses a microaxial blood pump to provide up to 4 L/min of cardiac output and is typically placed via a percutaneous technique. The device is positioned retrograde across the aortic valve, with inlet in the left ventricle and outlet in the ascending aorta (Fig. 17.21 and Video 17.21). Echocardiography plays a critical role in not only the placement and management of these devices but also in troubleshooting (Fig. 17.22 and Video 17.22a, b). For TEE, assessment with midesophageal long-axis and four-chamber views should be used to evaluate for positioning of the device, any evidence of acute right heart failure, assessment of the intraventricular septum, new valvular lesions, and evidence of direct myocardial injury during device placement [50]. Similar information is available from the apical four- or five-chamber views via TTE, as a parasternal long-axis view is commonly used to evaluate the device position.

An intra-aortic balloon pump (IABP) may be used to augment hemodynamics, coronary perfu-

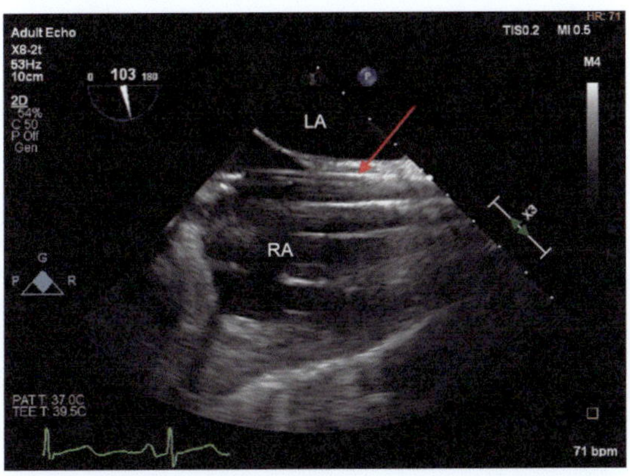

Fig. 17.20 Midesophageal bicaval view in a patient after placement of an Avalon Elite® VV-ECMO cannula (*red arrow*) placement through the right atrium. *LA* left atrium, *RA* right atrium

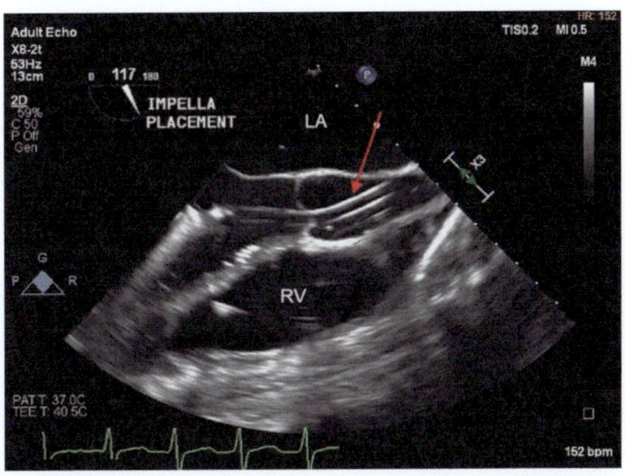

Fig. 17.21 Midesophageal AV long-axis view in a patient after placement of an Impella® LVAD (*red arrow*) placement. *LA* left atrium, *RV* right ventricle

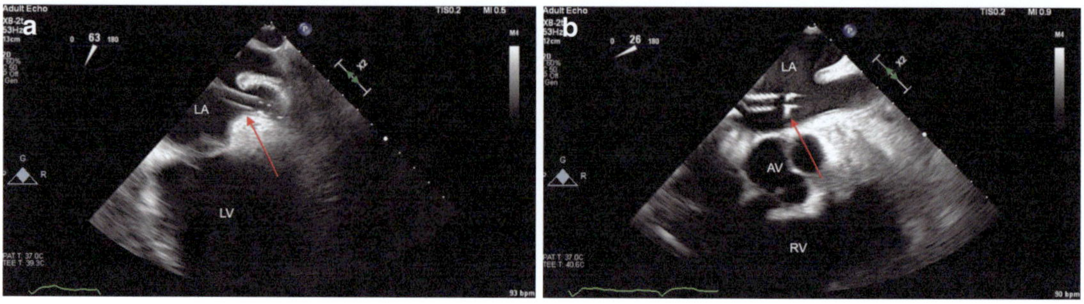

Fig. 17.22 (**a**) Midesophageal left atrial appendage view with a transseptal TandemHeart® inflow cannula malpositioned within the left atrial appendage (*red arrow*). (**b**) Midesophageal aortic valve short-axis view in the same patient demonstrating the appropriate positioning (via withdrawal; *red arrow*) of the TandemHeart® inflow cannula into the left atrium. *LA* left atrium, *LV* left ventricle, *AV* aortic valve, *RV* right ventricle

sion, and cardiac output in cases of cardiogenic shock. An IABP is typically inserted through the femoral artery, and the tip is placed distal to the takeoff of the left subclavian artery. The IABP inflation during diastole augments diastolic coronary artery perfusion, while deflation during systole decreases afterload and promotes forward flow. TEE is helpful in the correct positioning and placement of the IABP. The helium gas in the balloon during inflation causes significant artifact during imaging. The visualization and positioning of the balloon occurs with the upper esophageal and descending thoracic aortic views.

Long-term mechanical circulatory support is used in the setting of end-stage heart failure refractory to medical management, typically in the form of a left ventricular assist device (LVAD). Although a variety of these devices exist, the most commonly implanted devices are the HeartMate II™ (Abbott, Abbott Park, Illinois), HeartMate 3™ (Abbott, Abbott Park, Illinois), and HeartWare HVAD™ (Medtronic, Framingham, Massachusetts). The technical design of these devices is different, but they share basic components: a surgically implanted left ventricular inflow cannula, pump system outside of the heart, an outflow graft typically into the ascending aorta, and a tunneled line for connection with an external controller for adjustment and charging of the device [51]. The primary function of such a device is to move blood from the ventricular apex into the systemic circulation.

These pumps can generate flows between 4 and 7 L/min with pump speed as the fundamental parameter that can be altered. Echocardiography plays an essential role in managing patients with these devices. Although many of these patients are followed at specialized centers that have vast experience in managing ventricular assist devices, with the increasing number of implanted devices, it is important for clinicians to be familiar with their management. The TTE exam is the first step in evaluation of these patients; however acoustic windows may be challenging to obtain due to significant postoperative changes and implanted materials. TEE may allow for better visualization if TTE is inadequate. The goal of echocardiographic evaluation is to assess the structure and function of the left and right chambers, position of the intraventricular septum, and assessment of the valves [52] (Fig. 17.23 and Video 17.23). Commonly encountered life-threatening pathology that may be evident with

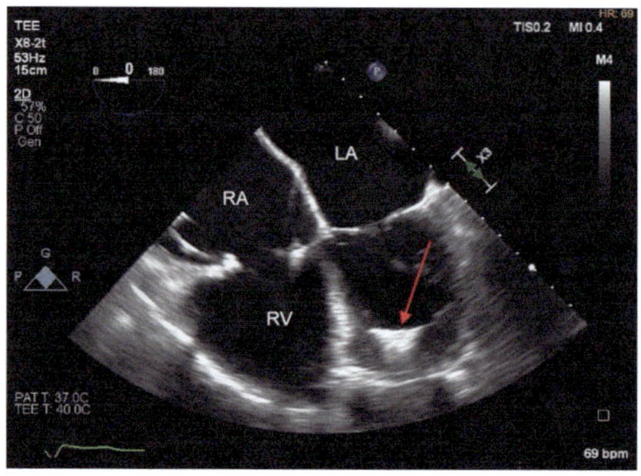

Fig. 17.23 Midesophageal four-chamber view in a patient after LVAD placement. The inflow cannula (*red arrow*) is visualized at the apex of the left ventricle. *LA* left atrium, *RA* right atrium, *RV* right ventricle

echocardiography includes hypovolemia, tamponade, RV failure, and dysrhythmias.

Conclusion

Echocardiography is a valuable tool in recognizing intracardiac masses and foreign bodies. It can be used to identify the location, shape, size, mobility, and any hemodynamic derangements associated with the intracardiac mass. While vegetations and thrombus are the most commonly encountered cardiac masses, benign and malignant tumors may be identified, as well. With the advancement of noninvasive cardiac intervention techniques and devices, it is increasingly common to note intracardiac devices and foreign bodies and guide their placement. Recognition and evaluation of these devices is important in management of the perioperative and critically ill patient.

Questions

1. Thrombus in which of the following cardiac chambers is most likely to result in stroke?

   A. Right atrium
   B. Right atrial appendage
   C. Left atrium
   D. Left atrial appendage

2. Vegetations associated with infective endocarditis are most likely to be found on which of the following surfaces of the valve?

   A. Ventricular side of the tricuspid valve
   B. Atrial side of the mitral valve
   C. Ventricular side of the mitral valve
   D. Aortic side of the aortic valve

3. Infective endocarditis is *least* likely to result in which of the following?

   A. Valvular prolapse
   B. Valvular stenosis
   C. Flail leaflet
   D. Leaflet perforation

4. Which of the following is the most frequently encountered type of intracardiac malignancy?

   A. Myxoma
   B. Lipoma
   C. Metastatic tumor
   D. Sarcoma

5. Which of the following is the most common type and location of primary benign intracardiac tumor in adults?

   A. Myxoma – right atrium
   B. Myxoma – left atrium
   C. Papillary fibroelastoma – right ventricle
   D. Papillary fibroelastoma – left ventricle

6. Which of the following manifestations is most likely as the result of carcinoid syndrome?

   A. Tricuspid stenosis
   B. Mitral regurgitation
   C. Mitral stenosis
   D. Aortic stenosis

7. Which of the following TEE views is best to confirm PA catheter position in the pulmonary artery?

   A. Midesophageal RV inflow-outflow view
   B. Midesophageal four-chamber view
   C. Midesophageal bicaval view
   D. Midesophageal ascending aorta short-axis view

8. At which point during cardiac cycle should an intra-aortic balloon pump inflate?

   A. Before aortic valve closure
   B. After aortic valve closure
   C. Before mitral valve closure
   D. After mitral valve closure

9. Renal cell carcinoma with intracardiac involvement is most likely to be extended into which of the following cardiac chambers?

   A. Left ventricle
   B. Left atrium

C. Right ventricle
D. Right atrium

10. Across which of the following valves is Impella CP® device placed?

A. Tricuspid valve
B. Pulmonic valve
C. Mitral valve
D. Aortic valve

References

1. Strandberg M, Marttila RJ, Helenius H, et al. Transoesophageal echocardiography in selecting patients for anticoagulation after ischaemic stroke or transient ischaemic attack. J Neurol Neurosurg Psychiatry. 2002;73:29–33.
2. Kamel H, Healey JS. Cardioembolic stroke. Circ Res. 2017;120:514–26.
3. Bogiatzi C, Hackam DG, McLeod AI, et al. Secular trends in ischemic stroke subtypes and stroke risk factors. Stroke. 2014;45:3208–13.
4. Turhan S, Ozcan OU, Erol C. Imaging of intracardiac thrombus. Cor Vasa. 2013;55:e176–83.
5. Manning WJ, Weintraub RM, Waksmonski CA, et al. Accuracy of transesophageal echocardiography for identifying left atrial thrombi. A prospective, intraoperative study. Ann Intern Med. 1995;123:817–22.
6. de Bruijn SF, Agema WR, Lammers GJ, et al. Transesophageal echocardiography is superior to transthoracic echocardiography in management of patients of any age with transient ischemic attack or stroke. Stroke. 2006;37:2531–4.
7. Shively BK, Gelgand EA, Crawford MH. Regional left atrial stasis during atrial fibrillation and flutter: determinants and relation to stroke. J Am Coll Cardiol. 1996;27:1722–9.
8. Pepi M, Evangelista A, Nihoyannopoulos P, et al. Recommendations for echocardiography use in the diagnosis and management of cardiac sources of embolism: European Association of Echocardiography (EAE) (a registered branch of the ESC). Eur J Echocardiogr. 2010;11:461–76.
9. Li JS, Sexton DJ, Mick N, et al. Proposed modifications to the Duke criteria for the diagnosis of infective endocarditis. Clin Infect Dis. 2000;30:633–8.
10. Bai AD, Steinberg M, Showler A, et al. Diagnostic accuracy of transthoracic echocardiography for infective endocarditis findings using transesophageal echocardiography as the reference standard: a meta-analysis. J Am Soc Echocardiogr. 2017;30:639–646.e638.
11. Sordelli C, Fele N, Mocerino R, et al. Infective endocarditis: echocardiographic imaging and new imaging modalities. J Cardiovasc Echogr. 2019;29:149–55.
12. Habib G, Badano L, Tribouilloy C, et al. Recommendations for the practice of echocardiography in infective endocarditis. Eur J Echocardiogr. 2010;11:202–19.
13. Hill EE, Herijgers P, Claus P, et al. Abscess in infective endocarditis: the value of transesophageal echocardiography and outcome: a 5-year study. Am Heart J. 2007;154:923–8.
14. Baddour LM, Wilson WR, Bayer AS, et al. Infective endocarditis in adults: diagnosis, antimicrobial therapy, and management of complications: a scientific statement for healthcare professionals from the American Heart Association. Circulation. 2015;132:1435–86.
15. Lam KY, Dickens P, Chan AC. Tumors of the heart. A 20-year experience with a review of 12,485 consecutive autopsies. Arch Pathol Lab Med. 1993;117:1027–31.
16. Markel ML, Waller BF, Armstrong WF. Cardiac myxoma. A review. Medicine (Baltimore). 1987;66:114–25.
17. Burke AP, Virmani R. Cardiac myxoma. A clinicopathologic study. Am J Clin Pathol. 1993;100:671–80.
18. Kaplan JA. Kaplan's cardiac anesthesia. 7th ed. Philadelphia: Elsevier; 2017.
19. Gowda RM, Khan IA, Nair CK, et al. Cardiac papillary fibroelastoma: a comprehensive analysis of 725 cases. Am Heart J. 2003;146:404–10.
20. Jain D, Maleszewski JJ, Halushka MK. Benign cardiac tumors and tumorlike conditions. Ann Diagn Pathol. 2010;14:215–30.
21. Vittala SS, Click RL, Challa S, et al. Multiple papillary fibroelastomas. Circulation. 2012;126:242–3.
22. Klarich KW, Enriquez-Sarano M, Gura GM, et al. Papillary fibroelastoma: echocardiographic characteristics for diagnosis and pathologic correlation. J Am Coll Cardiol. 1997;30:784–90.
23. Shapiro LM. Cardiac tumours: diagnosis and management. Heart. 2001;85:218–22.
24. Beghetti M, Gow RM, Haney I, et al. Pediatric primary benign cardiac tumors: a 15-year review. Am Heart J. 1997;134:1107–14.
25. Mankad R, Herrmann J. Cardiac tumors: echo assessment. Echo Res Pract. 2016;3:R65–r77.
26. Cohen RA, Loarte P, Navarro V, et al. Mature cardiac teratoma in an adult. Cardiol Res. 2012;3:97–9.
27. Mayer F, Aebert H, Rudert M, et al. Primary malignant sarcomas of the heart and great vessels in adult patients--a single-center experience. Oncologist. 2007;12:1134–42.
28. Meng Q, Lai H, Lima J, et al. Echocardiographic and pathologic characteristics of primary cardiac tumors: a study of 149 cases. Int J Cardiol. 2002;84:69–75.
29. Ambrus N, Havasi K, Kalapos A, et al. Primary cardiac angiosarcoma: a case report. Echocardiography. 2018;35:267–71.
30. Reynen K, Köckeritz U, Strasser RH. Metastases to the heart. Ann Oncol. 2004;15:375–81.
31. Miyasaka R, Mehta A, Pettersson GB, et al. Carcinoid tricuspid valve disease: applications of three dimen-

sional transesophageal echocardiography. Circ Cardiovasc Imaging. 2019;12:e009555.
32. Connolly HM. Carcinoid heart disease: medical and surgical considerations. Cancer Control. 2001;8:454–60.
33. Miles LF, Leong T, McCall P, et al. Carcinoid heart disease: correlation of echocardiographic and histopathological findings. BMJ Case Rep. 2014;2014:bcr2014207732.
34. Thoenes W, Störkel S, Rumpelt HJ. Histopathology and classification of renal cell tumors (adenomas, oncocytomas and carcinomas). The basic cytological and histopathological elements and their use for diagnostics. Pathol Res Pract. 1986;181:125–43.
35. McDougal AJW, Kavoussi L, Novick A, Partin A, Peters C, Ramchandani P. Urology. 1st ed. Philadelphia: Saunders; 2011.
36. Souki FG, Demos M, Fermin L, et al. Transesophageal echocardiography-guided thrombectomy of intracardiac renal cell carcinoma without cardiopulmonary bypass. Ann Card Anaesth. 2016;19:740–3.
37. Ahn JH, Kim IS, Yang JH, et al. Transoesophageal echocardiographic evaluation of central venous catheter positioning using Peres' formula or a radiological landmark-based approach: a prospective randomized single-centre study. Br J Anaesth. 2017;118:215–22.
38. Vesely TM. Central venous catheter tip position: a continuing controversy. J Vasc Interv Radiol. 2003;14:527–34.
39. Cronin B, Robbins R, Maus T. Pulmonary artery catheter placement using transesophageal echocardiography. J Cardiothorac Vasc Anesth. 2017;31:178–83.
40. Lancellotti P, Pibarot P, Chambers J, et al. Recommendations for the imaging assessment of prosthetic heart valves: a report from the European Association of Cardiovascular Imaging endorsed by the Chinese Society of Echocardiography, the Inter-American Society of Echocardiography, and the Brazilian Department of Cardiovascular Imaging. Eur Heart J Cardiovasc Imaging. 2016;17:589–90.
41. Mond HG, Proclemer A. The 11th world survey of cardiac pacing and implantable cardioverter-defibrillators: calendar year 2009--a World Society of Arrhythmia's project. Pacing Clin Electrophysiol. 2011;34:1013–27.
42. Gripari P, Maffessanti F, Tamborini G, et al. Patients selection for MitraClip: time to move to transthoracic echocardiographic screening? Int J Cardiol. 2014;176:491–4.
43. Aman E, Smith TW. Echocardiographic guidance for transcatheter mitral valve repair using edge-to-edge clip. J Echocardiogr. 2019;17:53–63.
44. Wolf PA, Abbott RD, Kannel WB. Atrial fibrillation as an independent risk factor for stroke: the Framingham Study. Stroke. 1991;22:983–8.
45. Mitrev L, Trautman N, Vadlamudi R, et al. Anesthesia and transesophageal echocardiography for WATCHMAN device implantation. J Cardiothorac Vasc Anesth. 2016;30:1685–92.
46. Homma S, Messé SR, Rundek T, et al. Patent foramen ovale. Nat Rev Dis Primers. 2016;2:15086.
47. Giblett JP, Abdul-Samad O, Shapiro LM, et al. Patent foramen ovale closure in 2019. Interv Cardiol. 2019;14:34–41.
48. Han Y, Zhang X, Zhang F. Patent foramen ovale closure by using transesophageal echocardiography for cryptogenic stroke: single center experience in 132 consecutive patients. J Cardiothorac Surg. 2020;15:11.
49. Griffee MJ, Zimmerman JM, McKellar SH, et al. Echocardiography-guided dual-lumen venovenous extracorporeal membrane oxygenation cannula placement in the ICU-A retrospective review. J Cardiothorac Vasc Anesth. 2020;34:698–705.
50. Crowley J, Cronin B, Essandoh M, et al. Transesophageal echocardiography for impella placement and management. J Cardiothorac Vasc Anesth. 2019;33:2663–8.
51. DeVore AD, Patel PA, Patel CB. Medical management of patients with a left ventricular assist device for the non-left ventricular assist device specialist. JACC Heart Fail. 2017;5:621–31.
52. Gargani L. Left ventricular assist device and echocardiography: no more sadness. Eur Heart J Cardiovasc Imaging. 2020.

Adult Congenital Heart Disease

18

Swapnil Khoche

Abbreviations

ASD	Atrial septal defect
CFD	Color flow Doppler
CHD	Congenital heart disease
IAS	Interatrial septum
IJ	Internal jugular
LAX	Long-axis
LVOT	Left ventricular outflow tract
ME	Midesophageal
PA	Pulmonary artery
PASP	Pulmonary artery systolic pressure
PDA	Patent ductus arteriosus
PFO	Patent foramen ovale
RV	Right ventricle
RVOT	Right ventricular outflow tract
SAX	Short-axis
SVC	Superior vena cava
TEE	Transesophageal echocardiography
ToF	Tetralogy of Fallot
TTE	Transthoracic echocardiography
VSD	Ventricular septal defect

Supplementary Information The online version of this chapter (https://doi.org/10.1007/978-3-030-84349-6_18) contains supplementary material, which is available to authorized users.

S. Khoche (✉)
Department of Anesthesiology, University of California San Diego Health, La Jolla, CA, USA
e-mail: skhoche@health.ucsd.edu

Introduction

With the advancement of technology, transesophageal echocardiography (TEE) has quickly become invaluable in pediatric congenital heart surgery, both as a diagnostic tool and to assess repair [1]. With more congenital heart disease (CHD) patients now surviving longer, it is not difficult to imagine that these patients will ultimately need further anesthesia for noncardiac and cardiac procedures [2]. Echocardiography has remained the cornerstone for diagnosing and managing these conditions. The basic perioperative transesophageal echocardiography consensus statement suggests that the echocardiographer should be familiar with, and able to recognize, simple congenital heart disease lesions. Complex lesions are beyond the scope of a basic echocardiographer, and if suspected, consultation with an advanced echocardiographer or a switch to another diagnostic technique is warranted. Perioperatively, TEE provides useful information about the real time monitoring of ventricular filling, myocardial performance, and identification of intracardiac shunting, in addition to optimization of hemodynamic management strategies. A brief outline of the major congenital cardiac lesions and their echocardiographic correlates is provided here. There is also an introduction to the applicability of transthoracic echocardiography (TTE) to these lesions as well. The bicuspid aortic valve, which is the most common congenital

T. M. Maus, C. R. Tainter (eds.), *Essential Echocardiography*,
https://doi.org/10.1007/978-3-030-84349-6_18

heart disease in adulthood, is discussed separately in Chap. 9.

Atrial Septal Defect (ASD) (Highlight Box 18.1)

Highlight Box 18.1

Atrial septal defects	
2D	• Echogenic defect of tissue in interatrial septum ∘ Secundum – ME four-chamber or bicaval views ∘ Primum – ME four-chamber view ∘ Sinus venosus – ME bicaval view ∘ Unroofed coronary sinus – difficult to visualize on 2D • Associated findings ∘ Cleft anterior mitral leaflet (primum) ∘ Anomalous pulmonary venous return (sinus venosus) ∘ Atrial enlargement ∘ Ventricular dilation
CFD	• Interatrial flow – note directionality ∘ May or may not be turbulent (dependent on ASD size)
Spectral	• Calculate pulmonary to systemic flow ratio (Qp/Qs)

ME midesophageal, *ASD* atrial septal defect

Atrial septal defects (ASDs) account for 7–8% of all congenital heart disease and, thus, are relatively common, either in combination with other lesions or by themselves. The location and size, which are related to its embryonic origin, often determine the magnitude of the hemodynamic effects. Due to the proximity of the left atrium to the probe, TEE results in excellent imaging of the inter-atrial septum (IAS) and is superior to TTE in this respect.

A patent foramen ovale (PFO), present in up to 27% of the population, can cause an intracardiac shunt if right atrial pressure exceeds the left atrial pressure [3]. Although a PFO represents a possible communication between the atria, it is technically not considered an ASD, as there is no actual defect or tissue missing. A PFO may be more easily identified with the help of color flow Doppler (CFD). While the flow through a PFO may be small, lowering the aliasing velocity on CFD scale may help to identify the lower flow (Fig. 18.1 and Video 18.1). An agitated saline study with identification of "microbubbles" moving across the foramen during a Valsalva maneuver can also help identify a PFO. The use of a Valsalva maneuver is important as the release of the Valsalva maneuver temporarily increases right atrial pressure in comparison to left atrial pressure, thereby creating right-to-left flow, allowing visualization of the agitated saline crossing the interatrial septum [3] (Fig. 18.2 and Video 18.2).

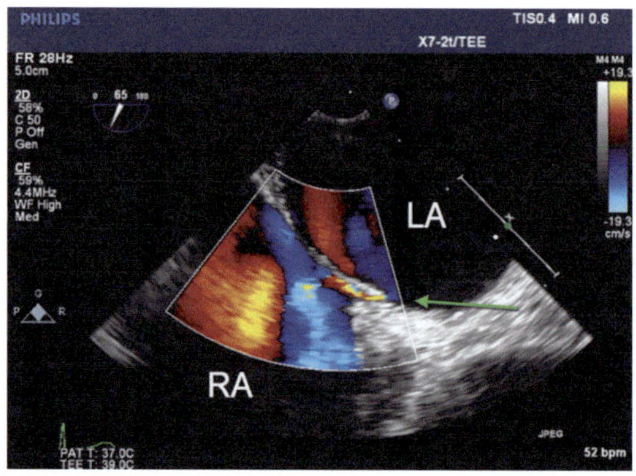

Fig. 18.1 Midesophageal view of the interatrial septum with color flow Doppler. The *green arrow* indicates a left-to-right shunt across a patent foramen ovale (PFO). *LA* left atrium, *RA* right atrium

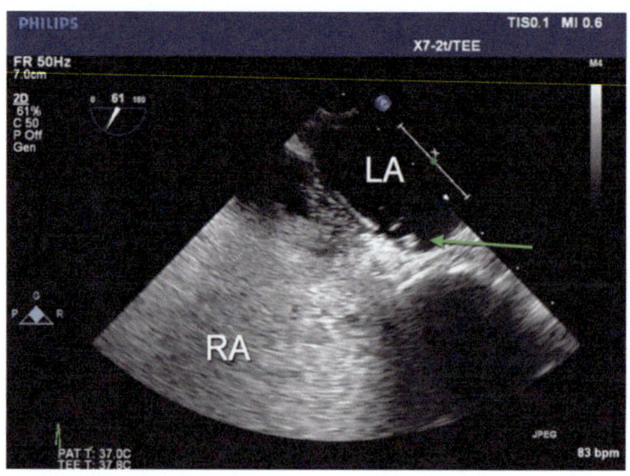

Fig. 18.2 Midesophageal view of the interatrial septum during agitated saline injection. The *green arrow* indicates transseptal flow of agitated saline from the right atrium (RA) to left atrium (LA)

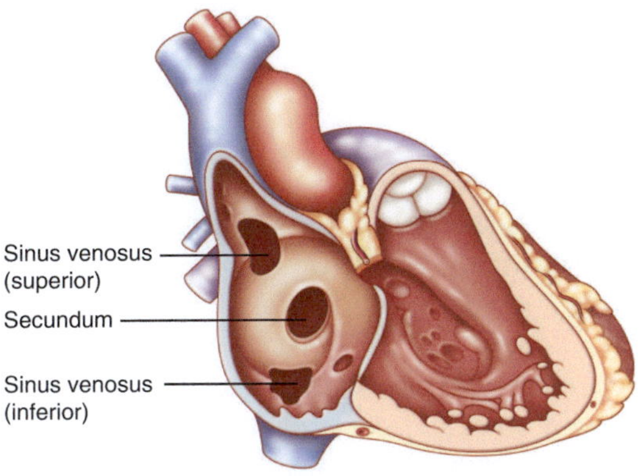

Fig. 18.3 Diagram of interatrial septum from the perspective of the right atrium and right ventricle

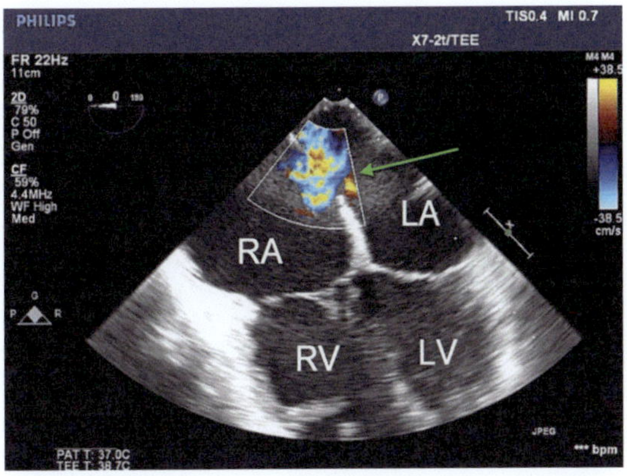

Fig. 18.4 Midesophageal four-chamber view demonstrating an ostium secundum ASD (*green arrow*) with left-to-right flow noted on color flow Doppler. *RA* right atrium, *LA* left atrium, *RV* right ventricle, *LV* left ventricle

The defects or gaps truly classified as ASDs involve some degree of absent tissue, allowing the potential for various degrees of intracardiac shunting. The ASDs are classified based upon their location which relates to the defect during embryologic development. The subdivided defects are described below (Fig. 18.3).

Ostium Secundum ASD

This is the most common ASD (approximately 70%) and generally occurs in the area contained in the limbus of the fossa ovalis [4]. During embryologic development, the septum primum grows toward the atrioventricular canal. An ostium develops centrally (termed the ostium secundum) which allows oxygenated blood in utero to cross the interatrial septum. Subsequently a septum secundum develops to cover this ostium yet still allows flow through as the foramen ovale. After birth with the increase in left atrial pressure from increased pulmonary blood flow, the foramen ovale is functionally pushed closed. Fusion of the two septae finalizes the process, leaving a fossa ovalis. A defective closure of the ostium secundum leads to the ostium secundum ASD (Fig. 18.4 and Video 18.3). It may be circular in shape or may be a series of fenestrations associated with an aneurysmal interatrial septum.

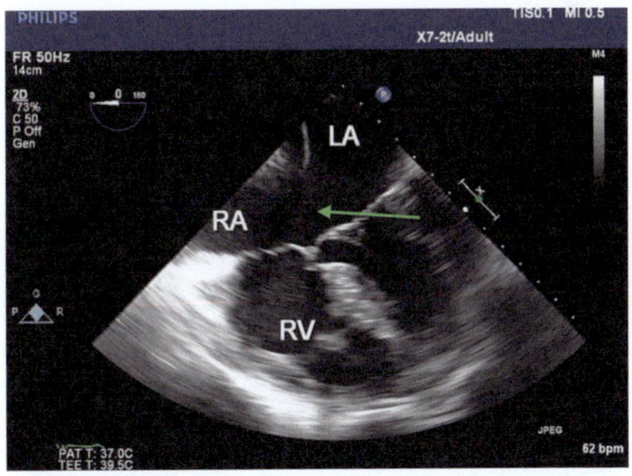

Fig. 18.5 Midesophageal four-chamber view demonstrating an ostium primum ASD (*green arrow*). *RA* right atrium, *LA* left atrium, *RV* right ventricle

Ostium Primum ASD

These defects are the second most common ASD (approximately 20%) and occur in the inferior and anterior portion of the IAS, near the atrioventricular valves. This defect generally represents the smallest degree of an atrioventricular canal defect. During embryologic development, the septum primum develops in the direction of the atrioventricular valves leaving the ostium primum to be covered by the septum secundum. Failure of this closure leaves the ostium primum atrial septal defect (Fig. 18.5 and Video 18.4). As

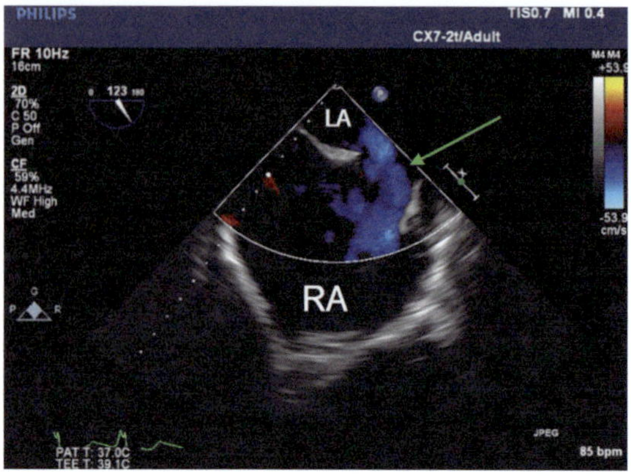

Fig. 18.6 Midesophageal bicaval view in a patient with a superior sinus venosus ASD and a grossly dilated right atrium (RA). The *green arrow* indicates left-to-right flow from the left atrium (LA) to the RA near the superior vena cava and RA junction

the endocardial cushion is also involved in the development of the atrioventricular valves, ostium primum defects can be associated with a cleft in the anterior mitral leaflet.

Sinus Venosus ASD

This defect represents an atrial communication adjacent to the attachment of either the superior or inferior vena cava, and results in the respective vena cava over-riding the defect. Sinus venosus defects account for about 8% of all ASDs [4]. Embryologically, the vena cavae are derived from the sinus venosus. Abnormal resorption of the sinus venosus leads to a defect between the cavae and the left atrium (Fig. 18.6 and Video 18.5). The defect is often associated with partial anomalous pulmonary venous return (i.e., anomalous right upper pulmonary vein draining into the left atrium).

Coronary Sinus ASD (Unroofed Coronary Sinus)

These rare defects (< 1%) result from a partial or complete defect in the separation between the LA and the coronary sinus, resulting in "unroofing" and causing communication between the right and the left atria.

Transesophageal Echocardiographic Examination for ASDs

The midesophageal (ME) four-chamber view can interrogate the majority of the interatrial septum, though probe withdrawal and insertion may be required for superiorly and inferiorly located ostium secundum defects as well as sinus venosus defects. Advancing the probe to the AV groove allows detection of ostium primum defects, evaluation of the coronary sinus, and Doppler evaluation of atrioventricular valves. Rotation of the probe to right and left is recommended to thoroughly interrogate the area. The ME aortic valve short-axis (SAX) or ME right ventricular inflow-outflow views can also be used to evaluate the septum, TV, and PV. In addition, these views can be used to quantify tricuspid regurgitation, estimate pulmonary artery systolic pressure (PASP) and right ventricular (RV) function, and search for abnormalities of venous return. The ME bicaval view provides a good cross-sectional display of the septum (superior to inferior), aligns the Doppler beam perpendicular to the septum, and is also an excellent view for agitated saline studies. This view is not particularly suited for detection of ostium primum defects but can be modified by clockwise or counterclockwise rotation and multiplane manipulation to detect and evaluate all other ASDs. The transgastric midpapillary SAX views can be used to detect flattening of the interventricular septum and help diagnose RV pressure or volume overload (see Chap. 10). While beyond the scope of this textbook, TEE, especially 3D TEE, can be invaluable during device closure of ASDs by identifying the site and size of the defect, evaluating adequacy of the tissue ring around the defect (generally 5 mm) to hold the device, and following the deployment of the device in real time.

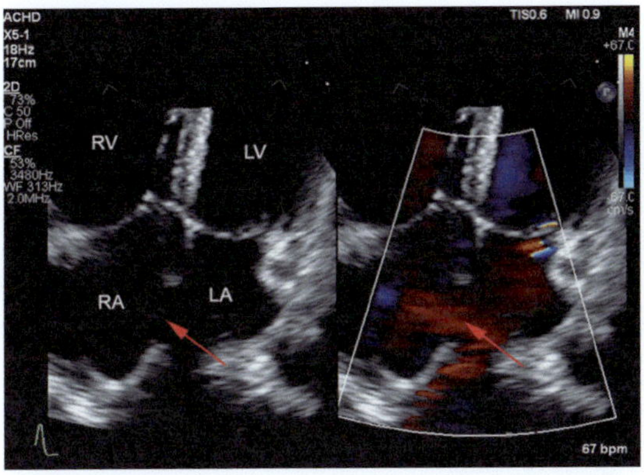

Fig. 18.7 Apical four-chamber view with a zoomed perspective of the interatrial septum with color compare feature (two-dimensional image on left; color flow Doppler applied on the right). The *red arrow* indicates a secundum ASD on both images. *RA* right atrium, *LA* left atrium, *RV* right ventricle, *LV* left ventricle

Transthoracic Echocardiographic Examination for ASDs

Factors that alert the clinician to the possibility of an ASD (during a TTE exam) include a hypermobile interatrial septum, abrupt septal irregularity, right atrial and ventricular volume overload, and pulmonary artery dilatation. A subcostal window, if it can be obtained, is ideal for examination of the IAS since the septum is mostly perpendicular to the Echo beam, and any existing shunt should be parallel to it. The apical four-chamber view, although satisfactory, suffers from the flow being perpendicular to the beam, limiting the sensitivity of Doppler evaluation (Fig. 18.7 and Video 18.6). Out of the subtypes, TTE is the most sensitive in detecting primum ASDs (100%) and the least sensitive when it comes to sinus venosus ASDs (44%) [5]. This is probably a reflection of distance from the probe and the variability in anatomy. TEE is considered superior to diagnose and quantify ASDs and is needed when TTE is either indeterminate or technically limited.

Ventricular Septal Defect (VSD) (Highlight Box 18.2)

Highlight Box 18.2

Ventricular septal defects	

2D	• Echogenic defect of tissue in interventricular septum
	  ◦ ME or apical four-chamber views (muscular and inlet)
	  ◦ ME AV SAX or PSAX basal level view (perimembranous and outlet)
	• Associated findings
	  ◦ Atrial enlargement
	  ◦ Ventricular dilation

CFD	• Presence of interventricular flow ◦ May or may not be turbulent (dependent on VSD size)
Spectral	• Calculate pulmonary to systemic flow ratio (Qp/Qs) • Estimate pulmonary arterial systolic pressure (TR jet)

ME midesophageal, *AV* aortic valve, *SAX* short-axis, *PSAX* parasternal short-axis, *VSD* ventricular septal defect

Ventricular septal defects (VSDs) are present in approximately 10% of all adults with congenital heart disease and can occur in isolation or associated with other disorders. The ventricular septum can be divided into four components, each with its distinct morphology: membranous, inlet, trabecular (muscular), and outlet [6] (Fig. 18.8). VSDs follow similar nomenclature but can span more than one segment. Spontaneous closure is more likely for VSDs of the membranous or muscular type.

The most common of the four subtypes is the perimembranous VSD, occurring in 75–80% of all VSDs. This defect is found in the membranous portion of the septum beneath the tricuspid valve and allows a connection to the left ventricular outflow tract immediately beneath the aortic valve [6]. It is best seen in the ME right ventricular

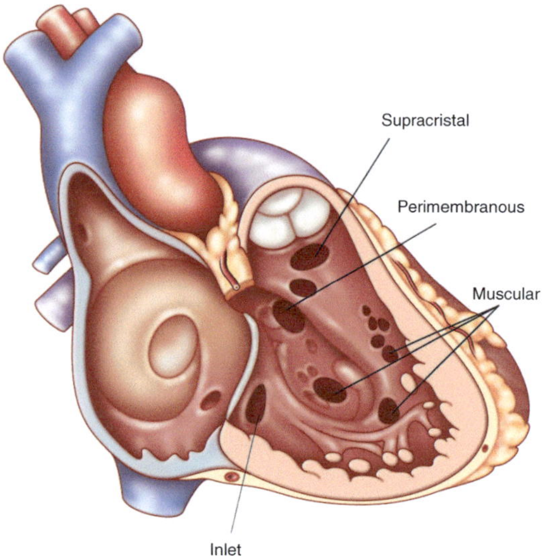

Fig. 18.8 Diagram of the interventricular septum from the perspective of the right atrium and right ventricle

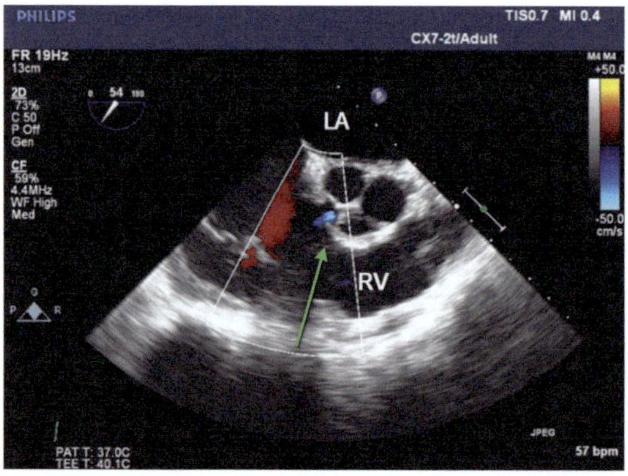

Fig. 18.9 Midesophageal right ventricular inflow-outflow view in a patient with a perimembranous ventricular septal defect (VSD) indicated by the *green arrow*. *LA* left atrium, *RV* right ventricle

inflow-outflow or ME aortic valve SAX views (Fig. 18.9 and Video 18.7). Associated aneurysm of the membranous septum or accessory tricuspid tissue may be visualized. Perimembranous defects that occur high in the left ventricular outflow tract (LVOT) can result in aortic regurgitation due to cusp herniation through the defect (most commonly the right coronary cusp).

Inlet VSDs, also part of the endocardial cushion defect spectrum, are located in the posterior portion

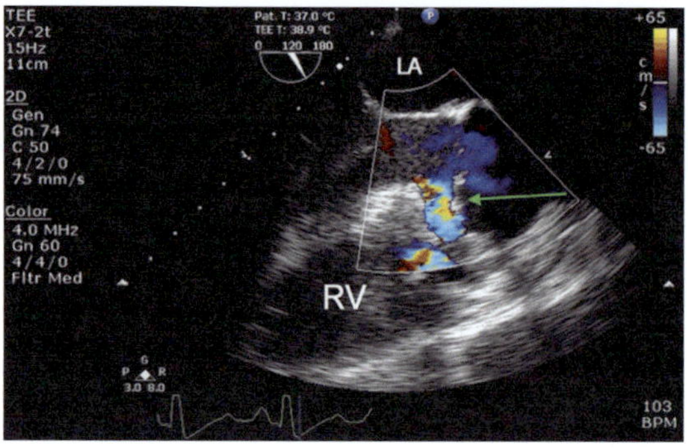

Fig. 18.10 Midesophageal aortic valve long-axis view in a patient with an outlet VSD (*green arrow*). *LA* left atrium, *RV* right ventricle

of the interventricular septum immediately below the mitral and tricuspid valves [6]. Echocardiographically, these two valves tend to be located at the same level; however the normal insertion of the tricuspid valve is typically a few millimeters inferiorly. These defects are large and generally do not close spontaneously. Multiple configurations of the atrioventricular valves can occur, the details of which are outside the scope of this text. Endocardial cushion defects represent defects in the separation of the right and the left heart chambers and can have complete absence of the septae, one common atrioventricular valve, and an ostium primum ASD, among other abnormalities.

Muscular defects, approximately 5–20% of all VSDs, occur centrally or apically in the trabecular portion and can have multiple openings ("Swiss cheese" appearance). Apical VSDs may occur after myocardial infarctions [7]. Color flow Doppler is invaluable to detect multiple defects in the muscular septum.

Outlet VSDs are also known by several terms: supracristal, infundibular, doubly committed, or subarterial VSDs. Irrespective of the nomenclature used, they occur in the region just below the aortic and pulmonic valves and can have associated aortic insufficiency (related to the herniation of the right coronary cusp). Interrogation of the outflow tracts side by side, done as a modification of the ME aortic valve long-axis (LAX) view or the ME right ventricular inflow-outflow view, is used to detect these defects (Fig. 18.10 and Video 18.8).

Transesophageal Echocardiographic Examination of VSDs

The complexity of the interventricular septum requires multiple views as well as rotation and use of the multiplane angle at nonstandard imaging planes. The ME four-chamber, ME aortic valve short-axis and long-axis, ME RV inflow-outflow, and deep transgastric long-axis views are recommended for a focused interrogation. Apart from number, size, location, and nature of the defect(s), other pertinent findings to look for include additional congenital lesions, aortic valve abnormalities, signs of RV pressure and volume overload, and functional consequences of the VSD. Doppler interrogation can quantify the nature and magnitude of the intracardiac shunt, estimate valvular regurgitation, and estimate PASP (see Chap. 4).

High velocity through the defect as evidenced by Doppler interrogation is indicative of a restrictive shunt, whereas low, non-turbulent flow denotes a nonrestrictive defect. Generally, a nonrestrictive defect indicates a more severe lesion [8, 9]. The ratio of pulmonary-to-systemic blood flow (Qp/Qs) should be measured since it has diagnostic and therapeutic implications. A high Qp/Qs indicates that there is a significant left-to-right shunt, which may eventually lead to pulmonary overcirculation and Eisenmenger's syndrome. A low Qp/Qs (< 1) is indicative of a right-to-left shunt.

Transthoracic Echocardiographic Examination for VSDs

Most patients with VSDs are investigated initially with a TTE for a murmur or other clinical indications. The ventricular septum is closer to the transthoracic probe, favoring this mode of imaging. Atrioventricular valves that lie on the same level or unusual LVOT shape can provide a clue to the presence of a VSD. Certain syndromes, such as trisomy 21 (Down syndrome, associated with an inlet VSD), CHARGE and Noonan syndromes, or VACTERL syndrome, are associated with VSDs as well. Abnormal flow detection with CFD is the first step to detection of a VSD. The parasternal long-axis view (and small variations thereof) is very helpful to detect perimembranous and outlet VSDs. The parasternal short-axis view with CFD box applied over the conal septum helps both in detection and identification (Fig. 18.11 and Video 18.9). Inlet VSDs are best visualized in the apical four-chamber view with CFD interrogation of the septum in the region of the atrioventricular valves. Muscular VSDs can be best detected in the apical four-chamber view but requires an off-axis view and sweeping loops since their trajectory can be convoluted (Fig. 18.12 and Video 18.10). Small jets of flow within the trabecula (especially in the RV) can occur that need to be distinguished from true flow across the septum. Restriction across the defect (usually a gradient exceeding 20–30 mm Hg), the direction of flow during the cardiac cycle, effect on other structures (dilation of chambers), and presence of pulmonary hypertension are all important parts of a thorough examination [10].

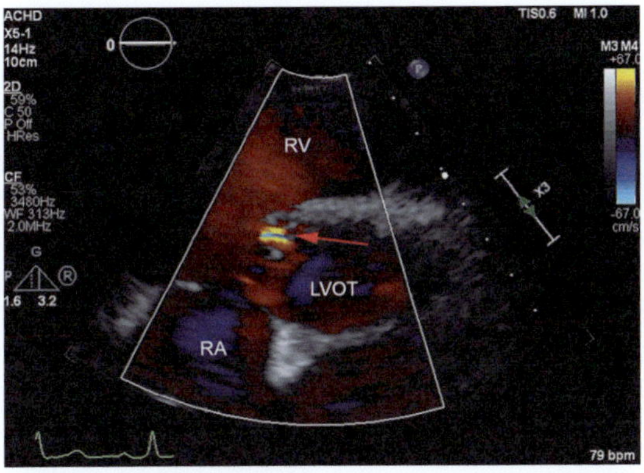

Fig. 18.11 Parasternal short-axis view at a basal level with color flow Doppler demonstrating a perimembranous VSD (*red arrow*). *RV* right ventricle, *RA* right atrium, *LVOT* left ventricular outflow tract

Persistent Left Superior Vena Cava (SVC)

Approximately 0.5% of the population has a persistent left SVC, which drains into the coronary sinus 90% of the time. It is uncommonly

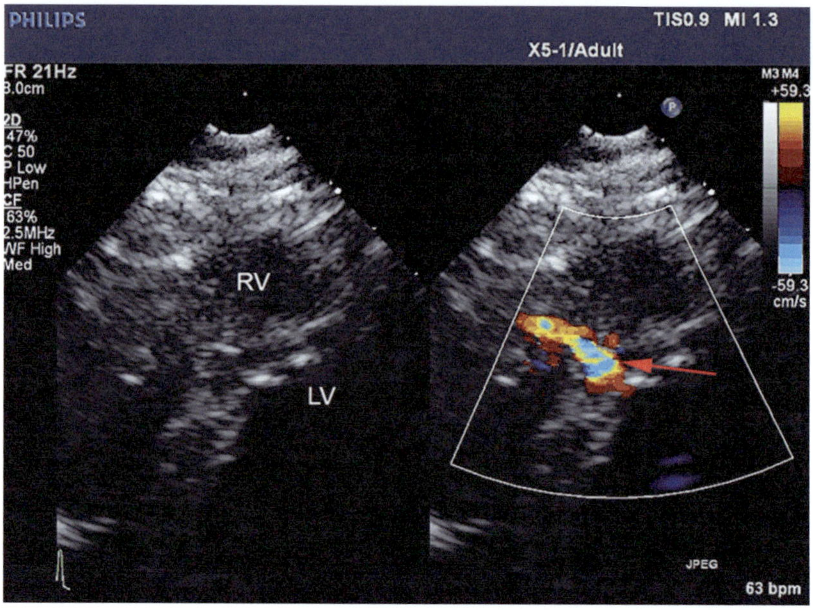

Fig. 18.12 Apical four-chamber view with an RV focus, zoomed perspective on interventricular septum with color compare feature (two-dimensional image on left; color flow Doppler applied on the right). Color flow Doppler demonstrates a muscular VSD (*red arrow*). *RV* right ventricle, *LV* left ventricle

associated with an absent right SVC. During embryologic development, there are two superior vena cavae. Normally the left-sided SVC regresses with blood from the internal jugular (IJ) and left subclavian returning to the heart via the innominate vein. In the setting of a persistent left SVC, the left IJ and subclavian typically return blood flow to the heart via the left SVC into the coronary sinus. In its presence, central venous cannulae and pacemakers can take an abnormal orientation. In cardiac surgery, retrograde cardioplegia can prove ineffective and venous cannulation strategies may need to be adjusted.

The coronary sinus can be imaged by pushing the probe in from a ME four-chamber view, a modified bicaval view, or in the posterior atrioventricular groove on the ME two-chamber view (Fig. 18.13 and Video 18.11). Dilatation of the coronary sinus (> 10 mm in diameter) should arouse suspicion for a persistent left SVC. Other causes such as elevated right atrial pressures from heart failure, atresia or stenosis of the ostium, or a coronary artery fistula to the coronary sinus are alternative causes for coronary sinus dilatation and should be evaluated as well. The suspicion can then be confirmed with agitated saline injection into the left upper extremity and resultant

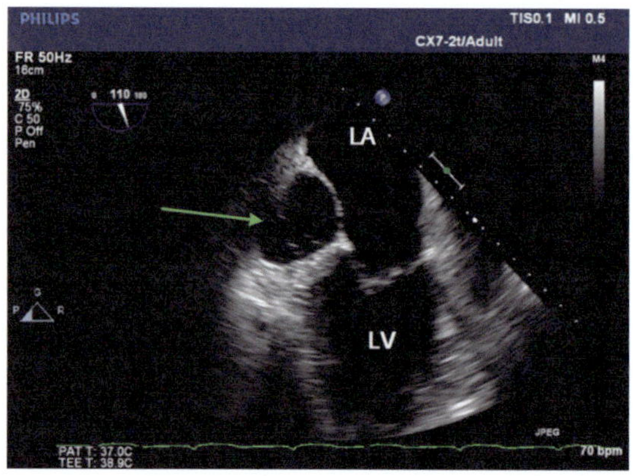

Fig. 18.13 Midesophageal two-chamber view with the dilated coronary sinus (*green arrow*) in cross section to the posterior aspect of the top of the left ventricle in a patient with a persistent left superior vena cava. *LA* left atrium, *LV* left ventricle

coronary sinus opacification. A large coronary sinus and its drainage into the right atrium have been mistaken for an ASD in some patients, and this makes thorough imaging essential [11]. The principles of identification and characterization for this condition remain similar with TTE and require agitated saline injection into the left arm resulting in opacification of the coronary sinus prior to the right atrium. Visualization of a dilated coronary sinus is done in the parasternal long-axis view (where it lies adjacent to the posterior mitral annulus) [12].

Patent Ductus Arteriosus/ Aorticopulmonary Window

The ductus arteriosus is a vascular communication between the proximal descending aorta and the main or the left pulmonary artery in its roof. It closes spontaneously after birth but can persist to adulthood in rare cases causing a left-to-right shunt. It is usually a co-incidental finding picked up due to a murmur that leads to echocardiography [13]. Echocardiography is helpful not only to diagnose the lesion but also to evaluate the shunt magnitude and volume load, estimate pulmonary artery pressures, and identify associated cardiac pathology. Some patients may present with endarteritis (endocarditis of the ductus), which is responsible for almost half of the deaths in adult patients with a patent ductus arteriosus (PDA) [14]. The pulmonary side of the ductus is more commonly the site of infection. The patent ductus can be closed either surgically or with a transcatheter device with excellent results. Upper esophageal views have been used to visualize a PDA, with nonstandard orientation of the multiplane angles. Since the connection between the aortic isthmus and the main pulmonary artery (PA) hides anterior to the left mainstem bronchus, it is often difficult to visualize with TEE. The demonstration of flow abnormality in the PA using color flow Doppler is excellent supportive evidence, but by itself not diagnostic of a PDA. Proper parallel alignment of the Doppler beam with the flow is even more difficult. It is important to note the FiO_2 during the shunt calculation since hyperoxia leads to reduction in PA pressures and an increase in the shunt [14]. Using a transthoracic approach, the PDA is imaged from the parasternal short-axis view at the base of the heart, suprasternal long-axis view, and high left parasternal long-axis views. Detailed description of the techniques is outside the scope of this text and can be found elsewhere [15]. The aorticopulmonary window represents a more proximal communication between the ascending aorta and the PA and can be easier to visualize with TEE. Hemodynamic consequences tend to be similar to a PDA.

Transesophageal Echocardiographic Evaluation of Tetralogy of Fallot (Highlight Box 18.3)

Highlight Box 18.3

Tetralogy of Fallot	
2D	• Pulmonic stenosis ◦ Narrowed RVOT in ME RV inflow-outflow or PSAX view
	• Right ventricular hypertrophy ◦ Measure in ME or apical four-chamber view • Overriding aorta ◦ Observed in ME LAX or PLAX view • Ventricular septal defect ◦ Typical perimembranous VSD in ME AV SAX or PSAX view
CFD	• Presence of interventricular flow ◦ May or may not be turbulent (dependent on VSD size) • Turbulence in RVOT/pulmonary artery
Spectral	• Calculate pulmonary to systemic flow ratio (Qp/Qs) • Estimate pulmonary arterial systolic pressure (TR jet)

RVOT right ventricular outflow tract, *ME* mid-esophageal, *RV* right ventricular, *PSAX* parasternal short-axis, *LAX* long-axis, *PLAX* parasternal long-axis view, *VSD* ventricular septal defect, *TR* tricuspid regurgitation

Classically, tetralogy of Fallot (ToF) patients manifest a VSD, pulmonic stenosis, an overriding aorta, and RV hypertrophy. Addition of an ASD makes it a pentalogy (present in about a third of cases). Multiple other congenital cardiac lesions can accompany a ToF, such as right aortic arch, systemic venous abnormalities, and LVOT obstruction, among others. Most patients require surgery early in life due to cyanosis from right-to-left shunt; thus patients that survive into adulthood generally have little RV obstruction. The goals of echocardiography should include (apart from confirming the diagnosis) quantification of the RV obstruction, VSD shunt magnitude, and direction and detection of associated anomalies.

The large, perimembranous VSD is best seen in the ME aortic valve LAX or SAX views. The defect is located between the right and the noncoronary cusps of the aortic valve. This generally permits shunt interrogation by Doppler (either color or spectral). The entire septum should be carefully interrogated to rule out additional defects. The ME aortic valve LAX view can also demonstrate the aortic override, which can be variable in presentation. In the post-repair adult, the repair of the VSD using a patch still permits identification of the override (Fig. 18.14 and Video 18.12). Involvement of the aortic valve, either as part of the primary lesion or during repair, needs to be carefully evaluated.

Manipulation of the multiplane angle from either the ME aortic valve LAX or ME right ventricular inflow-outflow view can be used to interrogate the RV outflow tract (RVOT). Obstruction is suggested (using color flow Doppler) by the presence of aliasing and turbulence in the RVOT. Transgastric views can be used to examine the RVOT as well. These views can help detect abnormalities of the pulmonic valve, if present. RV wall thickness can be measured in the ME right ventricular inflow-outflow to quantify the hypertrophy. Interrogation of the RV outflow and the pulmonary artery with 2D, color flow Doppler, and spectral Doppler is helpful after repair since stenosis can persist and even worsen as the patient continues to grow into adulthood.

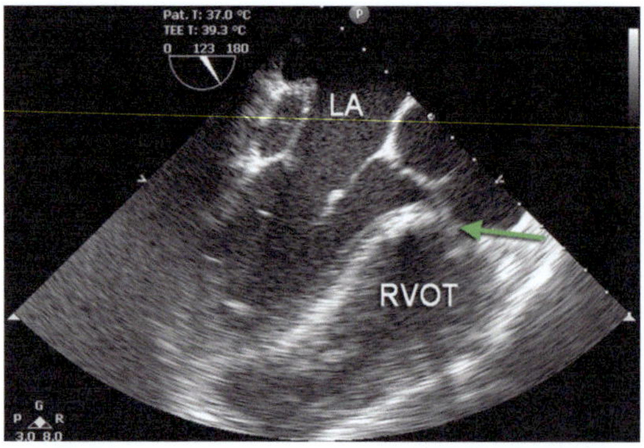

Fig. 18.14 Midesophageal long-axis view in a patient with tetralogy of Fallot after VSD repair. Note the overriding aorta (*green arrow*) that remains and the evidence of right ventricular hypertrophy. Incidentally, there is a dilated coronary sinus resulting from a persistent left-sided superior vena cava. *LA* left atrium, *RVOT* right ventricular outflow tract

After repair, left and right ventricular outflow obstruction and valvular regurgitation remain the focus. Assessment of RV systolic pressure, size, and function is vital to the exam. Tricuspid and pulmonic regurgitation is not uncommon, and their quantification can be useful for future comparison.

Transthoracic Echocardiographic Examination of Tetralogy of Fallot

Noninvasive fetal echocardiography can detect ToF as early as at 14 weeks of gestation. In early childhood, TTE is invaluable in the diagnosis and follow-up of ToF. The subcostal views (long- and short-axis) are utilized to evaluate the atrial septum and connections in the heart at the level of the valves. They can also help in assessing the VSD, RVOT obstruction, and potential ASDs. An apical four-chamber view can visualize both the atrioventricular valves and the VSD. The parasternal long-axis view is the best to identify the type of VSD and the degree of the aortic override (Fig. 18.15 and Video 18.13). The aorta overrides the VSD by less than 50% of the aortic diameter

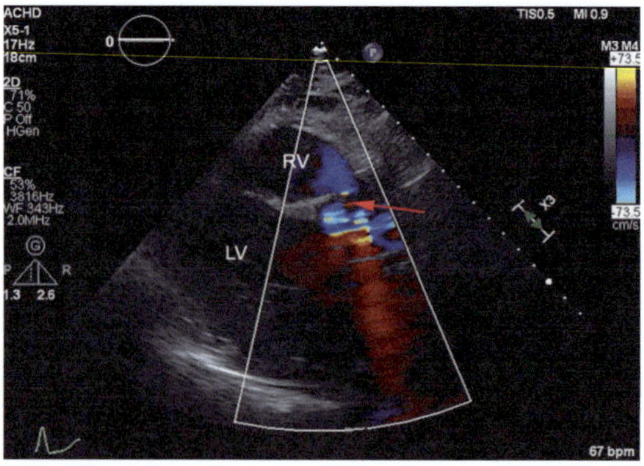

Fig. 18.15 Parasternal long-axis view in a patient with tetralogy of Fallot. The *red arrow* indicates the overriding aorta and a perimembranous VSD detected on color flow Doppler. *RV* right ventricle, *LV* left ventricle

in ToF, whereas the override is more than 50% in double-outlet right ventricle. The parasternal short-axis view can provide information regarding the coronary arterial configuration, VSD margins, and the RVOT anatomy. The suprasternal view is vital to assess the right- or left-sidedness of the aortic arch, as well as visualizing the branching from the aortic arch [16].

Conclusion

With more congenital heart disease patients now surviving longer, these patients will increasingly require clinical management related to or unrelated to their heart. Echocardiography has remained the cornerstone of diagnosing and managing these conditions. The basic echocardiographer should be familiar with and able to recognize simple congenital heart disease. Complex lesions should involve consultation with an advanced echocardiographer. Perioperative TEE or point-of-care TTE can provide useful information about the real-time monitoring of ventricular filling, myocardial performance, and identification of intra-cardiac shunting, in addition to optimization of hemodynamic management strategies.

Questions

1. Which of the following views provides the best visualization to detect shunt across a patent foramen ovale?

   A. Apical four-chamber view
   B. Transgastric midpapillary short-axis view
   C. Midesophageal bicaval view
   D. Midesophageal AV long-axis view

2. Which of the following is the most common kind of ventricular septal defect?

   A. Perimembranous
   B. Inlet
   C. Outlet
   D. Muscular

3. Which of the following congenital conditions in adults are amenable to device closure?

   A. Sinus venosus ASD
   B. Patent ductus arteriosus
   C. Complete AV cushion defect
   D. Situs inversus

4. Which of the following is a reason to use a Valsalva maneuver during a bubble study to detect a patent foramen ovale?

   A. To increase the turbulence of the blood across a shunt
   B. To induce a right-to-left shunt
   C. To enable positioning of the echo probe closer to the interatrial septum
   D. To reduce transit time of the echo contrast to reach the atrium

5. A 25-year-old woman is diagnosed with a ventricular septal defect, moderate tricuspid regurgitation, and no other valvular abnormalities. The peak velocity across the VSD is measured at 4 m/s. Her right atrial pressure (or CVP) is 4 mmHg, and her systolic BP is 110/70 mmHg. What is the peak systolic pulmonary pressure?

   A. 46 mmHg
   B. 50 mmHg
   C. 64 mmHg
   D. 94 mmHg

6. Which of the following is most true regarding restrictive VSDs?

   A. Compared to a nonrestrictive defect, they are easier to detect using 2D imaging.
   B. Reduction in the Nyquist limit using color flow Doppler aids in detection.

C. Restrictive VSDs are generally less severe than nonrestrictive defects.
D. Restrictive VSDs exhibit non-turbulent flow.

7. In the midesophageal bicaval view, following release of a Valsalva maneuver, which of the following would be expected regarding flow through a patent foramen ovale?

A. Flow should be toward the probe and the right side of the display.
B. Flow does not occur due to closure of the flap between the septum secundum and septum primum.
C. Flow is more difficult to detect with the color scale reduced to 30 cm/s.
D. Flow can only be detected with bubble contrast.

8. Which of the following conditions does not result in the dilation of the coronary sinus?

A. Unroofed coronary sinus
B. Persistent left SVC
C. Severe right ventricular pressure or volume overload
D. Presence of a Eustachian valve

9. Which of the following is most true regarding detection of VSDs with echocardiography?

A. Transthoracic views are not sensitive for small VSDs.
B. A low Qp/Qs indicates that there is a right-to-left shunt.
C. Bubble studies are generally not used for detection due to the risk for air emboli.
D. Flow is usually right to left.

10. Which of the following describes an ostium primum ASD?

A. It is the most common type of ASD.
B. It results from failure of fusion between the septum primum and the septum secundum.
C. It is the result of incomplete fusion between the septum primum and the endocardial cushion.
D. It is a communication between the ostium primum and the ostium secundum.

References

1. Miller-Hance WC, Russell IA. Intraoperative and postoperative transesophageal echocardiography in congenital heart disease. In: Wong PC, Miller-Hance WC, editors. Transesophageal echocardiography for congenital heart disease [Internet]. Springer London; 2014 [cited 2015 Jan 4]. p. 383–97. Available from: http://link.springer.com/chapter/10.1007/978-1-84800-064-3_15.
2. Webb G, Mulder BJ, Aboulhosn J, Daniels CJ, Elizari MA, Hong G, et al. The care of adults with congenital heart disease across the globe: current assessment and future perspective: a position statement from the International Society for Adult Congenital Heart Disease (ISACHD). Int J Cardiol [Internet]. [cited 2015 May 8]; Available from: http://www.sciencedirect.com/science/article/pii/S016752731500964X.
3. Hara H, Virmani R, Ladich E, Mackey-Bojack S, Titus J, Reisman M, et al. Patent foramen ovale: current pathology, pathophysiology, and clinical status. J Am Coll Cardiol. 2005;46(9):1768–76.
4. Craig RJ, Selzer A. Natural history and prognosis of atrial septal defect. Circulation. 1968;37(5):805–15.
5. Martin SS, Shapiro EP, Mukherjee M. Atrial septal defects – clinical manifestations, echo assessment, and intervention. Clin Med Insights Cardiol. 2015;8(Suppl 1):93–8.
6. Minette MS, Sahn DJ. Ventricular septal defects. Circulation. 2006;114(20):2190–7.
7. Kamran M, Attari M, Webber G. Ventricular septal defect complicating an acute myocardial infarction. Circulation. 2005;112(22):e337–8.
8. Ishii M, Hashino K, Eto G, Tsutsumi T, Himeno W, Sugahara Y, et al. Quantitative assessment of severity of ventricular septal defect by three-dimensional reconstruction of color Doppler–imaged vena contracta and flow convergence region. Circulation. 2001;103(5):664–9.
9. Backer CL, Winters RC, Zales VR, Takami H, Muster AJ, Benson DWJ, et al. Restrictive ventricular septal defect: how small is too small to close? Ann Thorac Surg. 56(5):1014–9.
10. Deri A, English K. EDUCATIONAL SERIES IN CONGENITAL HEART DISEASE: echocardiographic assessment of left to right shunts: atrial septal defect, ventricular septal defect, atrioventricular septal defect, patent arterial duct. Echo Res Pract. 2018;5(1):R1–16.

11. Sarodia BD, Stoller JK. Persistent left superior vena cava: case report and literature review. Respir Care. 2000;45(4):411–6.
12. Irwin RB, Greaves M, Schmitt M. Left superior vena cava: revisited. Eur Heart J Cardiovasc Imaging. 2012;13(4):284–91.
13. Wiyono SA, Witsenburg M, de Jaegere PPT, Roos-Hesselink JW. Patent ductus arteriosus in adults. Neth Heart J. 2008;16(7–8):255–9.
14. Rigby ML. Closure of a large patent ductus arteriosus in adults: first do no harm. Heart. 2007;93(4):417–8.
15. Snider AR, Serwer GA. Echocardiography in pediatric heart disease; 1990.
16. Bedair R, Iriart X. EDUCATIONAL SERIES IN CONGENITAL HEART DISEASE: tetralogy of fallot: diagnosis to long-term follow-up. Echo Res Pract. 2018;6(1):R9–23.

Part III

Critical Care Ultrasonography

19 Abdominal and Vascular Ultrasound

Kenneth Chen, Christopher R. Tainter, Ian Joel, and Gabriel Wardi

Abbreviations

ARDS	Acute (Adult) respiratory distress syndrome
CT	Computed tomography (scan)
CXR	Chest x-ray
DVT	Deep vein thrombosis
eFAST	Extended-Focused Assessment with Sonography in Trauma (exam)
FAST	Focused Assessment with Sonography in Trauma (exam)
LUQ	Left upper quadrant
PE	Pulmonary embolism
POCUS	Point-of-care ultrasound
RUQ	Right upper quadrant
SFJ	Saphenofemoral junction

Supplementary Information The online version of this chapter (https://doi.org/10.1007/978-3-030-84349-6_19) contains supplementary material, which is available to authorized users.

K. Chen
Department of Medicine, Division of Pulmonary, Critical Care, and Sleep Medicine, University of California San Diego Health, La Jolla, CA, USA
e-mail: gwardi@health.ucsd.edu

C. R. Tainter
Department of Anesthesiology, University of California San Diego Health, La Jolla, CA, USA

I. Joel
Department of Medicine, Los Robles Regional Medical Center, Thousand Oaks, CA, USA

G. Wardi (✉)
Department of Emergency Medicine and Department of Medicine, Division of Pulmonary, Critical Care, and Sleep Medicine, University of California San Diego Health, La Jolla, CA, USA
e-mail: gwardi@health.ucsd.edu

Introduction

Point-of-care ultrasound (POCUS) has established itself as a rapid, safe, and accurate diagnostic modality applicable to the care of critically ill patients. While many uses of POCUS exist in the acute care environment, scanning protocols for unexplained hypotension are based on some of the most well-established applications of ultrasound. In this chapter, we focus on three POCUS examinations relevant to the care of critically ill patients: the Focused Assessment with Sonography in Trauma (FAST) examination, detection of deep vein thrombosis (DVT), and evaluation of the abdominal aorta.

Focused Assessment with Sonography for Trauma (Highlight Box 19.1)

Background

One of the earliest uses of POCUS was for the detection of hemoperitoneum and hemopericardium in patients with blunt traumatic injuries [1].

T. M. Maus, C. R. Tainter (eds.), *Essential Echocardiography*,
https://doi.org/10.1007/978-3-030-84349-6_19

Highlight Box 19.1

Focused assessment with sonography in trauma (FAST)	
2D	• Evaluation for free peritoneal fluid (hemoperitoneum) ∘ Anechoic/hypoechoic area in hepatorenal space (right) ∘ Anechoic/hypoechoic area in splenorenal space (left) ∘ Anechoic/hypoechoic area in rectovesical (male) or rectouterine (female) space • Evaluation for pericardial fluid/ tamponade (hemopericardium) ∘ Anechoic area surrounding RA/RV ∘ Evaluate for chamber collapse
	• Evaluation for pleural fluid (hemothorax) ∘ Anechoic area above diaphragm noted in RUQ/LUQ views • M-mode assessment for pneumothorax with eFAST exam ∘ Absence of lung sliding and lung pulse
CFD	• Typically not utilized
Spectral	• Typically not utilized

Abbreviations: *RA* right atrium, *RV* right ventricle, *RUQ* right upper quadrant, *LUQ* left upper quadrant

The Focused Assessment with Sonography for Trauma (FAST) exam gained acceptance as a rapid and noninvasive alternative to diagnostic peritoneal lavage to help prioritize imaging and the need for operative management in hemodynamically unstable patients with blunt abdominal trauma. The original FAST examination included four views: a subxiphoid pericardial view, a right upper quadrant view, a left upper quadrant view, and a suprapubic view (Fig. 19.1). A “positive” FAST indicates free fluid in the peritoneum or pericardial space, presumed to be blood in the acute trauma patient. The sensitivity of the FAST examination is acceptable (69–98%), which increases with the volume of the fluid present, and it is highly specific (94–100%) for detection of free fluid in the peritoneum [2, 3]. More recently, the “extended FAST” (eFAST) has been described, which includes additional thoracic views to evaluate for pneumothorax and pleural effusion (hemothorax). The FAST is also a component of various ultrasound protocols to evaluate for undifferentiated hypotension. In this chapter, we focus on the abdominal components of the original FAST examination, as lung evaluation with ultrasound is described in detail in Chap. 21, and pericardial effusion is described in Chap. 14.

Anatomy

The FAST examination relies upon free fluid accumulation in gravity-dependent regions of the peritoneum and pelvis. While the pelvis is the most dependent space in the abdominopelvic space, the most dependent peritoneal space in the supine position is the hepatorenal space. The peritoneum is a serous membrane that lines the abdominal cavity and covers the abdominal and pelvic organs and normally contains a trace amount of free fluid to allow for the movement of internal organs. It does not contain retroperitoneal structures, such as the abdominal aorta or kidneys. The peritoneal cavity consists of the greater and lesser peritoneal sacs. The greater peritoneal sac contains two compartments: the supramesocolic (upper peritoneal) space and inframesocolic (lower peritoneal) space, which are separated by the transverse mesocolon. The right peri-colic gutter allows for free fluid to traverse from the supramesocolic to inframesocolic space, and vice versa, based on a patient’s position. The phrenicocolic ligament prevents fluid movement from the supramesocolic to inframesocolic space via the left peri-colic gutter, shunting free fluid from the perisplenic space to the hepatorenal space, rather than to the pelvis.

Epidemiology and Pathophysiology

An estimated 2.8 million Americans are hospitalized for injury each year [4]. Furthermore, approximately 214,000 people die each year from injury, which remains the number one cause of death in persons 1–44 years old in the United States [4]. Hemorrhage resulting from abdominal and thoracic injuries remains a common mechanism for death in these patients. In critically ill

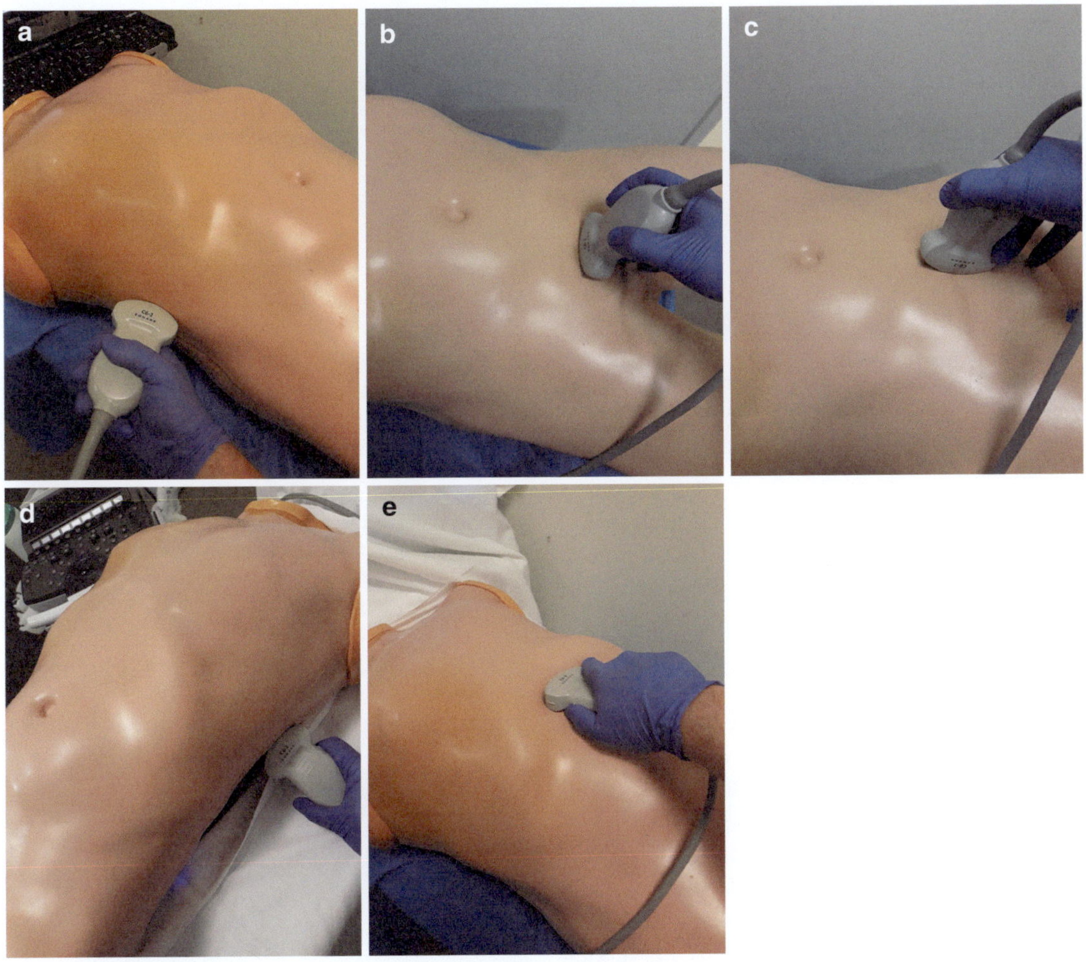

Fig. 19.1 Probe positions for the original FAST examination. The four views include the right upper quadrant view (**a**), with the probe in a coronal plane along the right mid-axillary line, with the indicator pointing cephalad; the supra-pubic view, with the probe immediately above the pubic symphysis, in axial (**b**) and sagittal (**c**) planes, with the indicator pointing to the patient's right and cephalad, respectively; the left upper quadrant view (**d**), with the probe in a coronal plane along the left posterior-axillary line, with the indicator pointing cephalad; and the subcostal view (**e**), with the probe in the subxiphoid position, in a modified axial plane, fanned cephalad, and the indicator pointing to the patient's right

patients without traumatic injury, hemorrhage into the peritoneum (e.g., ruptured ectopic pregnancy or inferior hypogastric artery laceration during paracentesis) is an uncommon but important cause of undifferentiated hypotension.

Ultrasound Technique

The abdominal FAST examination consists of an evaluation of three potential locations in the peritoneum: the right upper quadrant, the left upper quadrant, and the pelvis (Fig. 19.1). Using a low frequency (1–5 MHz) phased-array or curvilinear probe is recommended. Patients can be positioned in the supine position or angled (e.g., Trendelenburg when scanning the right and left upper quadrant or reverse Trendelenburg when evaluating the pelvis) to increase the sensitivity for free fluid. A subcostal view of the heart is the fourth and final view in the FAST exam and is intended to evaluate for hemopericardium. An

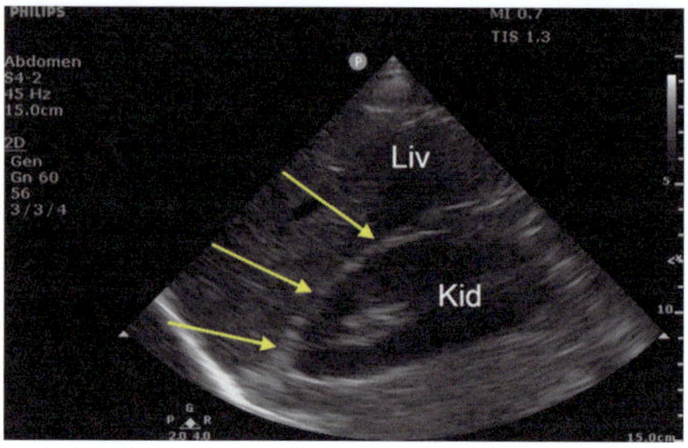

Fig. 19.2 A normal right upper quadrant view. The *yellow arrows* indicate the hepatorenal potential space (Morison's pouch), between the liver (Liv) and right kidney (Kid), without anechoic fluid seen

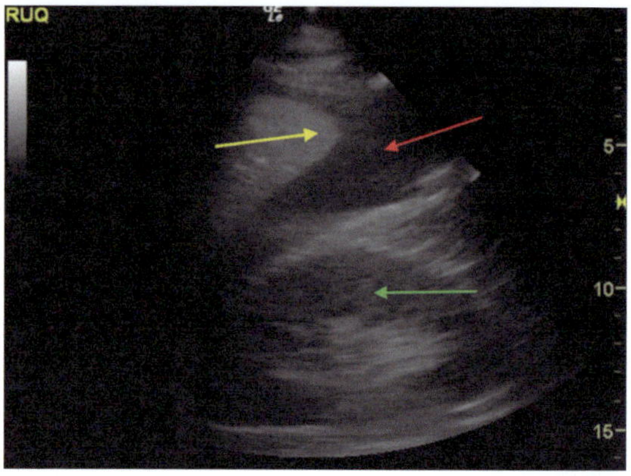

Fig. 19.3 An abnormal right upper quadrant view from a positive FAST exam. The *yellow arrow* indicates the inferior pole of the liver, which should always be visualized when examining the right upper quadrant, because intra-abdominal fluid tends to accumulate in this area before propagating to other potential spaces. The *red arrow* indicates anechoic/hypoechoic free fluid and a positive FAST exam. The kidney is visualized in the far field (*green arrow*)

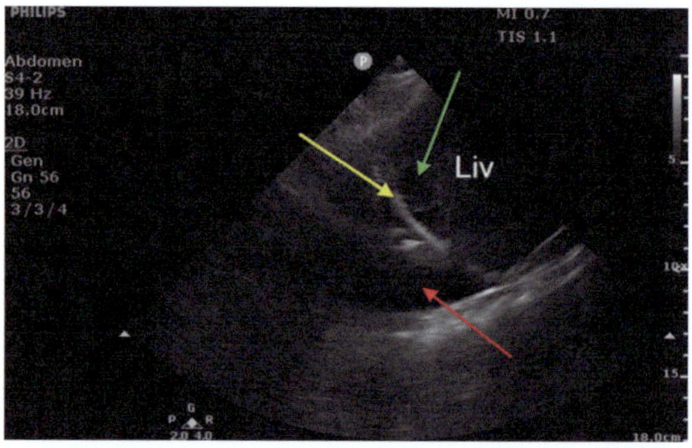

Fig. 19.4 An abnormal right upper quadrant view from a positive FAST exam, showing anechoic fluid both above and below the diaphragm (*yellow arrow*), representing free fluid in the abdomen (*green arrow*), and in the chest (*red arrow*)

extended FAST (eFAST) exam also includes evaluation for pneumothorax via the anterior chest and hemothorax via the posterolateral chest.

Right Upper Quadrant

The RUQ is typically the preferred initial site for detection of peritoneal free fluid, as the liver serves as a convenient acoustic window to evaluate the perihepatic and hepatorenal space. It is also the most sensitive region to evaluate for free fluid in some studies [5]. Three locations should be assessed from the right upper quadrant: the hepatorenal space (Morison's pouch), the subdiaphragmatic space, and the inferior pole of the right kidney. The transducer should be placed between the 9th and 11th rib spaces in the mid-axillary line, with the probe indicator pointing to the patient's head. The angle should be adjusted until the hepatorenal space is found (Fig. 19.2, Video 19.1), which sometimes may also necessitate moving up or down into a different rib space, depending on the patient's anatomy. Next, the imaging plane is fanned from anterior to posterior to ensure that small pockets of free fluid are not missed (Fig. 19.3, Video 19.2). The probe is moved cephalad to evaluate the area between the dome of the liver and diaphragm and above the diaphragm to evaluate for hemothorax (Fig. 19.4, Video 19.3). Finally, slide the probe caudally to evaluate the inferior pole of the right kidney and paracolic gutter. In addition to free peritoneal fluid, it may be possible to visualize solid organ injury to the liver or right kidney from this view.

Left Upper Quadrant

Three locations should be evaluated in the LUQ: the splenorenal space, the left subdiaphragmatic space, and the inferior pole of the left kidney. The splenorenal space is more posterior and superior than the hepatorenal space, which can be visualized by placing the transducer, with the indicator towards the patient's head, between the sixth and ninth rib along the posterior axillary line to identify this region (Fig. 19.5, Video 19.4). Slide or angle the probe cranially to evaluate for fluid in the space just below or above the diaphragm, identifying the tip of the spleen. Finally, slide or angle the probe caudally to evaluate the inferior pole of the left kidney.

Pelvis

Free fluid in the pelvis can be reliably found in the rectovesical space in males and the rectouterine space (pouch of Douglas) in females. A full bladder provides an excellent acoustic window and improves the ability to detect free fluid. The probe is placed over the pubic symphysis, with indicator to the patient's right, and fanned caudally to identify the bladder in the axial plane (Fig. 19.6, Video 19.5). Once this has been accomplished, fan the probe to evaluate the entire bladder for any evidence of free fluid in the rectovesical or rectouterine space. Next, rotate the probe 90 degrees clockwise into a sagittal plane, scanning from the patient's right to left (Fig. 19.7, Video 19.6). This improves the sensitivity to detect a small amount of pelvic fluid, which may be obscured by posterior acoustic enhancement from a full bladder.

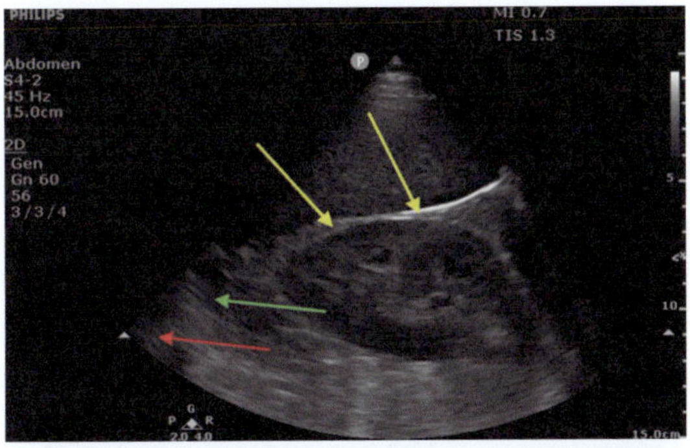

Fig. 19.5 A normal left upper quadrant view. The *yellow arrows* indicate the splenorenal potential space. The *green arrow* indicates the subdiaphragmatic potential space, and the *red arrow* indicates the pleural space above the diaphragm. The subdiaphragmatic space should always be interrogated when examining the LUQ, since fluid tends to accumulate early at this location in the left upper quadrant

Subcostal (Subxiphoid) View

The fourth area of investigation during a FAST exam is the pericardium, evaluated from a subxiphoid window, with the same technique as a subcostal four-chamber view (Chap. 3). A focus is on evaluation for hemopericardium and possible tamponade, but some assessment of cardiac function or hypovolemia can also be made from this view (Fig. 19.8, Video 19.7).

Image Interpretation

The minimum amount of free fluid in the abdomen that the FAST exam is able to detect has been reported as low as 100 mL, although this depends on patient positioning, operator experi-

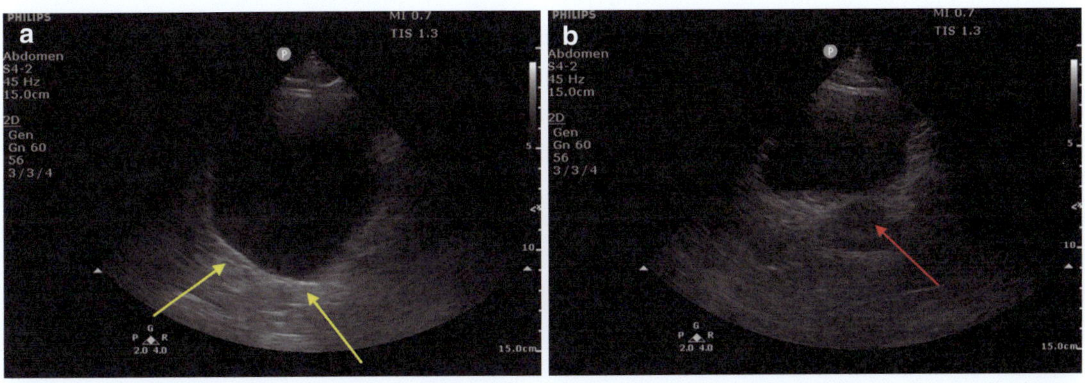

Fig. 19.6 (**a**) A normal suprapubic view, showing a distended bladder in an axial plane, with the probe indicator pointing to the patient's right. The brighter signal deep to the bladder is caused by posterior acoustic enhancement (*yellow arrows*). (**b**) An axial view of the pelvis with the probe fanning more inferiorly. The *red arrow* indicates the prostate in a transverse view, which is sometimes mistaken for pelvic free fluid

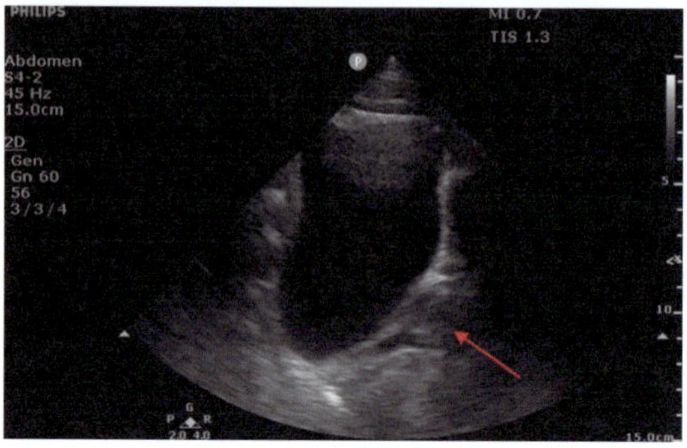

Fig. 19.7 The bladder in a sagittal view with the probe indicator pointing cephalad. In this view, the prostate (*red arrow*) is better recognized as a circular, midline structure posteroinferior to the bladder

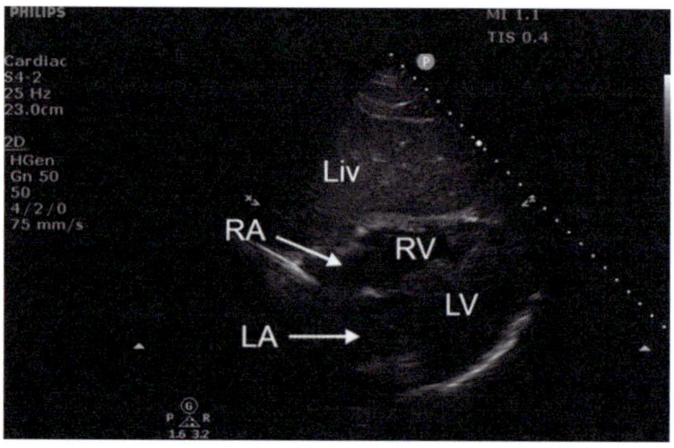

Fig. 19.8 A subcostal four-chamber view of the heart during a FAST exam. The right atrium (RA) and right ventricle (RV) can be seen adjacent to the liver (Liv), and the left atrium (LA) and left ventricle (LV) can be seen in the far field. There is no evidence of pericardial effusion

ence, and the rate of fluid accumulation [6]. While it is possible to miss a small volume of fluid initially, serial exams increase sensitivity as more blood volume accumulates, and the exam is very sensitive to a hemodynamically significant volume of hemorrhage (> 500 mL). Thus, if a patient is too unstable to perform CT, FAST can reliably exclude hemoperitoneum as the cause for the hemodynamic instability. In addition, FAST does not reliably exclude subtle solid organ injuries or hollow viscous injuries. Therefore, CT is the preferred test for a stable patient with suspected intraabdominal injuries.

Free fluid in the abdomen appears anechoic and ultrasound cannot differentiate between blood, ascitic fluid, peritoneal dialysate, or urine. Rarer etiologies of peritoneal free fluid leading to false-positive FAST examinations include large-volume fluid resuscitation (resulting in hydrostatic translocation of fluid into the peritoneum), ventriculoperitoneal shunt presence, ruptured ovarian cysts, and ovarian hyperstimulation syndrome. Females of reproductive age may have up to 50 mL of physiologic free fluid in the recto-uterine space that is not pathologic. Perinephric fat, which widens the splenorenal and hepatorenal space, can also result in a false-positive interpretation. Coagulated blood has mixed echogenicity, which may result in errors in interpretation due to the lack of an anechoic appearance, especially after a delayed presentation. A hematocrit sign (layering of separated blood layers) may also be visible. Often, complex fluid collections (infected ascites, purulent material) have septations or visible debris, and potentially layering, which should prompt providers to strongly consider paracentesis for definitive diagnosis.

Deep Venous Thrombosis (Highlight Box 19.2)

Highlight Box 19.2

Deep venous thrombosis (DVT)	
2D	• Direct visualization of thrombus • Compression evaluation of common femoral vein/saphenofemoral junction and popliteal vein ∘ Non-compression without visualization = fresh thrombus ∘ Non-compression with visualization of clot = older organized thrombus
CFD	• Confirmation of arterial and venous flow
Spectral	• Evaluation for proximal respirophasic variation • Evaluation for augmentation of flow with distal compression

Background

Deep vein thrombosis (DVT) is a major cause of morbidity and mortality in critically ill patients. It has an incidence rate ranging between 5% and

15%, despite the presence of thromboprophylaxis [7]. Clinician-performed point-of-care ultrasound (POCUS) allows timely recognition and management of DVT. It has been shown that POCUS assessment of DVT can be performed rapidly and accurately by bedside clinicians, with up to 96% of sensitivity and specificity with relatively little training [8, 9].

Anatomy

Lower Extremity Veins

Peripheral veins in the extremities (Fig. 19.9) can be divided into deep veins and superficial veins. Deep veins are accompanied by arteries, while superficial veins are not. The common femoral vein becomes the external iliac vein proximally as it passes the inguinal ligament, and the deep venous system in the lower extremities starts at this point. The common femoral vein is joined by the great saphenous vein (a superficial vein) at the saphenofemoral junction (SFJ). Further distally, the common femoral vein is created at the junction of the deep femoral vein (also known as profunda femoris) and femoral vein (previously called the superficial femoral vein, but new nomenclature has eliminated "superficial" to avoid confusion, as it is a deep vein). Distal to the adductor canal, the femoral vein is contiguous with the popliteal vein, posterior to the knee joint. The popliteal vein receives tributaries from three deep veins immediately below the knee. The deep venous system proximal to the trifurcation of the popliteal vein is considered "proximal," while distal to this landmark is referred to as the "distal" deep venous system. Below the knee, the deep venous system can be divided into axial veins (the "true deep veins") and muscular veins (also collectively called "sural veins"). Below-the-knee axial veins include the anterior tibial vein, posterior tibial vein, and peroneal vein. Deep vein thromboses in these veins bear a higher risk of propagation into proximal DVT compared with the muscular veins. Below-the-knee muscular veins include the gastrocnemius and soleal veins. Deep vein thromboses in these veins are considered to be of less clinical significance due to a lower probability of propagation and higher rates of spontaneous resolution, although some sources still recommend treatment.

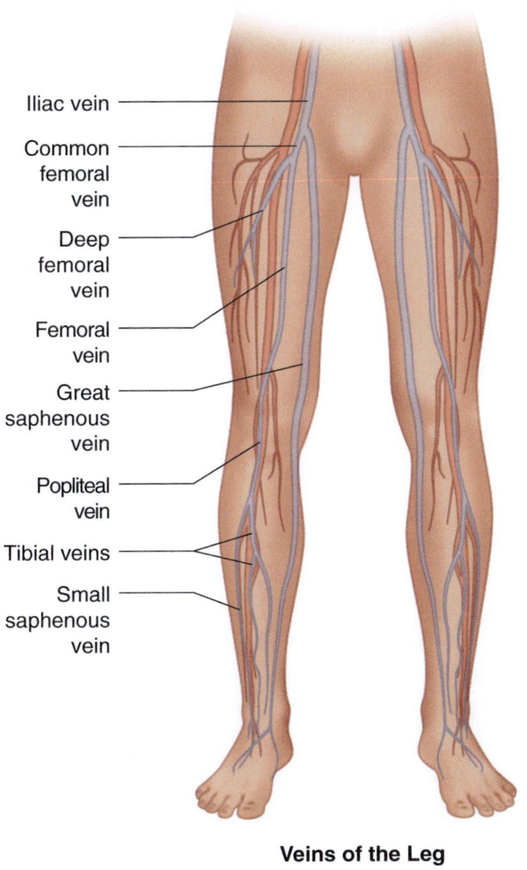

Fig. 19.9 Anatomy of lower extremity venous system

Upper Extremity Veins

The deep venous system in the upper extremities starts proximally at the confluence of the internal jugular and subclavian veins (Fig. 19.10). The subclavian vein is contiguous with the axillary vein after it passes the later border of the first rib. The axillary vein receives the drainage from the cephalic vein (a superficial vein) and originates distally at the inferior aspect of the teres minor muscle, at the confluence of the brachial vein (a deep vein) and basilic vein (a superficial vein). The brachial vein, basilic vein, and cephalic vein are all common access sites for peripherally inserted central catheters (PICCs). Catheter-

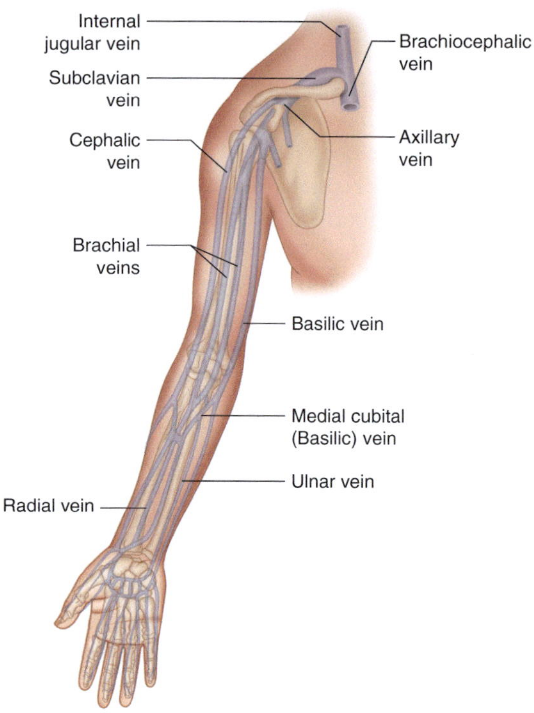

Fig. 19.10 Anatomy of the upper extremity venous system

associated thromboses at these sites carry a risk of propagation into a proximal DVT. Distally, the brachial vein starts at the confluence of the radial and ulnar veins, which are considered the "distal" deep veins of the upper extremity.

Pathophysiology and Epidemiology

Virchow's triad described three major risk factors for venous thromboembolism (VTE): venous stasis, endothelial injury, and hypercoagulability. Other predisposing conditions for VTE include indwelling catheters or devices, infection (e.g., Lemierre's syndrome), inflammatory conditions and vasculitis (e.g., Buerger's disease), and anatomical obstruction (e.g., thoracic outlet syndrome). About 260,000 cases of DVT are diagnosed in the US annually, and 90% are in the lower extremities. Up to 60% of untreated DVTs progresses to pulmonary embolism (PE).

Proximal DVTs are treated with therapeutic anticoagulation, with a duration determined by risk factors and the clinical scenario. For isolated below-the-knee (distal) DVT, The American College of Chest Physicians (ACCP) guideline recommends serial surveillance over 2 weeks, if asymptomatic [10]. However, anticoagulation may be considered for patients with risk factors for propagation: multiple vein involvement, length greater than 5 cm, diameter greater than 7 mm, location close to proximal deep veins, or the presence of persistent non-modifiable VTE risk factors. Superficial venous thromboses (also called superficial thrombophlebitis) are often managed conservatively with anti-inflammatory medications. However, accumulating epidemiologic data suggest that superficial venous thromboses originating within 3–5 cm of the saphenofemoral junction, or those greater than 5 cm in length, have a higher risk of propagation. The ACCP guideline for antithrombotic therapy suggests treating these with anticoagulation for 45 days [10]. For patients who were found to have superficial venous thromboses, studies have shown a prevalence of 18–50% with concurrent DVT, and 5–6.9% of these patients also had PE [11–14]. Male gender, a history of cancer or VTE, and the absence of varicose vein are risk factors for developing complications from superficial venous thromboses.

Ultrasound Technique

In the early 2000s, a two-point scanning technique was most commonly used for its simplicity and speed. The two-point technique interrogates only the common femoral and popliteal veins and reported a sensitivity of 89% and a specificity of 76%, compared with color duplex scanning in the vascular laboratory [15]. However, newer data reported a 4.6–22% rate of missed DVT with the two-point method and recommended a three-point exam, evaluating the common femoral and saphenofemoral junction (SFJ), femoral vein (formerly known as superficial femoral vein), and popliteal vein (Fig. 19.11). A prospective study demonstrated a significant increase in sensitivity with the three-point technique compared to using only two

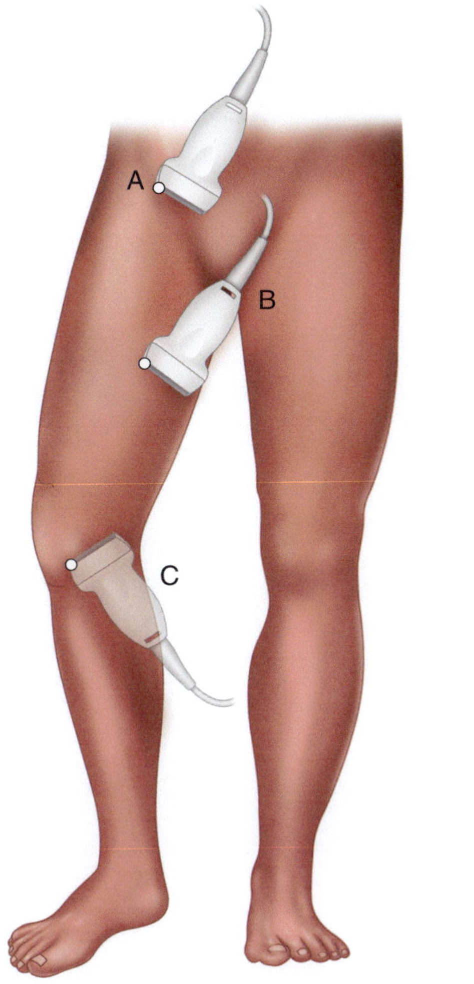

Fig. 19.11 The three-point lower extremity compression ultrasound to evaluate for DVT. The points of interrogation are (**a**) the common femoral and saphenofemoral junction (SFJ), (**b**) the femoral vein (formerly known as the superficial femoral vein), and (**c**) the popliteal vein. Note that the probe should be perpendicular to the skin during compression

points [16]. To further improve sensitivity, some clinicians advocate tracing the femoral vein with compression ultrasonography as far distally as possible and tracing the popliteal vein to the level of its trifurcation. It is conceivable that more comprehensive methods will have higher sensitivity, but complexity and the time burden must be balanced when it is performed by bedside clinicians. It is recommended to perform the three-point technique at a minimum, with visualization of the remainder of the proximal deep vein, if possible.

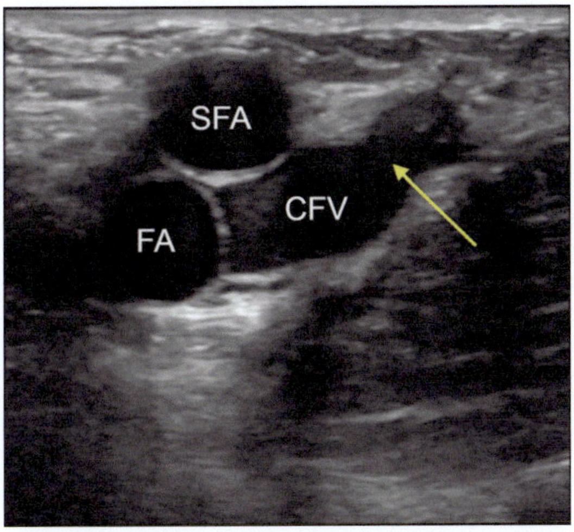

Fig. 19.12 Ultrasound imaging of the lower extremity vessels in the proximal right leg, showing the normal anatomy of the superficial femoral artery (SFA), femoral artery (FA), and common femoral vein (CFV) at the saphenofemoral junction (*yellow arrow*). Note that the arterial walls appear thicker, and the outline of arteries are typically more rounded compared with the adjacent veins

To perform the three-point DVT exam of the lower extremities, position the patient's hip with slight flexion, external rotation, and abduction to expose the inguinal area, with the knee slightly flexed to access the popliteal vein. A 20- to 30-degree reverse Trendelenburg position may be used to engorge the veins of the lower extremity, but this is not required. A high-frequency linear array probe should be used, although rarely a curvilinear probe may be necessary to visualize very deep veins in an obese patient. The probe should be maintained perpendicular to the skin to best define the vessel walls, with the veins imaged along their short axis.

Sweeping the probe along the length of vessels allows serial cross-sectional images to identify anatomical landmarks and distinguish arteries (deeper, thicker walled, pulsatile, and often with calcification in older patients) from veins (Fig. 19.12). At each site, identify the vessel of interest and apply gentle but firm pressure. Compress until the anterior and posterior wall of the vein are in contact with each other. The venous lumen should be completely obliterated before the arterial lumen is deformed by compression. Videos 19.8 and 19.9 provide examples of deep vein thromboses in the common femoral vein and popliteal vein, respectively. Older clots typically appear hyperechoic, whereas fresh clots appear hypoechoic or even anechoic. A noncompressible anechoic lumen represents the presence of a thrombus (Fig. 19.13).

When performing compression ultrasound, there are some pitfalls that may yield false-positive results. Enlarged lymph nodes can appear as a noncompressible, hyperechoic, and round structure with or without a hypoechoic

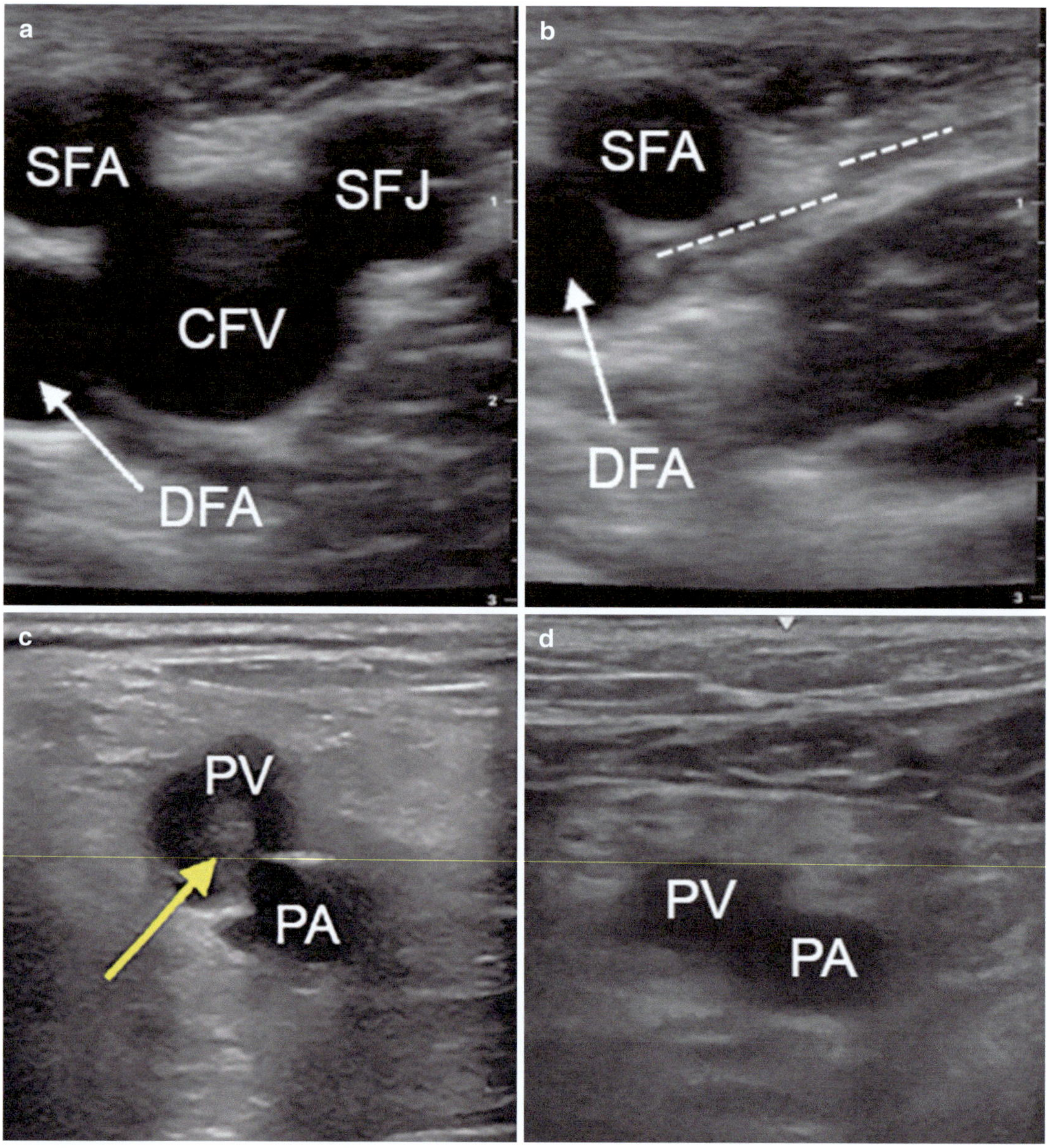

Fig. 19.13 Compression ultrasonography of the lower extremity. (**a**) Normal anatomy of the common femoral vein (CFV), saphenofemoral junction (SFJ), superficial femoral artery (SFA), and deep femoral artery (DFA). (**b**) The same location, but with application of compression, showing normal obliteration of the CFV and SFJ when there is no clot present (dotted lines). (**c**) A popliteal vein (PV) clot with echogenicity, likely an older clot. (**d**) A noncompressible PV with an anechoic clot, likely a fresher clot. Fresh anechoic clot can be identified through a properly performed compression examination, not by direct visualization. (With permission from Sukhdeep Singh, M.D.)

ring. Enlarged lymph nodes can be distinguished from veins by sliding the probe proximally and distally and seeing that they are not congruent with a blood vessel. Other situations that may be mistaken for DVT include inadequate compression, hematoma, abscess, Baker's cyst, and superficial venous thrombosis.

Color Doppler can be superimposed on 2D (B-mode) imaging to assess if the interrogated lumen is fully filled by color signals (Fig. 19.14). If the interrogated segment is not completely filled with Doppler signal, there is likely thrombus obstructing part or all of the lumen. When interrogating with Doppler signal, the sonographer should adjust the angle of insonation (Fig. 19.15) to less than 90 degrees (fan the probe closer to the skin), so that the Doppler shift produced by blood flow can be more reliably detected as flow toward or away from the transducer (see Chap. 4). Augmentation of blood flow by manually compressing the distal limb may also be used to increase the Doppler signal.

Pulsed-wave Doppler can also be used to evaluate the presence of spontaneous flow, respiratory phasicity, and augmented flow in response to manual distal limb compression to ensure vessel patency in the areas not directly visualized. Again, adjust the angle of insonation to less than 90 degrees to improve accuracy of the Doppler shift measurement, and place the sampling gate within the lumen of the vessel of interest. Respiratory variation should be apparent in veins all the way

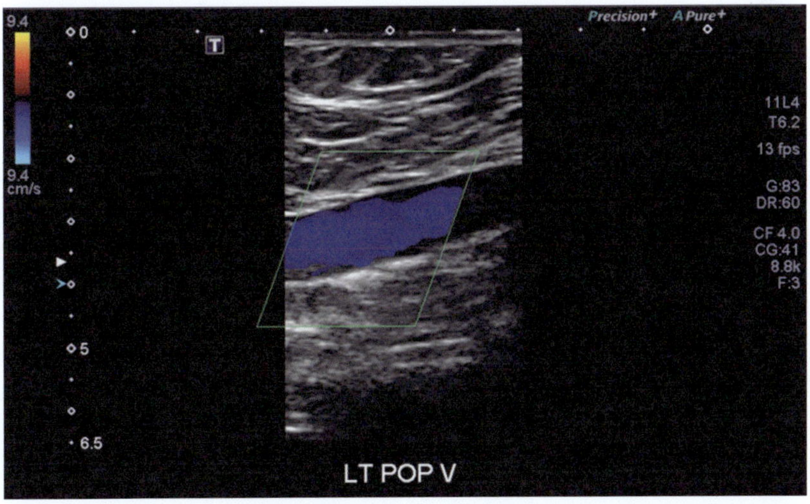

Fig. 19.14 Color Doppler assessment for deep vein thrombosis. The left popliteal vein is interrogated with color Doppler in longitudinal view. The lumen is completely filled with color, indicating vessel patency in the interrogated segment

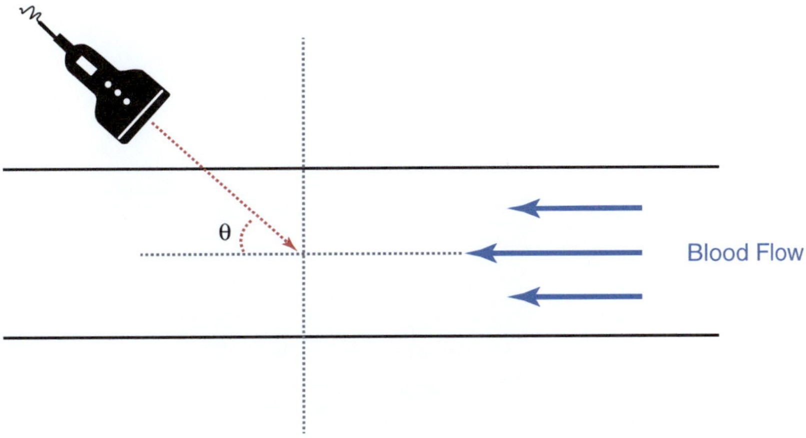

Fig. 19.15 Angle of insonation of the ultrasound beam. The angle of insonation is the angle between the ultrasound bean and the direction of the velocity of interest. The angle should be less than 60 degrees so that the velocity measurement is not significantly underestimated

distally until the popliteal fossa (Fig. 19.16). If respiratory variation is not seen, it raises suspicion for a more proximal thrombus. Similarly, flow variation should be observed with compression of the distal extremity (Fig. 19.16). If absent, this raises concern for a segmental thrombus distal to the image.

Differentiation Between Acute and Chronic Deep Vein Thromboses

In critically ill patients with a history of DVT, it may be difficult to differentiate between acute DVT and chronic venous scarring with ultrasound. Multiple findings are suggestive of acute venous thrombosis: (1) intraluminal material that is deformable during compression, (2) dilatation of the vein, and (3) smooth intraluminal material or a free tail floating proximally from the attachment of the clot on the vein wall [17]. Over time, acute DVTs may evolve with ultrasonographic signs of chronic scarring. These findings are largely dependent on the evolution of the thrombus, including lysis, thrombectomy, or embolic phenomena. Residual thrombosis may form chronic scarring and is more likely to be firmly adherent to the wall of the vein.

Abdominal Aorta (Highlight Box 19.3)

Highlight Box 19.3

Abdominal aorta	

2D	• Short-axis and long-axis imaging
	  ∘ Evaluation of size (aneurysm detection)
	  ∘ Observation for undulating intimal flap (aortic dissection)
	• Aortic rupture is often difficult to identify

CFD	• Confirmation of arterial flow • Differentiation between aortic lumen and thrombosis • Differentiation between true and false lumens
Spectral	• Typically not utilized

Background

Abdominal aortic pathology is an uncommon but devastating cause of morbidity and mortality. The most catastrophic is the ruptured abdominal aortic aneurysm (AAA), which carries an overall mortality rate exceeding 90% [18]. Unfortunately, ruptured AAAs are initially misdiagnosed in almost one-third of cases [19, 20]. Importantly, the detection of AAA with POCUS can be done

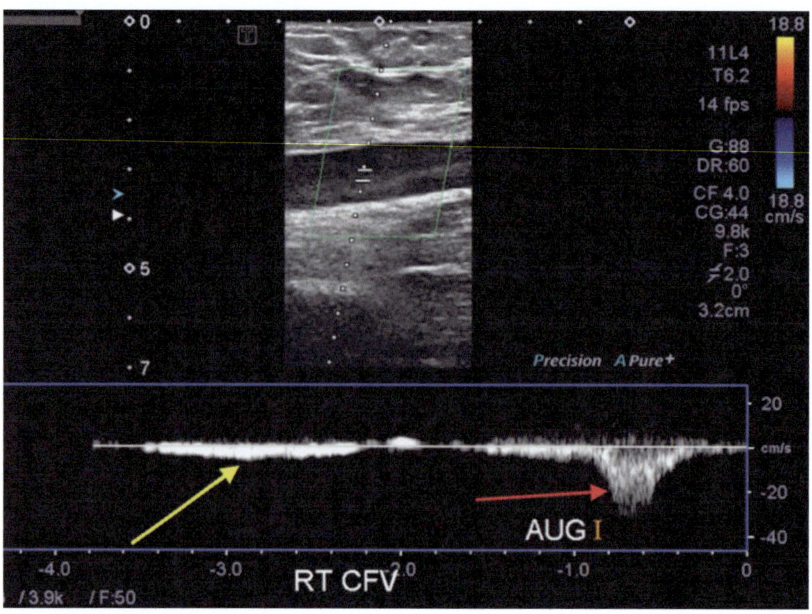

Fig. 19.16 Pulsed-wave Doppler interrogation for deep vein thrombosis. The right common femoral vein is interrogated in a longitudinal view with the pulsed-wave Doppler sample volume (gate) in the center of the lumen. The *yellow arrow* shows spontaneous venous flow with respiratory phasicity (proximally). The *red arrow* shows an augmented flow in response to manual limb compression (distally). The findings indicate patency of the vessel proximal and distal to the interrogated segment, respectively

rapidly by non-radiologists with a pooled sensitivity and specificity or 97.5% and 98.9%, respectively [21]. Abdominal aortic dissection may also be detected with POCUS, although with a significantly lower sensitivity. Abdominal aortic assessment has become an integral part of ultrasound protocols designed for rapid assessment of patients with undifferentiated shock and hypotension.

Anatomy

The abdominal aorta is a retroperitoneal structure that enters the abdomen through the posterior diaphragm just below the xiphoid process at the level of the 12th thoracic vertebra and bifurcates into the left and right common iliac arteries around the umbilicus at the level of the 4th lumbar vertebra. The aorta gives off a predictable series of branches (Fig. 19.17) as it descends through the abdomen. The first major branch is the celiac trunk, followed by the superior mesenteric artery (SMA), the left and right renal arteries, and finally branches of the gonadal and inferior mesenteric arteries. The celiac trunk divides into three vessels: the splenic artery, the common hepatic artery, and the left gastric artery. However, only the splenic artery and common hepatic artery are typically visualized with ultrasound. The SMA branches anteriorly from the aorta and then turns to run inferiorly parallel and anterior to the aorta. While the left and right renal arteries may sometimes be visualized with ultrasound, the gonadal and inferior mesenteric arteries, as well as the many smaller aortic branches, are not typically seen.

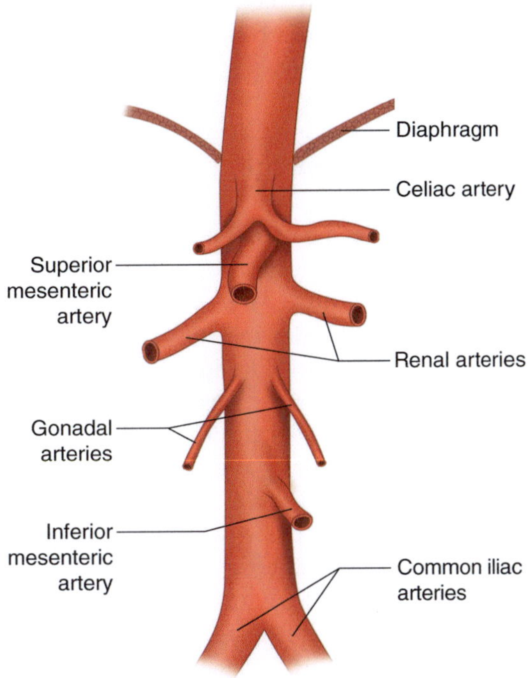

Fig. 19.17 Anatomy of the abdominal aorta and its major branches

Epidemiology and Pathophysiology

Abdominal aortic aneurysms are common in the general population, with an overall prevalence of approximately 3% in women and 4.7% in men [22]. Risk factors include male gender, white race, a history of smoking, pulmonary vascular disease, increased age, and family history [23]. A higher risk of AAA *rupture*, on the other hand, is found in females, hypertensive patients, smokers, and aneurysmal diameter of greater than 5.5 cm [24, 25]. Signs and symptoms that raise suspicion for AAA with potential rupture are abdominal pain, flank pain, back pain, a pulsatile abdominal mass on exam, and undifferentiated hypotension.

In most adults, the average diameter of the abdominal aorta is approximately 2 cm in diameter from outer wall to outer wall, and it tapers distally, although this varies by age, sex, and body habitus. A measured diameter of greater than 3 cm is considered aneurysmal, and likewise any aorta that fails to taper distally should be considered aneurysmal as well. The most common type of aneurysm encountered is a fusiform aneurysm, which represents dilatation of the entire circumference of the aneurysmal segment. The other type of aneurysm that may be encountered is the saccular aneurysm, which appears as a saclike asymmetric outpouching of an aortic segment. Saccular aneurysms may be more easily missed if the scanning technique is not methodical and comprehensive in both planes. Both types of aneurysms occur much more commonly below the level of the renal arteries [26].

Ultrasound Technique

The patient should be positioned to optimize the view of the abdominal aorta by ensuring they are laying supine with their hips and knees slightly flexed to relax the abdominal musculature. Bowel gas often interferes with portions of the scan, and this can be managed by applying firm steady downward pressure with the probe or by using the probe to directly move bowel aside. If initial visualization is still not optimized, consider lowering the frequency of the probe, which may allow for better visualization of deeper structures.

The exam typically starts at the proximal abdominal aorta by placing either the phased array probe (1–5 MHz) or the curvilinear probe (2–5 MHz) in an axial orientation, just below the xiphoid process in the center of the abdomen, with the probe indicator pointed to the patient's right. This produces a transverse (short-axis) view of the aorta, which should be identified as the anechoic circular structure immediately anterior and slightly to the left of the vertebral body (Fig. 19.18). The vertebral body should be the most posterior structure on the screen and will be noted by its intensely hyperechoic anterior surface which produces an anechoic shadow immediately posteriorly. The examiner should be cautious to not confuse the aorta with the inferior vena cava (IVC) which sits adjacent to the aorta but slightly to the right of midline. These structures can be further differentiated by the brighter, thicker walls and the presence of anterior branches of the aorta, and if needed, pulsed-wave and/or color flow Doppler. Once the aorta has been clearly identified in the transverse plane, it should be centered on the screen, and the probe then fanned or swept inferiorly down the abdominal wall in a methodical, contiguous fashion, sequentially identifying the celiac trunk (Fig. 19.19, Video 19.10), the SMA (Fig. 19.20), and the aortic bifurcation into the iliac arteries (Fig. 19.21, Video 19.11).

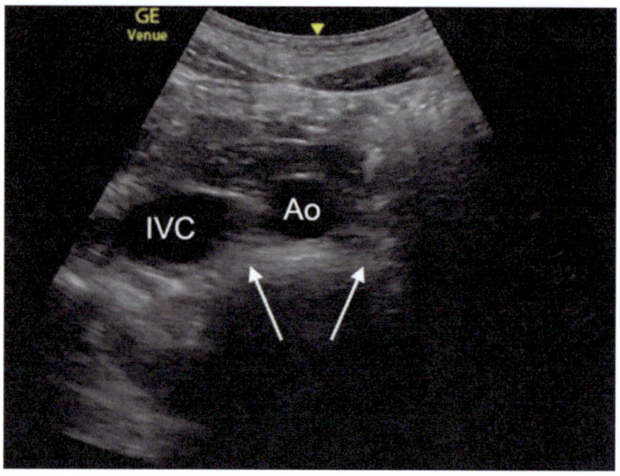

Fig. 19.18 Normal ultrasound imaging of the abdominal aorta in the axial plane just below the xiphoid process with the indicator pointing to the patient's right (left side of the image, by convention). The abdominal aorta (Ao) and inferior vena cava (IVC) are slightly anterior to the vertebral body (*white arrows*) at the level of upper abdomen, to the patient's left and right, respectively

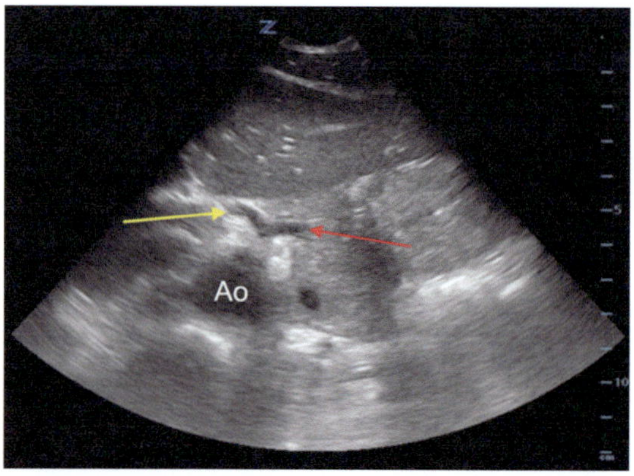

Fig. 19.19 An axial (short-axis) view of the proximal abdominal aorta (Ao), showing the celiac trunk as it bifurcates into the common hepatic artery (*yellow arrow*) and the splenic artery (*red arrow*), representing the "seagull sign"

It is crucial that the aortic diameter is measured in the transverse plane from outer wall to outer wall, so as not to underestimate the diameter by accidentally mistaking mural thrombus for the aortic wall (Fig. 19.22 and Video 19.12). Calipers should ideally be used to measure at the proximal, mid, and distal aorta without skipping any sections of the aorta during real-time visualization, which may overlook smaller or saccular aneurysms. Scanning in the axial plane is complete when the aorta is interrogated through the aortic bifurcation, as aneurysms may commonly extend into the iliac arteries.

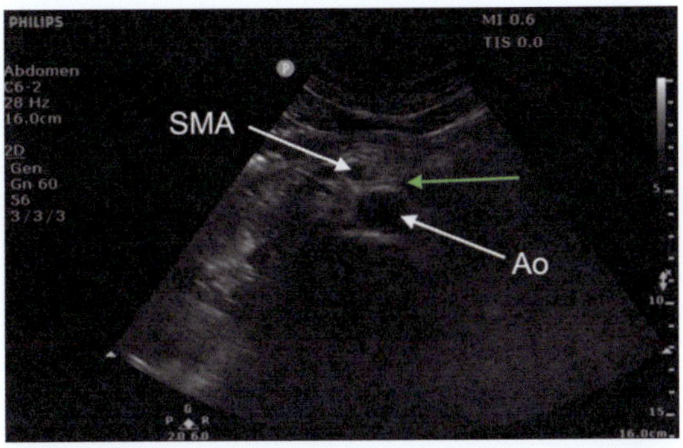

Fig. 19.20 An axial (short-axis) view of the abdominal aorta, showing the superior mesenteric artery (SMA) coursing anterior to the aorta (Ao). The left renal vein (*green arrow*) is typically between the SMA and aorta

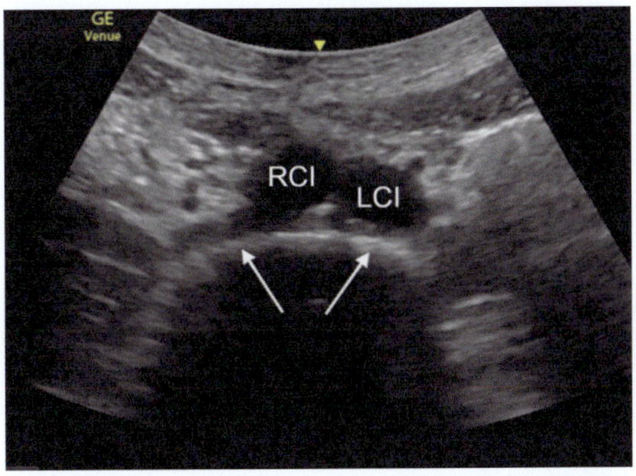

Fig. 19.21 An axial (short-axis) view of the abdominal aortic bifurcation into the left common iliac (LCI) and right common iliac (RCI) arteries, anterior to the L4 vertebral body (*white arrows*)

Next, interrogate the longitudinal plane of the aorta by placing the probe inferior to the xiphoid process and first centering the aorta on the screen in the transverse plane, as above. The probe should then be rotated clockwise so the indicator is oriented cephalad (Fig. 19.23, Video 19.13). Although calipers can be used to measure along the longitudinal plane, this plane is better-suited for visual inspection of aneurysms missed in the transverse plane, as scanning in the longitudinal plane is more prone to underestimation of diameter if inadvertently off-axis (the cylinder tangent effect, Fig. 19.24).

If usable diagnostic images of the abdominal aorta cannot be obtained anteriorly despite use of the troubleshooting techniques described above, the abdominal aorta can often be imaged laterally from the patient's left or right midaxillary line using either the liver or spleen as the acoustic window. However, it may be more challenging to acquire images in this plane due to the depth of imaging. To perform the exam in this fashion, the probe should be placed just below the costal margin with the probe marker oriented toward the patient's head. This will allow for interrogation of the aorta in the longitudinal plane. The probe can be rotated 90-degrees into an axial plane to obtain transverse views.

The risk of rupture of an aneurysm is directly related to its size. Referral to a vascular surgeon should be made for unruptured aneurysms greater

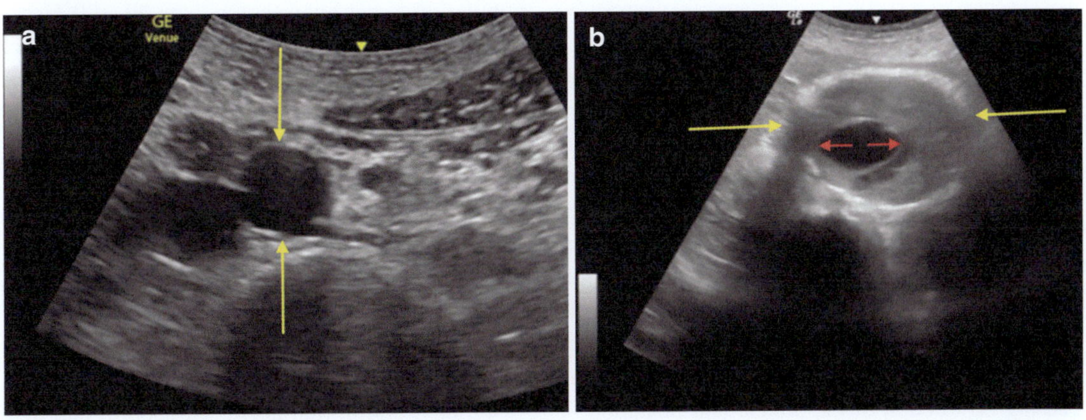

Fig. 19.22 The diameter of the abdominal aorta should always be measured from outer edge to outer edge. (**a**) A normal abdominal aorta measured from outer edge to outer edge (*yellow arrows*). (**b**) An abdominal aortic aneurysm with a large intramural hematoma. Measurement of only the inner diameter of the true lumen (*red arrows*) would significantly underestimate the size of the aortic aneurysm (*yellow arrows*)

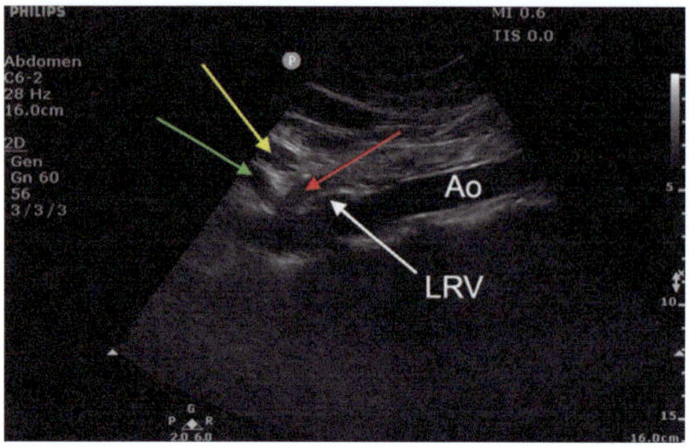

Fig. 19.23 A long-axis view of the descending abdominal aorta (Ao). The celiac artery (*green arrow*) and superior mesenteric artery (*red arrow*) originate anteriorly. The splenic vein (*yellow arrow*) and left renal vain (LRV) are visible in cross section

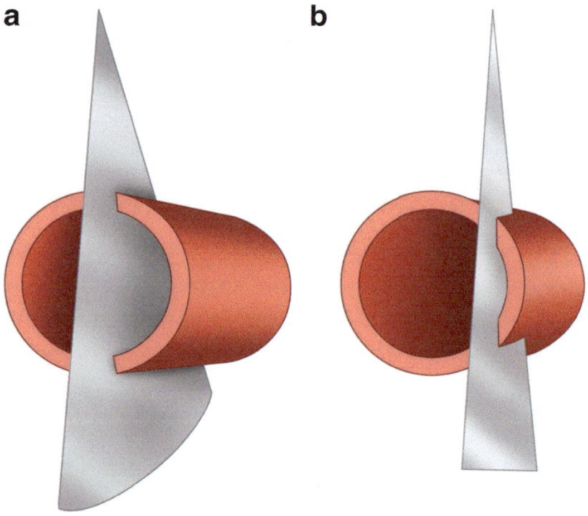

Fig. 19.24 The cylinder tangent effect. A longitudinal imaging plane that does not traverse the widest portion of the cylindrical vessel (**a**) will underestimate the diameter (**b**)

than 4 cm and are often followed for surveillance. Aneurysms with a diameter greater than 5.5 cm should undergo elective surgical repair without further surveillance, even without signs of rupture (Video 19.14). While ultrasound is quite sensitive for the detection of aneurysms, it is less sensitive for aneurysmal rupture, as these are most frequently retroperitoneal. They can be intraperitoneal, and the FAST examination can be used to identify intraperitoneal blood or, rarely, a retroperitoneal hematoma causing obstruction of the ureters and dilatation of the renal collecting system. If an AAA is identified in a patient with clinical symptoms, emergent vascular surgery consultation should be sought, with or without CT imaging, depending on patient stability.

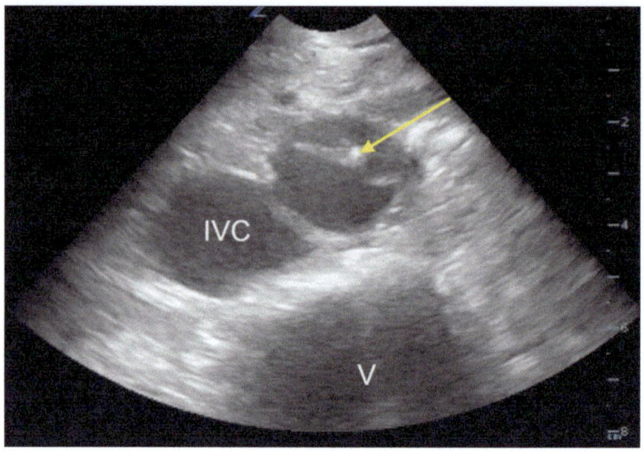

Fig. 19.25 This transverse (axial) view of the abdominal aorta shows an undulating intimal flap (*yellow arrow*) confirming the diagnosis of an aortic dissection. Also visible are an enlarged inferior vena cava (IVC) and a vertebral body (V). (With permission from Alex Anshus, MD and Dennis Liu, MD)

Aortic dissection, which is classified by involvement of the ascending (Stanford Type A) or isolated to the descending (Stanford Type B) thoracic aorta, is another aortic emergency that can be identified on abdominal aortic ultrasonography, by detecting the presence of a floating intimal dissection flap when it extends distally into the abdomen (Fig. 19.25 and Video 19.15). Identification of an intimal flap with ultrasonography should be confirmed in both the transverse and longitudinal plane since some artifacts may mimic its appearance. Typically, an undulating motion of the flap is observed, which is congruent with pulsatile blood flow. If an intimal flap is detected in a high-risk population, it has been shown to be 99–100% specific for dissection [27]. While the sensitivity of detecting a dissection flap when scanning only the abdominal aorta will be limited, in a recent study when abdominal, transthoracic, and suprasternal aortic scanning was integrated in high-risk patients, it achieved an 86.4% sensitivity, and a shorter time to diagnosis (10.5 vs. 79 minutes) [28]. If the suspicion for aortic dissection remains high despite negative ultrasonography, CT angiography or potentially TEE (for thoracic aortic dissections) should be pursued.

Finally, abdominal aortic ultrasound can also be used to guide and/or confirm placement of numerous intra-aortic cannulas or devices including intra-aortic balloon pumps, resuscitative endovascular balloon occlusion devices, and

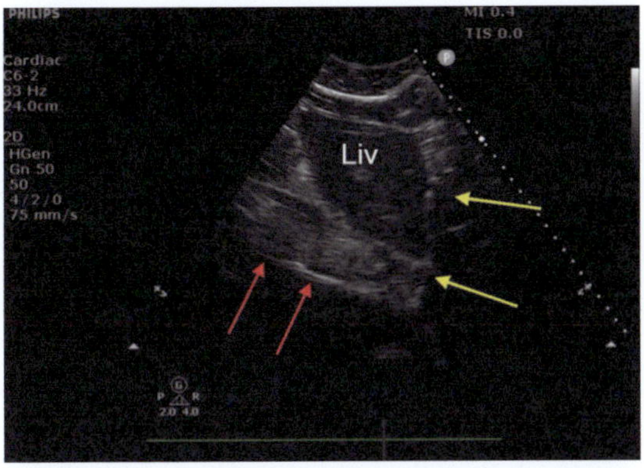

Fig. 19.26 Confirmation of an intra-aortic balloon pump (IABP) in the descending aorta by point-of-care ultrasound. The bright reflection from the air-filled IABP can be seen in the descending aorta to the left of the image (*red arrows*), deep to the liver (Liv), and below the diaphragm (*yellow arrows*)

extracorporeal membranous oxygenation (ECMO) cannulas (Fig. 19.26 and Video 19.16).

Conclusion

Abdominal and vascular applications of ultrasound are among the many important uses of POCUS in critically ill patients. In particular, the FAST exam, ultrasound assessment for DVT, and evaluation of the abdominal aorta can be done rapidly, and all have high sensitivity for certain life-threatening pathology. These examinations can be done as part of a protocol for undifferentiated hypotension, or individually as the clinical scenario dictates. Incorporation of these scanning techniques into the evaluation of unstable patients may decrease the time to diagnosis and help prioritize essential interventions.

Questions

1. A 67-year-old woman has been admitted to the ICU for acute hypoxemic respiratory failure requiring tracheal intubation and mechanical ventilation. Shortly after admission, the patient is noted to be febrile, tachycardic, and hypotensive. An ultrasound examination is performed, and free fluid is noted in the left upper quadrant. The following image in the left upper quadrant is obtained with a linear probe (Figure Q19-1). Which of the following is the MOST appropriate next step in management?

   A. Evaluate for other causes of the patient's hypotension
   B. Obtain a CT of the patient's abdomen
   C. Perform a diagnostic paracentesis and initiate intravenous antibiotics
   D. Transfer to the OR for operative intervention

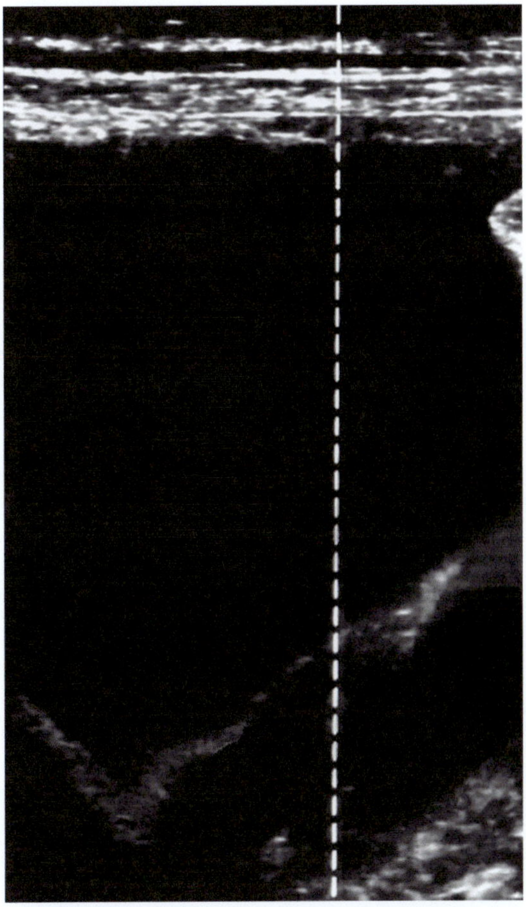

2. Which of the following best describes the test characteristics of the FAST examination for the detection of peritoneal free fluid?

   A. High specificity and high sensitivity
   B. Moderate specificity and high sensitivity

C. High specificity and moderate sensitivity
D. Moderate specificity and moderate sensitivity

3. A 34-year-old man presents to the trauma bay after being struck by a motor vehicle. His blood pressure is 83/43 mmHg and his heart rate is 112 beats per minute. Bruising is noted over the abdomen and pelvis. A FAST examination is performed, and the following image of the right upper quadrant is obtained (Figure Q19-3). Which is the next best step in the management of this patient?

   A. Evaluate for other causes of the patient's hypotension
   B. Obtain a CT of the patient's abdomen to evaluate for the source of bleeding
   C. Repeat the FAST examination in 30 minutes
   D. Transfer to the OR for operative intervention

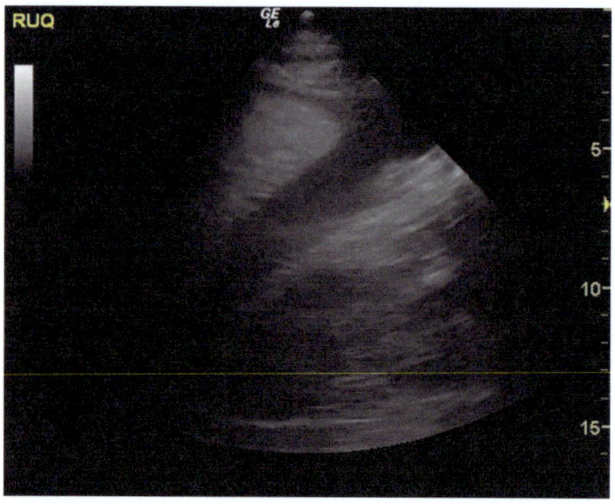

4. The FAST examination is best suited for detecting injury to which of the following?

   A. Aorta
   B. Diaphragm
   C. Hollow organs
   D. Solid organs

5. Which of the following can be managed by serial examinations (rather than therapeutic anticoagulation) in an asymptomatic patient?

   A. A thrombus in the distal one third segment of the femoral vein
   B. A thrombus in the great saphenous vein that is 3 centimeters away from the saphenofemoral junction
   C. A thrombus in the mid-segment of the soleal vein
   D. A thrombus in the popliteal vein that is proximal to the trifurcation

6. Which of the following maneuvers can augment blood flow to the desired region when using Doppler signal to perform a DVT examination?

   A. Place the patient in Trendelenburg position
   B. Apply firm compression with the ultrasound probe to narrow the proximal vein
   C. Squeeze the muscle bulk distal to the ultrasound probe
   D. Decrease Nyquist limit to amplify the Doppler signal

7. Where are the points of interrogation in the three-point compression ultrasonography protocol of the lower extremity DVT examination?

   A. Common femoral vein at the saphenofemoral junction, femoral vein, and popliteal vein
   B. Common femoral vein at the saphenofemoral junction, deep femoral vein, and popliteal vein
   C. Common femoral vein above the saphenofemoral junction, femoral vein, and popliteal vein
   D. Common femoral vein at the saphenofemoral junction, femoral vein, and deep femoral vein

8. Which of the following is true regarding the test characteristics of abdominal aortic ultrasonography for the diagnosis of aortic dissection?

   A. It is highly specific but not sensitive
   B. It is highly sensitive but not specific
   C. It is both highly sensitive and specific
   D. It is neither sensitive nor specific

9. Which type of abdominal aortic aneurysm would be MOST likely to be missed when failing to scan the aorta in both the transverse and longitudinal planes?

   A. Fusiform
   B. Saccular
   C. Obtuse
   D. All of the above

10. A patient is admitted for unexplained hypotension. A point-of-care ultrasound of the abdominal aorta is performed and reveals the following image (Figure Q19-10). Which of the following is the MOST appropriate next step in management?

    A. Immediate discussion with a vascular surgeon
    B. Computed tomography to better assess the aorta
    C. Evaluate for other causes of hypotension
    D. Outpatient referral with a vascular surgeon

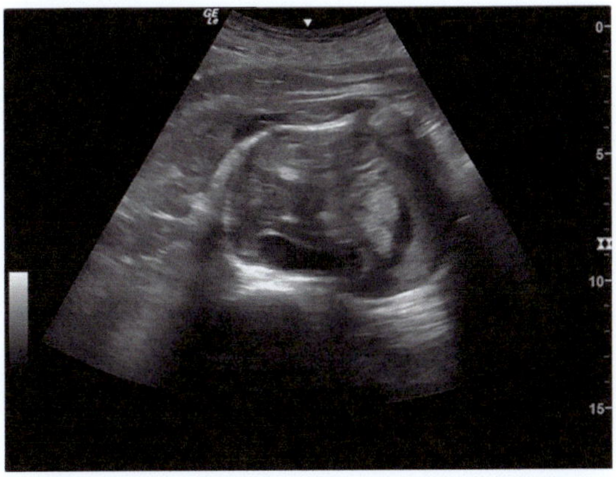

References

1. Kristensen JK, Buemann B, Kühl E. Ultrasonic scanning in the diagnosis of splenic haematomas. Acta Chir Scand. 1971;137:653–7.
2. Von Kuenssberg JD, Stiller G, Wagner D. Sensitivity in detecting free intraperitoneal fluid with the pelvic views of the FAST exam. Am J Emerg Med. 2003;21:476–8.
3. Pearl WS, Todd KH. Ultrasonography for the initial evaluation of blunt abdominal trauma: a review of prospective trials. Ann Emerg Med. 1996;27:353–61.
4. Web-based Injury Statistics Query and Reporting System (WISQARS) Nonfatal Injury Data: Centers for Disease Control and Prevention, National Center for Injury Prevention and Control. vol 20202017.
5. Lobo V, Hunter-Behrend M, Cullnan E, et al. Caudal edge of the liver in the right upper quadrant (RUQ) view is the most sensitive area for free fluid on the FAST exam. West J Emerg Med. 2017;18:270–80.
6. Branney SW, Wolfe RE, Moore EE, et al. Quantitative sensitivity of ultrasound in detecting free intraperitoneal fluid. J Trauma. 1995;39:375–80.
7. Boddi M, Peris A. Deep vein thrombosis in intensive care. Adv Exp Med Biol. 2017;906:167–81.
8. Burnside PR, Brown MD, Kline JA. Systematic review of emergency physician-performed ultrasonography for lower-extremity deep vein thrombosis. Acad Emerg Med. 2008;15:493–8.
9. Crisp JG, Lovato LM, Jang TB. Compression ultrasonography of the lower extremity with portable vascular ultrasonography can accurately detect deep venous thrombosis in the emergency department. Ann Emerg Med. 2010;56:601–10.
10. Kearon C, Akl EA, Ornelas J, et al. Antithrombotic therapy for VTE disease: CHEST guideline and expert panel report. Chest. 2016;149:315–52.
11. Frappé P, Buchmuller-Cordier A, Bertoletti L, et al. Annual diagnosis rate of superficial vein thrombosis of the lower limbs: the STEPH community-based study. J Thromb Haemost. 2014;12:831–8.
12. Decousus H, Quéré I, Presles E, et al. Superficial venous thrombosis and venous thromboembolism: a large, prospective epidemiologic study. Ann Intern Med. 2010;152:218–24.
13. Galanaud JP, Genty C, Sevestre MA, et al. Predictive factors for concurrent deep-vein thrombosis and symptomatic venous thromboembolic recurrence in case of superficial venous thrombosis. The OPTIMEV study. Thromb Haemost. 2011;105:31–9.
14. Di Minno MN, Ambrosino P, Ambrosini F, et al. Prevalence of deep vein thrombosis and pulmonary embolism in patients with superficial vein thrombosis: a systematic review and meta-analysis. J Thromb Haemost. 2016;14:964–72.
15. Wakai A. Emergency department compression ultrasound to diagnose proximal deep vein thrombosis. J Emerg Med. 2001;21:444–5.

16. Zuker-Herman R, Ayalon Dangur I, Berant R, et al. Comparison between two-point and three-point compression ultrasound for the diagnosis of deep vein thrombosis. J Thromb Thrombolysis. 2018;45:99–105.
17. Needleman L. Update on the lower extremity venous ultrasonography examination. Radiol Clin N Am. 2014;52:1359–74.
18. Ernst CB. Abdominal aortic aneurysm. N Engl J Med. 1993;328:1167–72.
19. Smidfelt K, Nordanstig J, Davidsson A, et al. Misdiagnosis of ruptured abdominal aortic aneurysms is common and is associated with increased mortality. J Vasc Surg. 2021;73(2):476–483.e3.
20. Marston WA, Ahlquist R, Johnson G Jr, et al. Misdiagnosis of ruptured abdominal aortic aneurysms. J Vasc Surg. 1992;16:17–22.
21. Concannon E, McHugh S, Healy DA, et al. Diagnostic accuracy of non-radiologist performed ultrasound for abdominal aortic aneurysm: systematic review and meta-analysis. Int J Clin Pract. 2014;68: 1122–9.
22. Bengtsson H, Sonesson B, Bergqvist D. Incidence and prevalence of abdominal aortic aneurysms, estimated by necropsy studies and population screening by ultrasound. Ann N Y Acad Sci. 1996;800:1–24.
23. Kent KC, Zwolak RM, Egorova NN, et al. Analysis of risk factors for abdominal aortic aneurysm in a cohort of more than 3 million individuals. J Vasc Surg. 2010;52:539–48.
24. Chaikof EL, Dalman RL, Eskandari MK, et al. The Society for Vascular Surgery practice guidelines on the care of patients with an abdominal aortic aneurysm. J Vasc Surg. 2018;67:2-77.e72.
25. Thompson AR, Cooper JA, Ashton HA, et al. Growth rates of small abdominal aortic aneurysms correlate with clinical events. Br J Surg. 2010;97:37–44.
26. Golledge J, Muller J, Daugherty A, et al. Abdominal aortic aneurysm: pathogenesis and implications for management. Arterioscler Thromb Vasc Biol. 2006;26:2605–13.
27. Fojtik JP, Costantino TG, Dean AJ. The diagnosis of aortic dissection by emergency medicine ultrasound. J Emerg Med. 2007;32:191–6.
28. Wang Y, Yu H, Cao Y, et al. Early screening for aortic dissection with point-of-care ultrasound by emergency physicians: a prospective pilot study. J Ultrasound Med. 2020;39:1309–15.

20 Volume Assessment and Fluid Responsiveness

Suraj Trivedi, Christopher R. Tainter, and E. Orestes O'Brien

Abbreviations

ASE	American Society of Echocardiography
CO	Cardiac output
CVP	Central venous pressure
HR	Heart rate
IVC	Inferior vena cava
LVEDP	Left ventricular end-diastolic pressure
LVOT	Left ventricular outflow tract
MAP	Mean arterial pressure
PCWP	Pulmonary capillary wedge pressure
PVV	Peak velocity variation
RAP	Right atrial pressure
SV	Stroke volume
SVR	Systemic vascular resistance
TEE	Transesophageal echocardiography
TTE	Transthoracic echocardiography
VTI	Velocity time integral

Supplementary Information The online version of this chapter (https://doi.org/10.1007/978-3-030-84349-6_20) contains supplementary material, which is available to authorized users.

S. Trivedi (✉) · C. R. Tainter · E. O. O'Brien
Department of Anesthesiology, University of California San Diego Health, La Jolla, CA, USA
e-mail: sutrivedi@health.ucsd.edu

Introduction

Echocardiography is an essential tool in the assessment and hemodynamic management of a critically ill patient, and assessment of preload and prediction of volume responsiveness is an integral component of this. The purpose of volume resuscitation is primarily to increase oxygen delivery to tissues through an increase in stroke volume, and thereby cardiac output. Cardiac output (CO) is the product of the stroke volume (SV) and the rate at which this volume is delivered (heart rate, HR):

$$CO = SV \times HR$$

The factors which influence the stroke volume are preload, afterload, and the intrinsic function of the heart (including contractility, valvular competency, and structural abnormalities).

The delivery of oxygen to tissues does not depend solely on cardiac output. Anemia, hypoxemia, and tissue edema can compromise oxygen delivery by decreasing the oxygen content in the blood or by impeding the diffusion of oxygen into cells. Because excess volume can result in hemodilution or tissue (including pulmonary) edema, excessive volume administration may be deleterious [1]. When evaluating methods to predict preload response, we must also consider whether the patient will be *tolerant* of additional volume, even if it would increase cardiac output. This "volume tolerance" is often confused with

T. M. Maus, C. R. Tainter (eds.), *Essential Echocardiography*,
https://doi.org/10.1007/978-3-030-84349-6_20

volume responsiveness, but the two concepts are distinct. A patient is fluid responsive if additional volume augments his stroke volume, but a patient is fluid tolerant if the net effect of additional fluid does not decrease end-organ perfusion and tissue delivery of oxygen. Transthoracic and transesophageal echocardiography (TTE and TEE, respectively) have been widely utilized to predict which patients will be fluid responsive, but in many cases, fluid tolerance will be a more important consideration. Determination of fluid tolerance requires consideration of additional clinical data and usually must be made on a case-by-case basis. This chapter focuses on the ultrasound evaluation of preload and appraises methods to predict whether changes in preload will affect cardiac output, tissue perfusion, and ultimately tissue oxygen delivery.

Physiology

According to the Frank-Starling law of the heart, as sarcomeres within the cardiac myocytes are stretched, they will contract more forcefully, thus increasing stroke volume [2]. This relationship is not linear. As myocytes receive more tension from a higher end-diastolic filling volume, there is less of an increase in contractility that occurs with further myocyte stretch (Fig. 20.1) [3].

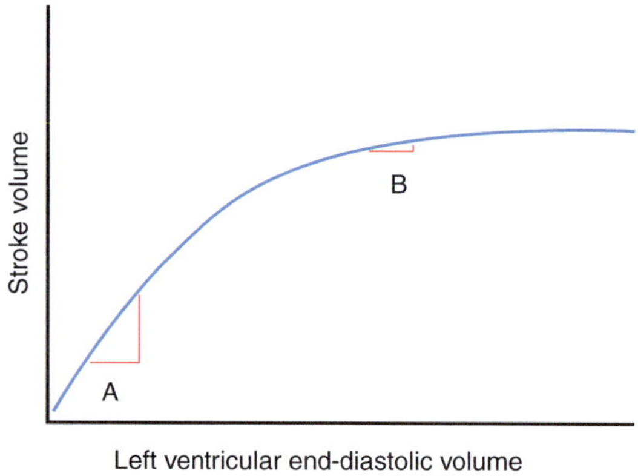

Fig. 20.1 Frank-Starling curve. Patients on the left portion of the curve will see a significant increase in stroke volume with an increase in preload (A). Patients on the right portion of the curve will only see minimal increases in stroke volume as the cardiac myocytes become maximally stretched (B)

Patients on the more steeply ascending portion of this Frank-Starling curve demonstrate a greater increase in stroke volume per unit of end-diastolic volume increase (increase in preload). Thus, increasing end-diastolic volume for patients with an already higher preload will result in a smaller increase in stroke volume [4].

"Volume responsiveness" or "fluid responsiveness" is a simplified description of this phenomenon, which has been defined in some settings as an increase in stroke volume by more than 15% in response to a 500 mL intravascular volume bolus [3]. Volume responsiveness describes where a given patient's preload lies along the Frank-Starling curve and claims to predict whether additional fluids will significantly augment stroke volume, and thereby cardiac output.

Predicting Preload Responsiveness (Highlight Box 20.1)

Highlight Box 20.1

Volume assessment	

2D	• Apical 4-chamber (TTE)
	• Parasternal short-axis
	  ∘ End-diastolic diameter (area)
	• Midesophageal 4-chamber (TEE)
	• Transgastric short-axis
	  ∘ End-diastolic diameter (area)
	• Subcostal IVC
	  ∘ Size and respiratory variation

CFD	• Not typically utilized
Spectral	• LVOT VTI and stroke volume variation • Mitral inflow velocity • Diastolic function assessment • Aortic and peripheral arterial velocity variation

TTE transthoracic echocardiography, *TEE* transesophageal echocardiography, *LVOT* left ventricular outflow tract, *VTI* velocity time integral

Preload, the stretching of cardiac myocytes prior to contraction, is determined by end-diastolic pressure or volume and is broadly described as venous return to the heart. Venous return to the right side of the heart (blood flow = cardiac output) is a function of total right atrial pressure (RAP) and the venous pressure driving flow toward the right atrium, which is largely influenced by the mean arterial pressure (MAP) and the systemic vascular resistance (SVR).

$$CO = \frac{MAP - RAP}{SVR}$$

The MAP and RAP are influenced by the volume of circulating blood and the smooth muscle tone in the walls of the venous system. Increasing blood volume increases atrial pressure, and thereby end-diastolic ventricular pressure. Vascular resistance is normally manipulated by the sympathetic nervous system's effect on the splanchnic venous system, which serves as a reservoir of the body's blood and can change its pressure to maintain venous return to the heart [5–7].

Static markers of preload such as central venous pressure (CVP), pulmonary capillary wedge pressure (PCWP), or global end-diastolic ventricular volumes are frequently measured, but can be unreliable when predicting volume responsiveness, in part because of endogenous compensation mechanisms. These static markers may correspond to preload responsiveness or unresponsiveness, depending on the relative position on the Frank-Starling curve, which varies from patient to patient and even varies within the same patient at different points in time. That is not to say that static markers of preload are useless in predicting volume responsiveness, but that they should be interpreted with caution [8].

Dynamic markers of preload can predict fluid responsiveness more effectively [9]. A dynamic marker of preload is a measured response to a provoked change in preload. This provoked change in preload is most commonly in the form of cardiopulmonary interactions, where changes in intrathoracic pressure with the respiratory cycle create the effect of a small "volume challenge" to the ventricles with each breath.

In a spontaneously breathing patient, negative intrathoracic pressure created during inspiration will result in increased venous return to the right heart and decreased venous return to the left heart. The effect of this small change in volume (preload) may be observed relative to the small opposite change in preload occurring during expiration. In contrast, a patient receiving positive pressure ventilation will have an increase in intrathoracic pressure during inspiration, resulting in a decrease in venous return to the right heart (increase to the left heart, as pulmonary capillary blood is forced into the pulmonary veins) and a change in preload. During expiration, the intrathoracic pressure decreases, producing the opposite change in preload.

We can interpret the hemodynamic effects of these small changes in preload by assessing changes in stroke volume (stroke volume variation) or by evaluating surrogate measurements for stroke volume variation, such as pulse pressure variation, systolic pressure variation, or systolic velocity variation. These measures predict volume responsiveness better than static measurements, but are subject to several important limitations

Table 20.1 Limitations to predicting volume responsiveness with dynamic measures

The patient should be in a sinus rhythm, as beat-to-beat stroke volume variation occurs with irregular atrial contraction (e.g., atrial fibrillation)
Changes in ventricular preload may be exaggerated in patients with increased respiratory effort or high tidal volumes, and conversely, changes in preload may be diminished with decreased respiratory effort or low tidal volumes
Increased intra-abdominal pressure, or IVC compression (e.g., pregnancy) may exaggerate changes in preload and stroke volume variation
Changes in intrathoracic pressure will alter preload. For example, a patient with an open chest may have less observed stroke volume variation, while a patient with high intrathoracic pressure may have increased variation
An increase in intrapericardial pressure (i.e., tamponade) will cause exaggerated respiratory variation in stroke volume and should not be attributed to hypovolemia alone
In patients with known or suspected left interventricular outflow obstruction, systolic anterior motion of the anterior leaflet of the mitral valve can be accentuated by hypovolemic or hyperkinetic states. Significant narrowing of the outflow tract occurs during these hemodynamic states and careful assessment of the outflow tract is required to determine if additional volume alone will correct this derangement [10]

IVC inferior vena cava

(Table 20.1) [10]. Despite these limitations, predicting preload responsiveness by dynamic measures may be quite useful in the management of hemodynamically unstable patients.

Assessment of Ventricular Volumes

Intraventricular volume has some predictive value regarding volume responsiveness. Ventricular volume can be most easily approximated via the cross-sectional area observed from the transgastric short-axis midpapillary view or the midesophageal four-chamber view with TEE. Using TTE, the parasternal short-axis view or apical four-chamber view are the most useful.

A very low end-systolic volume with ventricular walls contacting each other ("kissing papillaries") may suggest either low ventricular filling pressure (low preload) or low resistance to ejection of the stroke volume (low afterload). Observation of the end-diastolic volume may help make this distinction. A low end-diastolic volume suggests inadequate ventricular filling and a low preload, i.e., hypovolemia (Fig. 20.2, Video 20.1). A normal end-diastolic volume with a low end-systolic volume suggests that preload is adequate, but low afterload is present (Fig. 20.3, Video 20.2) [10, 11]. Left ventricular hypertrophy, or a highly vasodilated state, can exaggerate these findings, and careful clinical judgment is required to determine if a hypovolemic state is truly present [12].

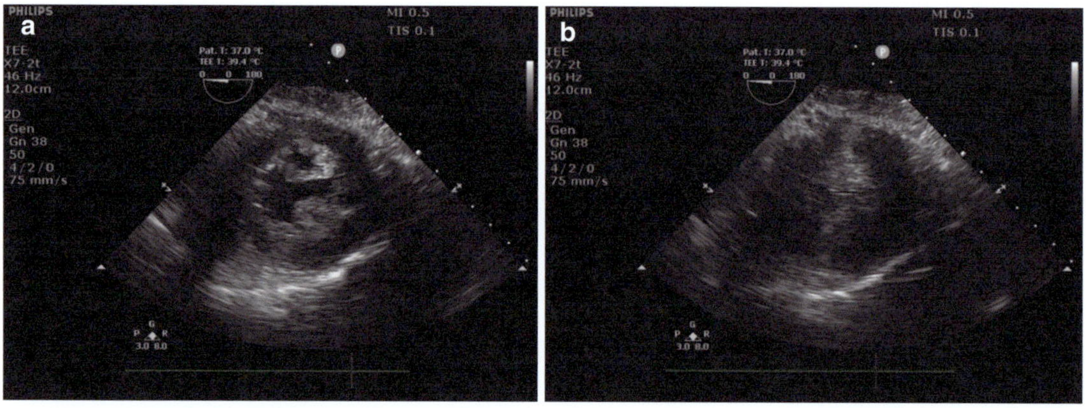

Fig. 20.2 Transgastric midpapillary short-axis view in a patient with hypovolemia. Note the small end-diastolic area (**a**) and small end-systolic area (**b**)

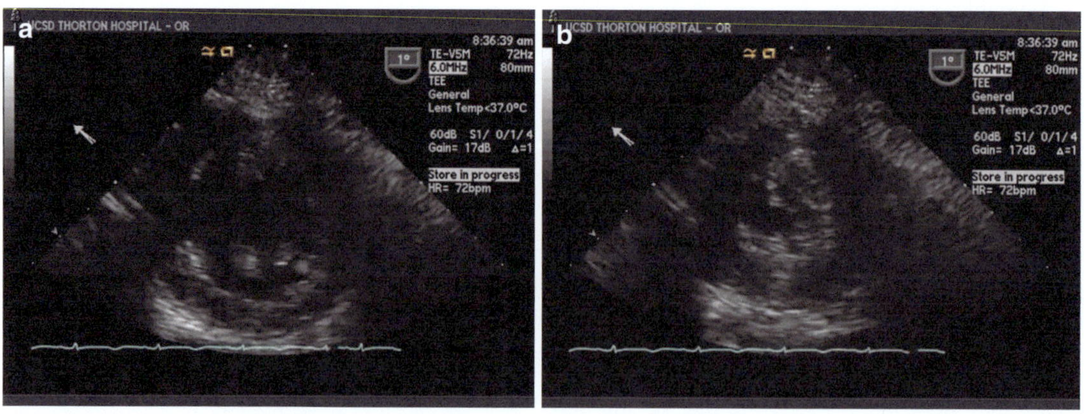

Fig. 20.3 Transgastric midpapillary short-axis view in a patient with low systemic afterload. Note the normal end-diastolic area (**a**) and a small end-systolic area (**b**)

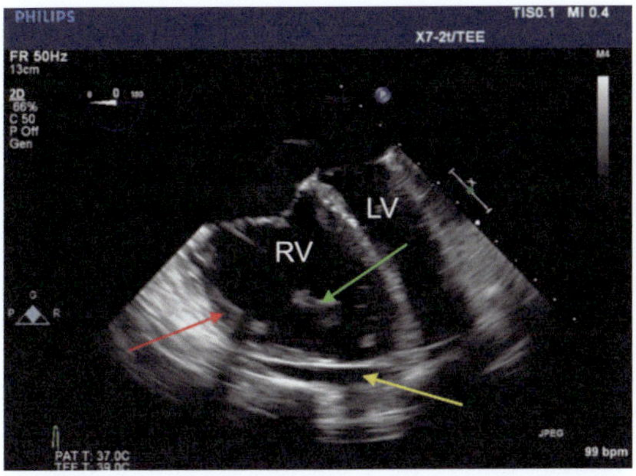

Fig. 20.4 A midesophageal four-chamber view demonstrating a dilated right ventricle in a patient with chronic thromboembolic pulmonary hypertension. Note that the right ventricular diameter (RV) is significantly larger than the left ventricle (LV). Right ventricular hypertrophy (*red arrow*) suggests a chronic process of pulmonary hypertension. The overloaded RV impairs diastolic filling of the left ventricle (ventricular interdependence). The moderator band and tricuspid apparatus are prominent (*green arrow*), and there is incidentally a small pericardial effusion visible near the apex (*yellow arrow*)

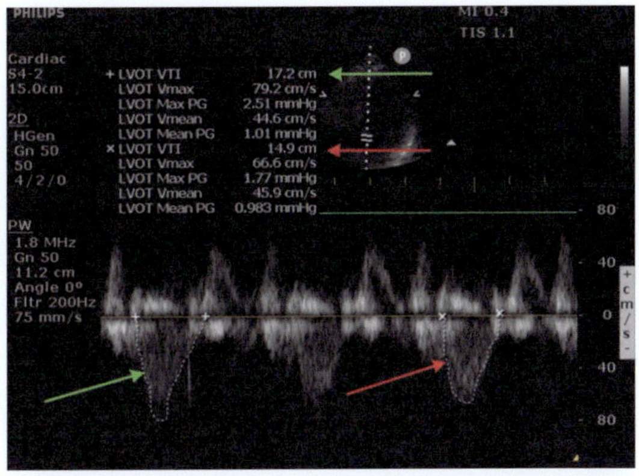

Fig. 20.5 Left ventricular outflow tract (LVOT) velocity time integral (VTI) via an apical five-chamber view in a spontaneously ventilating patient. The sampling gate is placed just below the aortic valve leaflets with the beam aligned with the flow through the LVOT. There is significant variation (13%) between the larger expiratory (*green arrows*) and smaller inspiratory (*red arrows*) VTI, showing that the stroke volume increases with more preload (volume responsive)

Using right ventricular volumes to assess preload and predict volume responsiveness should be done with caution. Right ventricular dysfunction can make these assessments less reliable and may exacerbate the deleterious effects of excessive preload. A dysfunctional right ventricle may be seen in patients with pulmonary hypertension, acute pulmonary embolism, right ventricular infarction, or high intrathoracic pressures (e.g., ventilator pressures required to ventilate "stiff" lungs) (Fig. 20.4, Video 20.3). The right ventricle has some ability to compensate for chronic dilatation; however, acute dilatation is poorly tolerated [13]. As both ventricles occupy a limited space, right ventricular distention may impair left ventricular filling (ventricular interdependence) and the ability to generate adequate stroke volumes and may confound observations of the respirophasic stroke volume changes used to predict volume responsiveness. Right ventricular failure can result in significant stroke volume variation, falsely suggesting a preload-responsive state [14].

Assessment of Left Ventricular Outflow Tract

Because the size of the left ventricular outflow tract (LVOT) remains relatively constant, the changes in left ventricular stroke volume occurring throughout the respiratory cycle can be simplified to the measurement of the LVOT velocity time integral (VTI) (see Chap. 4). Assessment of the LVOT VTI is most accurate when the imaging beam is parallel to the LVOT flow, from either an apical 5- or 3-chamber view (TTE) or a deep transgastric five-chamber view (TEE). The pulsed-wave Doppler gate should be positioned just proximal to the aortic annulus (within 0.5 cm), where the LVOT diameter is the most consistent. The largest and smallest VTI can be traced over the course of a respiratory cycle, and the percentage change can be calculated (Fig. 20.5) [9]. Table 20.2 shows the approximate values, and the corresponding likelihood of volume responsiveness.

A simplified version of the same concept is simply measuring variation in the peak systolic veloc-

Table 20.2 LVOT VTI variation to predict fluid responsiveness

VTI variation	Likelihood of volume responsiveness
< 10%	Low
10–14%	Indeterminate
> 14%	High

LVOT left ventricular outflow tract, *VTI* velocity time integral

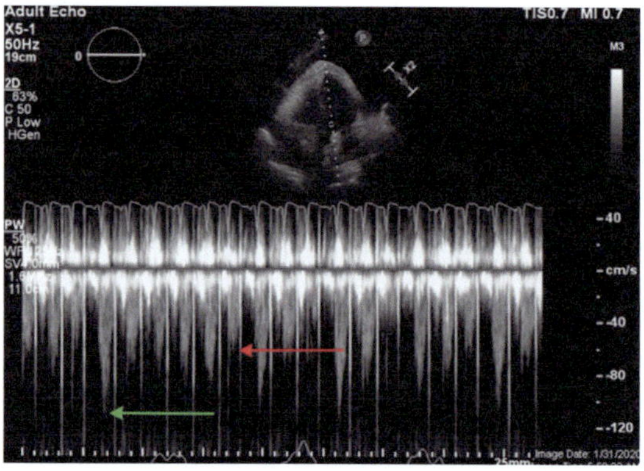

Fig. 20.6 Measurement of the peak systolic velocity variation through the left ventricular outflow tract (LVOT) from an apical five-chamber view, in a spontaneously ventilating patient. The sampling gate is placed just below the aortic valve leaflets, and the beam is aligned with the flow through the LVOT. There is significant variation between the maximal expiratory (*green arrow*) and the minimal inspiratory (*red arrow*) velocity, suggesting an increase in stroke volume with additional preload administration

ity through the LVOT during the respiratory cycle, rather than tracing the VTI (Fig. 20.6). Using pulsed-wave Doppler, and sampling at the level of the aortic valve, a peak velocity variation of greater than 12% suggests volume responsiveness [13, 15].

Assessment of Mitral Inflow Velocity

The left atrium is easily imaged with TEE, given its proximity to the esophagus. In contrast, it may be difficult to visualize from a transthoracic window, but either imaging mode can provide useful information about inflow from the left atrium into the left ventricle. Importantly, information from mitral inflow velocity and the left atrium are less influenced by systolic regional wall motion abnormalities than left ventricular imaging [16]. Pulsed-wave Doppler examination of the mitral inflow can provide estimation of diastolic filling patterns, which can be useful in estimating left ventricular filling pressures and sensitivity to changes in preload, as described in Chap. 12. As diastolic filling patterns progress "to the right," toward a more restrictive filling pattern, the ventricular compliance is reduced and is increasingly less likely to benefit from additional preload (see Chap. 12, Fig. 12.1).

Changes in left atrial and ventricular filling pressures alter the transmitral inflow velocity profile during both early and late diastolic filling. A reduction in acceleration and maximum flow velocity during early diastole occur as a result of a reduction in the pressure gradient across the mitral valve [17]. Akin to variation in LVOT VTI with the respiratory cycle as described above, similar respiratory variation may be observed through mitral valve inflow.

Notably, the ratio of early diastolic filling (*E*) to early diastolic lateral mitral annular velocity (*e*') correlates with left atrial pressure and can also help estimate left ventricular end-diastolic pressure (LVEDP) [18]. An *E*/*e*' ratio less than 8 suggests normal left ventricular filling pressures, which may improve stroke volume with additional preload, while a ratio > 14 suggests elevated pressures and would likely have no benefit from additional preload (Fig. 20.7) [19, 20].

When using mitral inflow velocities, it is important to remember potential pitfalls to this technique. Mitral stenosis, in particular, can dramatically alter the morphology of the inflow pattern. In addition, severe diastolic dysfunction with a restrictive filling pattern reflects elevated left ventricular diastolic pressures. The left ventricle can potentially be under filled despite high filling pressures, with an optimum filling range that is quite narrow, as it easily under- or overfills. Thus, in patients with significant diastolic dysfunction, fluid boluses must be administered cautiously.

Assessment of the Inferior Vena Cava

The size and variation of the inferior vena cava (IVC) during the respiratory cycle and its relation to a subject's right atrial pressure and volume responsiveness has been the subject of much debate [21]. IVC measurements can be used to estimate right atrial pressure in certain situations

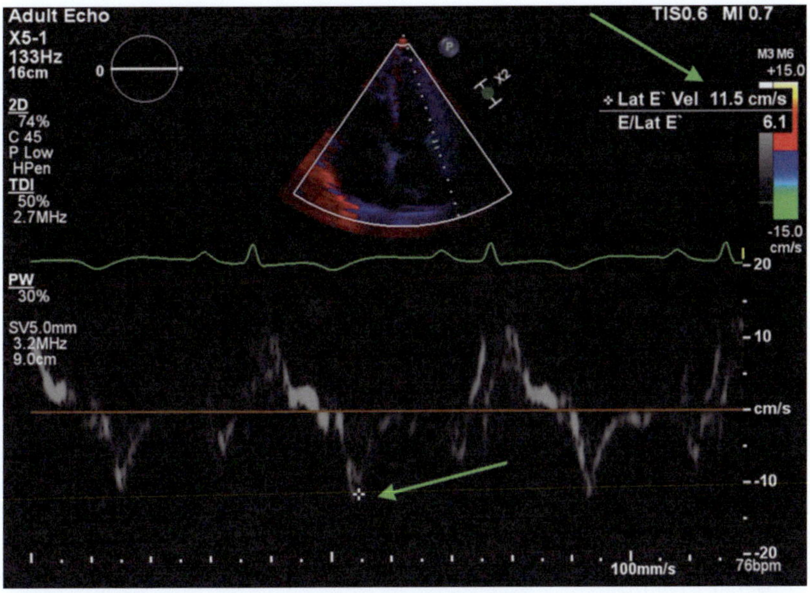

Fig. 20.7 A normal mitral annular velocity during early diastolic filling (e' = 11.5 cm/s, *green arrows*). The E/e' ratio (E wave velocity measurement not shown) is 6.1, and therefore suggests a low or normal left atrial pressure

and are therefore subject to the same limited predictive value for preload sensitivity as right atrial pressure itself. Studies evaluating IVC assessment are often difficult to compare or combine, as they have different reference standards, measure the IVC at different points during the cardiac or respiratory cycle, use positive or negative pressure ventilation, or use different outcome measures [22].

In patients receiving positive pressure ventilation, increased intrathoracic pressure during inspiration results in an increase in the pressure in the IVC, causing its volume to increase relative to its compliance and decrease during exhalation. For patients who are spontaneously breathing, the IVC diameter decreases with negative intrathoracic pressure during inspiration and increases during expiration [23–25].

The average diameter of the IVC is 1.7 cm, but varies between individuals, and the absolute diameter of the IVC does not correlate well with right atrial pressures or volume responsiveness, unless it is very small or very large [26]. Dynamic changes in the IVC diameter can be quantified as a percent change of the diameter over the respiratory cycle, called the IVC collapsibility index (CI):

$$\mathrm{CI} = \left[\frac{\left(\text{IVC diameter}_{\max} - \text{IVC diameter}_{\min}\right)}{\text{IVC diameter}_{\max}}\right] \times 100$$

Table 20.3 IVC collapsibility index, CVP, and volume response in mechanically ventilated patients

CI	CVP	Predicted response
> 50%	0–5 mm Hg	Likely to respond to volume
20–50%	5–10 mm Hg	Indeterminate
< 20%	> 10 mm Hg	Unlikely to respond to volume

CI collapsibility index, *CVP* central venous pressure

Table 20.4 Estimation of right atrial pressure from IVC diameter and collapse (spontaneous breathing)

IVC diameter	Change with respiration	Estimated right atrial pressure
≤ 2.1 cm	Decrease by > 50%	0–5 mmHg
> 2.1 cm	Decrease by > 50%	5–10 mmHg
> 2.1 cm	Decrease by < 50%	> 10 mmHg

The collapsibility index has been shown to correlate with central venous pressure in mechanically ventilated patients [26–28] (Table 20.3) and may also be a useful predictor for volume responsiveness when interpreted correctly in spontaneously breathing patients, although it is more difficult to control for the degree of change in intrathoracic pressure.

Table 20.4 summarizes recommendations for estimating right atrial pressure with IVC size and respiratory variation in spontaneously breathing patients [29]. These estimates are most accurate with low or high right atrial pressure (RAP). A small IVC diameter (≤ 2.1 cm) with a large degree of respiratory variation (> 50%) suggests a normal RAP of 0–5 mmHg. An IVC diameter > 2.1 cm with respiratory variation > 50% suggests a RAP 5–10 mmHg, and an IVC diameter > 2.1 cm with < 50% collapse suggests a high RAP, over 10 mmHg. If there is unclear variation with respiration, the patient can be asked to inhale rapidly, by "sniffing" to augment the interpretation.

The IVC can be best measured in long axis (sagittal), from the subcostal window (Fig. 20.8, Video 20.4, Fig. 20.9, Video 20.5). Measurements of the IVC should be made 2 cm from the right atrial junction (approximately 1 cm past the middle hepatic vein confluence). More proximal to this location, the IVC has a relatively fixed position, and variation might be underestimated. More distal to this location, the IVC will be smaller and more mobile, overestimating its size variation. Size and positioning of the patient also

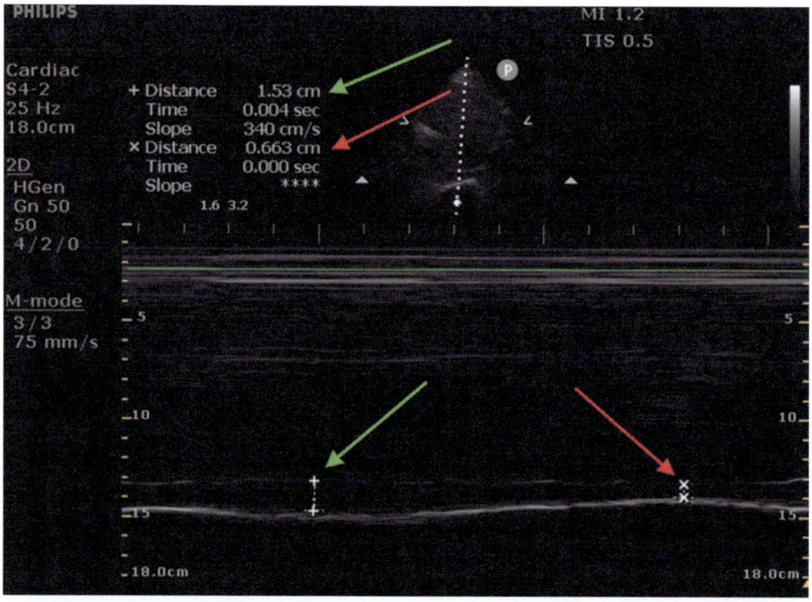

Fig. 20.8 Measurement of the IVC via M-mode imaging, demonstrating a small IVC (1.53 cm), with significant variation (57%) during inhalation, suggesting a low right atrial pressure, and likely volume responsiveness

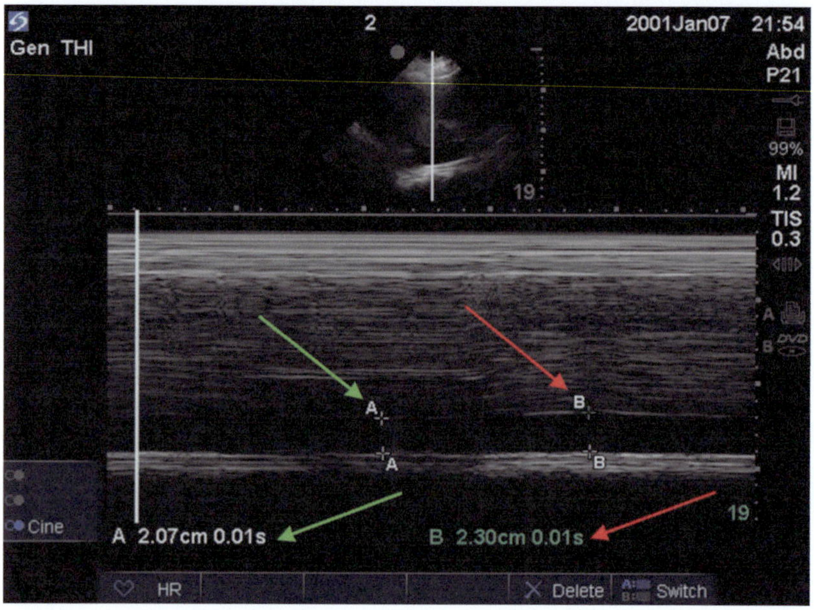

Fig. 20.9 Measurement of the IVC via M-mode imaging, demonstrating a large IVC (2.3 cm), with little variation (10%), suggesting a high right atrial pressure, and unlikely volume responsiveness

influence IVC measurements. IVC diameter is consistently largest in the right lateral or upright position and smallest in the left lateral position. The 2015 American Society of Echocardiography (ASE) guidelines recommend measuring IVC in the neutral supine position [29]. In obese patients, this can be challenging, and a transhepatic view of the IVC can be obtained instead. Using TEE, the IVC is best imaged by advancing the probe from a midesophageal bicaval view.

In addition to the problems with using RAP to predict volume responsiveness, IVC measurement has several limitations, which are important to consider when making interpretations. Right ventricular dysfunction and tricuspid regurgitation can alter venous return and result in a plethoric IVC, which shows no correlation with volume responsiveness. Increased abdominal pressure, large intrathoracic pressure swings, pressure-supported breathing, and high PEEP can also impact the IVC analysis. Technically, measuring the IVC in a position too close or too far from the right atrium may result in inaccuracy. And lastly, two-dimensional measurements of the IVC are likely more accurate than measurements taken in M-mode, as this can result in translational error, but still may be inaccurate for an irregularly shaped IVC.

Assessment of Arterial Velocity

Dynamic changes in stroke volume with changes in preload from respiratory variation will manifest as beat-to-beat changes in pulse pressure [9, 17]. Because the size of the vessels does not change considerably between cardiac cycles, these changes in pressure can also be measured as changes in velocity. The velocity of blood flow can be measured in the aorta or the main pulmonary artery as they exit the heart, or in more peripheral arteries, including the carotid arteries and the brachial arteries, which may be easier to visualize [13, 30]. Peak velocity variation (PVV) correlates with pulse pressure variation and has diagnostic value for predicting fluid responsiveness, particularly when PVV is above 12% (the difference between maximum and minimum values of peak velocity, divided by the maximum value) over one respiratory cycle (Fig. 20.10) [15]. However, it is important to remember that as the arterial flow becomes more peripheral, these changes may be affected by additional confounding elements like vascular compliance, thus more central measurements are more accurate.

These techniques do come with limitations, similar to those found when measuring other dynamic predictors of fluid responsiveness (Table 20.1). They are most accurate when

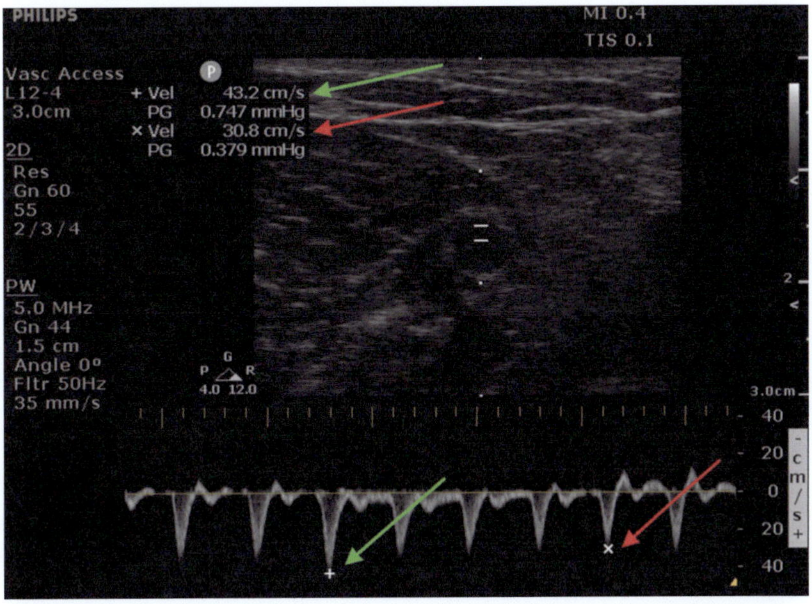

Fig. 20.10 Peak velocity variation in the brachial artery. The difference between maximum (43.2 cm/s, *green arrows*) and minimum (30.8 cm/s, *red arrows*) peak systolic velocity divided by the maximum velocity results in a 29% variation with respiration. A percentage variation over 12% indicates a likely volume-responsive state

patients are in sinus rhythm, breathing with consistent changes in intrathoracic pressure, have normal intra-abdominal pressures, and do not have vascular stenosis proximal to the site of investigation.

Assessing Response to Volume Challenge

Ultimately, determination of volume responsiveness is based on measuring an increase in stroke volume in response to a volume challenge [8]. The size of a volume challenge has been debated, but has generally been defined as a rapid administration of 250–500 mL of intravenous fluid [31]. Recently, Muller and colleagues reported that a mini-fluid challenge of only 100 mL accurately predicted fluid responsiveness using variations in aortic VTI [23]. Although significant improvements in stroke volume may not be reflected by changes in blood pressure, blood flow and consequent oxygen delivery may be improved.

Direct measurement of the stroke volume via the LVOT VTI before and after a volume challenge is an accurate way to determine changes in cardiac output. Because the size of the LVOT remains relatively constant, changes in the VTI correlate directly with changes in stroke volume. An increase of 15% in VTI measurement reflects an increase in 15% cardiac output, assuming the heart rate and LVOT size remain constant. Measurements of a VTI should ideally occur immediately before and after a fluid challenge, and be measured at end-expiration, or averaged over several beats.

Another method of increasing preload to the ventricles is to change the patient's position into a less gravity-dependent (more recumbent) position, allowing for increased venous return to the heart. The passive leg raise is accomplished by tilting the patient from a 45-degree head-up position to a 45-degree leg-up position and should effectively transfer up to 300 mL of intravascular volume into the central circulation. Tipping the whole bed and not just elevating the legs avoids compression of the femoral veins. Stroke volume or VTI is measured across the left ventricular outflow tract 1 minute before and after the passive leg raise. A change of 10% in stroke volume (or VTI) suggests a volume-responsive state [8, 12].

The passive leg raise has less risk of excessive fluid administration, as it is essentially "reversible" and can be performed quickly without additional resources. Downsides to a passive leg raise maneuver include patient discomfort, changes in respiratory mechanics, and elevated intracranial pressure. Passive leg raise maneuvers are generally less reliable in patients with severe peripheral vascular disease or lower limb amputation.

Conclusion

A thorough understanding of methods to assess preload and predict volume responsiveness is essential to manage a critically ill patient, and ultrasound affords several ways to achieve this. Because both hypovolemia and hypervolemia can compromise delivery of oxygen to tissues, the decision to administer intravascular volume should be made judiciously. Static measures of pressures and volumes, although common, are less reliable than dynamic measures, which take advantage of changes in intrathoracic pressure associated with mechanical or spontaneous ventilation. Ultrasound-based interrogation of VTI from the LV outflow tract, mitral inflow velocity, the collapsibility of the IVC, and peripheral arterial velocity changes can, if used appropriately, predict which patients will benefit from additional intravascular volume. A passive leg raise or a volume challenge can be combined with ultrasound interrogation to measure the effect of increased preload to further support this prediction. Despite well-described limitations, these techniques provide valuable tools to a clinician to enhance patient care.

Questions

1. Which of the following are possible effects of intravascular volume administration?
   A. Increase organ dysfunction
   B. Increase cardiac output

C. Decrease tissue oxygen delivery
D. All the above

2. Which of the following are considered dynamic measures of preload? (select all that apply)

A. Central venous pressure
B. Pulmonary capillary wedge pressure
C. Left ventricular end-diastolic pressure
D. Systolic velocity variation

3. Which of the following variables are unnecessary in the calculation of cardiac output with echocardiography?

A. Velocity time integral
B. Left ventricular outflow tract diameter
C. Peak mitral valve inflow velocity
D. Heart rate

4. Which of the following improves the predictive value for dynamic measures of preload?

A. Tidal volume ventilation of 6–8 mL/kg
B. No arrhythmias present
C. Open chest
D. High intraabdominal pressure

5. Which of the following conditions would be most likely to be increased in patients with hypovolemia?

A. Systolic anterior motion of the mitral valve (SAM)
B. Aortic insufficiency
C. Mitral stenosis
D. Diastolic dysfunction

6. What is the lowest percentage variation of the LVOT velocity time integral (VTI) above which a patient is likely to be volume responsive?

A. > 4%
B. > 9%
C. > 14%
D. > 19%

7. Which of the following is most likely to result in significant stroke volume variation, falsely indicating a volume-responsive state?

A. Right ventricular failure
B. Distributive shock
C. Aortic stenosis
D. Aortic regurgitation

8. What central venous pressure is suggested by the following image from a patient breathing spontaneously?

A. < 5 mmHg
B. 5–10 mmHg
C. 10–20 mmHg
D. > 20 mmHg

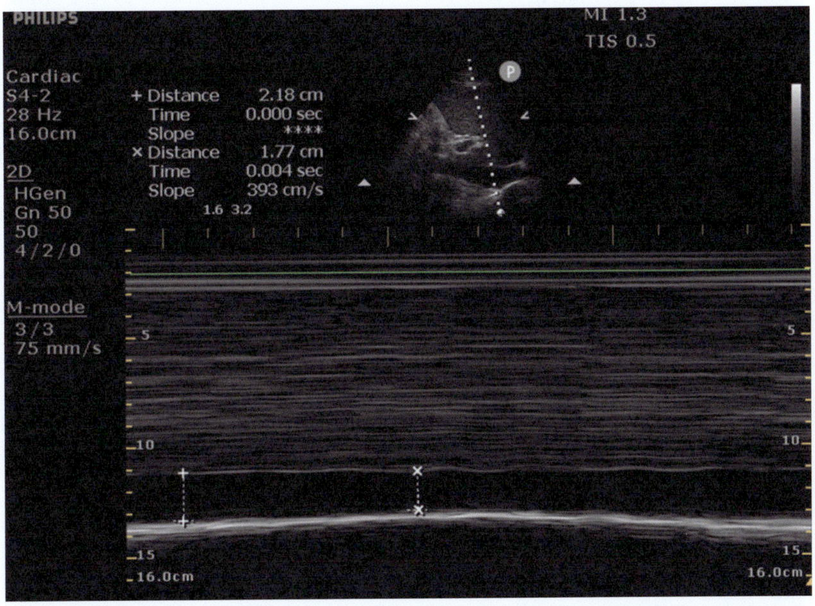

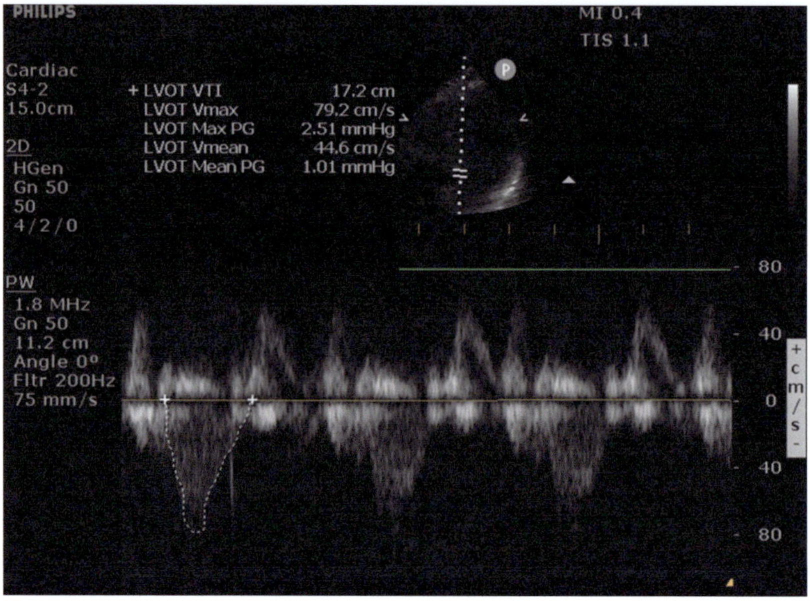

9. Which of the following factors are most likely to overestimate volume responsiveness from IVC measurements?

    A. Restrictive pericarditis
    B. Open abdomen
    C. PEEP 15 cmH_2O
    D. Positive pressure ventilation with tidal volume 6 mL/kg ideal body weight

10. A 70-year-old man presents with cough and fever for 3 days. His temperature is 38.6 °C, BP 80/45 mmHg (MAP 57 mmHg), HR 100 bpm, RR 25/min, and SpO_2 95% on room air. A point-of-care echocardiogram measures a cardiac output of 5.4 liters per minute, and a LVOT diameter of 2 cm. He is given appropriate antibiotic coverage and an IV bolus of 30 mL/kg lactated Ringer's solution. On repeat assessment, BP is 90/45 mmHg (MAP 60 mmHg), HR is 100 bpm, RR is 25, and SpO_2 is unchanged. A point-of-care echocardiography is repeated, and the following image is obtained. What is the most appropriate next step in management?

    A. Repeat IV fluid bolus 30 mL/kg.
    B. Initiate dobutamine 3 mcg/kg/min.
    C. Initiate norepinephrine, titrated to MAP > 65 mmHg.
    D. Perform passive leg raise maneuver and assess response.

References

1. Marik PE. Iatrogenic salt water drowning and the hazards of a high central venous pressure. Ann Intensive Care. 2014;4:21.
2. Katz AM. Ernest Henry Starling, his predecessors, and the "Law of the Heart". Circulation. 2002;106:2986–92.
3. Miller A, Mandeville J. Predicting and measuring fluid responsiveness with echocardiography. Echo Res Pract. 2016;3:G1–G12.
4. Jalil BA, Cavallazzi R. Predicting fluid responsiveness: a review of literature and a guide for the clinician. Am J Emerg Med. 2018;36:2093–102.
5. Magder S, De Varennes B. Clinical death and the measurement of stressed vascular volume. Crit Care Med. 1998;26:1061–4.
6. Monnet X, Marik PE, Teboul J-L. Prediction of fluid responsiveness: an update. Ann Intensive Care. 2016;6:111.
7. Gelman S. Venous function and central venous pressure. Anesthesiology. 2008;108:735–48.
8. Marik PE. Fluid responsiveness and the six guiding principles of fluid resuscitation. Crit Care Med. 2016;44:1920–2.

9. Marik PE, Cavallazzi R, Vasu T, et al. Dynamic changes in arterial waveform derived variables and fluid responsiveness in mechanically ventilated patients: a systematic review of the literature*. Crit Care Med. 2009;37:2642–7.
10. Bentzer P, Griesdale DE, Boyd J, et al. Will this hemodynamically unstable patient respond to a bolus of intravenous fluids? JAMA. 2016;316:1298.
11. Cecconi M, Hofer C, Teboul J-L, et al. Fluid challenges in intensive care: the FENICE study. Intensive Care Med. 2015;41:1529–37.
12. Tousignant CP, Walsh F, Mazer CD. The use of transesophageal echocardiography for preload assessment in critically ill patients. Anesth Analg. 2000;90:351.
13. Ranucci M, Pazzaglia A, Tritapepe L, et al. Fluid responsiveness and right ventricular function in cardiac surgical patients. A multicenter study. HSR Proc Intensive Care Cardiovasc Anesth. 2009;1:21–9.
14. Wiesenack C, Fiegl C, Keyser A, et al. Continuously assessed right ventricular end-diastolic volume as a marker of cardiac preload and fluid responsiveness in mechanically ventilated cardiac surgical patients. Crit Care. 2005;9:R226.
15. Feissel M, Mangin I, Ruyer O, et al. Respiratory changes in aortic blood velocity as an indicator of fluid responsiveness in ventilated patients with septic shock. Chest. 2001;119:867–73.
16. Bouhemad B, Nicolas-Robin A, Benois A, et al. Echocardiographic Doppler assessment of pulmonary capillary wedge pressure in surgical patients with postoperative circulatory shock and acute lung injury. Anesthesiology. 2003;98:1091–100.
17. Courtois M, Vered Z, Barzilai B, et al. The transmitral pressure-flow velocity relation. Effect of abrupt preload reduction. Circulation. 1988;78:1459–68.
18. Nagueh SF, Smiseth OA, Appleton CP, et al. Recommendations for the evaluation of left ventricular diastolic function by echocardiography: an update from the American Society of Echocardiography and the European Association of Cardiovascular Imaging. J Am Soc Echocardiogr. 2016;29:277–314
19. Jacques DC, Pinsky MR, Severyn D, et al. Influence of alterations in loading on mitral annular velocity by tissue Doppler echocardiography and its associated ability to predict filling pressures. Chest. 2004;126:1910–8.
20. Marques NR, De Riese J, Yelverton BC, et al. Diastolic function and peripheral venous pressure as indices for fluid responsiveness in cardiac surgical patients. J Cardiothorac Vasc Anesth. 2019;33:2208–15.
21. Long E, Oakley E, Duke T, et al. Does respiratory variation in inferior vena cava diameter predict fluid responsiveness: a systematic review and meta-analysis. Shock. 2017;47:550–9.
22. Orde S, Slama M, Hilton A, et al. Pearls and pitfalls in comprehensive critical care echocardiography. Crit Care. 2017;21:279.
23. Muller L, Bobbia X, Toumi M, et al. Respiratory variations of inferior vena cava diameter to predict fluid responsiveness in spontaneously breathing patients with acute circulatory failure: need for a cautious use. Crit Care. 2012;16:R188.
24. Preau S, Bortolotti P, Colling D, et al. Diagnostic accuracy of the inferior vena cava collapsibility to predict fluid responsiveness in spontaneously breathing patients with sepsis and acute circulatory failure. Crit Care Med. 2017;45:e290–7.
25. Brennan JM, Blair JE, Goonewardena S, et al. Reappraisal of the use of inferior vena cava for estimating right atrial pressure. J Am Soc Echocardiogr. 2007;20:857–61.
26. Feissel M, Michard F, Faller J-P, et al. The respiratory variation in inferior vena cava diameter as a guide to fluid therapy. Intensive Care Med. 2004;30:1834–7.
27. Moreno FLL, Hagan AD, Holmen JR, et al. Evaluation of size and dynamics of the inferior vena cava as an index of right-sided cardiac function. Am J Cardiol. 1984;53:579–85.
28. Beigel R, Cercek B, Luo H, et al. Noninvasive evaluation of right atrial pressure. J Am Soc Echocardiogr. 2013;26:1033–42.
29. Porter TR, Shillcutt SK, Adams MS, et al. Guidelines for the use of echocardiography as a monitor for therapeutic intervention in adults: a report from the American Society of Echocardiography. J Am Soc Echocardiogr. 2015;28:40–56.
30. Yao B, Liu J-y, Sun Y-b. Respiratory variation in peripheral arterial blood flow peak velocity to predict fluid responsiveness in mechanically ventilated patients: a systematic review and meta-analysis. BMC Anesthesiol. 2018;18:168.
31. Vincent J-L, Weil MH. Fluid challenge revisited. Crit Care Med. 2006;34:1333–7.

21 Lung Ultrasonography

Andrew Goodrich and Christopher R. Tainter

Abbreviations

ARDS	Acute (adult) respiratory distress syndrome
BLUE	Bedside lung ultrasound in emergency (protocol)
CT	Computed tomography (scan)
CXR	Chest x-ray
DVT	Deep vein thrombosis
PE	Pulmonary embolism
PLAPS	Posterolateral alveolar-pleural syndrome (point)

Introduction

Ultrasound is ideal for the rapid bedside evaluation of respiratory distress [1–6]. Much of the pioneering work with the interpretation of lung ultrasound was done by Daniel Lichtenstein in the 1980s, at a time when it was mostly felt that useful imaging was not possible with ultrasound due to the attenuation of the ultrasound waves from air in the lungs. He described several principles that we now consider central to the interpretation of lung ultrasound [2]. The lung and pleura contain both air and fluid, which will rise and fall with gravity, respectively. Almost all lung signs will start at the pleural line, and normal aerated lung tissue will not be visualized directly. Instead, the use of simple equipment allows for the presence of artifacts, which enable the deduction of useful clinical information.

Ultrasound has several distinct advantages for lung imaging. First, it is usually available at the bedside more rapidly than CXR or CT scan. Second, when correctly interpreted, it has better sensitivity than CXR for many conditions, including pneumothorax and pleural effusion. Third, the ultrasound exam does not expose the patient to the potential harms of ionizing radiation.

Equipment

Lung ultrasound has been described using a variety of ultrasound transducers. Lichtenstein and others prefer a 5 MHz microconvex probe with 8–10 cm depth, which can also be used for cardiac, venous, abdominal, and ocular exams [1]. Other authors report using a linear array probe of 13–4 MHz [4, 7, 8], a curvilinear probe of

Supplementary Information The online version of this chapter (https://doi.org/10.1007/978-3-030-84349-6_21) contains supplementary material, which is available to authorized users.

A. Goodrich (✉) · C. R. Tainter
Department of Anesthesiology, University of California San Diego Health, La Jolla, CA, USA
e-mail: asgoodrich@health.ucsd.edu

T. M. Maus, C. R. Tainter (eds.), *Essential Echocardiography*,
https://doi.org/10.1007/978-3-030-84349-6_21

8–2.5 MHz [4, 5, 7], or a phased array probe of 2.5 MHz [5, 8]. Because lung ultrasound relies heavily on artifacts, all filters and image processing should be turned off. Some ultrasound machines will have a "lung" setting for this purpose, or a "null" setting, which is also acceptable. Doppler is not needed for lung ultrasound, although M-mode may be useful. A small, portable machine has obvious advantages in a crowded environment and may be more feasible, since many of the more advanced imaging functions are generally not required.

Performing the Examination

The optimal positioning and placement of the ultrasound probe for a lung exam depends on the area of interest and the specific question at hand. A limited exam in an area of interest may be adequate to answer a clinical question with a single view (e.g., identifying a large pleural effusion or excluding a large pneumothorax), or a more comprehensive evaluation may be needed. In general, fluid will be more dependent than lung tissue, so a pleural effusion may be posterior in a supine patient, or inferior in a patient who is more upright. Conversely, a pneumothorax may be more "anti-dependent," i.e., anterior or apical. For this reason, patient positioning may help optimize visualization even further.

The Bedside Lung Ultrasound in Emergency (BLUE) protocol [1, 2] is designed for the rapid evaluation of an acutely ill patient and evaluates three points on each side. Two points are located on the anterior chest, referred to as the upper and lower BLUE points. The third point is located on the posterolateral chest and is referred to as the posterolateral alveolar-pleural syndrome (PLAPS) point. These points can be identified by placing the provider's hands on the patient's chest side by side, just below the ipsilateral clavicle (Fig. 21.1). The upper BLUE point is located between the base of the third and fourth fingers, at approximately the third intercostal space in the midclavicular line. The lower BLUE point is located at the middle of the palm of the lower hand, approximately the fifth intercostal space, just lateral to the nipple. The PLAPS point is located by tracing the lower BLUE point laterally to the posterior axillary line.

The PLAPS point should be scanned perpendicularly to the skin, and evaluation of this point in a critically ill patient may require some movement. Lifting the ipsilateral arm across the chest may assist in exposure. If evaluation of the PLAPS point is initially negative, the next lower rib spaces can be evaluated to produce higher sensitivity.

A more thorough examination may use 6 points on each side: 4 anterior quadrants and upper and lower lateral portions [8]. Other systems are also reported including a 2-point anterolateral-posterior scan [4] and 28 rib interspaces [9]. Finally, a comprehensive TEE exam can visualize portions of the lungs and pleura as well, essentially providing an "internal" PLAPS view.

The probe should be oriented in the longitudinal plane to optimize visualization of the pleura. The subcutaneous tissue will be seen on the image, including the ribs and intercostal muscles. The dense ribs will appear very bright at the periosteum, with dark shadows deeper. The pleural line will be seen in between the ribs at their deep border

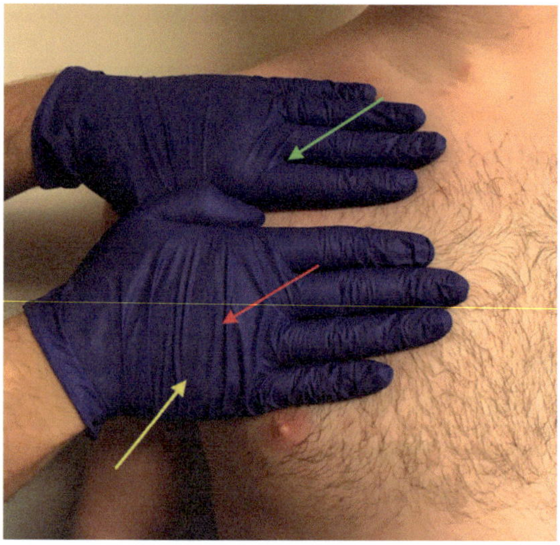

Fig. 21.1 BLUE points of examination for lung ultrasound. With hands aligned adjacent to the clavicle, the upper BLUE point is between the base of the third and fourth fingers down from the clavicle (*green arrow*), at approximately the third intercostal space in the midclavicular line. The lower BLUE point is at the middle of the palm of the lower hand, approximately the fifth intercostal space, just lateral to the nipple (*red arrow*). The PLAPS point is lateral to the lower BLUE point in the posterior axillary line (*yellow arrow*)

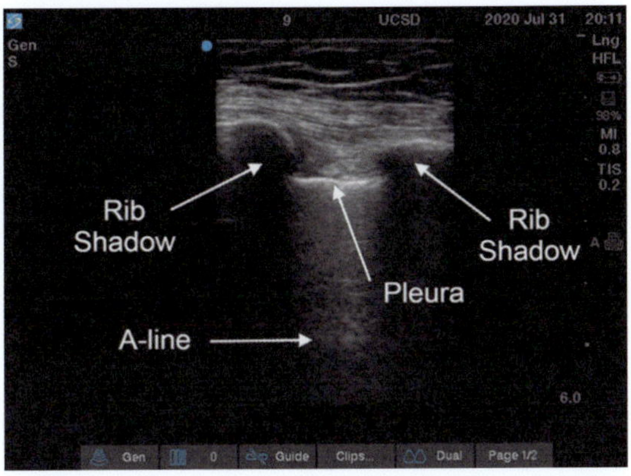

Fig. 21.2 The pleura is visualized between rib shadows, revealing the "bat sign." A normal A-line is also present

(Fig. 21.2, Video 21.1). This normal appearance has been termed the "bat sign," as the curved surface of the ribs resembles the underside of the wings of a flying bat, and the intercostal tissues provide the form of its body. It provides a useful landmark for identification of the pleura, and a window for visualization. In the case of subcutaneous emphysema, compression with the probe may be sufficient to still identify the rib and pleural landmarks.

Artifacts and Findings (Highlight Box 21.1)

Highlight Box 21.1

Lung ultrasound	

2D	• Lung sliding suggestive of pneumothorax
	  ◦ "Barcode" instead of "Sandy Beach" on M-mode imaging
	• A-lines suggestive of normally aerated lung
	  ◦ Reverberation artifact twice the depth from probe to pleural line
	• B-lines suggestive of thickened interlobular septa (e.g., pulmonary edema)
	  ◦ "Comet tail" artifact extending from pleural line away from the probe
	• Visualization of lung parenchyma is suggestive of lung consolidation
	  ◦ "Hepatization" or air bronchograms may be present

CFD	• Evaluation of DVT – see Chap. 19
Spectral	• Not typically utilized

As lung ultrasound relies on artifacts for much of its use, a brief discussion of ultrasound artifacts is warranted. The ultrasound machine relies on several assumptions of the behavior of the sound waves. It assumes that the sound travels in a straight line, directly to the tissue and back, and at a constant speed. However, the heterogeneous nature of human tissue can bend these assumptions and cause unexpected signals to return to the probe.

Shadowing

When an ultrasound wave encounters an object of significantly different density than the surrounding tissue (e.g., bone surrounded by muscle fibers), it will reflect nearly all of the ultrasound waves. The periosteum is highly reflective leaving very little ultrasound signal available to penetrate distally past the bone. With more ultrasound waves being reflected, fewer will continue deeper into the tissue, and no waves will be reflected from beyond that object, casting a shadow-like artifact. In the case of bone, almost all of the ultrasound waves are reflected, so imaging of the lung or pleura must be achieved between the rib spaces (Fig. 21.2).

Lung Sliding

The layers of pleura are sufficiently thin that it is not possible to distinguish whether one or both layers are being visualized with ultrasound. The appearance of lung sliding indicates that the visceral pleura is in close contact with the parietal pleura and there is movement between them [10]. This motion and appearance as been described as "to-and-fro," "twinkling," or "ants marching." In fact, in normal aerated lung tissue, the entire space displayed below the pleura is an artifact generated at the level of the pleura, as the lung tissue itself reflects the ultrasound wave almost completely. Lichtenstein now defines normal lung sliding by this "sparkling" of the entire space rather than just motion of the pleural line itself (Video 21.2) [1].

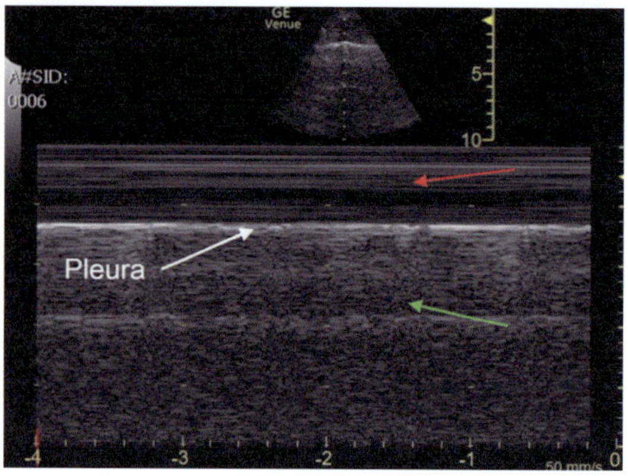

Fig. 21.3 Normal lung sliding with M-Mode imaging, generating a "seashore sign" appearance. There is very little motion above the pleural line (*red arrow*), and significant movement below the pleura (*green arrow*)

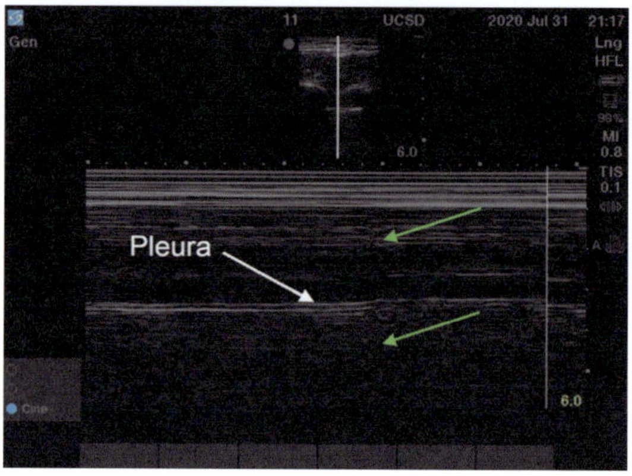

Fig. 21.4 Absence of lung sliding, causing the "barcode sign" on M-Mode. There is motion artifact (*green arrows*), which extends above and below the pleural line

Lung sliding may be more difficult to detect when the lung motion itself is decreased, such as in the case of low tidal volume ventilation or in the apices of the lunges. M-mode may help enhance this visualization by demonstrating the "seashore sign" (Fig. 21.3). The movement at and below the pleura create a "sandy beach" appearance, in contrast to the relatively static tissues above the pleural line.

If lung sliding is absent, there will not be any "sparkling" of either the pleural line or the pleural/artifact space on live two-dimensional ultrasound. M-mode imaging will display the "barcode" or "stratosphere" sign, where there is little variation of the pleural/artifact space (Fig. 21.4). In this particular image, there are several lines noted below the pleural line. However, these lines represent reverberation artifact from lines in the subcutaneous tissue.

Absent lung sliding can be a sign of a pneumothorax, indicating that the visceral and parietal pleura have lost contact. However, other conditions can cause a loss of lung sliding as well. Generally, these conditions result in a loss of ventilation and consequent lung movement (apnea, impaired lung compliance, complete atelectasis, severe acute asthma, esophageal or mainstem intubation, jet ventilation, abdominal compartment syndrome, or prior pneumonectomy). Additionally, inflammatory or exudative processes can abolish lung sliding due to subsequent adhesion to the pleural wall. Such conditions can include empyema, pleural adhesions, pleurisy, prior pleurodesis, ARDS, and pneumonia.

T-Lines and Lung Pulse

In the absence of significant respiratory movement of the pleura, more subtle movements between the pleural layers can still be appreciated. Because the signs of lung sliding are generated at the pleura, motion that is observed on both sides of the pleura is not related to pleural movement and instead represents movement of the entire chest wall relative to the transducer. Figure 21.5 demonstrates a patient without significant respiratory lung motion and without a clear "seashore sign" on M-mode. Intermittent small lung movements will create "T-lines" as a result of minimal movement between the layers of pleura. The T-shaped appearance between the pleura and this vertical artifact confirm that both pleural layers are visualized. In contrast, Fig. 21.5 also shows a motion artifact generated by patient movement, occurring both above and below the pleural line.

Another subtle version of lung sliding is the lung pulse. If the heart, pericardium, pleura, and lung tissue are all contiguous, the motion of the heartbeat can be transmitted to the lung and detected at the pleura, creating T-lines at intervals

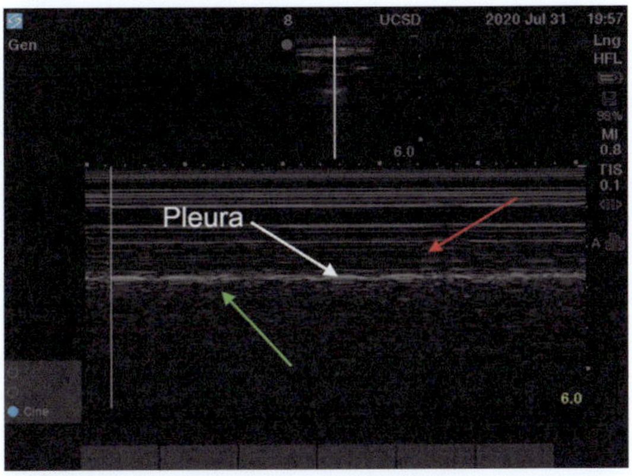

Fig. 21.5 T-lines on M-mode indicate the presence of subtle movements between the layers of pleura (*green arrow*). The presence of these movements below the pleura excludes the presence of pneumothorax at that location. Movement that occurs both above and below the pleura (*red arrow*) is an artifact from motion of the chest wall relative to the transducer

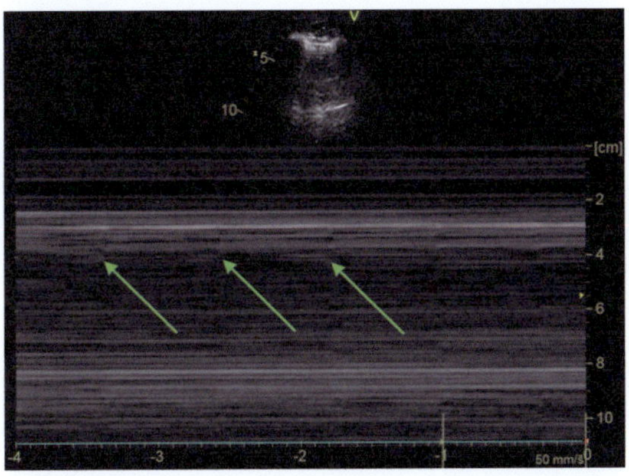

Fig. 21.6 Motion from heartbeats can be transmitted to the pleura as a specific type of T-line artifact, termed a "lung pulse" (*green arrows*)

consistent with cardiac motion (Fig. 21.6, Video 21.3). This finding also shows that the visceral and parietal pleura are in contact appropriately, excluding pneumothorax at that location, even if there is no respiratory movement.

Lung Point

A pneumothorax can also be confirmed by identifying a "lung point," i.e., the precise point at which the lung loses contact with the pleura [11].

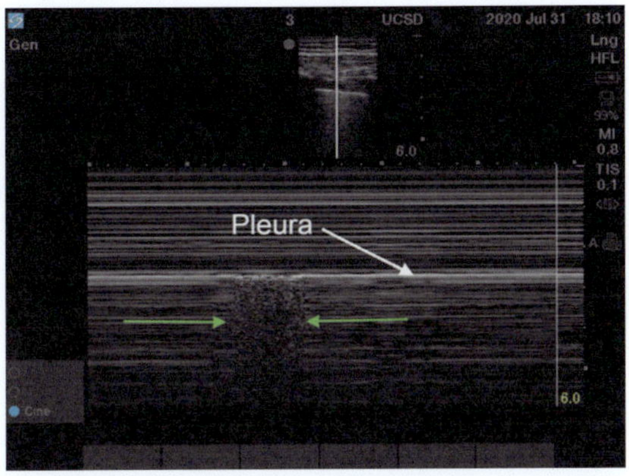

Fig. 21.7 A "lung point" demonstrated on M-Mode in a patient with a pneumothorax. The visceral pleural layer makes intermittent contact with the parietal pleura during inspiration, creating a transient "seashore sign" (between *green arrows*)

On live two-dimensional ultrasound, this will appear as an image where only part of the lung shows lung sliding, and another part does not. The point commonly moves with respiration, and this movement will also cause an intermittent "seashore sign" on M-mode (Fig. 21.7, Video 21.4). The lung point is typically found more laterally as the pneumothorax will rise to the front of the chest while the lung will fall with gravity toward the back of the chest.

A-Lines (Reverberation Artifact)

Reverberation is caused when two strong reflectors are in the path of the ultrasound beam. Most commonly in lung ultrasound, this will be the pleural line and the surface of the transducer itself. Normally, the ultrasound beam will be reflected off the pleural line and then be absorbed by the transducer upon its return, causing the ultrasound machine to sense the pleural line. However, some of the reflected beam may again bounce off the skin or probe surface, sending the beam back down toward the pleural line. The pleural line again reflects the beam back toward the probe, having taken twice the expected amount of time to return to the ultrasound probe. Therefore, the machine interprets another reflector (tissue layer or pleural line) twice as deep,

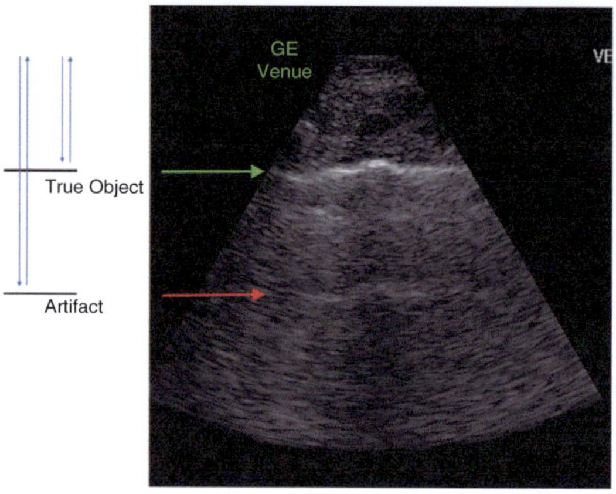

Fig. 21.8 A reverberation artifact occurs between strong reflectors, in this case the two strong reflectors are the pleura (*green arrow*) and the transducer surface. The ultrasound energy traverses the path twice between the transducer and pleura, creating the duplicate appearance of the pleural line at twice the distance from the transducer providing the appearance of an "A-line" (*red arrow*)

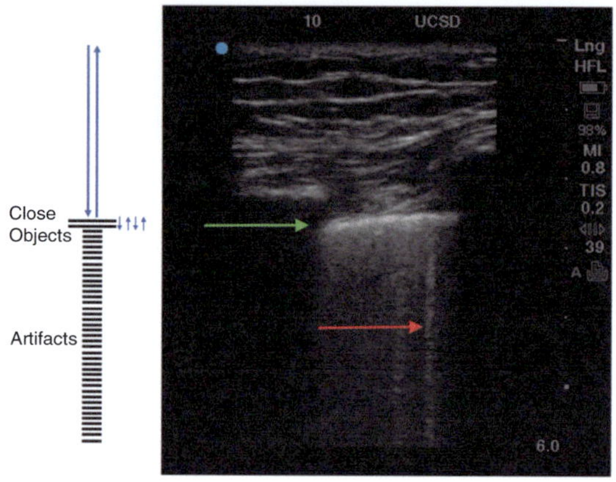

Fig. 21.9 Reverberation artifact from the pleural layers (*green arrow*), causing B-lines extending to the bottom of the screen (*red arrow*)

which is called an A-line (Fig. 21.8, Video 21.1 and 21.2).

A-lines are parallel to the pleural line and signify a strong reflection (air) below the pleura, which can either be normal aerated lung or potentially a pneumothorax. The lack of any A- (or B-) lines can be referred to as an O-line, which may also be a normal finding or may occur with the lack of a strong reflector (e.g., pleural effusion). Multiple A-lines may occur in a single imaging plane at intervals equidistant to the pleural line, with decreasing brightness as less and less signal is reflected to the transducer.

B-Lines (Comet Tails)

B-lines, also known as "comet tails," "lung rockets," or "ring down" artifact, are effectively a very tight series of reverberation artifacts starting at the pleural line, and continuing to the end of the image. B-lines will occur in the axis parallel to the ultrasound beam and can be differentiated from a probe malfunction (e.g., broken crystal) because they do not originate at the probe and will move with movement of the pleura. When two strong reflectors are in close proximity (e.g., pleura and nearby aerated alveoli separated by interstitial edema [1, 12]), the resulting reverberation artifact will appear almost as a continuous beam, rather than separate lines (Figs. 21.9 and 21.10, Video 21.5).

B-lines start at the pleura and move with lung sliding. Almost always, they will obliterate A-lines and extend to the edge of the screen. A Z-line is a normal artifact, appearing as a short vertical line originating from the pleura, but not extending beyond 3–4 cm, and should not be counted as a B-line. Occasional B-lines are a normal finding, likely due to a lung fissure. Three or more B-lines in any one rib space are considered abnormal, signifying diseased interlobular septa and pulmonary edema. Diffuse symmetric pulmonary edema suggests a transudative cause such as heart failure or fluid overload. Unilateral or irregular pulmonary edema suggests an exudative/inflammatory cause such as pneumonia or ARDS.

Interlobular septa are 6–7 mm apart, coincidentally the distance between initial B-lines. Typically, there will be 3–4 B-lines with early pulmonary edema, representing septal thickening. Progression of the pulmonary edema will generate 6–8 B-lines approximately 3 mm apart, corresponding to a ground-glass pattern on CT. Extreme edema will generate confluent B-lines, which may be difficult to differentiate; however, the entire pleural/artifact space will be bright like the pleural line.

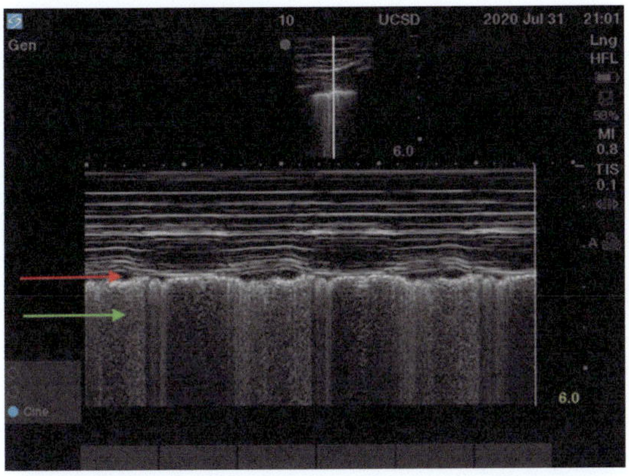

Fig. 21.10 B-lines visualized in M-mode. Movement of the B-lines causes intermittent brightness of the pleural/artifact space (*green arrow*), as well as intermittent visualization of a small pleural effusion (*red arrow*)

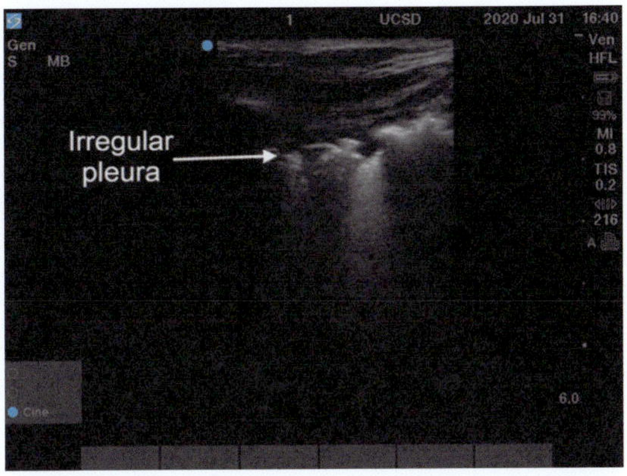

Fig. 21.12 The pleura has an irregular appearance, labeled a C-profile, consistent with an underlying pneumonia

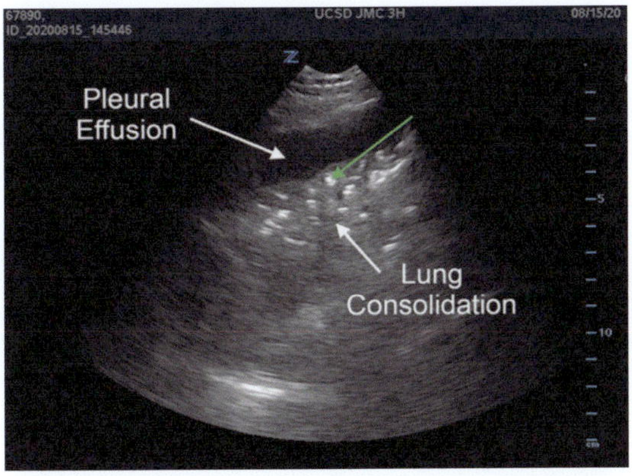

Fig. 21.11 Lung consolidation from pneumonia, with pleural effusion. The consolidated lung tissue has as a similar appearance to soft tissue, i.e., "hepatization." In addition, air bronchograms are visible within the consolidated lung (*green arrow*)

Consolidation

Normal, aerated lung tissue will reflect ultrasound waves almost entirely, as previously discussed. The ability to visualize lung parenchyma therefore represents an abnormality. Consolidation and consequent de-aeration of the lung tissue may provide an appearance similar to soft tissue like the liver, earning the moniker "hepatization" (Fig. 21.11, Video 21.6). In addition, it may be possible to visualize air bronchograms, which have the same clinical significance with ultrasound as they do with radiography (consolidation next to patent airways). If the consolidation involves only a portion of the lobe, the aerated tissue may reflect waves, casting a bright appearance deep to the consolidation. This abrupt transition has been labeled the "shred sign" and suggests a focal or non-lobar pneumonia [1, 3]. More subtle consolidations may contain aerated lung, but generate an irregular appearance of the pleura (Fig. 21.12, Video 21.7). Consolidations are often associated with adjacent pleural effusions, which are visualized as hypoechoic or anechoic fluid in the pleural space.

Profiles

These various findings, representing different lung pathologies, have been organized into a system of "profiles," described by Dr. Lichtenstein (Table 21.1) [2]. These profiles are separated based on the appearance of the pleural space and the presence or absence of lung sliding. Absence of lung sliding is noted by a "prime" or " ' " next to the profile letter. An A-profile will demonstrate normal aerated lung with A-lines and lung sliding, while an A'-profile will demonstrate A-lines without lung sliding, suggesting a pneumothorax. A B-profile will demonstrate B-lines with lung sliding, which most commonly relates to simple pulmonary edema (e.g., CHF exacerbation), while a B'-profile has the presence of multiple

Table 21.1 Lung ultrasound profiles

Profile	Findings	Physiology	Clinical significance
A	A-lines +lung sliding	Aerated space Both layers of pleura	Normal aerated lung No pneumothorax
A'	A-lines No lung sliding	Aerated space No pleural movement	Pneumothorax or non-ventilated lung (e.g., airway obstruction)
B	B-lines +lung sliding	Interstitial edema Pleural movement	Pulmonary edema (e.g., CHF)
B'	B-lines No lung sliding	Interstitial edema Restricted pleural movement	Pneumonia ARDS
C	Irregular pleura or visible lung tissue +lung sliding	Consolidation Pleural movement	Pneumonia
C'	Visible lung tissue no lung sliding	Consolidation Restricted lung movement	Severe pneumonia

B-lines, but without lung sliding, as occurs with an inflammatory process like pneumonia or ARDS. A C-profile will demonstrate an irregular pleura or visible consolidation, in which part of the lung can be seen directly, also consistent with pneumonia. Restricted lung sliding (C'-profile) may also be present, depending on the severity of the disease.

Diagnoses

Pneumothorax

Lung ultrasound has robust data showing much better sensitivity for pneumothorax than CXR. Lichtenstein studied 115 patients and concluded that A-lines with no lung sliding (A'-profile, Fig. 21.4) was 100% sensitive and 96.5% specific for pneumothorax [13]. In an earlier study, he found a sensitivity of 95.3% and specificity of 91.1% [10], although he later explained that this should have been 100% due to the exclusion of patients with subcutaneous emphysema. His 2005 study of 200 patients showed that the A'-profile had a sensitivity of 95% and specificity of 94%, while the lung point had a sensitivity of 79% and specificity of 100% [14]. Soldati et al. studied 109 trauma patients and found that ultrasound had a sensitivity of 92% and specificity of 99.5%, compared to CXR which had a sensitivity of 52% and specificity of 100% [15]. A meta-analysis by Alrajab et al. demonstrated a sensitivity of 79% and specificity of 98% for ultrasound evaluation for pneumothorax, compared to a sensitivity of 40% and specificity of 99.3% for CXR [16].

Because the specificity of the A'-profile is only 91–95% and the treatment is an invasive chest tube, further confirmation may be sought in the form of the lung point, which is the visualization of the location where the lung separates from the pleura. It has a sensitivity of 66% and a specificity of 100% [11]. The location of the lung point can also be used to estimate the size of the pneumothorax, as air tends to move against gravity. If the lung point is located on the superior chest, the pneumothorax is smaller. If the lung point is located more laterally, the pneumothorax is larger. In very large pneumothoraces, there may not be a lung point at all, as the lung is completely separated from the chest wall.

Pulmonary Edema

Transudative pulmonary edema is usually diagnosed with the B-profile (Fig. 21.9, Fig. 21.10, Video 21.5), which Lichtenstein found to be 93% sensitive and specific compared to CXR in a study of 250 patients [12], although later claimed 100% due to misinterpretation of Z-lines. In an Emergency Department study, Koh et al. found that ultrasound was 71.4% sensitive and 80.9% specific for pulmonary edema [7]. As a sign of pulmonary edema, B-lines have also been correlated with extravascular lung water on CXR, [17] as well as pulmonary artery occlusion pressure (PAOP) [18]. The A-profile (lack of B-lines) was

67% sensitive and 90% specific for a PAOP ≤ 13 mmHg. It was 50% sensitive and 93% specific for a PAOP ≤ 18 mmHg [19]. In patients with acute decompensated heart failure, the severity of the B-profile correlated with the CXR appearance, clinical score, and BNP. Furthermore, the sonographic lung appearance correlated with improvement in the CXR and clinical scores as the patients improved with treatment [20].

While the B-profile is normally associated with transudative edema, it can also be seen in early exudative processes like pneumonia. Transudative edema is more likely to be symmetric and dependent, although posterior consolidation, atelectasis, and effusions are common in patients with pulmonary edema due to gravity and immobility.

Pleural Effusion

A pleural effusion will appear as an anechoic or hypoechoic area between the pleural line and lung. Septations or debris within the effusion suggest complex fluid (i.e., empyema). A four-sided "quad sign" may help identify a pleural effusion (Fig. 21.13, Video 21.6). The four borders are the two rib shadows, the pleural line, and the lung border. M-mode may also demonstrate movement of the lung distal to the effusion (Fig. 21.14).

Pulmonary edema is common in the setting of a pleural effusion (and vice versa), and B-lines may be seen at the lung edge below an effusion (Fig. 21.15). When appearing below a pleural effusion, they may also be called "sub B-lines."

Chest X-ray may miss significant pleural effusions, even some of those requiring intervention [21]. Lichtenstein studied 32 patients and found that ultrasound was 92% sensitive and 93% specific for pleural effusion compared to CT scan, while CXR was only 39% sensitive and 85% specific [22]. In another study, ultrasound was used to evaluate for pleural effusion and a thoracente-

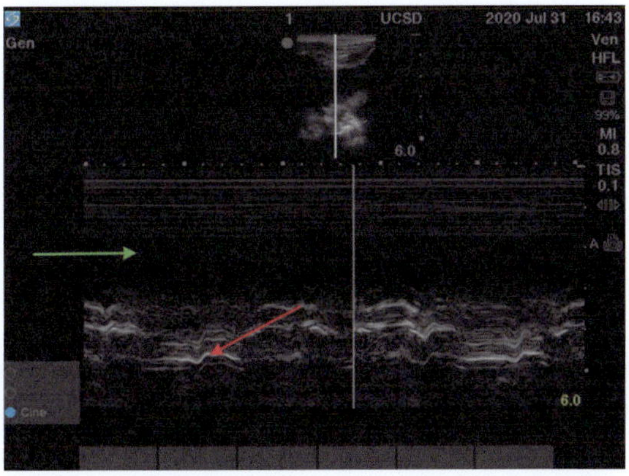

Fig. 21.14 M-mode displaying a pleural effusion (*green arrow*), with underlying lung motion. The *red arrow* highlights the movement of an air bronchogram within an area of consolidated lung tissue

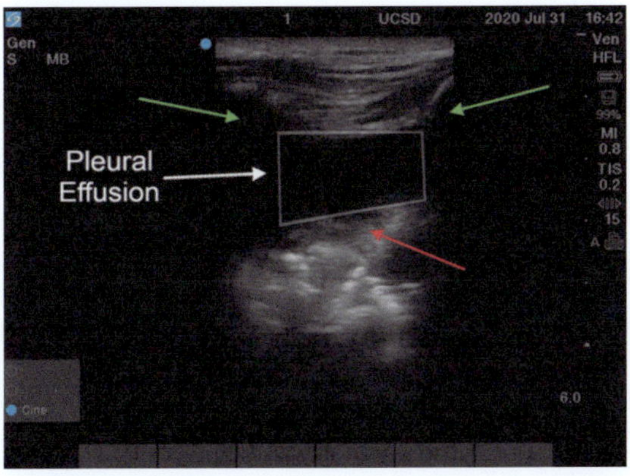

Fig. 21.13 A four-sided "quad sign" identifying a pleural effusion. The four borders are the two rib shadows (*green arrows*), the pleural line, and the edge of the consolidated lung (*red arrow*)

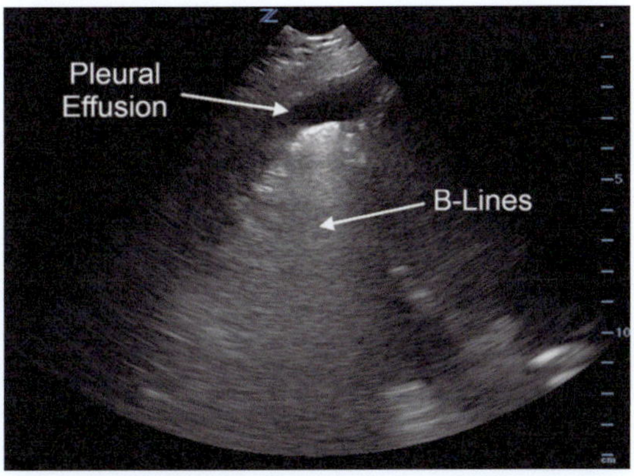

Fig. 21.15 Confluent B-lines occurring below a pleural effusion, indicating severe interstitial edema. When occurring below an effusion, these may also be called "sub B-lines"

sis was performed if the interpleural distance was ≥ 15 mm. Out of 45 effusions seen with ultrasound, fluid was obtained in 44. Of note, only 60% of those were visible on CXR [23].

Pneumonia

Unlike other findings with lung ultrasound, effusions and consolidations are directly visualized, rather than relying on interpretation of artifacts. Due to the dependent nature of these processes, the appropriately named PLAPS point is the highest yield when evaluating for both processes. Consolidated lung will appear like soft tissue, similar to hepatic tissue (Fig. 21.11, Video 21.6). Air bronchograms may be visible as bright hyperechoic regions, which may expand with inspiration, suggesting a patent airway and making obstructive atelectasis an unlikely cause. In the anterior lung, there may be sufficient aeration to prevent direct visualization of consolidation, but the pleural line may appear thickened and irregular (Fig. 21.12, Video 21.7). Interestingly, ultrasonographic evaluation of consolidation and B-lines can also be used to evaluate lung recruitment and optimize PEEP in ventilated patients [24].

As a focal or heterogeneous disease, pneumonia can have different sonographic appearances. The BLUE protocol (described below) concludes with pneumonia in the following cases: B'-profile anywhere (11% sensitive, 100% specific), C-profile anywhere (21% sensitive, 99% specific), unilateral B-profile (14% sensitive, 100% specific), and PLAPS effusion/consolidation in the absence of both B-profiles and DVT (42% sensitive, 96% specific) [25]. Combined, ultrasound had a sensitivity of 89% and specificity of 94% for detection of pneumonia. An earlier study by Lichtenstein et al. found that ultrasound was 90% sensitive and 98% specific for alveolar consolidation [26]. A study by Bourcier et al. in the Emergency Department compared ultrasound and CXR to discharge diagnosis [27]. Ultrasound had a sensitivity of 95% and specificity of 57%, while CXR had a sensitivity of 60% and specificity of 76%. Of note, ultrasound was much more sensitive than CXR for patients with symptoms less than 24 hours. In another Emergency Department study, Koh et al. found that ultrasound was 65.3% sensitive and 82% specific for pneumonia [7].

Lung Contusion

Much like pneumonia, ultrasound can evaluate for pulmonary contusions. Soldati et al. studied 121 blunt chest trauma patients [28]. B-lines were 94.6% sensitive and 96.1% specific, while the C-profile was 18.9% sensitive but 100% specific for pulmonary contusions in this population.

Pulmonary Embolism

Diagnosis of pulmonary embolism by lung ultrasound alone is difficult. Unless the PE is large enough to cause lung infarction, the lung usually appears normal (A-profile). Thus, indirect signs such as right heart strain or DVT are used. Even small DVTs are significant in this setting, because most of the thrombus may have already embolized. Lichtenstein et al. found that a normal (A-profile) lung in combination with a positive DVT was 81% sensitive and 99% specific for pulmonary embolism in patients that are acutely short of breath [25]. The PLAPS point will have a positive finding in approximately 52% of PE cases, which is why a DVT scan may be considered first. Additionally, approximately 5% of C-profile cases will be a PE rather than pneumonia [1]. Mathis et al. studied 194 patients with confirmed pulmonary embolism and found that there were an average of 2.3 subpleural lesions (C-profile) in each. A small pleural effusion was found in 49%. He estimated that finding 2 of these lesions, or 1 plus a pleural effusion, was 74% sensitive and 95% specific in a population with suspected PE and a 55% prevalence [29].

Diaphragmatic Weakness

Ultrasound may also be used to quantify the distance of diaphragmatic excursion in the evaluation of diaphragmatic weakness. This may be a useful adjunct to ventilator measurements such as tidal volume, forced vital capacity, and negative inspiratory force. It can still be measured in non-ventilated patients as well when evaluating for critical illness myopathy, neuropathy, phrenic nerve injury, or other cause of diaphragm weakness. The diaphragm is imaged using the liver and spleen as sonographic windows at the anterior axillary lines (Fig. 21.16) [30]. When measuring at the posterior third of the diaphragm, quiet breathing generated an average of 1.8 cm excursion in men and a 1.6 cm excursion in women [31]. Diaphragmatic excursion can also be used as a ventilator weaning measure. One study using a cutoff of 14 mm on the right and 12 mm on the left generated a similar "area under the curve" as the Rapid Shallow Breathing Index (RSBI), although the agreement between the two measures was poor [32].

Asthma/COPD

Asthma and COPD will have a normal A-profile on lung ultrasound, although the diaphragm may be displaced downward due to air trapping. The diagnosis relies on additional clinical information, including history and wheezing on examination. However, pulmonary embolism will also frequently show an A-profile, although the prevalence of a PE in this scenario is much lower in general. Lichtenstein estimates that approximately one A-profile patient will have a PE for every 40 that have COPD or asthma in the Emergency Department [1]. Koh et al. found that ultrasound was 64.5% sensitive and 89.8% specific for asthma/COPD [7]. Ultrasound alone cannot confirm obstructive airway disease, but it can help eliminate other causes of dyspnea.

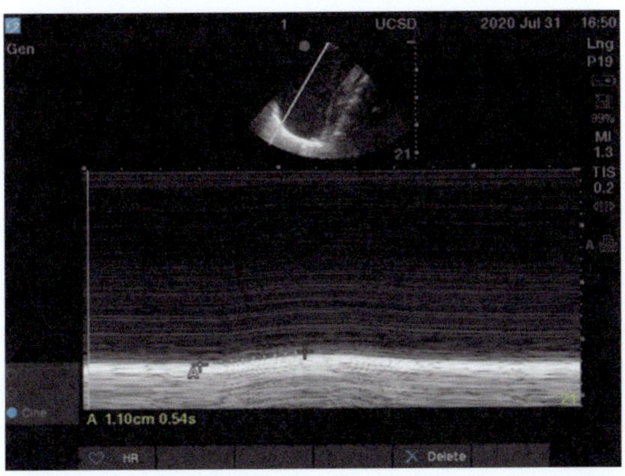

Fig. 21.16 Diaphragmatic excursion measured through the liver using M-mode. The excursion measurement of 1.1 cm is below normal and indicates diaphragmatic weakness in a spontaneously breathing patient

Thromboembolic Disease

Lung ultrasound is unable to directly visualize pulmonary emboli in most cases, and more commonly relies on adjunctive examinations. Portions of the pulmonary arteries may be visualized in several views by both TTE (e.g., parasternal short-axis view) and TEE (e.g., midesophageal ascending aorta short-axis view), or venous ultrasound scanning may be used to evaluate for the presence of DVT. The technique for evaluation for DVT is discussed in detail in Chap. 20.

Protocols

Several protocols have been developed to organize the ultrasound evaluation of lung pathology. None have been established as particularly superior, each with relative advantages and disadvantages, and they share many of the same elements.

BLUE Protocol

Lichtenstein's Bedside Lung Ultrasound in Emergency (BLUE) protocol [1, 2, 25] is one of the first and likely most prosperous systems of evaluating lung pathology with ultrasound (Fig. 21.17). In the initial study, the case mix was 31% pneumonia, 24% CHF, 18% COPD, 12% asthma, 8% PE, and 3% pneumothorax. The

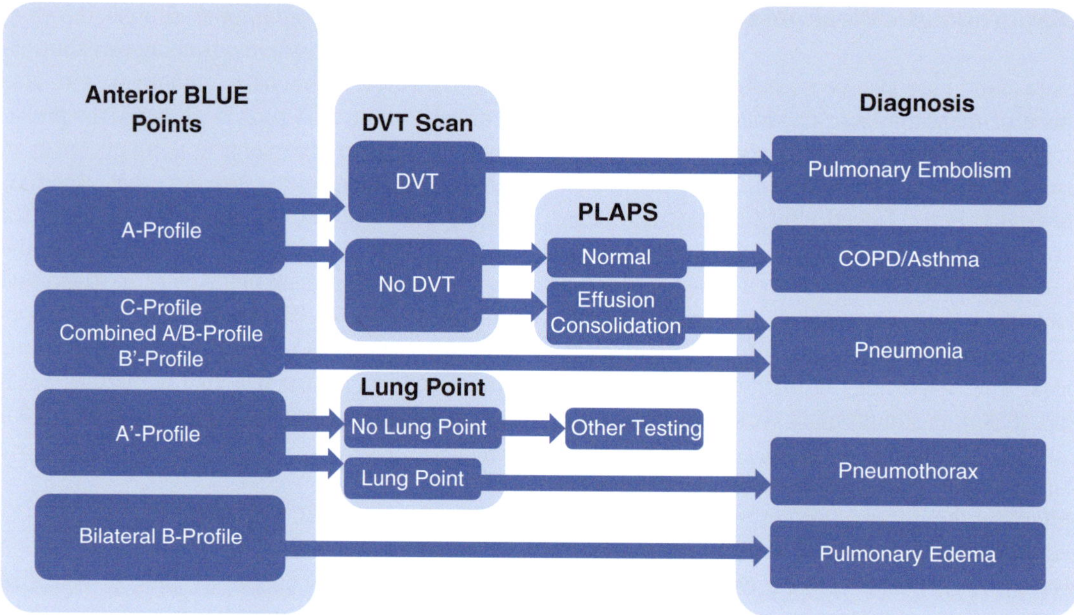

Fig. 21.17 The Bedside Lung Ultrasound in Emergency (BLUE) Protocol [25]

BLUE protocol reached the correct diagnosis in 90.5% of cases. An Emergency Department study of a similar but expanded protocol found that it was > 90% specific for most conditions, but only 40% sensitive for PE and 77–88% sensitive in other conditions [4]. An even more recent study involving 383 patients presenting to the Emergency Department with dyspnea showed sensitivity and specificity of 87.6% and 96.2% for pulmonary edema, 85.7% and 99.0% for pneumonia, 98.2% and 67.3% for asthma/COPD, 46.2% and 100% for pulmonary embolism, and 71.4% and 100% for pneumothorax [33].

There are several limitations to this protocol. The diagnosis of PE relies on some residual DVT, and the protocol will miss a PE when the entire DVT has embolized with none remaining peripherally, although this is uncommon. Early bilateral pneumonia can have a B-profile and may be diagnosed as pulmonary edema instead. Although it relies on provider familiarity, it does provide a useful framework for the ultrasound evaluation of dyspnea and has shown impressive test characteristics in the hands of an experienced provider.

Extended BLUE Protocol

When more clinical data and time is available, a more comprehensive assessment of the patient can take place. The Extended BLUE protocol is not strictly a protocol itself, but rather encourages the physician to include additional information outside the ultrasound [1]. For example, in the context of fever, a bilateral B-profile likely represents pneumonia rather than pulmonary edema. In true cardiogenic pulmonary edema, the B-lines should improve with medical treatment, and lack of improvement would prompt a continued search for a diagnosis. Wheezing on examination would support the diagnosis of asthma or COPD. A small pleural effusion or C-profile with otherwise normal lungs would usually be diagnosed as pneumonia, but could represent a pulmonary embolism, especially if the dyspnea is out of proportion to the ultrasound findings. The addition of cardiac ultrasound may help diagnose an interstitial lung disease if right-sided abnormalities are found. It may also support the diagnosis of pneumonia if a bilateral

B-Profile is seen, but the left ventricular function is maintained. As a final example, aspiration of pleural fluid or even lung abscesses [34] will yield additional information and may be therapeutic.

PINK Protocol

The PINK protocol was designed to quantitate the findings in a patient already diagnosed with ARDS. The name "PINK" is in distinction to those in whom the "BLUE" protocol is used, because the etiology of their dyspnea is known, and generally they are being ventilated, thus not "blue." With this protocol, patients with ARDS had a pneumonia (B', C, A/B, or PLAPS) pattern 86% of the time, and a pulmonary edema (B-profile) pattern the remaining 14% [19, 25]. Lung sliding may be quantified as normal (> 2 cm per breath), decreased (5–10 mm), impaired (1 mm), or abolished. The volume of pleural effusion may be estimated based on the interpleural distance measured with ultrasound using a variety of potential methods. One simple estimate of the volume in mL is 20 times the interpleural distance in millimeters [35], and another uses 5 cm as a cutoff for an estimate of 500 mL of pleural fluid [36]. Lichtenstein recommends measuring the interpleural distance at the PLAPS point at expiration and estimates pleural fluid volume as follows: 1 cm = 75–100 mL, 2 cm = 300–600 mL, 3.5 cm = 1.2–2.5 L [1].

Thoracentesis of > 500 mL has been shown to improve the patient's oxygenation [36]. The use and safety of ultrasound-guided thoracentesis has been well documented, with one study of 232 procedures generating only three pneumothoraces, without other major complications [37].

Other estimations include the volume of lung consolidations calculated as the length of the consolidation taken to the third power [1] as well as pneumothoraces by the location of the lung point. In one study, only 8% of patients with an anterior lung point needed a chest tube, while one was needed in 90% of patients with a lateral lung point (indicating a larger pneumothorax) [14]. Another study showed good concordance between CT scanning and the location of the ultrasound lung point [15].

CLOT Protocol

The incidence of catheter-associated DVTs has been reported in the range of 2–67% [38]. An Indian study of internal jugular lines found a 33% incidence at 6 days [39]. The Catheter-Linked Occult Thrombosis (CLOT) protocol therefore is a method of monitoring for DVT and subsequent PE [1]. Initially, the patient is scanned for catheter-associated DVT on a daily basis. If a thrombus is identified and then subsequently disappears abruptly on daily monitoring, it can be reasonably assumed to have migrated toward the lung given insufficient time for natural fibrinolysis.

FALLS Protocol

The Fluid Administration Limited by Lung Sonography (FALLS) protocol uses lung ultrasound for hemodynamic evaluation in hypotensive patients [1]. As mentioned earlier, pulmonary edema and subsequent B-Lines can predict the pulmonary artery occlusion pressure [18, 19]. Initially, an obstructive shock is ruled out by evaluating the pericardium (for tamponade), lungs (for pneumothorax), and deep veins and RV (for pulmonary embolism). Next, the lungs are evaluated for signs of pulmonary edema subsequent to cardiogenic causes. If the findings are negative and the lungs show an A-profile, the PAOP is likely equal to or less than 13 mmHg. The patient is then administered fluid while monitoring for the development B-lines. Once B-lines appear, the patient has likely reached their limit of fluid tolerance and vasopressors are started instead.

Conclusion

Ultrasound is ideal for the rapid bedside evaluation of dyspnea. In the right hands, it has sufficient sensitivity and specificity to guide management of acute pulmonary pathology, including pneumothorax, pulmonary edema, and pneumonia, and with adjunctive information may help identify COPD/asthma or pulmonary embolism. With additional time and detail, the findings can also be quantified to follow the disease course. Additionally, lung ultrasound can contribute information regarding the patients' hemodynamics and volume status and is a valuable tool for the acute care provider.

Questions

1. You are called to evaluate a 64-year-old man for sudden-onset dyspnea. He has a history of COPD, CHF, and type 2 diabetes. His heart rate is 114, his respiratory rate is 28, his blood pressure is 144/96, and his oxygen saturation is 93% on 4L nasal cannula. You see 2 B-lines with lung sliding on the anterior right lung, and A-lines without lung sliding on the anterior left lung. What is the next step?

   A. Initiate nitroglycerin, furosemide, and CPAP
   B. Initiate inhaled albuterol, ipratropium, and systemic methylprednisolone
   C. Locate a positive lung point on the left, then insert a percutaneous chest tube
   D. Insert a percutaneous chest tube on the left

2. You are called to evaluate a 59-year-old man for sudden-onset dyspnea. He has a history of COPD, CHF, and DM type 2. His heart rate is 123, his respiratory rate is 34, his blood pressure is 173/112, and his oxygen saturation is 92% on 4L NC. You see 5 B-lines in the bilateral anterior lungs. What is your next step?

   A. Initiate nitroglycerin, furosemide, and noninvasive positive pressure ventilation
   B. Initiate inhaled albuterol, ipratropium, and systemic methylprednisolone
   C. Search for a lung point, and then insert a chest tube if present
   D. Initiate piperacillin/tazobactam, azithromycin, and vancomycin

3. How are A-lines created?

   A. Reverberation artifact between the pleural line and fluid-filled alveoli
   B. Reverberation artifact between the skin and pleural line
   C. Complete blocking of ultrasound waves by rib bone
   D. Subtle lung movement on M-Mode

4. You are called to evaluate a 56-year-old woman for sudden-onset dyspnea. She has a history of COPD, CHF, and DM type 2. Her heart rate is 123, her respiratory rate is 31, her blood pressure is 110/74, and her oxygen saturation is 93% on 4L NC. You see A-lines with lung sliding in the bilateral anterior lungs. What is your next step?

   A. Initiate nitroglycerin, furosemide, and CPAP
   B. Initiate inhaled albuterol, ipratropium, and systemic methylprednisolone
   C. Scan veins for sign of DVT
   D. Initiate piperacillin/tazobactam, azithromycin, and vancomycin

5. You are using ultrasound to guide the resuscitation of a hypotensive patient. You have ruled out pneumothorax, pericardial tamponade, and pulmonary embolism. You see A-lines in the bilateral lungs. Which is true?

   A. PAOP is likely > 18; start inotropes and pressors
   B. CVP is likely > 13; start inotropes and pressors
   C. PAOP is likely < 18; continue fluid resuscitation
   D. CVP is likely < 13; continue fluid resuscitation

6. You are called to evaluate a 66-year-old woman for dyspnea. She has a history of COPD, CHF, and DM type 2. Her heart rate is 107, her respiratory rate is 29, her blood pressure is 108/71, and her oxygen saturation is 92% on 4L NC. You see A-lines with lung sliding on the left, and 4 B-lines without lung sliding on the right. What is your next step?

   A. Initiate nitroglycerin, furosemide, and CPAP
   B. Initiate a heparin infusion
   C. Search for a lung point, and then insert a chest tube if present
   D. Initiate piperacillin/tazobactam, azithromycin, and vancomycin

7. You locate a pleural effusion in a patient. There is a distance of 2 cm between the parietal pleura and visceral pleura. What is the approximately volume of the effusion?

   A. 50 mL
   B. 100 mL
   C. 400 mL
   D. 1000 mL

8. You are evaluating an intubated patient for hypoxia. You see an entire lobe of lung that has the appearance of tissue or liver. Within the lung are air bronchograms, which do not move at all with inspiration and expiration. What is the next step?

   A. Broaden antibiotics
   B. Increase PEEP
   C. Bronchoscopy
   D. Chest tube

9. What ultrasound settings should be used for lung ultrasound?

   A. Tissue harmonic imaging
   B. Doppler
   C. Filters to reduce artifacts
   D. None

10. How can motion artifact be differentiated from true lung sliding?

   A. Motion artifact will only occur deep to the pleura
   B. Motion artifact will only occur superficial to the pleura
   C. Lung sliding will only occur deep to the pleura
   D. Lung sliding will only occur superficial to the pleura

References

1. Lichtenstein DA. Lung Ultrasound in the Critically Ill: The BLUE Protocol. Softcover reprint of the original 1st ed. 2016 edition. Springer; 2018.
2. Lichtenstein DA. Lung ultrasound in the critically ill. Ann Intensive Care. 2014;4:1.
3. Mojoli F, Bouhemad B, Mongodi S, et al. Lung ultrasound for critically ill patients. Am J Respir Crit Care Med. 2019;199:701–14.
4. Zanobetti M, Scorpiniti M, Gigli C, et al. Point-of-care ultrasonography for evaluation of acute dyspnea in the ED. Chest. 2017;151:1295–301.
5. Yin W, Li Y, Zeng X, et al. The utilization of critical care ultrasound to assess hemodynamics and lung pathology on ICU admission and the potential for predicting outcome. PLoS One. 2017;12:e0182881.
6. Manno E, Navarra M, Faccio L, et al. Deep impact of ultrasound in the intensive care unit. Anesthesiology. 2012;117:801–9.
7. Koh Y, Chua MT, Ho WH, et al. Assessment of dyspneic patients in the emergency department using point-of-care lung and cardiac ultrasonography—a prospective observational study. J Thorac Dis. 2018;10:6221–9.
8. Chiumello D, Mongodi S, Algieri I, et al. Assessment of lung aeration and recruitment by CT scan and ultrasound in acute respiratory distress syndrome patients*. Crit Care Med. 2018;46:1761–8.
9. Volpicelli G, Elbarbary M, Blaivas M, et al. International evidence-based recommendations for point-of-care lung ultrasound. Intensive Care Med. 2012;38:577–91.
10. Lichtenstein DA, Menu Y. A bedside ultrasound sign ruling out pneumothorax in the critically Ill. Chest. 1995;108:1345–8.
11. Lichtenstein D, Mezière G, Biderman P, et al. The "lung point": an ultrasound sign specific to pneumothorax. Intensive Care Med. 2000;26:1434–40.

12. Lichtenstein D, MÉZiÈRe G, Biderman P, et al. The comet-tail artifact. Am J Respir Crit Care Med. 1997;156:1640–6.
13. Lichtenstein D, Mezière G, Biderman P, et al. The comet-tail artifact: an ultrasound sign ruling out pneumothorax. Intensive Care Med. 1999;25:383–8.
14. Lichtenstein DA, Mezière G, Lascols N, et al. Ultrasound diagnosis of occult pneumothorax*. Crit Care Med. 2005;33:1231–8.
15. Soldati G, Testa A, Sher S, et al. Occult traumatic pneumothorax. Chest. 2008;133:204–11.
16. Alrajab S, Youssef AM, Akkus NI, et al. Pleural ultrasonography versus chest radiography for the diagnosis of pneumothorax: review of the literature and meta-analysis. Crit Care. 2013;17:R208.
17. Jambrik Z, Monti S, Coppola V, et al. Usefulness of ultrasound lung comets as a nonradiologic sign of extravascular lung water. Am J Cardiol. 2004;93:1265–70.
18. Agricola E, Bove T, Oppizzi M, et al. "Ultrasound comet-tail images": a marker of pulmonary edema. Chest. 2005;127:1690–5.
19. Lichtenstein DA, Mezière GA, Lagoueyte J-F, et al. A-lines and B-lines. Chest. 2009;136:1014–20.
20. Volpicelli G, Caramello V, Cardinale L, et al. Bedside ultrasound of the lung for the monitoring of acute decompensated heart failure. Am J Emerg Med. 2008;26:585–91.
21. Brixey AG, Luo Y, Skouras V, et al. The efficacy of chest radiographs in detecting parapneumonic effusions. Respirology. 2011;16:1000–4.
22. Lichtenstein D, Goldstein I, Mourgeon E, et al. Comparative diagnostic performances of auscultation, chest radiography, and lung ultrasonography in acute respiratory distress syndrome. Anesthesiology. 2004;100:9–15.
23. Lichtenstein D, Hulot JS, Rabiller A, et al. Feasibility and safety of ultrasound-aided thoracentesis in mechanically ventilated patients. Intensive Care Med. 1999;25:955–8.
24. Bouhemad B, Brisson H, Le-Guen M, et al. Bedside ultrasound assessment of positive end-expiratory pressure–induced lung recruitment. Am J Respir Crit Care Med. 2011;183:341–7.
25. Lichtenstein DA, Mezière GA. Relevance of lung ultrasound in the diagnosis of acute respiratory failure*: the BLUE protocol. Chest. 2008;134:117–25.
26. Lichtenstein DA, Lascols N, Mezière G, et al. Ultrasound diagnosis of alveolar consolidation in the critically ill. Intensive Care Med. 2004;30:276–81.
27. Bourcier J-E, Paquet J, Seinger M, et al. Performance comparison of lung ultrasound and chest x-ray for the diagnosis of pneumonia in the ED. Am J Emerg Med. 2014;32:115–8.
28. Soldati G, Testa A, Silva FR, et al. Chest ultrasonography in lung contusion. Chest. 2006;130:533–8.
29. Mathis G, Blank W, Reißig A, et al. Thoracic ultrasound for diagnosing pulmonary embolism. Chest. 2005;128:1531–8.
30. Matamis D, Soilemezi E, Tsagourias M, et al. Sonographic evaluation of the diaphragm in critically ill patients. Technique and clinical applications. Intensive Care Med. 2013;39:801–10.
31. Boussuges A, Gole Y, Blanc P. Diaphragmatic motion studied by M-mode ultrasonography. Chest. 2009;135:391–400.
32. Kim WY, Suh HJ, Hong S-B, et al. Diaphragm dysfunction assessed by ultrasonography: influence on weaning from mechanical ventilation*. Crit Care Med. 2011;39:2627–30.
33. Bekgoz B, Kilicaslan I, Bildik F, et al. BLUE protocol ultrasonography in Emergency Department patients presenting with acute dyspnea. Am J Emerg Med. 2019;37:2020–7.
34. Wali S. An update on the drainage of pyogenic lung abscesses. Ann Thorac Med. 2012;7:3.
35. Balik M, Plasil P, Waldauf P, et al. Ultrasound estimation of volume of pleural fluid in mechanically ventilated patients. Intensive Care Med. 2006;32:318.
36. Roch A, Bojan M, Michelet P, et al. Usefulness of ultrasonography in predicting pleural effusions > 500 mL in patients receiving mechanical ventilation. Chest. 2005;127:224–32.
37. Mayo PH, Goltz HR, Tafreshi M, et al. Safety of ultrasound-guided thoracentesis in patients receiving mechanical ventilation. Chest. 2004;125:1059–62.
38. Rooden CJ, Tesselaar MET, Osanto S, et al. Deep vein thrombosis associated with central venous catheters - a review. J Thromb Haemost. 2005;3:2409–19.
39. Rao S, Kujur R, Badwaik G, et al. Thrombosis associated with right internal jugular central venous catheters: a prospective observational study. Indian J Crit Care Med. 2012;16:17–21.

Shock and Cardiac Arrest

22

Eric Tzeng, Christopher R. Tainter,
and Diana Hylton

Abbreviations

CI	Collapsibility index
EKG	Electrocardiogram
IVC	Inferior vena cava
LUQ	Left upper quadrant
LVIDd	Left ventricular inner diameter in diastole
LVIDs	Left ventricular inner diameter in systole
LVOT	Left ventricular outflow tract
ME	Midesophageal
PASP	Pulmonary arterial systolic pressure
PE	Pulmonary embolism
PLAX	Parasternal long-axis
PSAX	Parasternal short-axis
RAP	Right atrial pressure
RUQ	Right upper quadrant
RV S'	Right ventricular (tissue) systolic velocity
RV	Right ventricle
RVIDd	Right ventricular inner diameter in diastole
SVC	Superior vena cava
TAPSE	Tricuspid annular plane systolic excursion
TEE	Transesophageal echocardiography
TG	Transgastric
TR	Tricuspid regurgitation
TTE	Transthoracic echocardiography
TV	Tricuspid valve

Introduction

Shock is a life-threatening and generalized maldistributive process of blood flow impeding oxygen delivery and/or use in the tissues. Prolonged shock can lead to irreversible tissue damage, resulting in multiorgan failure or death. Effective treatment relies on identification of the shock state and appropriate treatment of the underlying etiology, alongside other supportive measures to maintain end-organ perfusion. Shock can be considered a spectrum, ranging from mild hypotension to multiorgan failure and ultimately cardiac arrest.

Many different processes can lead to shock, but even without knowing the exact underlying process, identification of the physiologic derange-

Supplementary Information The online version of this chapter (https://doi.org/10.1007/978-3-030-84349-6_22) contains supplementary material, which is available to authorized users.

E. Tzeng (✉) · C. R. Tainter · D. Hylton
Department of Anesthesiology, University of California San Diego Health, La Jolla, CA, USA
e-mail: ertzeng@health.ucsd.edu

T. M. Maus, C. R. Tainter (eds.), *Essential Echocardiography*,
https://doi.org/10.1007/978-3-030-84349-6_22

ments can guide therapy. There are four physiologic patterns of shock: cardiogenic, obstructive, hypovolemic, and distributive, and more than one may occur simultaneously [1]. Overall, distributive shock from sepsis is the most frequent cause of shock (62%), followed by cardiogenic shock (16%), hypovolemic shock (16%), non-sepsis distributive shock (4%), and obstructive shock (2%) [2].

Early recognition and prompt treatment of different shock subtypes have been shown to decrease mortality in various types of shock [3]. Point-of-care echocardiography in patients with septic shock has been demonstrated to reduce mortality (22% relative reduction for in-hospital mortality) and facilitate earlier liberation from vasopressor therapy [4]. In general, this leads to more aggressive early resuscitation, with fluids, inotropes, and vasopressors, leading to a trend towards earlier reduction from these therapies.

Using Point-of-Care Echocardiography

Today, point-of-care ultrasound is a fundamental tool that is quick, safe, ubiquitous, and reproducible. In particular, transthoracic and transesophageal echocardiography (TTE and TEE, respectively) may provide insight into the mechanism for hemodynamic derangements. A provider with basic ultrasound skills can identify a variety of pathology and respond accordingly, and these skills can be learned quickly. In a group of physicians unfamiliar with TTE, Vignon et al. found that they were able to train participants to recognize a subset of basic views with only 8 hours of practical experience [5]. Many methods of systematic evaluation of shock with point-of-care ultrasound have been proposed and have repeatedly demonstrated a positive impact on patient care. The views and the orders in which they are obtained vary (see Table 22.1), but all revolve around the same principles.

Table 22.1 Selected ultrasound protocols for shock

Exam	Name	Views	Year described: data/comments
FATE	Focused Assessed Transthoracic Echocardiogram	Subcostal, apical, PLAX, PSAX, pleural	*1989:* 233 patients in shock, found useful in 97%, with 37% revealing new information and 24% resulting in decisive change[a]
eFAST	Extended Focused Assessment with Sonography in Trauma	Subcostal or PLAX, RUQ, pelvis, LUQ, pleural	*2004:* 24,350 trauma patients showing high sensitivity for pneumothorax, pericardial effusion, and abdominal free fluid leading to changes in management[b]
FEER	Focused Echocardiographic Evaluation during Resuscitation	Subcostal, PSAX, PLAX, apical	*2007:* 30 exams in field by EMS for suspect PEA, changed management in 24 cases with 19 having cardiac activity[c]
FOCUS	FOcused Cardiac UltraSound	PLAX, PSAX, apical, subcostal, IVC	*2010:* ASE consensus guidelines, with aggregate data demonstrating improved survival in trauma, shock, cardiac arrest, and dyspnea[d]
FEEL	Focused Echocardiographic Evaluation in Life support	Subcostal or parasternal or apical	*2010:* 204 exams in field by EMS, changed management in 66% with shock and 89% for cardiac arrest[e]
CLUE	Cardiopulmonary Limited Ultrasound Examination	PLAX, subcostal, pleural	*2011:* 1016 exams, "reasonable diagnostic accuracy"[f]
LTTE	Limited TransThoracic Echocardiogram	Subcostal, apical, PLAX, PSAX	*2013:* 148 exams in trauma bay, 41% resulted in therapies leading to decreased ICU stay (96% for age > 65)[g]

PLAX parasternal long-axis, *PSAX* parasternal short-axis, *RUQ* right upper quadrant, *LUQ* left upper quadrant, *IVC* inferior vena cava

[a]Feng, et al. [4]
[b]Netherton, et al. [16]
[c]Byhahn [2]
[d]Alrajhi, et al. [10]
[e]Breitkreutz, et al. [17]
[f]Kimura, et al. [18]
[g]Ferrada, et al. [19]

No one particular algorithm will be the most effective in all situations, as the clinical situation surrounding the onset of shock or cardiac arrest will dictate the priority of evaluating each etiology. In addition, patient factors may limit the utility of certain examinations. In the relative absence of clinical clues, we suggest pursuing a systematic course of investigation, focusing on reversible causes. In this chapter, we will outline relevant echocardiographic findings for the etiologies of shock: cardiogenic, obstructive, hypovolemic, and distributive.

Cardiogenic Shock (Table 22.2)

Decreased cardiac contractility from causes such as myocardial ischemia or cardiotoxicity can lead to impaired systemic perfusion. The body will attempt to compensate by raising vascular resistance to increase myocardial and systemic perfusion, which may increase afterload and paradoxically decrease cardiac output further. Echocardiography plays an important diagnostic role in estimating right and left ventricular function, identifying structural and valvular irregularities, and determining distributions of myocardial ischemia (i.e., regional wall motion abnormalities). The apical or subcostal four-chamber view (TTE) or the midesophageal four-chamber view (TEE) can rapidly assess global biventricular function and serve as excellent starting points for examining cardiac motion.

Table 22.2 Assessment of cardiogenic shock

Echo parameter	Echo view(s)	Abnormal
LV systolic function	TTE: apical, subcostal, parasternal SAX TEE: ME 4-chamber, TG	Fractional area change < 50% Fractional shortening < 25% Regional wall motion change
RV size	TTE: apical, subcostal TEE: ME 4-chamber	> 0.6 LV size: moderate dilatation > LV size: severe dilatation RVIDd > 0.9 LVIDd: RV dilatation
RV S'	TTE: apical TEE: ME 4-chamber or RV inflow-outflow	< 9.5 cm/s
TAPSE	TTE: apical TEE: ME 4-chamber or RV inflow-outflow	≤ 17 mm

SAX short-axis, *ME* midesophageal, *TG* transgastric, *RV* right ventricle, *RV S'* right ventricular tissue velocity during systole, *LV* left ventricle, *RVIDd* right ventricular inner diameter during diastole, *LVIDd* left ventricular inner diameter during diastole

Rate and Rhythm Abnormalities

Although cardiac rhythm monitors may be used primarily, echocardiography can readily visualize when extremes of rate (i.e., bradycardia and tachycardia) can lead to inadequate cardiac output. In addition, it can be used to detect symptomatic arrhythmias with aberrant atrial or ventricular contraction, such as atrial fibrillation or ventricular tachycardia. By maintaining the ultrasound view, dynamic changes to rate and/or rhythm following interventions can guide the need for further advanced therapies, like defibrillation, synchronized cardioversion, or exogenous pacing.

Global Systolic Function

At a glance, TTE and TEE can provide an estimate of ventricular wall thickening and assess whether or not there is adequate and coordinated concentric ventricular contraction. In a two-dimensional view, a normal fractional area change of the LV is 45–65% of the end-diastolic volume (Video 22.1). In cases where only a portion of the LV can be visualized, M-mode applied through a cross section can be used to measure fractional shortening, which should be greater than 25% of the end-diastolic diameter (Fig. 22.1). In most cases, an overall gestalt assessment may be adequate to make a determination about the immediate need for intervention (Video 22.2). The assessment of systolic function is described in further detail in Chap. 6.

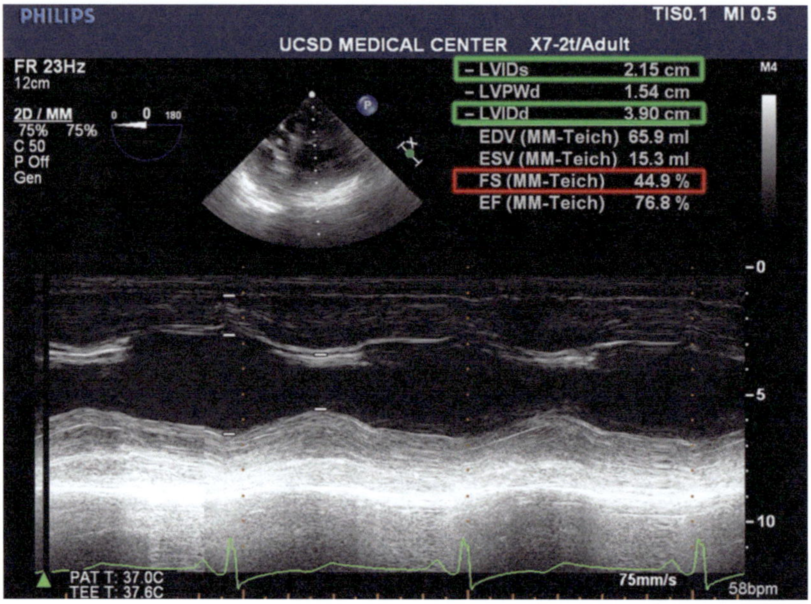

Fig. 22.1 Fractional shortening calculation based on M-mode imaging in a transgastric midpapillary short-axis view, along a one-dimensional axis from the inferior to anterior wall. The dark portions denote the LV cavity, while the echogenic lines indicate inferior and anterior wall motion over time. Note that care has been taken to exclude the papillary muscles, which encroach on the LV cavity during systolic measurement. Fractional shortening is obtained by noting the internal diameter in systole and diastole

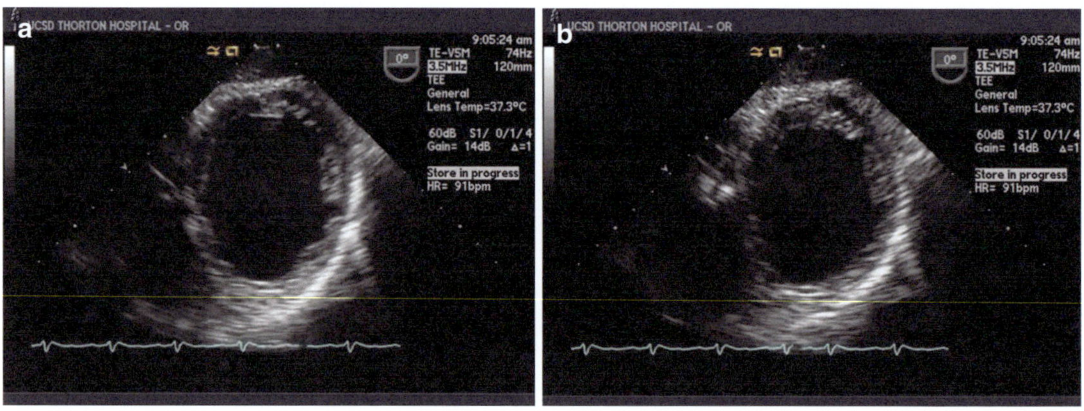

Fig. 22.2 Transgastric midpapillary short-axis view in a patient with an akinetic anterior wall secondary to a left anterior descending (LAD) coronary lesion. Note the lack of thickening and central wall excursion in the anterior portion of the left ventricle. (**a**) diastole. (**b**) systole

Regional Wall Motion Abnormalities

Segmental wall thickening < 30% suggests focal myocardial ischemia and can manifest even before EKG changes (Fig. 22.2). Akinesis or dyskinesis in the absence of other contributing factors can also suggest focal myocardial ischemia or infarction. Evolving echocardiographic findings in response to interventions may help determine whether these changes might benefit from percutaneous coronary intervention or, in extreme cases, mechanical circulatory support. Regional wall motion abnormalities are further described in Chap. 7.

Valvular Abnormalities

A limited Doppler evaluation of the cardiac valves can readily identify hemodynamically significant stenotic or regurgitant lesions. Most hemodynamically significant lesions should be readily identifiable with a brief color flow Doppler evaluation. Acute-onset tricuspid or mitral regurgitation may point to ischemia, ventricular failure or volume overload, or otherwise increased ventricular afterload (Fig. 22.3, Video 22.3). In general, regurgitant lesions respond favorably to decreased afterload and increased heart rate to decrease the regurgitant fraction, whereas stenotic lesions respond favorably to higher preload and a slower heart rate to optimize filling time (Fig. 22.4, Video 22.4). Dynamic left ventricular outflow tract obstruction, visualized with turbulent flow in a narrowed LVOT (i.e., systolic anterior motion of the mitral valve) should be treated similarly to aortic stenosis with optimization of afterload and increased filling time (slower heart rate) (Fig. 22.5, Video 22.5).

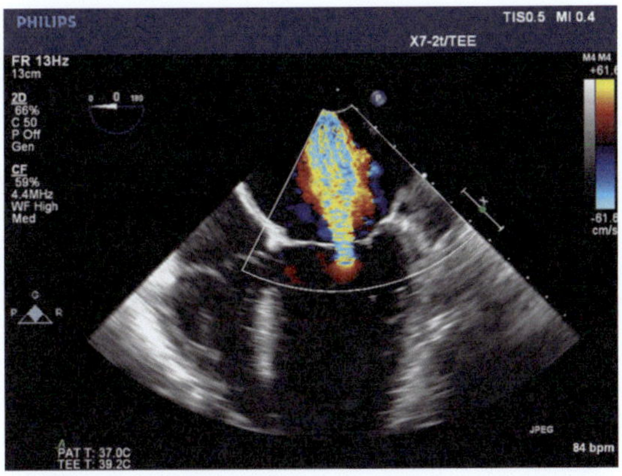

Fig. 22.3 Midesophageal four-chamber view with color flow Doppler showing severe mitral regurgitation

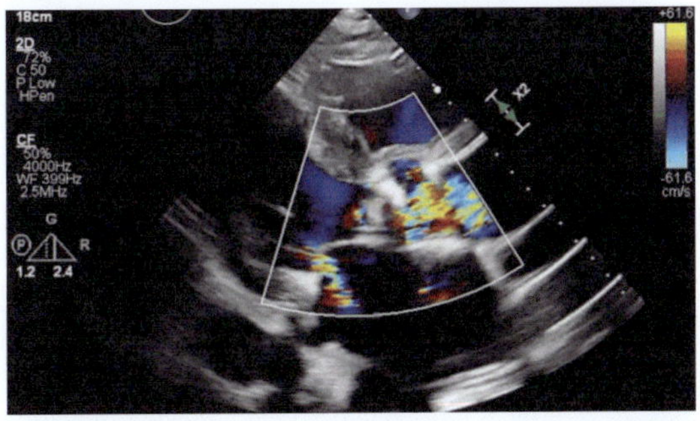

Fig. 22.4 Parasternal long-axis view with color flow Doppler showing severe aortic stenosis and mitral regurgitation

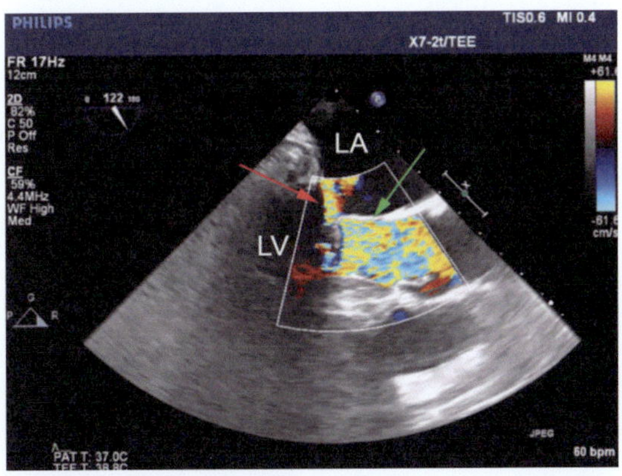

Fig. 22.5 Midesophageal long-axis view in a patient with dynamic left ventricular outflow tract obstruction. Note the aliasing on color flow Doppler in the left ventricular outflow tract (*green arrow*) and the posterior directed mitral regurgitation (*red arrow*). *LA* left atrium, *LV* left ventricle

Right Ventricular Dysfunction

Right ventricular (RV) dysfunction can indicate a problem primarily with the right ventricle (e.g., myocardial infarction) or may be secondary to another process (e.g., pulmonary embolism). Dysfunction may manifest as dilatation or elevated pressures, while failure suggests that the RV cannot produce forward flow. Evaluation for the structure and function of the right ventricle is described in detail in Chap. 10, but some general principles can be applied to help differentiate types of shock.

Imaging of the right and left ventricles concurrently can be achieved in either the apical four-chamber or subcostal four-chamber view with TTE, or in the midesophageal four-chamber view with TEE. A normal-sized right ventricle should be no more than 60% of the size of the left ventricle in cross-sectional area. A right ventricular area 70% of the left ventricular area suggests mild RV dilatation. A right ventricular area equal to the left ventricular area suggests moderate RV dilatation, and a right ventricular area exceeding the left ventricular area suggests severe dilatation (Fig. 22.6, Video 22.6). Right ventricular dilatation can more simply be assessed as a ratio of the right ventricular internal diameter at end-diastole (RVIDd) to left ventricular internal diameter at end-diastole (LVIDd) in a parasternal or transgastric midpapillary short-axis view. A value greater than 0.9 suggests RV dilatation. Measurements should be taken at the widest point of the right ventricle in its short axis [12].

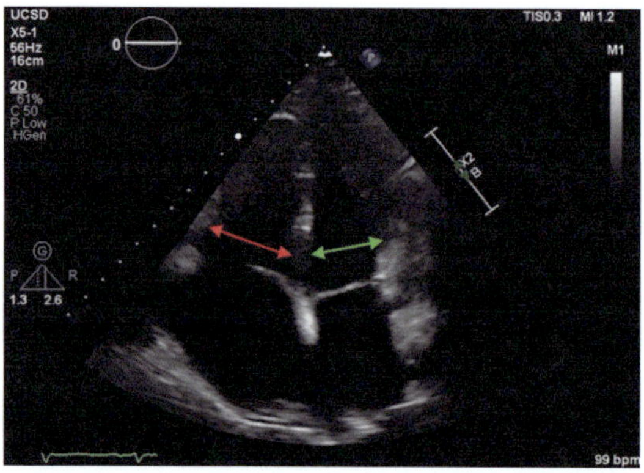

Fig. 22.6 Apical four-chamber view, showing dilatation of the right ventricle. The RV area and width (*red arrow*) exceed that of the left ventricle (*green arrow*), suggesting severe RV dysfunction

The distance of the tricuspid annular plane excursion (TAPSE) and right ventricular systolic velocity (RV S') are estimates of RV systolic dysfunction. These are both acquired in the apical four-chamber view (TTE) or the midesophageal four-chamber view (TEE), focusing on the lateral annulus of the tricuspid valve (TV). To calculate the TAPSE, use M-mode with the beam directed through lateral annulus of the TV, and measure the distance of annular motion longitudinally between end-diastole and end-systole (Fig. 22.7). Caution should be exercised in the use of M-mode for TAPSE assessment in the midesophageal four-chamber view with TEE, as the direction of annular motion is often not parallel with the ultrasound beam leading to underestimation of TAPSE. As discussed in Chap. 10, the RV S' uses tissue Doppler imaging through the lateral annulus of the TV and records the highest systolic velocity (Fig. 22.8). A TAPSE $\leq$ 17 mm or a RV S' $\leq$ 9.5 cm/s suggests RV dysfunction [6].

Pulmonary artery systolic pressure (PASP) can be estimated when there is tricuspid regurgitation (TR), which is frequently present in the

Fig. 22.7 Apical four-chamber view, measuring TAPSE at the lateral tricuspid annulus, with M-mode imaging. The measured value (1.06 cm) suggests RV dysfunction

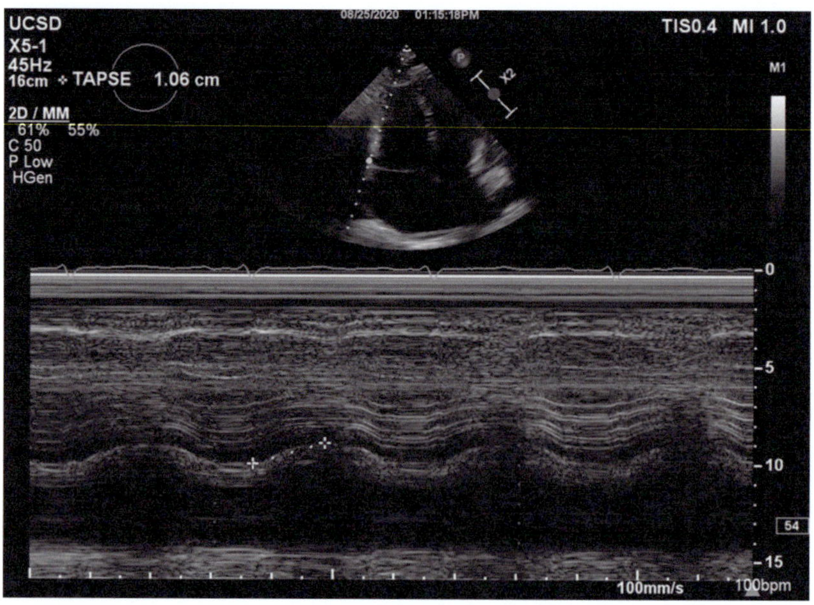

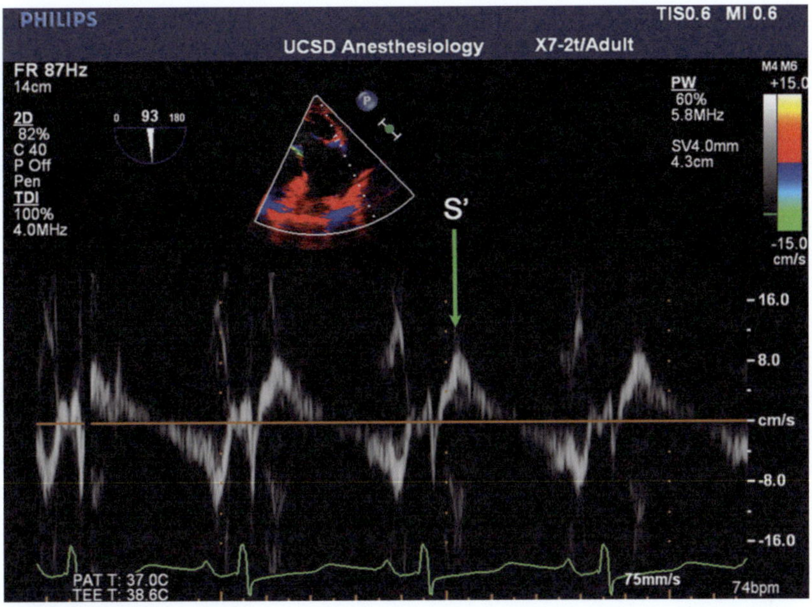

Fig. 22.8 Pulsed-wave tissue Doppler imaging of the basal right ventricular myocardium in a modified transgastric RV inflow view. Peak tricuspid annular systolic velocity (S') is identified by the *green arrow*

Table 22.3 Assessment of obstructive shock

Echo findings	Echo view(s)	Interpretation
IVC dilatation	TTE: subcostal IVC TEE: ME bicaval, TG IVC	> 2.1 cm considered dilated IVC obstruction or high RV afterload
Biventricular collapse	TTE: subcostal, apical TTE: ME 4-chamber	Low preload Impaired venous return or hypovolemia
New or worsening TR	TTE: subcostal, apical TEE: ME 4-chamber, RV inflow/outflow	Increased RV afterload e.g., PE or pneumothorax
Pericardial effusion	TTE: subcostal, apical, parasternal TEE: midesophageal	> 10 mm moderate > 20 mm severe
Right atrial collapse	TTE: subcostal, apical TEE: ME 4-chamber, RV inflow/outflow	Early tamponade If collapse > ⅓ of cardiac cycle AND effusion, strongly suggestive of tamponade
Ventricular interdependence	TTE: parasternal TEE: ME 4-chamber, TG SAX	M-mode through septum: towards LV in inspiration, towards RV in expiration; suggestive of tamponade

IVC inferior vena cava, *ME* midesophageal, *TG* transgastric, *TR* tricuspid regurgitation, *RV* right ventricle, *PE* pulmonary embolism, *SAX* short axis, *LV* left ventricle

setting of elevated right ventricular pressure. The RV-to-RA pressure gradient can be calculated by measuring the TR jet velocity during systole with continuous-wave Doppler, and applying the modified Bernoulli equation: 4 × (peak TR jet velocity)^2. Pulmonary artery systolic pressure is then estimated by adding the RV-to-RA pressure gradient to the central venous pressure. This is further described in Chap. 4.

Obstructive Shock (Table 22.3)

Obstructive etiologies of shock stem from extrinsic factors that impede blood flow, either affecting the vasculature or the heart itself. Identification and reversal of common etiologies of obstructive shock are overviewed here: pericardial disease, including pericardial tamponade and constrictive pericarditis; increased pulmonary vascular resistance, including pulmonary embolism and pulmonary hypertension; tension pneumothorax; and compression of the great vessels (IVC, SVC, or aorta).

Obstructive shock affecting the right heart usually presents with a dilated IVC (> 2.1 cm), which can be seen in a subcostal view with TTE or a transgastric perspective with TEE, although this may be a delayed finding in obstruction localized to the left side of the heart or aorta. Right ventricular dilatation indicates increased right ventricular afterload or excessive preload, while right-sided collapse or underfilling may indicate impeded venous return to the heart, or extrinsic compression of the RA or RV [9]. Of note, acute right ventricular dysfunction leading to RV dilatation may also be due to cardiogenic causes, such as a right-sided myocardial infarction or ischemia. Evaluation of the right ventricle is described in more detail in Chap. 10.

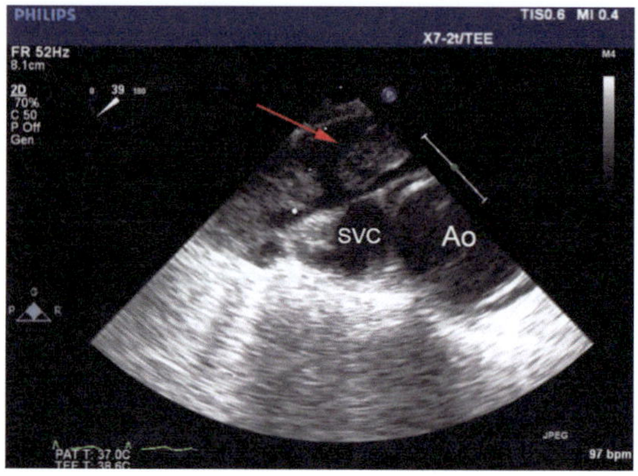

Fig. 22.9 Midesophageal ascending aortic short-axis view (right rotated) demonstrating a pulmonary embolus in the right pulmonary artery (*red arrow*). *Ao* aorta, *SVC* superior vena cava

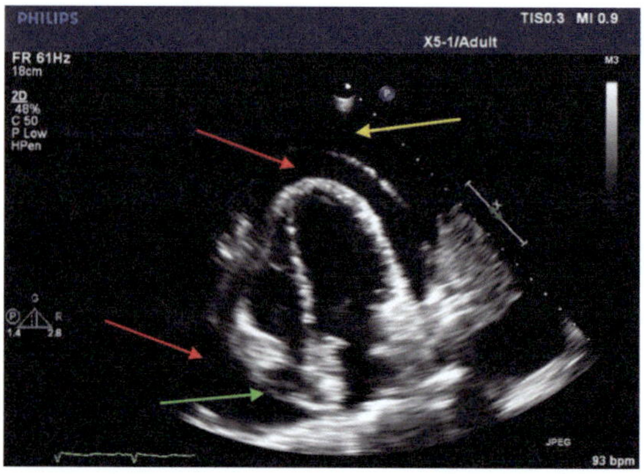

Fig. 22.10 Apical four-chamber view showing a large pericardial effusion (*red arrows*) causing collapse of the right atrium (*green arrow*). There is also a large left pleural effusion (*yellow arrow*)

Pulmonary Embolism

Right ventricular dilatation and hypokinesis with new or worsening tricuspid regurgitation is the most common constellation of findings associated with obstructive shock from pulmonary embolism (PE). A TAPSE of ≤ 17 mm may help to identify reduced RV longitudinal function. While it does not exclude all pulmonary emboli, a normal RV size and TAPSE suggests that this is likely not the cause of shock. McConnell's sign describes basal RV hypokinesis and dilatation, with preservation of apical function, which suggests an acute increase in RV afterload; however, it lacks specificity for PE. In extreme cases of pulmonary emboli, it may be possible to visualize thrombus within the RV outflow tract and into the pulmonary arteries (Fig. 22.9, Video 22.7).

Cardiac Tamponade

Extrinsic compression of the heart may impede filling of one or more chambers and lead to shock. A circumferential pericardial effusion will preferentially compress the lowest-pressure chamber first, which is generally the right atrium (Fig. 22.10), followed by the right ventricle (Video 22.8), although a localized process may affect only one area of the heart (e.g., a mediastinal hematoma compressing the left atrium). Chamber compression leads to fixed chamber filling volumes and impaired cardiac output, often displaying exaggerated respiratory stroke volume variation. There will be exaggerated ventricular interdependence as well, as the changes in relative pressures between the systemic and pulmonary systems have an amplified effect. Ultimately, pressures in all of the heart chambers (as well as central venous and pulmonary venous pressures) will equilibrate with the compression pressure (equalization of pressures), leading to cessation of blood flow. Pericardial disease is described in further detail in Chap. 14.

Tension Pneumothorax

Tension pneumothorax will result in movement of the mediastinum or direct compression of the heart. This may result in increased afterload for the right ventricle, or in decreased preload to either side of the heart due to rotational movement "kinking" the venous system entering the atria. This may result in IVC or SVC dilatation, left ventricular underfilling, and the right ventricle may appear either dilated or underfilled. Ultimately, a lack of left ventricular filling will result in decreased cardiac output and cardiac arrest. Ultrasound can quickly and accurately identify the presence of a pneumothorax by a lack of lung sliding or lung pulse, the presence of a lung point, or M-mode displaying a "barcode" or "stratosphere" sign [7]. Evaluation for pneumothorax is described in further detail in Chap. 21.

Great Vessel Compression

Acute obstruction of the great vessels can lead to cardiovascular collapse by drastically altering preload or afterload. In the case of venous compression, the affected chamber will appear underfilled, mimicking hypovolemia, but with systemic signs of venous engorgement. This may occur with IVC thrombosis or compression from a late-term pregnancy, intra-abdominal tumor, large-volume ascites, or significant bowel edema. SVC compression may result from a mediastinal hematoma following trauma or surgery, tumor, vessel stenosis/occlusion, or thrombosis.

Arterial compression leading to obstruction may occur in either the aorta or pulmonary arterial system, leading to left or right heart failure, respectively. Aortic compression or occlusion is relatively rare, in part due to the high pressure in the aorta, but may be suspected in a patient displaying signs of high LV afterload with decreased flow. Pulmonary arterial compression causing increased RV afterload will mimic the findings seen with a massive pulmonary embolism, namely, RV dilatation, tricuspid regurgitation, etc.

Hypovolemic Shock (Table 22.4)

Hypovolemia or intravascular depletion as a contributing factor to shock can sometimes be difficult to assess clinically, especially in the context of significant interstitial edema. Echocardiographic assessment can help assess preload and predict whether stroke volume (and thereby cardiac output) may increase with additional volume resus-

Table 22.4 Assessment of hypovolemic shock

Echo parameter	Echo view(s)	Interpretation
LVIDd and LVIDs	TTE: parasternal SAX or LAX TEE: ME 4-chamber, TG SAX	LVIDd < 4.2 cm in men and 3.9 cm in women: hypovolemia LVIDd normal and LVIDs < 2.6 cm in men and 2.3 cm in women: decreased SVR
IVC collapsibility	TTE: subcostal IVC TEE: TG IVC/hepatic vein	IVC ≤ 2.1 cm, > 50% variation or IVC CI > 50%: RAP < 5, likely volume-responsive IVC > 2.1 cm, < 50% variation or IVC CI < 20%: RAP > 10, likely not volume-responsive
LVOT VTI	TTE: apical 5-chamber or LAX TEE: deep TG 5-chamber or LAX	Variation < 10%: unlikely volume-responsive Variation > 14%: likely volume-responsive Increase in VTI > 10–15% during leg raise or small fluid bolus suggests a positive volume response

LVIDd left ventricular inner diameter during diastole, *LVIDs* left ventricular inner diameter during systole, *SAX* short axis, *LAX* long axis, *ME* midesophageal, *TG* transgastric, *IVC* inferior vena cava, *CI* collapsibility index, *RAP* right atrial pressure, *LVOT* left ventricular outflow tract, *VTI* velocity-time integral citation. TTE and TEE can assess left and right ventricular volumes, the left ventricular outflow tract flow, and/or the inferior vena cava collapsibility. Serial measurements may be particularly helpful in assessing the response to intravascular volume boluses. This is described in further detail in Chap. 20.

Left Ventricular Chamber Size

Left ventricular size can be most accurately evaluated in the parasternal short-axis or long-axis views or the apical four-chamber view by TTE; the corresponding views with TEE are the transgastric short-axis or midesophageal long-axis or four-chamber views. The left ventricular internal diameter at end-diastole (LVIDd) and left ventricular internal diameter at end-systole (LVIDs) are measured along the LV minor axis, 1 cm distal to the mitral valve annulus. Reference values for LVIDd are 4.2–5.9 cm in men and 3.9–5.3 cm in women. Reference values for LVIDs are 2.6–3.9 cm in men and 2.3–3.5 cm in women. A decrease in the LVIDd is generally due to decreased LV preload, while a decrease in LVIDs can be due to decreased preload, decreased systemic vascular resistance, or increased cardiac contractility. A decrease in both LVIDd and LVIDs suggests hypovolemia (Fig. 22.11, Video 22.9), while a decreased LVIDs with a preserved LVIDd suggests decreased SVR (Fig. 22.12, Video 22.10) [11].

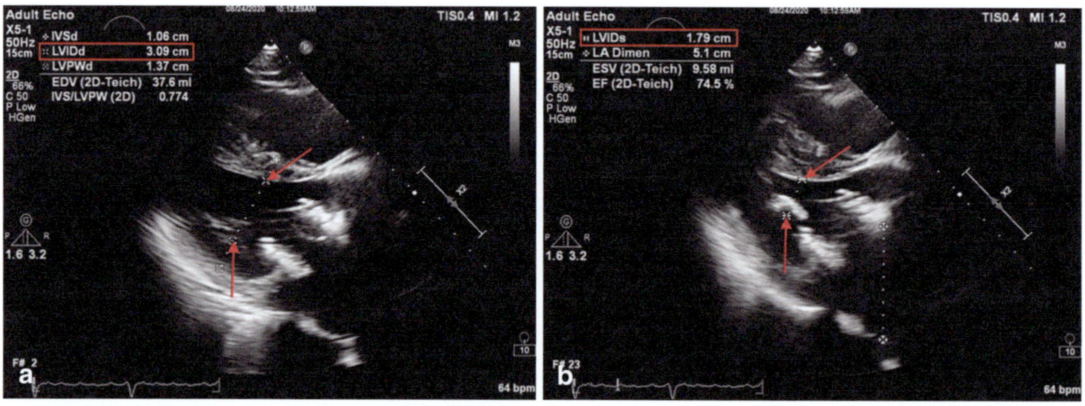

Fig. 22.11 Parasternal long-axis view of a hyperdynamic ventricle during diastole (**a**) and systole (**b**), showing a small LVIDd (*red arrows*), suggesting low preload (hypovolemia)

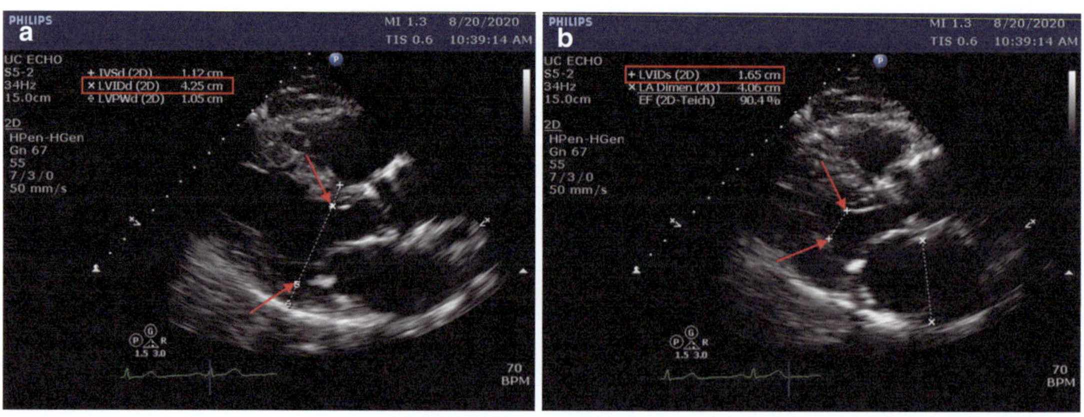

Fig. 22.12 Parasternal long-axis view of a hyperdynamic ventricle during diastole (**a**) and systole (**b**), showing a normal LVIDd (*red arrows*), suggesting adequate preload and low afterload

IVC Evaluation

Ultrasound imaging may help estimate the central venous pressure in the IVC, and thereby predict right atrial pressure. A low right atrial pressure may predict volume responsiveness, while a high right atrial pressure (RAP) suggests an increase in stroke volume is less likely in response to additional preload. The IVC can be viewed from the TTE subcostal window, rotating the probe counterclockwise from the subcostal four-chamber view to view the IVC in a sagittal plane as it enters the right atrium. With TEE, the IVC can be visualized from a transgastric position, with the probe rotated to the right and the multiplane set at 60°–90°. The ideal measurement should be 1–3 cm from the cavoatrial junction. M-mode may help with dynamic measurements.

In a spontaneously breathing patient, an IVC diameter ≤ 2.1 cm with > 50% collapse during inspiration predicts a RAP of 0–5 mmHg. An IVC diameter > 2.1 cm with > 50% collapse predicts a RAP 5–10 mmHg (Fig. 22.13, Video 22.11). An IVC diameter > 2.1 cm with < 50% collapse predicts a RAP more than 10 mmHg (Fig. 22.14, Video 22.12) [10, 13]. Changes in intrathoracic pressure during positive pressure ventilation may also be exploited to predict right atrial pressure [14]. The IVC collapsibility index (CI) may be a useful metric to use for this estimation, as described in Chap. 20: CI = [(IVC diameter_{max} − IVC diameter_{min}) / IVC diameter_{max}] × 100. An IVC CI > 50% predicts a RAP 0–5 mmHg, while an IVC CI < 20% predicts a RAP > 10 mmHg. Any estimates of right atrial pressure from IVC ultrasound are subject to several limitations, which are summarized in Table 20.1.

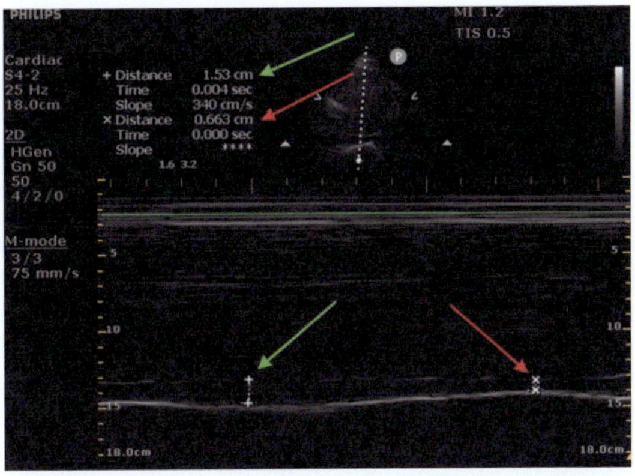

Fig. 22.13 Measurement of the IVC via M-mode imaging, demonstrating a small IVC (1.53 cm), with significant variation (57%) during inhalation, suggesting a low right atrial pressure, and likely volume responsiveness

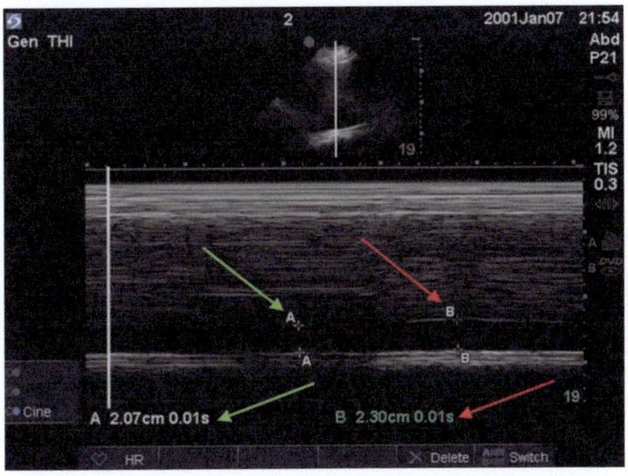

Fig. 22.14 Measurement of the IVC via M-mode imaging, demonstrating a large IVC (2.3 cm), with little variation (10%), suggesting a high right atrial pressure, and unlikely volume responsiveness

Stroke Volume Variation

The LV stroke volume can be measured through the LVOT, as described in Chap. 4. Small changes in stroke volume resulting from respirophasic changes in intrathoracic pressure suggest that increased intravascular volume will increase cardiac output. This can be quantified by measuring variation in the LVOT VTI, pulse pressure variation, or systolic velocity variation through the aorta or peripheral arteries.

Assessment of stroke volume before and after a volume bolus can confirm the effect. A significant increase in stroke volume (> 10–15%) suggests a favorable response, and additional volume may be considered, if indicated. Conversely, a small change in stroke volume suggests that additional volume resuscitation is unlikely to benefit. It is important to remember that even in a euvolemic state, increases of preload should result in increased cardiac output, so it does not guarantee that hypovolemia is the cause of shock. Additionally, there are many situations where cardiogenic, obstructive, and distributive shock may all improve stroke volume with increased preload.

Distributive Shock

Distributive shock (low systemic vascular resistance, SVR) is not readily visualized via ultrasound directly and instead is usually diagnosed sonographically by a process of elimination. The most common cause for distributive shock by far is sepsis, but other possibilities include adrenal insufficiency, anaphylaxis, neurogenic shock, and other endocrinological or drug-induced states. If the degree of shock is not completely explained by any of the previous etiologies, and there are echocardiographic signs suggestive of low afterload (e.g., decreased left ventricular volume or internal diameter at end-systole), then a component of distributive shock should be suspected. This is often confounded by the concurrent use of vasopressor support in the setting of ongoing resuscitation efforts. Serial reassessment may facilitate titration of vasopressor therapy relative to other interventions (intravascular volume boluses, inotropic therapy, etc.) [8].

Point-of-Care Ultrasound During Cardiac Arrest

Cardiac arrest may be considered the most extreme form of shock. The same principles apply when evaluating for reversible causes of cardiac arrest, and identification of the physiologic derangements may help guide interventions. In the case of ongoing chest compressions, it is imperative that diagnostic evaluation does not interrupt the circulation supported by chest compressions for more than a few seconds. To limit the duration of pulse checks and avoid unnecessary interruptions, the ultrasound probe should be placed in the appropriate position while chest compressions are ongoing. In the setting of an intubated patient, TEE imaging allows continuous imaging during chest compressions and can assess the quality of chest compressions. Whether via TTE or TEE, early imaging in cardiac arrest is most useful. If imaging occurs after prolonged resuscitative efforts, confounding findings may exist, such as stunned myocardium and RV dysfunction from the cardiac arrest that are not the inciting cause of the arrest. Recording short clips of images can greatly facilitate this process, as they can then be reviewed after compressions have resumed. Directed, yes/no questions should be asked and answered quickly (e.g., is a pericardial effusion present?), rather than targeting a comprehensive evaluation. If the structure of interest cannot be visualized within a few seconds while the chest compressions are held, the ultrasound should be aborted and can be tried differently at the next appropriate interval. Often, it may be possible to answer pertinent questions without compromising chest compressions at all, through subcostal, apical, or TEE views.

If a shockable rhythm is identified, efforts should be focused on delivery of appropriate defibrillation/cardioversion, without delay by ultrasound interpretation. Echocardiography can guide additional resuscitation efforts after a stable rhythm is established, or if an alternative cause must be evaluated.

The concept of pulseless electrical activity (PEA) is inclusive of a variety of different scenarios, including any form of shock leading to a pulse pressure low enough that it is not palpable. If mechanical cardiac activity is present, but a pulse is not palpable, identification of reversible causes should again be focused on whether one or more cardiogenic, obstructive, hypovolemic, or distributive processes are present. True electrical activity without any mechanical cardiac motion is most commonly related to metabolic or ischemic conditions. The finding of true cardiac standstill with ultrasound is known to be associated with very poor outcomes when compared with presence of ventricular activity. Gaspari et al. showed that 0.6% of patients with PEA without mechanical activity survived to hospital discharge, compared with 3.6% of patients with some evidence of mechanical activity (pseudo-PEA) [15]. This evaluation may also help guide determinations regarding when to terminate resuscitative efforts.

Systematic Evaluation

Different clinical scenarios will suggest different methods for evaluation and management of shock and cardiac arrest. Systematic evaluation can help guide clinicians toward the most appropriate interventions and avoid missing important information (Fig. 22.15). From a view in which all four chambers of the heart can be clearly visualized (e.g., subcostal or apical four-chamber, or midesophageal four-chamber views), gross cardiac motion can be assessed. This may differentiate cardiac standstill (PEA/asystole), dysrhythmias (e.g., ventricular tachycardia/fibrillation), and whether there is a significant structural lesion present in the heart (e.g., papillary muscle rupture). Color flow Doppler can quickly assess for severe valvulopathies, and different views can focus on ventricular walls if there is gross hypokinesis or akinesis.

Following evaluation of cardiogenic contributors to shock, obstructive causes can be assessed. Tamponade can be visualized by fluid around the heart and chamber collapse, whereas RV failure can point towards pneumothorax, right-sided myocardial infarction, or pulmonary embolism. In contrast, an underfilled right ventricle or IVC may suggest a hypovolemic cause (e.g., hemorrhage, dehydration). Finally, if cardiogenic, obstructive, and hypovolemic contributors are addressed, there is likely an underlying distributive component.

Conclusion

Point-of-care echocardiography, when combined with appropriate clinical assessment and other clinical data, can help rapidly guide therapeutic measures for patients within the spectrum of circulatory failure. Many echocardiographic protocols have been described, though no one approach is definitively superior. Because the utility of each application varies by setting, clinicians (or institutions) must decide how they can best utilize ultrasound for each individual case, considering the clinical picture of the patient and the acuity of the environment.

In the case of cardiac arrest, emphasis should be placed on rapid and efficient scanning to ensure minimal interruption to other interventions, especially chest compressions and early defibrillation. A systematic approach can identify cardiogenic, obstructive, hypovolemic, and dis-

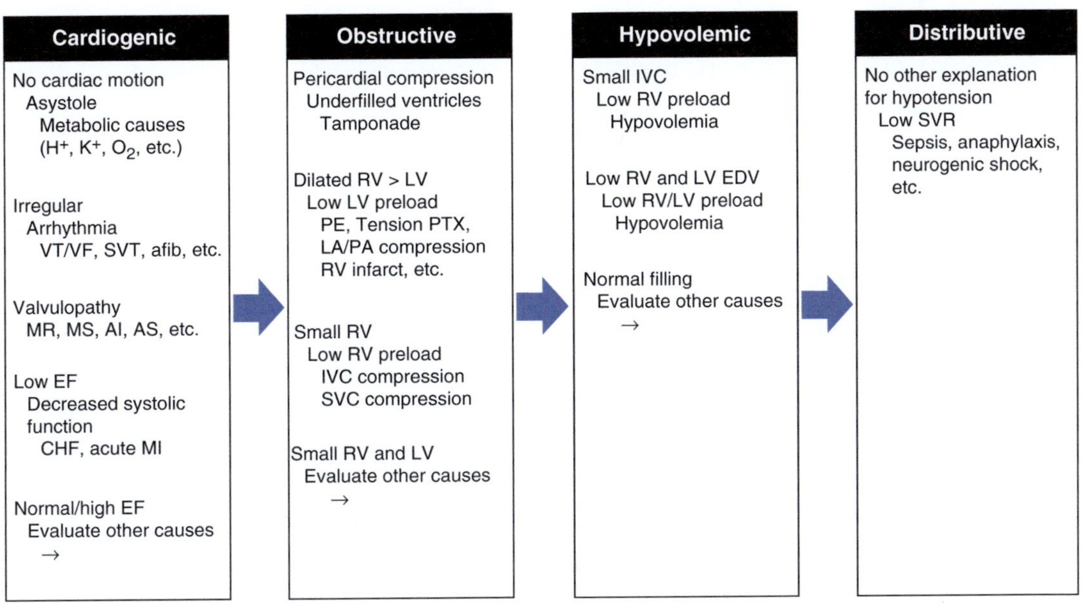

Fig. 22.15 Systematic approach to evaluation of shock

tributive contributions to shock and cardiac arrest.

Questions

1. A 72-year-old man is post-op day #3 from an aortic valve replacement. He was extubated 6 hours ago and is off all vasopressor agents. The pulmonary artery catheter was removed, but the epicardial pacing wires and chest tubes remain in place. Through the day, he develops shortness of breath and diaphoresis. His blood pressure in the morning was 115/75 and is now 90/45 mmHg. The heart rate was 80 and is now 120 beats per minute. On bedside evaluation, there is elevated jugular venous distension. Chest tube output remains low. Bedside ultrasound shows the following image. What is the most appropriate next step for the management of this patient?

   A. Initiate epinephrine infusion to increase the cardiac index
   B. Initiate phenylephrine infusion to increase mean arterial pressure
   C. Insert a chest tube at the bedside
   D. Manipulate the chest drains and prepare for possible intervention to relieve tamponade

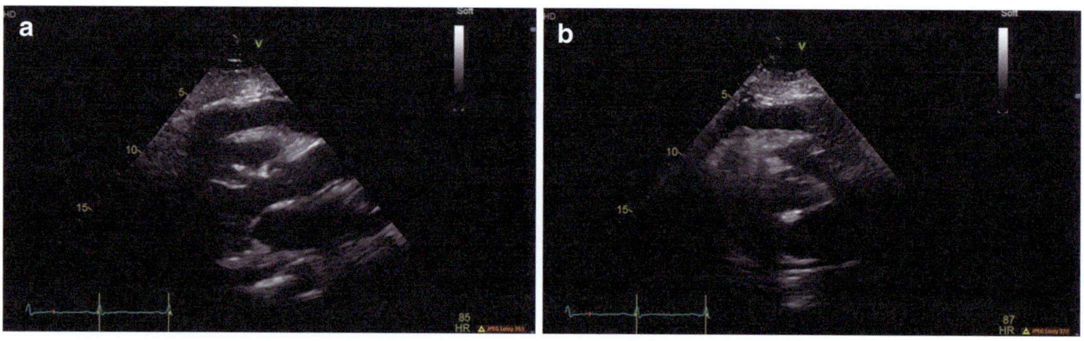

2. A 55-year-old man is admitted to the ICU for acute hypoxemic respiratory failure due to COVID-19 pneumonia and ARDS and has been intubated for 9 days. The respiratory therapist notes that the SpO_2 has decreased and the ventilator has been alarming with peak airway pressure of 60 cmH_2O. New crepitus is palpable on the anterior chest wall, and the blood pressure has decreased from 105/50 to 95/50 mmHg. Which of the following ultrasound findings would be most likely?

   A. Normal cardiac exam, with no lung sliding
   B. Dilated right ventricle with no lung sliding
   C. Dilated right ventricle with lung point
   D. Normal cardiac exam, with lung point

3. A 65-year-old woman presents with cough and fever for several days. She has a past medical history of a kidney transplant, type 2 diabetes mellitus and anemia. Her temperature is 39 °C, BP 90/45 mmHg, HR 100 bpm, RR 24/min, and SpO_2 95% on 6 L nasal cannula. Her serum lactate level is measured at 4.2 mmol/L. She receives 30 mL/kg bolus of lactated Ringer's, and repeat blood pressure is 100/50 mmHg, HR 95 bpm. Her RR has increased to 30/min, and SpO_2 has decreased to 90% on 6 L nasal cannula. The following image is obtained from a subcostal ultrasound exam. Which of

the following in the most appropriate next step in management?

A. Start norepinephrine infusion
B. Evaluate velocity time integral (VTI) through the left ventricular outflow tract (LVOT)
C. Obtain chest X-ray
D. Repeat intravascular fluid bolus

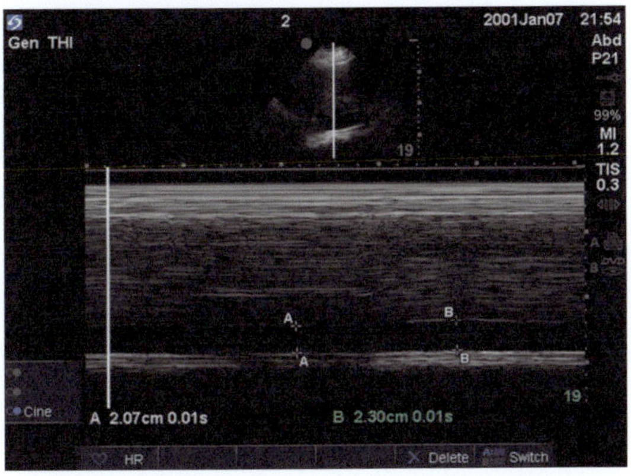

4. A 28-year-old-man presents to the ED with dizziness. The patient was recently involved in a motor vehicle collision and sustained a femur fracture, which was treated surgically. His BP is 96/51 mmHg, HR 117 bpm, RR 30/min, and SpO_2 91% on room air. Physical exam reveals a young male in moderate distress with a cast on his left leg. Chest x-ray demonstrates a right lower lobe infiltrate. The patient is given 30 mL/kg of lactated Ringer's for his septic shock and is started on broad spectrum antibiotics. On subsequent evaluation, his BP is now 86/40 mmHg, HR has increased to 130 bpm, and a point-of-care ultrasound exam is performed. Which of the following is the most likely cause of his shock?

A. Distributive shock from sepsis, attributable to pneumonia
B. Cardiogenic shock from septic cardiomyopathy and hypoxemia
C. Obstructive shock from massive pulmonary embolism
D. Hypovolemic shock from dehydration

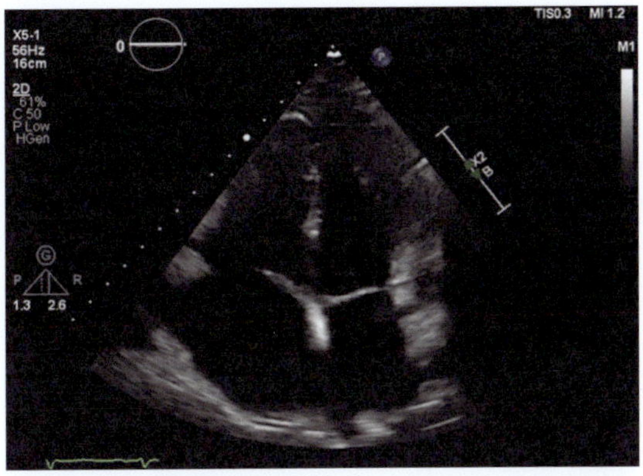

5. A 65-year-old man presents to the Emergency Department in cardiopulmonary arrest after he was found down at home. Chest compressions are ongoing by the paramedics on arrival. A wide-complex irregular rhythm is evident on the monitor between compressions. Which of the following would be the most appropriate to facilitate resuscitation attempts?

A. Ultrasound evaluation during pulse checks to evaluate for cardiac activity
B. Subcostal ultrasound examination during compressions to evaluate for pericardial effusion
C. Apical four-chamber evaluation during compressions to evaluate for right ventricular dilation
D. Ultrasound evaluation is not indicated

6. A 77-year-old man with a history of hypertension, dyslipidemia, and type 2 diabetes is found altered at home by a neighbor. Patient's wife reports that he has had chest pain for a few days and increasing dyspnea with minimal exertion. Upon arrival to the ED, blood pressure is noted to be 95/55 mmHg, HR 118 bpm, RR 23, and SpO_2 91% on 4 L of nasal cannula oxygen. Physical exam reveals bilateral crackles and a holosystolic murmur at the apex. The following image is obtained with point-of-care ultrasound. What is the most appropriate next step for the management of this patient?

A. Place the patient on non-rebreather mask or high-flow nasal cannula

B. Administer diuretics due to pulmonary edema and volume overload
C. Consult cardiac surgery emergently
D. Administer 30 mL/kg IV fluid bolus and broad-spectrum antibiotics

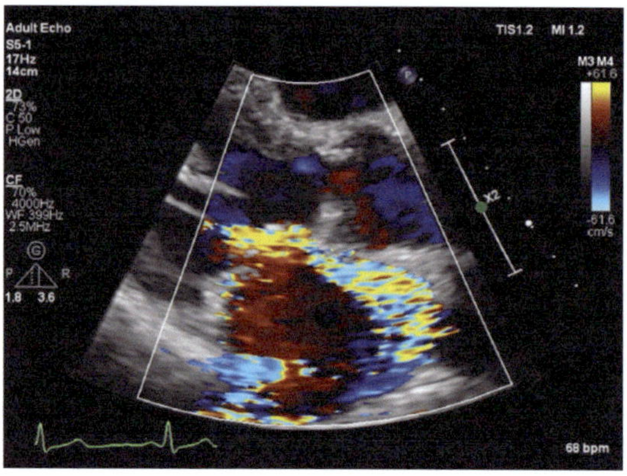

7. A 39-year-old man with past medical history of asthma and IV drug use presents to the ED with altered mental status, fever, and tachycardia. His temperature is 38.5 °C, BP 90/52 mmHg, HR 117 bpm, RR 22/min, and SpO_2 96% on room air. Point-of-care echocardiography demonstrates a hyperdynamic heart, and ultrasound evaluation of the IVC reveals the following image. Which of the following is the most appropriate next step in management for this patient?

A. Administer antibiotics and repeat IVC ultrasound
B. Administer antibiotics and 30 mL/kg IV fluid bolus, and then repeat echocardiography
C. Administer antibiotics and 30 mL/kg IV fluid bolus, and then repeat IVC ultrasound
D. Administer antibiotics and initiate norepinephrine infusion

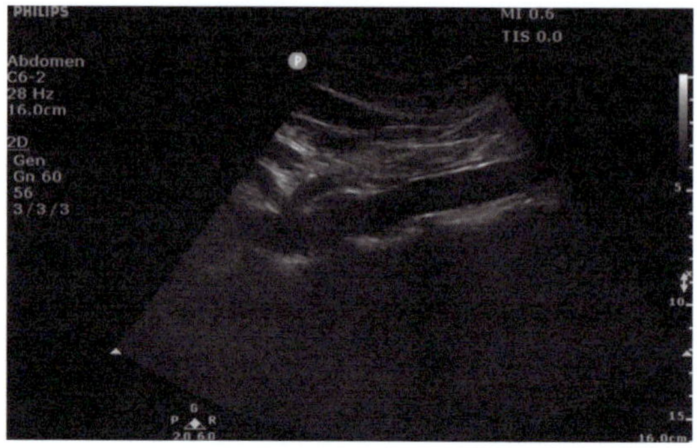

8. A 35-year-old woman develops shortness of breath after a normal spontaneous vaginal delivery. She had significant blood loss during the procedure and received 6 units of PRBCs. Her BP is 95/60 mmHg, HR 110 bpm, RR 24/min, and SpO_2 90% on 4 liters oxygen via nasal cannula. Point-of-care ultrasound reveals the following images. Which of the following is the most appropriate next step in her management?

A. Initiate dobutamine infusion and consult cardiology
B. Initiate norepinephrine infusion and start antibiotics for chorioamnionitis
C. Consult for possible mechanical circulatory support and consider heparin for amniotic fluid embolus
D. Give 1 gram calcium chloride for hypocalcemia from blood product transfusion

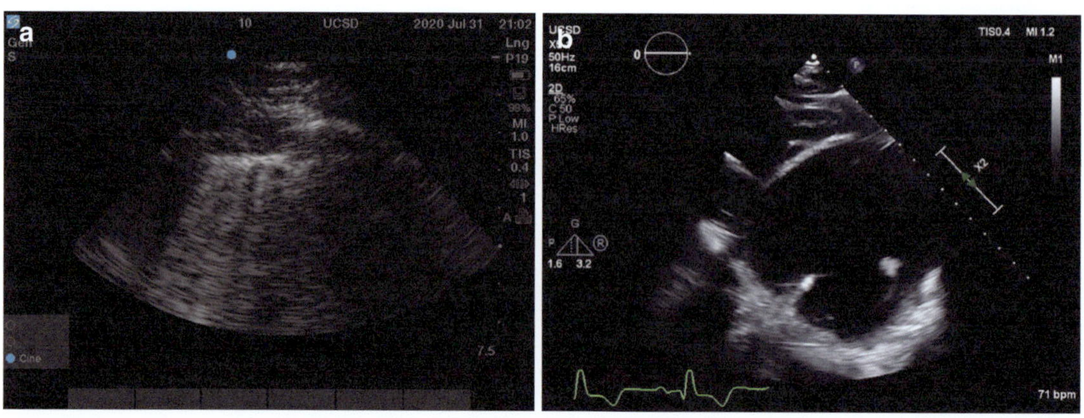

9. A 25-year-old man is brought in by EMS after he was found unconscious in the street with a laceration on his head. His BP is 85/45 mmHg, and his HR is 120 bpm. Point-of-care echocardiography reveals hyperdynamic left and right ventricles and a small IVC which collapses with respiration. FAST exam is negative for intraperitoneal fluid. His hemoglobin level is 14 g/dL (normal 13.5–17.5 g/dL). He is given 2 liters of lactated Ringer's solution, and BP improves to 110/65 mmHg, and he is intubated for poor neurologic status. One hour later, his BP is again 85/45 mmHg. What is the most appropriate next step in management?

    A. CT abdomen/pelvis to evaluate for occult injury
    B. Repeat FAST exam to evaluate for injury missed initially
    C. Proceed to emergent exploratory laparotomy
    D. Repeat hemoglobin level to evaluate for ongoing bleeding

10. A 75-year-old woman is recovering in the ICU following a pancreaticoduodenectomy (Whipple) procedure. She has a past medical history of heart failure with a reduced ejection fraction (30%), type 2 diabetes mellitus, and pancreatic cancer. The procedure lasted a total of 8 hours, and she received 3 liters of IV crystalloid resuscitation with 1200 mL of total urine output. Her BP is 93/42 mmHg, HR 114 bpm, RR 23/min, and SpO_2 96%. She appears anxious and in pain, and her urine output for the last hour was 10 mL. What is the most appropriate next step in her management?

    A. Give 30 mL/kg bolus of lactated Ringer's solution and assess change in LVOT VTI
    B. Give a 250 mL bolus of lactated Ringer's and reassess
    C. Order pain medication and reassess her RR and HR
    D. Initiate dobutamine infusion

References

1. Cecconi M, De Backer D, Antonelli M, et al. Consensus on circulatory shock and hemodynamic monitoring. Task force of the European Society of Intensive Care Medicine. Intensive Care Med. 2014;40:1795–815.
2. Byhahn C. Prehospital echocardiography in pulseless electrical activity victims using portable, handheld ultrasound. Crit Care. 2007;11(Suppl 2):P279.
3. Kolte D, Khera S, Aronow WS, et al. Trends in incidence, management, and outcomes of cardiogenic shock complicating ST-elevation myocardial infarction in the United States. J Am Heart Assoc. 2014;3:e000590.
4. Feng M, McSparron JI, Kien DT, et al. Transthoracic echocardiography and mortality in sepsis: analysis of the MIMIC-III database. Intensive Care Med. 2018;44:884–92.
5. Vignon P, Dugard A, Abraham J, et al. Focused training for goal-oriented hand-held echocardiography performed by noncardiologist residents in the intensive care unit. Intensive Care Med. 2007;33:1795–9.
6. Rudski LG, Lai WW, Afilalo J, et al. Guidelines for the echocardiographic assessment of the right heart in adults: a report from the American Society of Echocardiography endorsed by the European Association of Echocardiography, a registered branch of the European Society of Cardiology, and the Canadian Society of Echocardiography. J Am Soc Echocardiogr. 2010;23:685–713; quiz 786-688.
7. Perrino A, Reeves S. A practical approach to transesophageal echocardiography. 3rd ed. Philadelphia: Wolter Kluwer; 2008.
8. De Backer D, Biston P, Devriendt J, et al. Comparison of dopamine and norepinephrine in the treatment of shock. N Engl J Med. 2010;362:779–89.
9. Gillam LD, Guyer DE, Gibson TC, et al. Hydrodynamic compression of the right atrium: a new echocardiographic sign of cardiac tamponade. Circulation. 1983;68:294–301.
10. Alrajhi K, Woo MY, Vaillancourt C. Test characteristics of ultrasonography for the detection of pneumothorax: a systematic review and meta-analysis. Chest. 2012;141:703–8.
11. Ilercil A, O'Grady MJ, Roman MJ, et al. Reference values for echocardiographic measurements in urban and rural populations of differing ethnicity: the Strong Heart Study. J Am Soc Echocardiogr. 2001;14:601–11.
12. Brennan JM, Ronan A, Goonewardena S, et al. Handcarried ultrasound measurement of the inferior vena cava for assessment of intravascular volume status in the outpatient hemodialysis clinic. Clin J Am Soc Nephrol. 2006;1:749–53.
13. Porter TR, Shillcutt SK, Adams MS, et al. Guidelines for the use of echocardiography as a monitor for therapeutic intervention in adults: a report from the

American Society of Echocardiography. J Am Soc Echocardiogr. 2015;28:40–56.
14. Beigel R, Cercek B, Luo H, et al. Noninvasive evaluation of right atrial pressure. J Am Soc Echocardiogr. 2013;26:1033–42.
15. Gaspari R, Weekes A, Adhikari S, et al. Emergency department point-of-care ultrasound in out-of-hospital and in-ED cardiac arrest. Resuscitation. 2016;109:33–9.
16. Netherton S, Milenkovic V, Taylor M, et al. Diagnostic accuracy of eFAST in the trauma patient: a systematic review and meta-analysis. CJEM. 2019;21:727–38.
17. Breitkreutz R, Price S, Steiger HV, et al. Focused echocardiographic evaluation in life support and peri-resuscitation of emergency patients: a prospective trial. Resuscitation. 2010;81:1527–33.
18. Kimura BJ, Yogo N, O'Connell CW, et al. Cardiopulmonary limited ultrasound examination for "quick-look" bedside application. Am J Cardiol. 2011;108:586–90.
19. Ferrada P, Vanguri P, Anand RJ, et al. A, B, C, D, echo: limited transthoracic echocardiogram is a useful tool to guide therapy for hypotension in the trauma bay--a pilot study. J Trauma Acute Care Surg. 2013;74:220–3.

Ultrasound for Vascular Access

23

Seth T. Herway and Brett Cronin

Abbreviations

ASE	American Society of Echocardiography
CA	Carotid artery
CVC	Central venous catheter
CVP	Central venous pressure
FV	Femoral vein
IJ	Internal jugular (vein)
LAX	Long-axis
PAC	Pulmonary arterial catheter
SAX	Short-axis
SC	Subclavian (vein)
SCA	Society of Cardiovascular Anesthesiologists
TEE	Transesophageal echocardiography
TTE	Transthoracic echocardiography

Introduction

Proper vascular access is imperative for appropriate perioperative care and includes the use of peripheral venous access for fluid and drug administration, central venous access for vasoactive infusion and central venous pressure (CVP) monitoring, and lastly, arterial access for continuous blood pressure monitoring and arterial blood sampling. The indications of each type of access are outside of the scope of this text; however, the utility of ultrasound for obtaining vascular access will be discussed. Ultrasound imaging during vascular procedures can be used to "scout" the anatomy prior to skin puncture, provide needle guidance towards the intended structure, as well as confirm wire placement during the Seldinger technique. The intention of ultrasound imaging is often to reduce complications, reduce the time to vascular access, and aid in difficult cannulations; however, the magnitude of this benefit may vary depending upon the vessel selected and the patient's individual anatomy.

Supplementary Information The online version of this chapter (https://doi.org/10.1007/978-3-030-84349-6_23) contains supplementary material, which is available to authorized users.

S. T. Herway · B. Cronin (✉)
Department of Anesthesiology, University of California San Diego Health, La Jolla, CA, USA
e-mail: bcronin@health.ucsd.edu

Probe Orientation

Unlike the standard orientations found in echocardiography, ultrasound for vascular access can have varying probe and image orientations based on the vessel being cannulated and the operator's position. In general, it is recommended that the probe be oriented to display the same anatomy on the screen that would be visible to the operator from that vantage point. Thus, anatomic structures on the left side of the probe should appear

T. M. Maus, C. R. Tainter (eds.), *Essential Echocardiography*,
https://doi.org/10.1007/978-3-030-84349-6_23

on the left side of the screen, and right-sided structures should appear on the right side of the screen. Although it is common for ultrasound probes to have an indicator that denotes one side of the probe that correlates with a specific side of the screen, the user can also briefly confirm anatomic and screen orientation alignment by moving the probe left to right or by applying gentle external pressure on one side of the probe confirming correlation with the image on the screen.

Ultrasound may be used for vascular access both in the long (in-plane) axis (LAX) and in the short (out-of-plane) axis (SAX). Both views may be utilized to guide needle movement; however, the in-plane technique serves to keep the entire needle length in view while the out-of-plane technique catches a cross section of the needle. The advantage that an out-of-plane technique has over an in-plane technique is the ability to visualize surrounding structures during needle movement (e.g., carotid artery during internal jugular cannulation), and the imaging plane can be moved to follow the trajectory of the needle. Oblique views can also be obtained but are not conventionally used and are not addressed further here.

In the SAX view, the probe is placed perpendicular to the desired vessel, providing a cross section of the vessel and needle, which appears as a hyperechoic point (Fig. 23.1; Videos 23.1a, b). In the LAX view, the probe is placed parallel to the desired vessel, providing an image that shows the course of the vessel across the screen and the needle shaft as it is advanced (Fig. 23.2; Videos 23.2a, b). Again, the advantage of the SAX view is that it provides superior visualization of anatomic structures surrounding the vessel of interest. This advantage can be critical because ultrasound is often used to access central veins that run in close proximity to critical arteries. It appears that for novice users, the SAX view also results in faster cannulation times and is perceived to be an easier approach by the operator [1]. The LAX view provides the advantage of better visualization of the needle itself during its approach to and its course within the vessel. However, maintaining proper alignment of both the ultrasound transducer and the access needle can be challenging. Any malalignment results in the cannulating needle not being imaged and may lead to unsuccessful cannulation or inadvertent damage to surrounding structures.

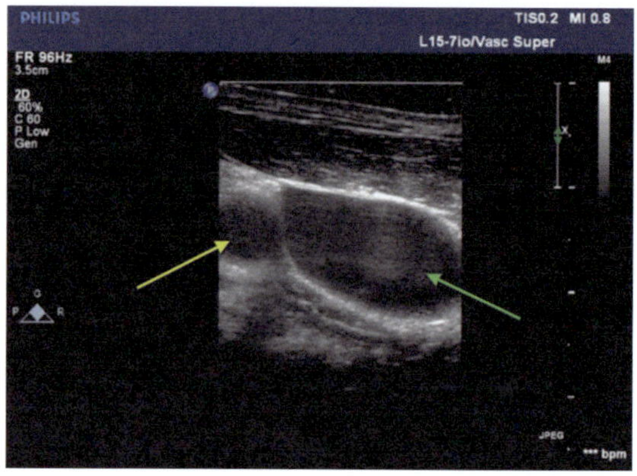

Fig. 23.1 Out-of-plane or short-axis (SAX) imaging of the right internal jugular vein (*green arrow*). The *yellow arrow* indicates the carotid artery just to the medial aspect of the larger, collapsible internal jugular vein

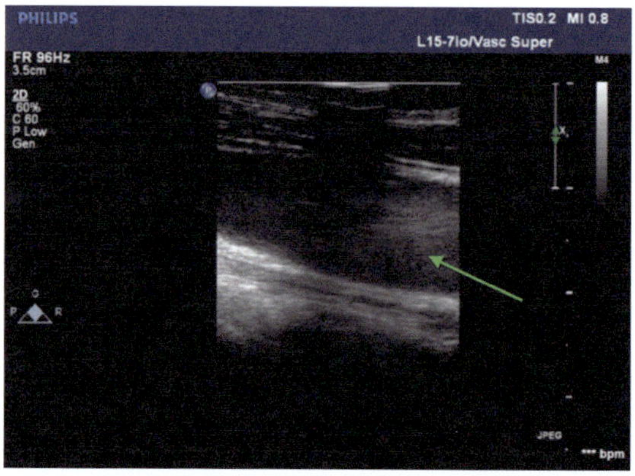

Fig. 23.2 In-plane or long-axis (LAX) imaging of the right internal jugular vein (*green arrow*) from the same patient in Fig. 23.1

Vessel Selection

There are a number of factors involved in selecting the site for vessel cannulation. Anatomic considerations, patient positioning, patient tolerance, venous drainage and vessel patency, and relative rates of complications should all be considered for arterial, peripheral, or central venous cannulation. In general, larger central venous catheters and those with more lumens have a higher risk for infections [2]. Subclavian central venous catheters have the lowest risk for infection (1.5–4%) and thrombosis (1.2–1.9%). Internal jugular catheters have an infection rate of 4–8% and a thrombosis rate of 7.6%. The femoral site has the highest incidence of both infection and thrombosis at 19.8% and 21.5%, respectively [3, 4].

Vessel Identification

Differentiation of veins from arteries is a critical aspect of the appropriate use of ultrasound for obtaining vascular access. Both have anechoic (black) lumens, but arteries generally have thicker walls that are more hyperechoic (white) than the walls of veins. Additionally, arteries are typically pulsatile and the higher pressure makes them less compressible than veins (though a completely noncompressible vessel suggests thrombosis).

With the vessel viewed in the short axis, as gentle pressure is applied, veins will compress, while nearby arteries should remain patent and pulsatile. However, with excessive pressure both arteries and veins can collapse. Color flow Doppler imaging may also be used to identify pulsatile flow (Figs. 23.3 and 23.4; Videos 23.3 and 23.4). Venous blood flow will be more uniform in color, have lower velocity, and may be present during systole and diastole, whereas arterial flow will be of higher velocity and detected predominantly during systole. The Doppler scale can be lowered and the color gain increased to detect flow if not initially observed. In addition, the probe should be oriented so that flow is toward or away from the transducer in order to register a Doppler signal. Flow perpendicular to the probe will not demonstrate a Doppler shift (see Chap. 4).

Because techniques for vessel identification can be rendered less reliable in low-flow states or cardiac arrest, it is crucial that the operator understands the normal anatomic relationships between arteries and veins surrounding the vessel selected for cannulation. Additionally, other confirmatory measures and verification of correct placement of the guidewire and/or catheter are necessary and will be covered in later sections.

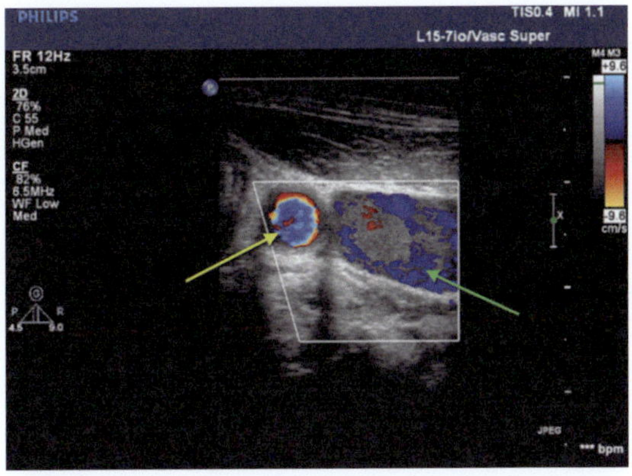

Fig. 23.3 Out-of-plane imaging (SAX view) of the right internal jugular vein (*green arrow*) with color flow Doppler. The *yellow arrow* indicates the carotid artery. Color flow Doppler imaging demonstrates faster pulsatile laminar flow in the carotid artery, with slower flow in the jugular vein

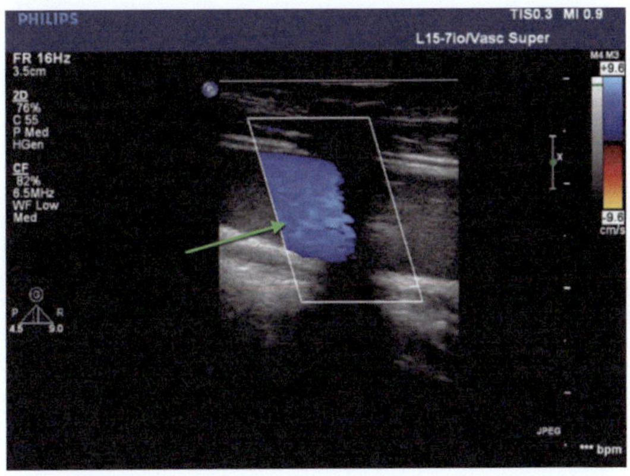

Fig. 23.4 In-plane imaging (LAX view) of the right internal jugular vein (*green arrow*) with color flow Doppler

Static Versus Dynamic Imaging

Static imaging uses ultrasound to identify the vessel selected for cannulation and the appropriate site of needle entry after which the ultrasound is no longer used to guide the procedure. The dynamic approach uses real-time ultrasound throughout the procedure to guide needle placement and vessel entry, either in a long-axis plane (in-plane) or with a stepwise series of movements of the short-axis imaging plane (out-of-plane). Dynamic imaging provides faster cannulation with fewer attempts, but reported complication rates for both techniques appear to be similar [5–7].

Performing the Procedure

Proper positioning of the patient will aid in vessel detection and in the performance of the procedure. Trendelenburg positioning during central venous cannulation of the internal jugular or subclavian veins may increase central venous pressure and thereby the size of the vessel on imaging. After identifying the appropriate vessel with ultrasound, the desired trajectory of the needle should be determined. Typically, the needle should be directed towards the middle of the vessel, which is best determined using the SAX view. If the LAX view is used, the needle should be visualized throughout its course towards and within the vessel.

The angle of approach should be such that the needle will avoid nearby structures, both during approach and in the event the needle penetrates through the posterior aspect ("backwall") of the target vessel. Care should be taken to avoid posterior wall puncture, but having the nearby structures away from the trajectory of the needle will minimize the risk of complication in the event of accidental posterior wall puncture.

In the SAX view, the needle tip can be visualized entering the imaging plane as a hyperechoic dot appearing on the screen, often with a ring-down artifact. The imaging plane can then be moved slightly ahead of the needle tip, and the needle can be advanced again to come into the new imaging plane. This careful, stepwise approach allows for small corrections in the needle trajectory, and almost continuous visualization of the needle tip. It is important to note that if the needle is advanced *through* the imaging plane, a cross section of the needle will be seen as a hyperechoic dot, but the needle tip is not visualized. A stepwise progression *ahead* of the needle tip, with visualization of the needle entering the imaging plane, can avoid inadvertent needle tip misplacement.

As the needle reaches the edge of the target vessel, it may be seen to indent the wall of the vessel. With gentle traction on the syringe connected to the needle, a flash of blood will be seen in the syringe as the needle enters the vessel. After placement of the guidewire, ultrasound can be used in both SAX and LAX to confirm that the guidewire is both in the target vessel and not in surrounding vessels (Fig. 23.5a, b; Videos 23.5a, b). Other techniques to aid in confirming appro-

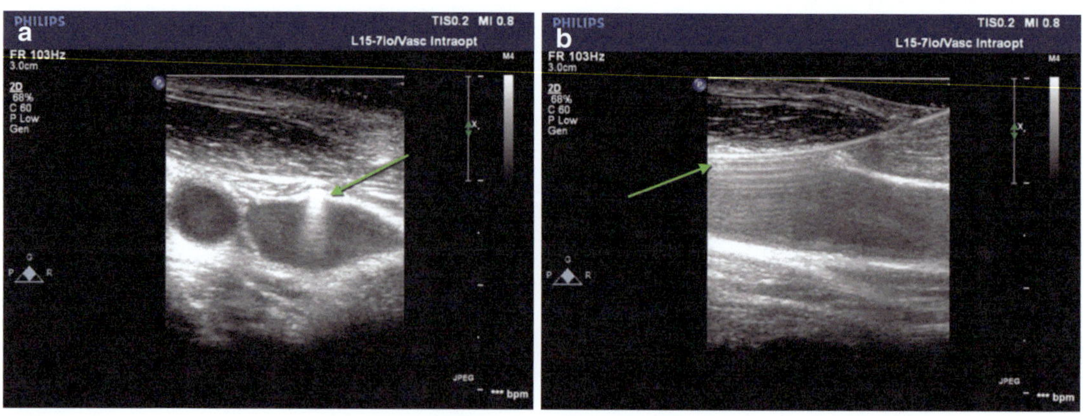

Fig. 23.5 (**a**) Short-axis imaging of right internal jugular vein with a wire within its lumen. (**b**) Long-axis imaging of the right internal jugular vein with a wire noted to be within its lumen (no evidence of "backwall"). The *green arrow* indicates the wire within the jugular vein

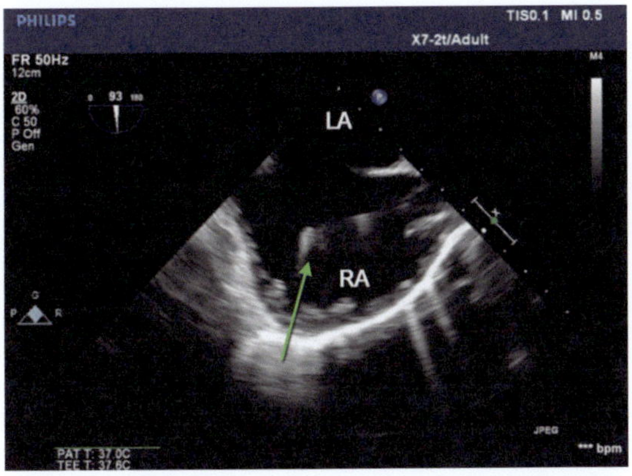

Fig. 23.6 Midesophageal bicaval view demonstrating the "J-tip" of the central access wire within the right atrium, confirming venous access. The *green arrow* indicates the "J-tip." *LA* left atrium, *RA* right atrium

priate vessel cannulation include direct pressure transduction, manometry, blood gas analysis, visualization of the wire with transesophageal echocardiography, and fluoroscopy. With the concurrent use of transesophageal echocardiography, a midesophageal bicaval view can confirm venous placement of the wire, noting the "J" tip of the wire in the right atrium (Fig. 23.6; Video 23.6). The American Society of Echocardiography (ASE) and the Society of Cardiovascular Anesthesiologists (SCA) recommend that real-time ultrasound be used to confirm vessel cannulation. The ASE/SCA recommendation is that if the combination of SAX and LAX is not utilized for confirmation of wire placement, manometry should be used [8].

Internal Jugular Vein Cannulation

The superiority of ultrasound guidance over landmark-based techniques for internal jugular (IJ) vein cannulation has been well documented [5, 9–11]. The use of ultrasound improves the overall and first-pass success rate, decreases time to cannulation and rate of arterial punctures, and decreases the total number of needle advances [11]. The ASE and SCA recommend that properly trained clinicians use real-time ultrasound for IJ cannulation whenever possible [8].

Any practitioner using ultrasound for IJ venous access should be familiar with the sonographic appearance of the local anatomy. The size of the IJ can be increased (potentially improving cannulation success) with Valsalva techniques and Trendelenburg positioning. These maneuvers also decrease the risk of air entrainment in the spontaneously ventilating patient [12, 13]. There is an intimate relationship between the IJ and the carotid artery (CA) at the location where IJ cannulation is typically pursued. This relationship explains the benefit of using ultrasound for IJ cannulation. Overlap between the IJ and the CA can lead to unintentional puncture and/or cannulation of the CA due to a through-and-through puncture of the vein. Ultrasound can be used to angle the approach such that CA puncture would be avoided in the event of accidental through-and-through puncture [14, 15]. Additionally, ultrasound can be used in both SAX and LAX to visualize the guidewire in the IJ and confirm that it is not in the CA, to avoid accidental CA dilation and cannulation [16]. Real-time ultrasound imaging can also potentially decrease the risk for pneumothorax by allowing for recognition of pleural tissue.

Subclavian/Axillary Vein Cannulation

While ultrasound-guided IJ vein access provides clear complication and success rate benefits over landmark-based techniques, evidence supporting ultrasound-guided subclavian (SC) vein cannulation is evolving. There are studies, however, that document higher success rates with ultrasound-guided cannulation of the SC vein compared to landmark techniques [17–19]. Obese patients and others with obscured external landmarks appear to benefit the most from the use of ultrasound for SC vein cannulation [20, 21].

The ASE and SCA state that the current literature does not support the routine use of ultrasound for uncomplicated patients undergoing SC vein cannulation. However, these associations do indicate that high-risk patients may benefit from the use of ultrasound to identify vessel location and patency prior to cannulation [8].

Although the supraclavicular approach is rarely used with landmark-based techniques because of the high incidence of pneumothorax, it is being used more frequently now as ultrasound identification of supraclavicular vessels is becoming more commonplace. Nevertheless, the infraclavicular approach remains the most common technique for SC vein cannulation with both landmark and ultrasound-guided techniques.

The middle third of the clavicle is typically chosen as the site for ultrasound imaging and needle insertion. The vein and artery should be identified just below the distal half of the clavicle (Fig. 23.7; Video 23.7). A short-axis approach is usually preferred due to the difficulty of differentiating vein and artery at this location in the LAX. A more lateral approach, targeting the axillary vein after it emerges from under the clavicle may also facilitate the use of ultrasound and minimize the risk for complications [22]. Trendelenburg position does not increase relative SC vein size to the same degree as with the IJ vein and thus, supine positioning is commonly used except in the case of a spontaneously breathing patient where Trendelenburg position will reduce the risk for air embolism [23].

Femoral Vein Cannulation

The benefit of ultrasound-guided femoral vein (FV) cannulation in reducing incidence of vascular-related complications to the femoral artery and FV, as well as improved first-pass and overall success rates has been established [24–26]. However, the evidence is insufficient to support a recommendation for routine use by the ASE and SCA, who recommend that ultrasound be used *when feasible* for FV cannulation to identify vessel overlap and patency [8], although other societal recommendations do support the routine use of ultrasound guidance for femoral arterial and venous cannulation [27–29].

Although infection and thrombosis are the most common serious complications related to femoral venous catheters, the most common complication related to the FV cannulation procedure itself is vascular injury. Of particular concern is common femoral artery puncture, which would occur when the needle is directed too laterally or when there is significant vessel overlap. The common femoral artery is typically located at the midpoint of the inguinal ligament connecting the anterior iliac spine to the pubic tubercle. The FV is located just medial to the common femoral artery, and it is this close anatomic relationship that makes the use of ultrasound-guided examination prior to cannulation beneficial (Fig. 23.8; Video 23.8).

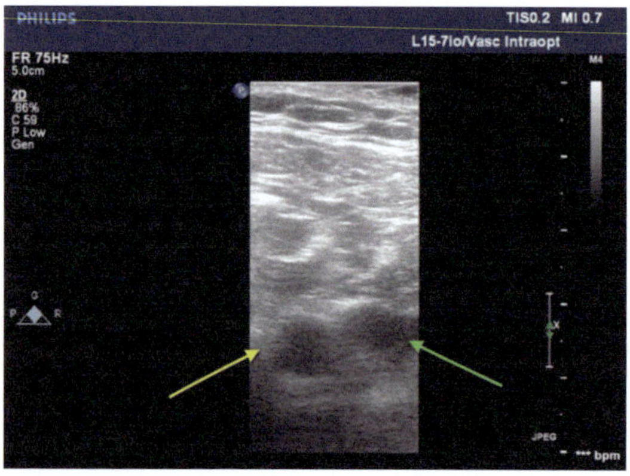

Fig. 23.7 Short-axis imaging of the right subclavian artery and vein. The *green arrow* indicates the vein and the *yellow arrow* indicates the artery

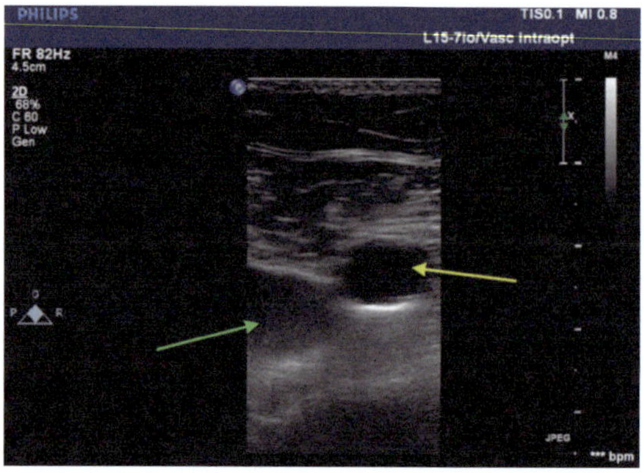

Fig. 23.8 Short-axis imaging of the left femoral artery and vein. The *green arrow* indicates the vein and the *yellow arrow* indicates the artery

Ultrasound for Arterial Access

Ultrasound can be used to guide arterial access at any site at which arterial access is typically obtained, including the radial, brachial, femoral, and dorsalis pedis arteries. The cannulation technique should not differ from the techniques used for ultrasound-guided venous access. The patient should be appropriately positioned, the orientation of the ultrasound probe and its correlation with the image on the screen should be confirmed, and measures such as a manual compression with the ultrasound probe and color flow Doppler should be taken to appropriately differentiate the target artery from surrounding vessels. Either the SAX or LAX can be used to cannulate the artery (Fig. 23.9a, b; Video 23.9a, b). The catheter can be inserted either over the needle or utilizing a guidewire.

Use of ultrasound for radial arterial access has been demonstrated to improve both first-attempt and overall success rates and reduce time to cannulation when compared with palpation-based techniques [30–32]. Ultrasound can be particularly useful in patients who are obese, who have low perfusion or non-pulsatile blood flow, or who have had previous unsuccessful cannulation attempts [33]. The ASE and SCA recognize the evidence supporting the use of ultrasound to improve first-pass success rates, but do not recommend routine use of real-time ultrasound for arterial access [8], although, again, several other societies do [27–29].

Ultrasound for Peripheral Venous Access

Ultrasound can be used to facilitate peripheral venous cannulation, particularly in deeper veins that are not palpable or visible. There are a number of reports of successful use of ultrasound in both the SAX and LAX for peripheral venous cannulation [34, 35]. Due to the collapsibility of peripheral veins, this can often be a difficult technique to achieve. The use of a tourniquet will increase peripheral venous pressure, improving success (Fig. 23.10; Video 23.10). It may be advantageous to advance the needle under direct ultrasound visualization, past the point where the "flash" of blood returns, as this may indicate the needle tip, but not the overlying catheter, is within the vessel. If the

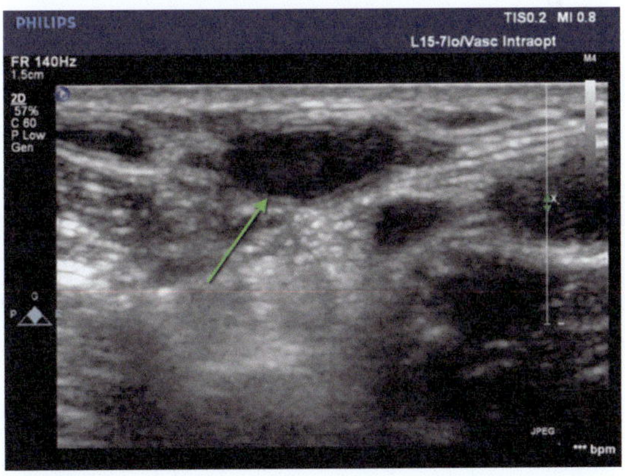

Fig. 23.10 Short-axis imaging of a left basilic peripheral vein (*green arrow*)

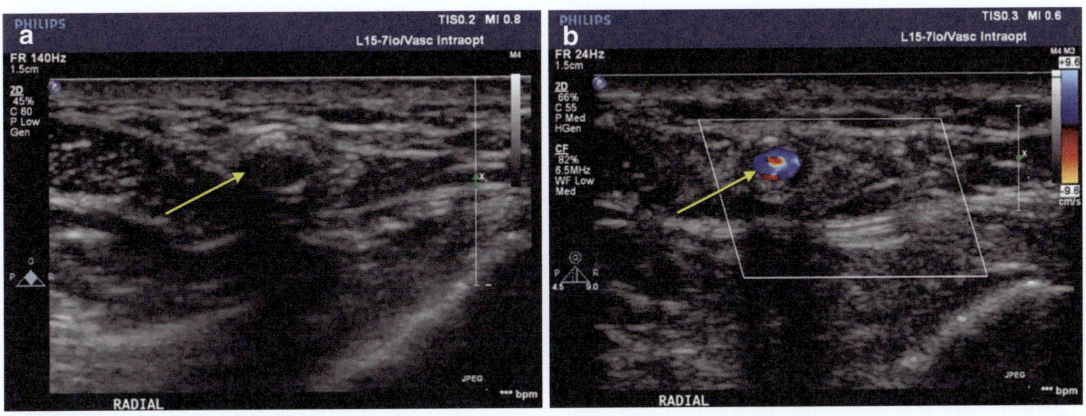

Fig. 23.9 (**a**) Short-axis imaging the radial artery. (**b**) Short-axis imaging of the same patient with color flow Doppler imaging. The *yellow arrow* indicates the radial artery

needle tip is continuously visualized within the vessel, the risk for "backwalling" or additional vascular injury is minimized. Some societies recommend the use of ultrasound guidance for difficult peripheral venous access [28, 29].

Ultrasound for Guidewire Confirmation and Pulmonary Arterial Catheter Placement

Guidewire Placement and Catheter Patency

As previously mentioned, there are multiple modalities by which a guidewire can be confirmed in the target vessel, including pressure transduction, manometry, radiography, and ultrasound. Visualization of the guidewire in the intended vessel in either the SAX or LAX view provides some evidence to the practitioner that the vessel has been appropriately accessed (Fig. 23.5; Videos 23.5a, b). However, visualization of the guidewire in the right atrium (RA) with either transesophageal echocardiography (TEE) (Fig. 23.6; Video 23.6) or transthoracic echocardiography (TTE) (Fig. 23.11; Video 23.11) further confirms proper venous placement of the guidewire prior to central venous catheter (CVC) placement. TTE or TEE can also be used to confirm patency of either a peripheral venous catheter or CVC via the presence of agitated saline in the right atrium or right ventricle shortly after injection (Fig. 23.12). While only two TTE views – a modified subcostal and parasternal RV inflow – have been provided as examples in this chapter, a number of other TTE and TEE views can be used to either confirm guidewire placement or catheter patency.

Finally, TTE or more commonly TEE, is frequently utilized in the operating room to confirm guidewire placement in the lumen of the central arterial system prior to arterial stent placement, femoral cannulation, or intra-aortic balloon pump insertion (Fig. 23.13; Video 23.12). A view of the descending aorta can be obtained by rotating the probe to the left from the midesophageal position. The distal and proximal descending aorta can then be interrogated in either the SAX or

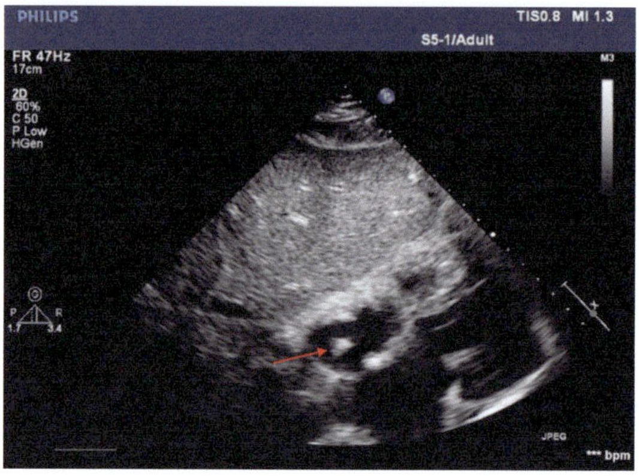

Fig. 23.11 Modified subcostal four-chamber view. A guidewire is visible in the right atrium (*red arrow*)

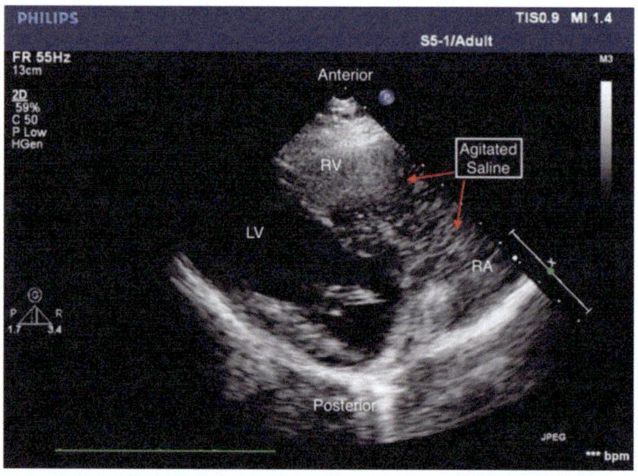

Fig. 23.12 Modified parasternal long-axis RV inflow view showing agitated saline in the right atrium (RA) and right ventricle (RV). In comparison, the left ventricle (LV), which is located in the far field, lacks agitated saline (Reproduced with permission from Fretwell et al. [39])

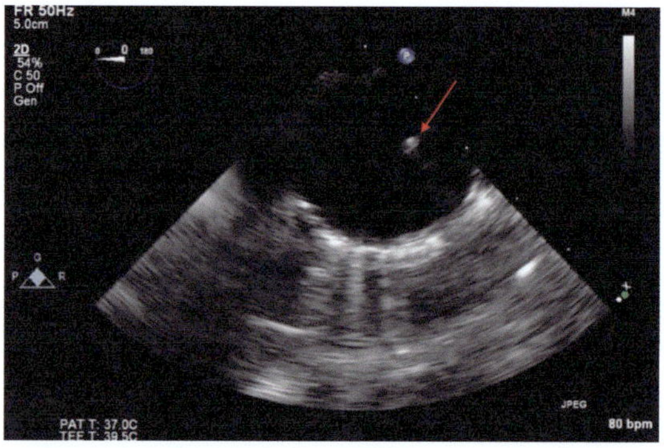

Fig. 23.13 Descending aorta short-axis view (depth reduced) with the distal tip of an intra-aortic balloon pump (*red arrow*) in the lumen of the aorta

LAX view by advancing and withdrawing the probe, respectively.

Pulmonary Arterial Catheter Placement with Ultrasound

Pulmonary arterial catheters (PACs) have traditionally been placed using pressure waveform tracings and length-insertion norms. With the increasing utilization of ultrasound (i.e., TTE and TEE) in the perioperative period, it is not surprising that ultrasound has also been integrated into this procedure. While it was theorized that ultrasound guidance would increase success rates, decrease the time to placement, and decrease associated complications, this has not been confirmed. However, TEE-guided placement did result in greater precision in the final location of the catheter in a study completed by the authors [36]. The authors contend that positioning the distal PAC in the proximal right pulmonary artery may reduce the incidence of pulmonary artery damage, accidental wedging, and arrhythmia generation.

Risk factors for difficult PAC placement and indications that ultrasound may be useful include low cardiac output states, right-sided chamber dilation, tricuspid valve regurgitation, tricuspid annuloplasty or replacement, and pulmonary hypertension [37]. In the authors' experience, the most common manipulation required is a counterclockwise turn to redirect the distal tip of the PAC from the right atrial appendage towards the tricuspid valve (Fig. 23.14) [38]. A midesophageal modified bicaval view is extremely useful for manipulations of the catheter in the RA, as it permits imaging of the superior vena cava, right atrial appendage, right atrium, and tricuspid valve (Fig. 23.15; Video 23.13).

Once the catheter passes through the tricuspid valve, a midesophageal RV inflow-outflow view can confirm orientation of the catheter towards the pulmonic valve and facilitates manipulations within the RV (Fig. 23.16; Video 23.14). Finally, the PAC can be positioned in the main pulmonary artery or proximal right pulmonary artery in the ascending aorta SAX view (Fig. 23.17). For a more detailed description of the TEE views and manipulations employed during TEE-guided PAC placement, please see the referenced article. In situations where TEE is either not indicated or contraindicated, TTE can also be used to guide placement and confirm the final position (e.g., left parasternal RV inflow, left parasternal basal SAX, and subcostal views) (Fig. 23.18; Video 23.15).

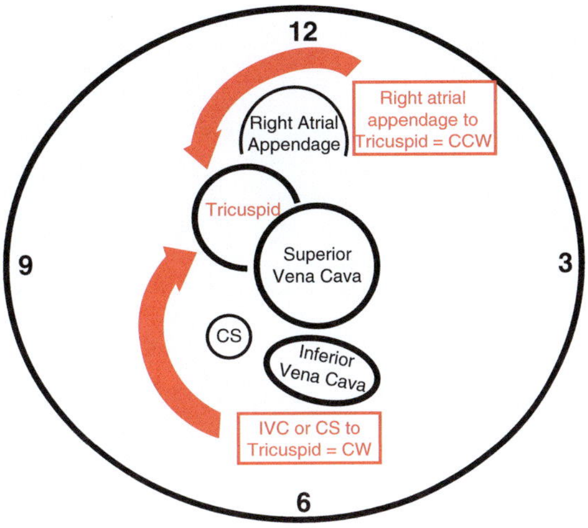

Fig. 23.14 Pulmonary artery catheter manipulations used to pass through the tricuspid valve (viewed from the superior vena cava). A catheter in the right atrial appendage should have counterclockwise torque applied to direct it towards the tricuspid valve. A catheter near the inferior vena cava or coronary sinus should have clockwise torque applied to direct it to the tricuspid valve. *CCW* counterclockwise, *CW* clockwise, *IVC* inferior vena cava, *CS* coronary sinus (Reproduced with permission from Cronin et al. [38])

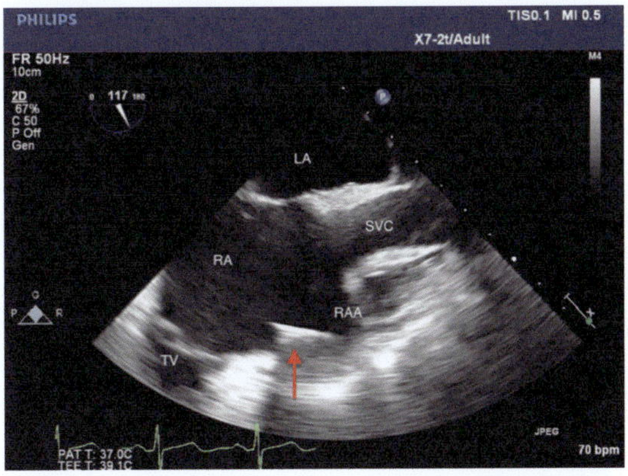

Fig. 23.15 Midesophageal modified bicaval view. A PAC with the balloon inflated (*red arrow*) is present in the right atrial appendage. *SVC* superior vena cava, *RA* right atrium, *LA* left atrium, *TV* tricuspid valve, *RAA* right atrial appendage (Reproduced with permission from Cronin et al. [38])

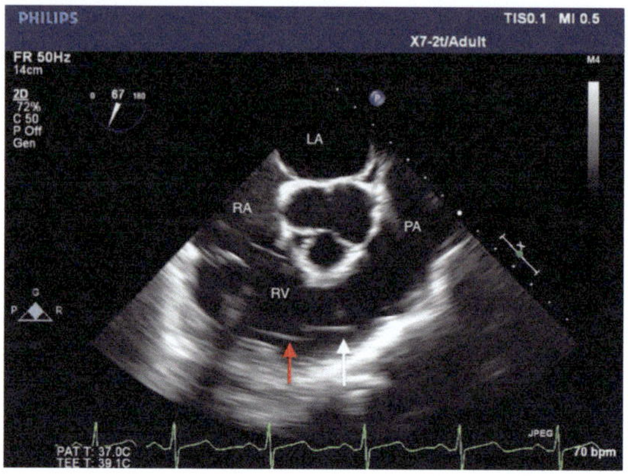

Fig. 23.16 Midesophageal RV inflow-outflow view (diastole). A PAC is seen traversing the RV with the catheter (*red arrow*) and balloon (*white arrow*) clearly visualized. *LA* left atrium, *RA* right atrium, *RV* right ventricle, *PA* pulmonary artery (Reproduced with permission from Cronin et al. [38])

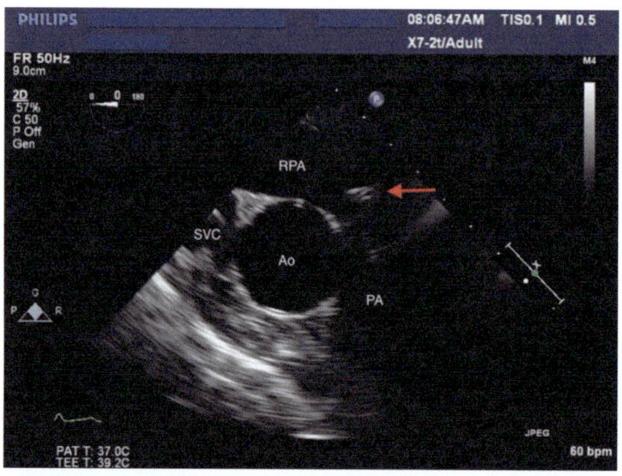

Fig. 23.17 Midesophageal ascending aorta short-axis view. The PAC balloon (*red arrow*) is visualized in the proximal right pulmonary artery. *SVC* superior vena cava, *Ao* aorta, *RPA* right pulmonary artery, *PA* pulmonary artery. (Reproduced with permission from Cronin et al. [38])

Conclusion

Ultrasound can facilitate central and peripheral venous and arterial access. It may increase success rates, decrease the time required for the procedure, and minimize the risk for complications. Additionally, echocardiography can be utilized to confirm proper guidewire placement and aid in the placement of aortic, central venous, or pulmonary artery catheters.

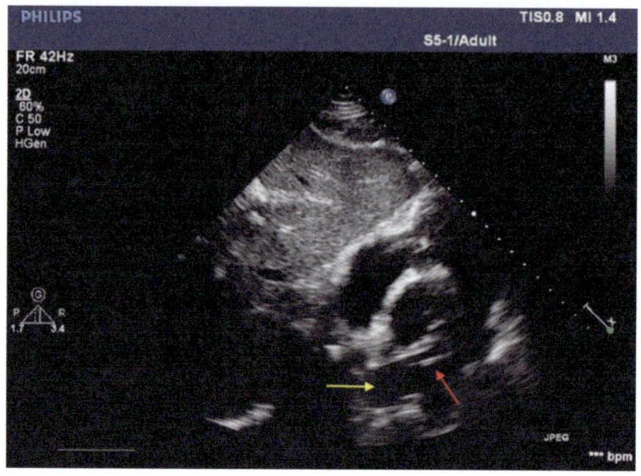

Fig. 23.18 Subcostal basal short-axis view. The distal tip of a PAC (*red arrow*) is located in proximal right pulmonary artery (*yellow arrow*)

Questions

1. The following image is obtained while attempting to place a radial arterial catheter. Which of the following is most true?

   A. This site is not suitable, because the radial artery is occluded
   B. The depth should be increased
   C. The angle of the probe should be adjusted
   D. This site is suitable for cannulation

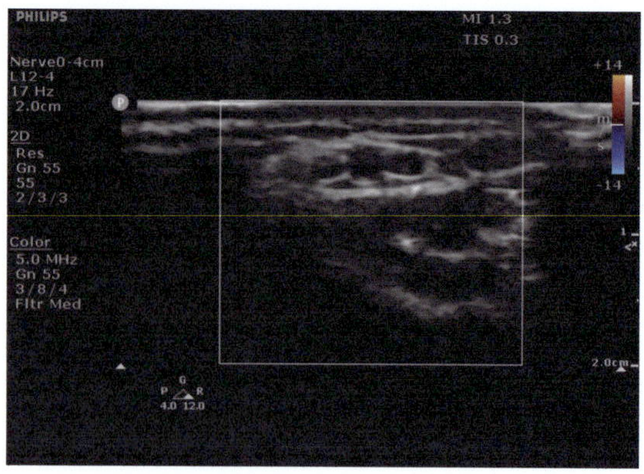

2. While attempting peripheral venous access, the following image is obtained. There is no return of blood in the catheter. What is the next best step?

   A. Withdraw the needle and advance again
   B. Advance the needle further into the vessel
   C. Rotate the probe to obtain a long-axis view
   D. Agitate the needle to confirm visualization

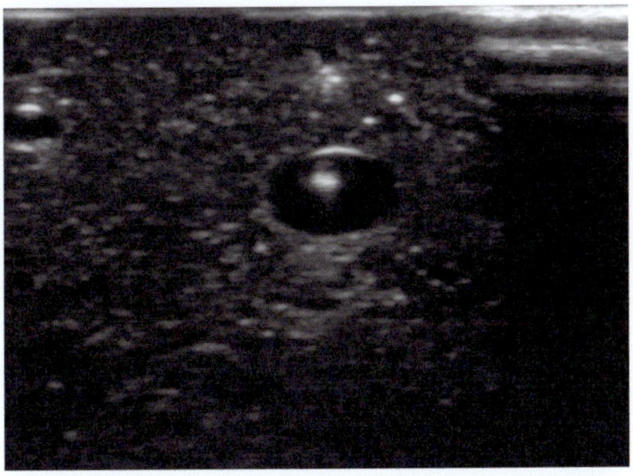

3. Which of the following statements is most accurate?

   A. Subclavian catheters have a lower infectious risk, but higher thrombotic risk than femoral catheters.
   B. Internal jugular catheters have the lowest risk for infection.
   C. Ultrasound cannot be used for guidance for subclavian cannulation.
   D. Femoral catheters have the highest risk for both thrombosis and infection.

4. Which of the following statements regarding pulmonary arterial catheter (PAC) placement is most true?

   A. A midesophageal ascending aorta SAX view can confirm appropriate catheter position.
   B. A midesophageal RV inflow-outflow view can confirm appropriate catheter position.
   C. Ultrasound decreases time to placement and the success rate of PACs.
   D. A midesophageal modified bicaval tricuspid valve view can confirm appropriate catheter position.

5. Which of the following sites would be most appropriate for insertion of a LEFT femoral venous catheter in the following image?

   A. A
   B. B
   C. C or D
   D. None of the above

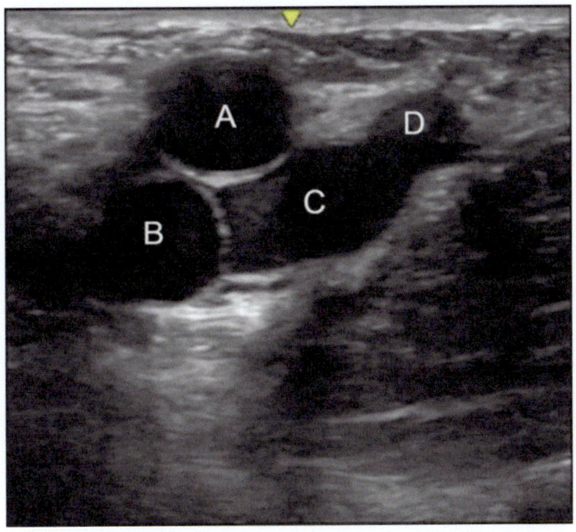

References

1. Blaivas M, Brannam L, Fernandez E. Short-axis versus long-axis approaches for teaching ultrasound-guided vascular access on a new inanimate model. Acad Emerg Med. 2003;10:1307–11.
2. Merrer J. Complications of femoral and subclavian venous catheterization in critically ill patients: a randomized controlled trial. JAMA. 2001;286:700.
3. McGee DC, Gould MK. Preventing complications of central venous catheterization. N Engl J Med. 2003;348:1123–33.
4. Parienti JJ, Mongardon N, Mégarbane B, et al. Intravascular complications of central venous catheterization by insertion site. N Engl J Med. 2015;373:1220–9.
5. Hosokawa K, Shime N, Kato Y, et al. A randomized trial of ultrasound image–based skin surface marking versus real-time ultrasound-guided internal jugular vein catheterization in infants. Anesthesiology. 2007;107:720–4.
6. Milling TJ, Rose J, Briggs WM, et al. Randomized, controlled clinical trial of point-of-care limited ultrasonography assistance of central venous cannulation: the Third Sonography Outcomes Assessment Program (SOAP-3) trial*. Crit Care Med. 2005;33:1764–9.
7. Schnadower D, Lin S, Perera P, et al. A pilot study of ultrasound analysis before pediatric peripheral vein cannulation attempt. Acad Emerg Med. 2007;14:483–5.
8. Troianos CA, Hartman GS, Glas KE, et al. Guidelines for performing ultrasound guided vascular cannulation. Anesth Analg. 2012;114:46–72.
9. Denys BG, Uretsky BF, Reddy PS. Ultrasound-assisted cannulation of the internal jugular vein. A prospective comparison to the external landmark-guided technique. Circulation. 1993;87:1557–62.

10. Karakitsos D, Labropoulos N, De Groot E, et al. Real-time ultrasound-guided catheterisation of the internal jugular vein: a prospective comparison with the landmark technique in critical care patients. Crit Care. 2006;10:R162.
11. Troianos CA, Jobes DR, Ellison N. Ultrasound-guided cannulation of the internal jugular vein. A prospective, randomized study. Anesth Analg. 1991;72:823–6.
12. Bellazzini MA, Rankin PM, Gangnon RE, et al. Ultrasound validation of maneuvers to increase internal jugular vein cross-sectional area and decrease compressibility. Am J Emerg Med. 2009;27:454–9.
13. Terai C, Anada H, Matsushima S, et al. Effects of mild Trendelenburg on central hemodynamics and internal jugular vein velocity, cross-sectional area, and flow. Am J Emerg Med. 1995;13:255–8.
14. Blaivas M, Adhikari S. An unseen danger: frequency of posterior vessel wall penetration by needles during attempts to place internal jugular vein central catheters using ultrasound guidance*. Crit Care Med. 2009;37:2345–9.
15. Stone MB, Hern HG. Inadvertent carotid artery cannulation during ultrasound guided central venous catheterization. Ann Emerg Med. 2007;49:720.
16. Moak JH, Lyons MS, Wright SW, et al. Needle and guidewire visualization in ultrasound-guided internal jugular vein cannulation. Am J Emerg Med. 2011;29:432–6.
17. Balls A, LoVecchio F, Kroeger A, et al. Ultrasound guidance for central venous catheter placement: results from the Central Line Emergency Access Registry Database. Am J Emerg Med. 2010;28:561–7.
18. Gualtieri E, Deppe SA, Sipperly ME, et al. Subclavian venous catheterization. Crit Care Med. 1995;23:692–7.
19. Lalu MM, Fayad A, Ahmed O, et al. Ultrasound-guided subclavian vein catheterization: a systematic review and meta-analysis. Crit Care Med. 2015;43:1498–507.
20. Beaulieu Y. Bedside ultrasonography in the ICU *. Chest. 2005;128:1766.
21. Hind D. Ultrasonic locating devices for central venous cannulation: meta-analysis. BMJ. 2003;327:361–0.
22. Maddali MM, Arora NR, Chatterjee N. Ultrasound guided out-of-plane versus in-plane transpectoral left axillary vein cannulation. J Cardiothorac Vasc Anesth. 2017;31:1707–12.
23. Tan B-K, Hong S-W, Huang MHS, et al. Anatomic basis of safe percutaneous subclavian venous catheterization. J Trauma. 2000;48:82.
24. Iwashima S, Ishikawa T, Ohzeki T. Ultrasound-guided versus landmark-guided femoral vein access in pediatric cardiac catheterization. Pediatr Cardiol. 2007;29:339–42.
25. Kwon T, Kim Y, Cho D. Ultrasound-guided cannulation of the femoral vein for acute haemodialysis access. Nephrol Dial Transplant. 1997;12:1009–12.
26. Seto AH, Abu-Fadel MS, Sparling JM, et al. Real-time ultrasound guidance facilitates femoral arterial access and reduces vascular complications. J Am Coll Cardiol Intv. 2010;3:751–8.
27. Timsit JF, Baleine J, Bernard L, et al. Expert consensus-based clinical practice guidelines management of intravascular catheters in the intensive care unit. Ann Intensive Care. 2020;10:118.
28. Lamperti M, Biasucci DG, Disma N, et al. European Society of Anaesthesiology guidelines on peri-operative use of ultrasound-guided for vascular access (PERSEUS vascular access). Eur J Anaesthesiol. 2020;37:344–76.
29. Frankel HL, Kirkpatrick AW, Elbarbary M, et al. Guidelines for the appropriate use of bedside general and cardiac ultrasonography in the evaluation of critically ill patients-part I: general ultrasonography. Crit Care Med. 2015;43:2479–502.
30. Levin PD, Sheinin O, Gozal Y. Use of ultrasound guidance in the insertion of radial artery catheters. Crit Care Med. 2003;31:481–4.
31. Shiloh AL. Ultrasound-guided catheterization of the radial artery. Chest. 2011;139:524.
32. Shiver S, Blaivas M, Lyon M. A prospective comparison of ultrasound-guided and blindly placed radial arterial catheters. Acad Emerg Med. 2006;13:1275–9.
33. Sandhu NS, Patel B. Use of ultrasonography as a rescue technique for failed radial artery cannulation. J Clin Anesth. 2006;18:138–41.
34. Keyes LE, Frazee BW, Snoey ER, et al. Ultrasound-guided brachial and Basilic vein cannulation in emergency department patients with difficult intravenous access. Ann Emerg Med. 1999;34:711–4.
35. Sandhu NPS. Mid-arm approach to basilic and cephalic vein cannulation using ultrasound guidance. Br J Anaesth. 2004;93:292–4.
36. Cronin B, Kolotiniuk N, Youssefzadeh K, et al. Pulmonary artery catheter placement aided by transesophageal echocardiography versus pressure waveform transduction. J Cardiothorac Vasc Anesth. 2018;32:2578–82.
37. Turnage WS, Fontanet H. Transesophageal echocardiography-guided pulmonary artery catheter placement. Anesth Analg. 1993;77:858–9.
38. Cronin B, Robbins R, Maus T. Pulmonary artery catheter placement using transesophageal echocardiography. J Cardiothorac Vasc Anesth. 2017;31:178–83.
39. Fretwell D, Smith M, Martin E, et al. Epidural intravascular injection detection by transthoracic echocardiography. J Cardiothorac Vasc Anesth. 2020;34:1288–91.

Appendix – Answers

Chapter 1

1. **Answer: C**
   Rationale: Certification in Basic Perioperative Transesophageal Echocardiography's scope of practice is limited to utilizing TEE in a nondiagnostic or monitoring-only manner except in emergency situations, while Certification in Advanced Perioperative Transesophageal Echocardiography's scope of practice includes diagnostic uses and the guidance of surgical interventions.
2. **Answer: C**
   Rationale: Absolute contraindications often involve esophageal pathology such as esophagectomy or esophageal strictures. Stable esophageal varices that are not actively bleeding are considered a relative contraindication. Mediastinal radiation and unstable cervical spines represent relative contraindications.
3. **Answer: D**
   Rationale: Transesophageal echocardiography probe manipulations include insertion/withdrawal, anteflexion/retroflexion (performed with clockwise and counterclockwise turn of the large knob, respectively), right/left flexion (performed with clockwise and counterclockwise turn of the small knob, respectively), right/left probe rotation (performed by turning the probe shaft to the right or left), and increasing or decreasing the multiplane angle (from 0° to 180°).
4. **Answer: C**
   Rationale: At zero degree of multiplane angle, the right side of the screen displays the left side of the patient's heart. For example, the midesophageal four-chamber view at zero degree displays the patient's right heart on the left side of the screen and the left heart on the right side of the screen.
5. **Answer: A**
   Rationale: The six probe manipulations with transthoracic echocardiography include sweeping (linear movement along the X-axis), fanning (rotational movement along the X-axis), sliding (linear movement along the Y-axis), rocking (rotational movement along the Y-axis), compression (movement into the patient along the Z-axis), and rotation (twisting movement along the Z-axis).

Chapter 2

1. **Answer: B**
   Rationale: The midesophageal four-chamber view displays both the mitral and tricuspid valves while also providing segmental analysis (base-mid-apex) of the left ventricular septal and lateral walls.
2. **Answer: C**
   Rationale: While the deep transgastric five-chamber view visualizes the left ventricular outflow tract and aortic valve annulus, these structures are in the far field and are not perpendicular to the ultrasound beam.

T. M. Maus, C. R. Tainter (eds.), *Essential Echocardiography*,
https://doi.org/10.1007/978-3-030-84349-6

The midesophageal aortic valve long-axis view orients these structures perpendicular to the ultrasound beam in the near field allowing better measurements.

3. **Answer: C**

   Rationale: For the opposite reasons of Question #2, the deep transgastric five-chamber view orients left ventricular outflow tract and aortic valve blood flow parallel to the ultrasound beam which is optimal for Doppler analysis.

4. **Answer: B**

   Rationale: While the pulmonic valve may be visualized in the midesophageal right ventricular inflow-outflow view and occasionally in the midesophageal aortic valve short-axis view, the orientation is rarely parallel to the ultrasound beam allowing adequate Doppler analysis. The upper esophageal aortic arch short-axis view however orients the right ventricular outflow tract, pulmonic valve, and proximal pulmonary artery in parallel to the ultrasound beam which allows appropriate Doppler interrogation.

5. **Answer: A**

   Rationale: While each of these views is important for the evaluation of wall motion abnormalities, the transgastric midpapillary short-axis view allows evaluation of the mid-segment territories of all three coronary arteries. The anterior and anteroseptal walls are perfused by the left anterior descending artery, the lateral walls are perfused by the left circumflex artery, and the inferior and inferoseptal walls are typically perfused by the right coronary artery.

6. **Answer: D**

   Rationale: All of these views are helpful in the guidance of pulmonary artery catheter (PAC) placement. The midesophageal modified bicaval tricuspid valve view assists with entering of the PAC into the right atrium from the superior vena cava and directing the catheter toward the right ventricle. The midesophageal right ventricular inflow-outflow view assists with the PAC traversing the right ventricle toward the pulmonic valve, while the midesophageal ascending aortic short-axis view displays the main and right pulmonary arteries to assist with final positioning of the PAC.

7. **Answer: A**

   Rationale: The transgastric basal short-axis view provides an image of the mitral valve in plane with the ultrasound beam. This provides the characteristic view of the mitral valve that appears like a fish mouth opening and closing allowing a view of all of the segments of the mitral valve leaflets at once.

8. **Answer: A**

   Rationale: There is often confusion between the difference between the midesophageal long-axis view (ME LAX) and the midesophageal aortic valve long-axis view (ME AV LAX). The ME LAX view contains the left atrium, mitral and aortic valves, and the left ventricle down to the left ventricular apex. The purpose of this view is severalfold including evaluation of the mitral valve (the view is perpendicular to the mitral valve coaptation line) and evaluation of segmental left ventricular function (anteroseptal and inferolateral walls). The ME AV LAX view is achieved by withdrawing the probe with a small right-hand turn of the TEE probe and will place the aortic valve perpendicular to the ultrasound probe for better visualization. The act of withdrawing and turning the probe often removes the left ventricular apex from the image.

9. **Answer: B**

   Rationale: There are several views that image the interatrial septum including the midesophageal four-chamber view, the midesophageal aortic valve short-axis view, and the midesophageal bicaval view. Of the listed views, only the midesophageal bicaval view will display the interatrial septum.

10. **Answer: B**

    Rationale: Knowledge of the imaged left ventricular walls in midesophageal views is important in the detection of ischemia. The midesophageal four-chamber view images the septal and lateral walls, and the midesophageal two-chamber view images the anterior and inferior walls, while the midesophageal long-axis view images the anteroseptal and inferolateral walls.

Chapter 3

1. **Answer: A**

   Rationale: From this parasternal short-axis midpapillary (mid ventricular) view (Fig. A.1), the midsection of the following walls of the left ventricle are visible: anterior (A), anteroseptal (AS), inferoseptal (IS), inferior (I), inferolateral (IL), and anterolateral (AL).

2. **Answer: C**

   Rationale: The first image is an apical long-axis (3-chamber) view, which is located along the same axis as the image on the right, the apical 2-chamber view, but about 30° counterclockwise. Therefore, from the image on the left, rotation 30° clockwise will obtain the image on the right. Tilting medially would move the image from the right to the left side of the screen. Fanning inferiorly would foreshorten the image by moving the imaging plane away from the axis of the heart.

3. **Answer: A**

   Rationale: The aortic valve and LVOT are visible in the apical long-axis (3-chamber) view. Both the apical 4-chamber view and the subcostal 4-chamber view should visualize the right and left atria, right and left ventricles, as well as the atrioventricular valves, but not the pulmonic or aortic valves.

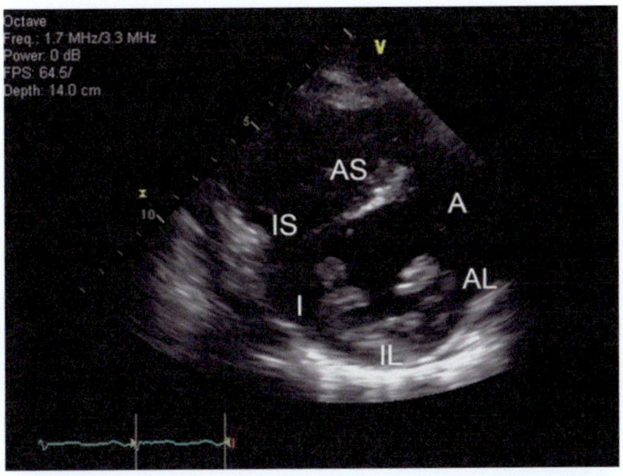

Fig. A.1 Parasternal short-axis midpapillary view, demonstrating the anterior (A), anteroseptal (AS), inferoseptal (IS), inferior (I), inferolateral (IL), and anterolateral (AL) walls

4. **Answer: D**

   Rationale: The indicated structure is the anterolateral papillary muscle. The other papillary muscle visible is the posteromedial papillary muscle (not labeled here). There is no inferolateral papillary muscle. An LV thrombus may appear hyperechoic, but would more likely be located in an area of hypokinesis and adherent to the ventricular wall.

5. **Answer: D**

   Rationale: The parasternal midpapillary short-axis view displays the mid-left ventricle in short-axis, and the right ventricle in short-axis more proximally, and slightly to the patient's right (away from the probe marker, to the left of the image). Image A shows the right ventricle to the patient's left, toward the probe marker, thus is oriented backward. Image B is a reversed transgastric short-axis view, which shows the right ventricle in the far field, toward the probe marker (backward), and image C is a transgastric short-axis view showing the RV in the far field to the patient's right.

6. **Answer: A**

   Rationale: The usual window used to obtain the parasternal long-axis view is just to the left of the sternal border, in the second or third intercostal space, with the ultrasound probe indicator pointing toward the patient's right shoulder. A 90-degree clockwise rotation, directing the probe marker toward the patient's left shoulder will obtain a parasternal short-axis view. The second or third intercostal space to the right of the sternal border may be useful in imaging some elements of the heart, in some patients, particularly with distorted anatomy, but it would not be expected to yield a parasternal window in most patients.

7. **Answer: C**

   Rationale: The image shows a suprasternal view of the aortic arch. The ascending aorta is to the left of the image, and the proximal descending aorta is to the right. The origins of the great vessels are visible at the top of the image. The right pulmonary artery is typically seen coursing below the aortic arch, in cross section. The superior vena cava is typically not visible from this view, though occasionally may be visualized by rotating the probe approximately 90°, and angling toward the right side of the patient.

8. **Answer: A**

   Rationale: An apical five-chamber or three-chamber view provides a line of interrogation very close to the direction of flow through the aortic valve, which decreases error in Doppler calculations. In contrast, TEE provides excellent imaging and alignment of the mitral valve through a midesophageal window. Although accurate Doppler measurements through the mitral valve may be possible with TTE, TEE generally provides superior imaging of the mitral valve. Transthoracic echocardiography is often limited by patient issues, including body habitus, positioning, or the use of mechanical ventilation, but in most cases, useful information is still available. While not all imaging windows may be available, using multiple sites of interrogation may be able to answer most clinical questions. The ascending aorta, aortic arch, and proximal descending aorta are visible from a suprasternal window using transthoracic echocardiography.

9. **Answer: C**

   Explanation: Positioning can play an important role in optimizing image acquisition for transthoracic echocardiography. Optimal positioning depends upon the specific imaging window and desired view and may be slightly different from patient to patient. Parasternal and apically located views often utilize the left lateral decubitus position to bring the heart closer to the chest wall. In addition, raising the patient's left arm above the head may help separate the rib spaces and decrease rib shadowing. Holding in a breath may help displace the heart toward the diaphragm, improving subcostal visualization, but by expanding the lungs, it is likely to worsen parasternal or apical visualization by causing more lung interference. Raising or lowering the bed may improve or worsen various views, depending on specific scenarios, but also remains a viable option for some patients.

10. **Answer: B**

    Rationale: The image on the left shows an apical four-chamber view, obtained in the fourth or fifth intercostal space, near the anterior axillary line. The image on the right is an apical five-chamber view, obtained by fanning the probe anteriorly from the same probe location, as evidenced by the continued visualization of the apex of the left ventricle. Translation along the chest wall would move away from the apex of the heart, and the apical segment would no longer be visualized in the near field. Rotational movement (clockwise or counterclockwise) would be expected to develop a plane which would still not pass through the LVOT and aortic valve until the apical long-axis view which places the LVOT and aortic valve on the right side of the screen.

Chapter 4

1. **Answer: C**

   Rationale: Ultrasound uses the energy reflected by sound waves to determine the position of reflectors, similar to SONAR. RADAR uses reflected radio waves to determine the position of reflectors. Global Positioning System (GPS) also uses radio wave signals from geosynchronous satellites to localize position relative to Earth's surface. Cellular triangulation uses the time delay between cellular telephone signals and towers to provide a location of the signal origination.

2. **Answer: A**

   Rationale: Ultrasound waves are longitudinal waves, which a frequency above the threshold for human hearing (> 20 kHz). Because they cause compressions and rarefactions, they cannot propagate through a vacuum. A portion of sound waves (including ultrasound) will reflect from surfaces with different densities.

3. **Answer: C**

   Rationale: Lateral resolution (the ability to distinguish two points next to each other equidistant from the transducer) depends on the density of waves, which is determined by the number of crystals on the transducer. The orientation of the waves can be adjusted to optimize lateral resolution at a convergence point (the focus). Longitudinal (axial) resolution is affected by pulse length, frequency, and wavelength. The signal amplitude affects the strength of the received signal, but not the resolution.

4. **Answer: C**

   Rationale: Longitudinal (axial) resolution is the ability to distinguish two points along the line of transmission of the ultrasound wave. It is improved (the distance one is able to distinguish is smaller) by a shorter pulse length, which is a consequence of higher frequency or shorter (decreased) wavelength. The number of piezoelectric crystals influences the lateral resolution, but does not affect the axial resolution.

5. **Answer: B**

   Rationale: The change in frequency (Δf) of a wave reflected from a moving object is directly proportional to the velocity of the object (v).

$$v = \frac{C\Delta f}{2f_T \cos\theta}$$

   The speed of sound in the medium (c) is directly proportional to the change in frequency of the reflected wave. The frequency shift is directly proportional to the cosine of the angle between the velocity of the reflector and the direction of the ultrasound wave (Θ), as well as the transmitted frequency (f_T).

6. **Answer: C**

   Rationale: The change in pressure can be related to the resultant velocity (in physiologic conditions) by the modified Bernoulli equation:

$$\Delta P = 4v^2$$

   where ΔP is the pressure gradient and v is the peak velocity in m/sec. If the "downstream" pressure in the right atrium during systole is 8 mmHg, then (RVSP – 8) = 4 $(3 \text{ m/s})^2$, and RVSP = 44 mmHg.

7. **Answer: C**

   Rationale: Cardiac output is equal to stroke volume times heart rate. Stroke volume is equal to the cross-sectional area of the LVOT ($\text{Area}_{\text{LVOT}}$) multiplied by the velocity time integral of the flow through the LVOT (VTI_{LVOT}). Because the diameter of the LVOT is 2 cm, the radius is 1 cm, and $\text{Area}_{\text{LVOT}} = \pi(1 \text{ cm})^2 \cong 3.14 \text{ cm}^2$. Stroke volume is therefore $3.14 \text{ cm}^2 \times 25 \text{ cm} = 78.5 \text{ cm}^3$, and cardiac output = $78.5 \text{ cm}^3 \times 76 \text{ bpm} = 5966 \text{ cm}^3/\text{min} \cong 6$ liters per minute.

8. **Answer: A**

   Rationale: The stroke volume through the LVOT must equal the stroke volume through the aortic valve orifice (assuming there is no blood flow diverted anywhere else). Then, according to the continuity equation, the cross-sectional area of the LVOT (A_{LVOT}) multiplied by the VTI through the LVOT (VTI_{LVOT}) must equal the area of the aortic valve orifice (A_{AV}) multiplied by the velocity of flow through the aortic valve (VTI_{AV}). Therefore, $A_{\text{AV}} \times 100 \text{ cm} = \pi(1 \text{ cm})^2 \times 25 \text{ cm}$, and $A_{\text{AV}} \cong 78.5 \text{ cm}^3/100 \text{ cm} = 0.79 \text{ cm}^2$.

9. **Answer: C**

   Rationale: The pressure difference between two chambers can be derived from the velocity of flow between them ($\Delta P = 4v^2$). If the left ventricular pressure during systole is known (systemic arterial systolic pressure), then a regurgitant velocity through the mitral valve would allow calculation of the left atrial pressure (LAP = LVSP – $4v^2$).

10. **Answer: D**

    Rationale: Ultrasound uses waves of energy passing through human tissue to develop images, and the effects of this energy should always be considered. The ALARA principle (As Low As Reasonably Achievable) suggests using the lowest level of energy possible to obtain the desired result. Thermal injury may occur from tissue distortion, and cavitation (nonthermal) injury may occur from expansion and collapse of air bubbles within the tissues. Increasing density of ultrasound waves increases the potential for injury. M-mode uses a single ultrasound beam, thus a small amount of energy relative to other modes of imaging. Color Doppler uses multiple pulsed waves, in addition to the waves used to produce a B-mode image "background," thus exposing the tissues to more energy and potential for injury.

Chapter 5

1. **Answer: C**

   Rationale: Optimal gain settings include the ability to see both high amplitude signals and low amplitude signals across the gray scale. Blood-filled spaces should appear black as blood does not reflect significant amounts of ultrasound. If the gain is reduced to the point that only the brightest structures are apparent, significant detail of low amplitude signals will be lost. Lastly, adjustment of the range of amplitudes displayed is adjustment of dynamic range (compression) as opposed to gain.
2. **Answer: A**

   Rationale: Time gain compensation involves adjusting the sliders that move left and right on the keyboard to either increase or decrease gain at specific depths from the ultrasound probe. As the speed of ultrasound in tissue is constant, time equals depth.
3. **Answer: D**

   Rationale: Autoscan or iScan is a computer algorithm that evaluates the brightness of the image on the screen and automatically adjusts the time gain compensation to obtain a more even brightness from the near to far field.
4. **Answer: C**

   Rationale: Lateral resolution is best obtained at the focal point. Lateral resolution is acceptable in the near field and very poor in the far field past the focal point. Therefore, it is best to place the focal point near the structure of interest. For example, if one is imaging the mitral valve, the focal point should be placed at or just beyond the depth of the mitral valve.
5. **Answer: A**

   Rationale: Reducing the sector width will reduce the number of total scan lines to generate one complete frame. With a reduction of the number of total scan lines, more frames can be generated per second which results in a higher frame rate otherwise known as increased temporal resolution.
6. **Answer: C**

   Rationale: As M-mode imaging only requires the generation of a single scan line, the frame rate is therefore extremely high. Only one scan line is necessary per "frame" and therefore hundreds to thousands of frames per second can be generated providing the highest temporal resolution. In contrast, three-dimensional imaging is utilizing multiple scan lines in multiple planes and therefore often has the lowest frame rate.
7. **Answer: B**

   Rationale: Pulsed-wave Doppler utilizes one crystal to both emit and receive ultrasound signals. The time delay between emitting and receiving allows the determination of velocities at a specific depth. The range of depths that the system is "listening" is termed a sample gate. The sample gate is therefore the area on the ultrasound screen where velocity measurements will be taken. Due to the time delay, there is a limit on the speed of blood flood that can be measured. This is termed the aliasing velocity.
8. **Answer: B**

   Rationale: Color flow Doppler is based upon pulsed-wave Doppler which allows the range specificity (knowing the velocity at a specific location) at the cost of aliasing (a limit to the measured velocity). The color flow Doppler box is a function of multiple pulsed-wave Doppler scan lines that are color-coded and overlaid on top of the two-dimensional image. This requires two sets of scanning lines over each area that the color flow box covers, one for the two-dimensional imaging and one for the color flow Doppler imaging. This requires a lot of computational power and therefore results in decreased temporal resolution.

9. **Answer: A**

   Rationale: Continuous-wave Doppler involves the use of two crystals where one emits and one receives on a continuous basis. This modality therefore is constantly measuring without the time-delay inherent in pulsed-wave Doppler. This leads to the ability to measure high velocities without aliasing. The downside to this modality is range ambiguity and therefore the inability to determine exactly along the interrogation line a specific measurement occurred.

10. **Answer: A**

    Rationale: When the freeze button is engaged such that imaging is paused, no further ultrasound generation is occurring. Therefore, the risk of thermal injury is substantially reduced. It is recommended to pause the imaging system when the modality is not being activity utilized. Three-dimensional imaging and color flow Doppler utilize additional scan lines over two-dimensional imaging and therefore potentially generate additional heat. The ALARA (As Low As Reasonably Achievable) principle involves utilizing the least amount of power and imaging resources that is needed to achieve the clinical information and result. Utilizing the least amount of power would reduce the chance of thermal injury.

Chapter 6

1. **Answer: A**

   Rationale: Tissue Doppler imaging provides relatively load-independent assessment of myocardial function. Fractional area change will be altered by various states of volume loading. Color flow-based propagation velocity and lateral *E*/*e*' assess left ventricular diastolic function and not directly systolic function.

2. **Answer: D**

   Rationale: The rate of rise of left ventricular pressure utilizes a continuous-wave Doppler interrogation of a mitral regurgitant jet and, assuming a negligible left atrial pressure, evaluates the rate of pressure rise during systole. The time to develop a left ventricular pressure from 4 to 36 mmHg is calculated to determine the d*P*/d*T*. The transgastric midpapillary short-axis view does not contain the mitral valve and therefore cannot be utilized for this technique.

3. **Answer: A**

   Rationale: The rate of rise of left ventricular pressure is calculated as the time required for a change in pressure from 4 to 36 mm Hg. 4 and 36 mmHg correlate to the pressure gradient across the mitral valve at 1 and 3 m/s, respectively. The calculation of d*P*/d*t* is therefore 32/*t* with *t* in seconds. 32/0.02 seconds = 1600 mmHg/s, which suggests normal LV systolic function.

4. **Answer: C**

   Rationale: While 3D echocardiography is not typically utilized in basic perioperative echocardiography, understanding its benefit helps to identify limitations of two-dimensional assessments of left ventricular systolic dysfunction. Three-dimensional echocardiography-based ejection fraction is not limited by alterations in left ventricular geometry, such as an apical aneurysm or a wall motion abnormality that may be missed by traditional midesophageal four- and two-chamber views.

5. **Answer: C**

   Rationale: The transgastric midpapillary short-axis or parasternal short-axis views are most commonly utilized for fractional area change measurements of the left ventricle. The midesophageal aortic valve short-axis view does not visualize the left ventricle, and the deep transgastric five-chamber view is not optimally aligned to appropriately calculate the fractional area of change.

6. **Answer: D**

   Rationale: Strain measurement is a load-independent assessment of left ventricular function. It is most commonly calculated utilizing speckle tracking techniques, but can also be calculated utilizing tissue Doppler techniques.

7. **Answer: B**

   Rationale: Simpson's biplane method of ejection fraction calculation is often referred to as Simpson's method of discs. Conceptually, it is the estimation of left ventricular volume by a "stack" of equal-height discs of varying diameters, determined by the width of the left ventricular cavity at that particular level. The volumes of the discs are summated to determine the estimated volume of the chamber. This is completed during both diastole and systole to calculate the estimated ejection fraction.

8. **Answer: C**

   Rationale: Left ventricular fractional shortening provides an estimate of left ventricular function. However, it extrapolates the movement of two walls to that of the entire left ventricle. Therefore, it is not accurate in the presence of altered LV geometry. Due to the assumption of the entire left ventricular function from the assessment of only two walls, it is not the recommended technique. The normal values are lower percentages than the normal range for ejection fraction; however, they do correlate well.

9. **Answer: A**

   Rationale: Left ventricular wall thickness is most commonly measured in the parasternal long-axis view, which provides a view of the anterior portion of the septum and the inferolateral walls. With TEE imaging, the transgastric midpapillary short-axis view can provide this measurement.

10. **Answer: C**

    Rationale: The Simpson's biplane method of ejection fraction measurement requires a diastolic and systolic frame in both the four- and two-chamber views. This may occur with either transesophageal or transthoracic imaging. Application of Simpson's method of discs volume estimate in both four- and two-chamber views allow a biplane evaluation of the left ventricle and a more accurate estimation of ejection fraction.

Chapter 7

1. **Answer: B**

   Rationale: One of the first clinical effects of acute myocardial ischemia is a new wall motion abnormality on echocardiography. The abnormality may precede electrocardiographic changes by minutes. Rising pulmonary capillary wedge pressures have been shown to be both insensitive and nonspecific. Hypotension may be a late finding in ischemia and is not specific to myocardial ischemia.

2. **Answer: C**

   Rationale: The most common coronary artery pattern is a left and right main coronary artery extending from their respective sinuses of Valsalva with the left main coronary branching relatively quickly into the left anterior descending artery and the left circumflex artery. Branches of the LAD include septal perforators and diagonals, branches of the left circumflex include obtuse marginal arteries, and branches of the right coronary artery include acute marginals and posterolateral and posterior descending arteries. A ramus intermedius is a trifurcation of the left main with a third branch that supplies the anterior and anterolateral wall and is present in approximately 25–30% of patients.

3. **Answer: B**

   Rationale: In most patients, the left anterior descending artery perfuses the anterior and anteroseptal walls, and the left circumflex supplies the lateral walls, while the right coronary artery perfuses the inferior wall and the right ventricle.

4. **Answer: D**

   Rationale: The midesophageal two-chamber view displays the basal, mid, and apical segments of the anterior and inferior walls of the left ventricle. These two walls are perfused by the left anterior descending and right coronary arteries, respectively.

5. **Answer: C**

   Rationale: The transgastric midpapillary short-axis view visualizes the territories of all three main coronary arteries: left anterior descending covering the anterior and anteroseptal walls, the left circumflex covering the lateral walls, and the right coronary artery covering the inferior wall and right ventricle. Both the left ventricle and right ventricle are visualized in this view; however, only the mid portions of the left ventricle are observed. Wall motion abnormalities of the base or apex will not be visualized and appreciated, potentially missing acute ischemia.

6. **Answer: B**

   Rationale: Wall motion abnormalities are graded upon two criteria: the degree of wall excursion toward the center of the chamber and the change in wall thickness during systolic contraction. Normal contraction involves a wall excursion of greater than 30% and an increase in wall thickness during systolic contraction of 30–50%.

7. **Answer: D**

   Rationale: There are several causes of abnormal wall motion that are not related to ischemia. Conduction abnormalities such as bundle branch blocks or exogenous ventricular depolarization lead to dyssynchrony, which may appear as a wall motion abnormality. Rhythm disturbances such as profound bradycardia may lead to the appearance of sluggish wall motion, and acute hemodynamic or volume changes can result in abnormal wall motion.

8. **Answer: C**

   Rationale: Left ventricular diastolic function is an energy-dependent process. As the myocardium becomes ischemic, the ventricle will begin to display an impaired relaxation pattern due to the ischemia-induced diastolic dysfunction. Diastolic dysfunction may present prior to the appearance of wall motion abnormalities. Posteromedial papillary muscle and ventricular septal rupture are post-infarct changes and are not directly reversible with the reestablishment of coronary blood flow. Additional surgical correction is necessary.

9. **Answer: C**

   Rationale: Stunned myocardium represents heart tissue that was recently ischemic (e.g., post-cardiac surgery after a cardioplegic episode) that possesses normal coronary blood flow but remains dysfunctional. The treatment of stunned myocardium includes inotropic agents and time. Hibernating myocardium, however, is chronically ischemic myocardium that also is dysfunctional (e.g., wall motion abnormalities), yet will improve with revascularization.

10. **Answer: B**

    Rationale: Left ventricular aneurysm formation most commonly occurs after a large myocardial infarction that leads to ventricular scar and the appearance of dyskinesis on echocardiography. The most common location is in the anterior or anteroseptal wall of the left ventricle. Dyskinesis will demonstrate a thinning of the myocardium and wall excursion away from the center of the chamber during systole. This is typically post-infarct and therefore does not present within minutes of an acute ischemic episode.

Chapter 8

1. **Answer: A**

   Rationale: The posterior leaflet has discrete scallops that are titled P1, P2, and P3 (moving from anterolateral to posteromedial). The posterior leaflet encompasses two-thirds of the circumference while the anterior leaflet encompasses one-third of the annular circumference. In terms of surface area, the posterior leaflet encompasses one-third of the area, while the anterior leaflet encompasses two-thirds of the surface area. The anterior leaflet is bordered by a rich network of fibrous tissue and the cardiac trigones, providing more support than the posterior leaflet.

2. **Answer: B**

   Rationale: The long-axis views on both midesophageal TEE imaging and parasternal TTE imaging will image through the anterior-posterior dimension of the mitral valve annulus. This often "slices" through the A2 and P2 segments and correlates to the high portions of the saddle-shaped mitral annulus. The midesophageal mitral commissural view will image through the anterolateral and posteromedial dimensions of the mitral annulus, while the remaining choices will cut orthogonally through the mitral valve annulus.

3. **Answer: D**

   Rationale: All of the answers are mechanisms of ischemic mitral regurgitation. With regional wall motion abnormalities, there is abnormal geometry of the papillary muscles and their attachments to the mitral leaflets leading to leaflet tethering. Frank infarction of the papillary muscles destroys the integrity of the chordae allowing the leaflet to prolapse or flail. Left ventricular dilation and dysfunction causes abnormal geometry of the mitral valve apparatus, leading to dilation of the annulus and apical tethering of the mitral valve leaflets.

4. **Answer: B**

   Rationale: The anterior leaflet always resides near the interatrial and interventricular septum in the four-chamber views, while the posterior leaflet always resides near the lateral aspect of the heart in this view. The pulmonary veins are not typically utilized to identify leaflet anatomy.

5. **Answer: C**

   Rationale: Often in diastole when the mitral valve opens, the anterior leaflet may approach or even touch the interventricular septum. The anterior leaflet is in the near field in this view close to the aortic valve and right ventricle. The posterior leaflet is always away from the aortic valve and is anatomically near the left atrial appendage. However, the left atrial appendage is not visualized in the parasternal long-axis view.

6. **Answer: C**

   Rationale: The Carpentier classification of mitral regurgitation is based upon distinguishing mechanisms of regurgitation by the leaflet motion. Type 2 is defined by excessive leaflet motion which includes prolapsed or flail leaflets, such as in myxomatous degeneration. Type 1 is normal leaflet motion which includes leaflet perforation, while Type 3 involves restricted leaflet motion, such as in rheumatic disease or functional mitral regurgitation.

7. **Answer: B**

   Rationale: Severe mitral regurgitation is defined by flow convergence on the ventricular side of the mitral valve on color flow Doppler with a large jet into the left atrium. Vena contracta measurements will exceed 7 mm, with evidence of systolic flow reversal on pulmonary venous Doppler. Mitral regurgitation is not associated with spontaneous echo contrast in the left atrium, due to fast-moving blood from the regurgitation.

8. **Answer: C**

   Rationale: Hemodynamic factors that reduce mitral regurgitation include increasing preload, decreasing afterload, and faster heart rates. Increased contractility, while increasing cardiac output, may also increase the amount of regurgitant volume. Therefore, during anesthesia, the degree of mitral regurgitation is often dynamic based upon changes in preload, afterload, and heart rate.

9. **Answer: C**

   Rationale: Mitral stenosis is identified on two-dimensional echocardiography with thickened and calcified leaflets with reduced opening, a dilated left atrium (often with spontaneous echo contrast), an underfilled left ventricle, color flow Doppler with aliasing velocities on the atrial side of the mitral leaflets, and low velocity blood flow in the left atrial appendage (measured with spectral Doppler).

10. **Answer: C**

    Rationale: Severe mitral stenosis is identified on continuous-wave Doppler interrogation with a prolonged pressure half-time measurement, significantly elevated peak *E* wave velocity (typically > 1.5 m/s), a mean gradient greater than 10 mmHg, and a prolonged deceleration time (> 75).

Chapter 9

1. **Answer: D**

   Rationale: Two-dimensional views of the aortic valve in the ME AV LAX or PLAX view can show the maximum distance between leaflet tips during systole. A distance less than 8 mm is 97% predictive of severe disease and 100% predictive of moderate or severe disease, whereas 12 mm or more is 96% predictive of mild disease or less.
2. **Answer: B**

   Rationale: The view shows a "double envelope" resulting from continuous-wave Doppler measurement across and aortic valve and LVOT with significant aortic stenosis. Because the direction of flow through the LVOT is directed away from the probe (below the baseline on spectral Doppler), it must be positioned near the apex of the heart with the flow exiting the heart away from the probe. From the options listed, only the deep transgastric long-axis view includes the LVOT from this orientation.
3. **Answer: D**

   Rationale: The use of systolic velocity measurements to grade the severity of aortic stenosis is subject to important limitations, most notably factors which decrease stroke volume (e.g., systolic dysfunction, hypovolemia). Because this patient has a history of significant systolic dysfunction, his left ventricle may not generate adequate pressure to create a velocity congruent with the severity of his aortic stenosis, which may underestimate its severity.
4. **Answer: A**

   Rationale: Associated anatomic findings in patients with AS are secondary to the change in physiology caused by the stenosis. Left ventricular hypertrophy develops to overcome the increase in afterload, which may lead to diastolic dysfunction and elevated pulmonary artery pressures. Downstream from the valve, turbulent flow exerts an outward pressure on the aortic wall and over time leads to aortic dilatation. Mitral valve stenosis may coexist with aortic stenosis in rheumatic heart disease; however, it is less common in calcific aortic stenosis.
5. **Answer: A**

   Rationale: This view shows a midesophageal AV short-axis view. This view, or a parasternal short-axis view, can be used to trace the perimeter of the leaflet tips during mid to late systole to measure the area of the aortic valve orifice (planimetry). Using color flow Doppler can help to identify the narrowest opening between the three leaflets during systole and optimizing tissue echogenicity by turning down the gain can help delineate the orifice. Quantitative measurements of aortic flow (peak systolic velocity, mean pressure gradient, etc.) will be unreliable from this view, as the flow is perpendicular to the ultrasound beam. The vena contracta is measured in a long-axis view of the aortic valve.
6. **Answer: A**

   Rationale: The continuity equation states that the volume of blood in a single beat ejected through the LVOT during systole must equal the same volume ejected through the aortic valve orifice during the same single beat:

   $$\text{LVOT}_{\text{CSA}} \times \text{LVOT}_{\text{VTI}} = \text{AV}_{\text{CSA}} \times \text{AV}_{\text{VTI}}$$

   The LVOT is assumed to be cylindrical in shape and the cross-sectional area (CSA) can be calculated as πr^2, in this case $\pi(1.0)^2 \cong 3.14\ \text{cm}^2$. Multiplying by the LVOT_{VTI} gives the stroke volume = $3.14\ \text{cm}^2 \times 32\ \text{cm} \cong 100\ \text{cm}^3$. This must be the same stroke volume that travels through the aortic valve orifice (AV_{CSA}); thus, $\text{AV}_{\text{CSA}} = 100\ \text{cm}^3/\text{AV}_{\text{VTI}} = 1.0\ \text{cm}^2$.
7. **Answer: C**

   Rationale: The ratio of the jet width to LVOT diameter is an easily employed quantitative measure of aortic regurgitation. A regurgitant jet that occupies more than 65% of the LVOT is severe, as in this case, which is nearly 100%. A jet occupying less than 25% is considered mild, and 25–65% is moderate.

8. **Answer: B**

   Rationale: Measuring a vena contracta is a simple and quick method of estimating the severity of aortic regurgitation. The neck of the regurgitant jet at its narrowest point as it crosses the aortic valve is measured. A diameter below 3 mm (0.3 cm) is considered mild, 3–6 mm is moderate, and measurements above 6 mm are considered severe regurgitation. A vena contracta is a relatively load-independent measurement, which is a valuable characteristic to this modality.

9. **Answer: A**

   Rationale: The image provided shows a continuous-wave Doppler tracing through the aortic valve from an apical three-chamber view (TTE). The flow toward the probe represents regurgitant flow. The pressure half-time is measured at 482 ms, which qualifies as moderate aortic insufficiency (200–500 ms). Values less than this is are considered severe (< 200 ms), and values greater than this are mild (> 500 ms).

10. **Answer: B**

    Rationale: The image shows mild flow reversal in the proximal descending aorta. Normally, aortic flow in the descending thoracic aorta should be antegrade during systolic ejection, as well as during the diastolic runoff. Holodiastolic reversal of flow in the lower descending thoracic aorta suggests severe regurgitation. Moderate regurgitant lesions may have reversal in the proximal descending aorta while mild regurgitant lesions typically will not have any reversal of flow within the descending aorta. However, the absence of diastolic flow reversal in the aorta does not rule out a severely regurgitant lesion.

Chapter 10

1. **Answer: C**

   Rationale: Assessment of right ventricular function should assess shape, area, thickness, and motion of the free wall and interventricular septum. The midesophageal RV inflow-outflow view provides good visualization of the free wall motion. The transgastric midpapillary short-axis view provides a cross-sectional view of the size of the RV (relative to the LV), as well as the septal and free wall motion. The apical four-chamber view provides a long-axis view of the RV, which may be useful to assess size and function via annular excursion, as well as movement of the free wall and septum.

2. **Answer: C**

   Rationale: Normal right ventricular systolic function is suggested by a tricuspid annular plane systolic excursion (TAPSE) of > 17 mm, a fractional area change (FAC) of > 35%, or a tissue Doppler peak systolic velocity (S′) ≥9.5 cm/s. Flattening of the interventricular septum at end-systole suggests RV dysfunction or pressure overload.

3. **Answer: D**

   Rationale: An eccentricity index > 1 at end-diastole would be expected in situations causing volume overload. These may include left-to-right shunt, pulmonary hypertension, or severe tricuspid regurgitation.

4. **Answer: C**

   Rationale: The right ventricular systolic pressure may be estimated using the modified Bernoulli equation ($\Delta \mathbf{P} = 4\boldsymbol{v}^2$), where ΔP = RVSP - RAP and v is the peak velocity in m/sec. If v = 2.74 m/s, then RVSP = $10 + 4(2.74)^2 \cong 40$ mmHg.

5. **Answer: D**

   Rationale: The moderator band is a muscular band traversing the right ventricle from the base of the anterior papillary muscle to the ventricular septum. It becomes prominent with RV hypertrophy or dilation and may be mistaken for a thrombus or mass. The midesophageal bicaval view does not provide good visualization of the apex of the right ventricle; thus, it would not be expected to demonstrate the moderator band.

6. **Answer: C**

   Rationale: Contraction of the right ventricle begins with the inlet portion, contracting toward the apex, and ending in the infundibulum. The vascular supply for the right ventricle is primarily the right coronary artery. In the absence of significant shunt, the stroke volume from the right ventricle is equal to the left ventricle. The interventricular septum is an important component of RV contraction.

7. **Answer: A**

   Rationale: Acute pulmonary embolism causing a sudden increase in RV afterload may impair RV function. It is expected to cause prolongation of both the isovolumic contraction and relaxation times. Dilation and decreased stroke volume from the RV may cause impaired left ventricular filling and decreased stroke volume. Cardiac output may decrease, which may result in elevated right atrial pressure and dilated IVC without significant respiratory variation. Basal function may be preferentially impaired, with some sparing of the apical function (McConnell's sign).

8. **Answer: B**

   Rationale: The right ventricle is crescentic, while the left ventricle is circular in a normal situation. While stroke volume and cardiac output are similar between the ventricles, afterload is significantly different. Normally, myocardial perfusion to the right ventricle is present in both systole and diastole, but with elevated right ventricular pressure in the setting of significant pulmonary hypertension, the majority of myocardial perfusion occurs during diastole. The RVOT is visible in cross section from the parasternal long-axis view, adjacent to the left ventricle. Trabeculations within the right ventricle are commonly observed with echocardiography.

9. **Answer: B**

   Rationale: Paradoxical motion of the intraventricular septum is commonly observed in situations causing pressure overload of the right ventricle. Tricuspid regurgitation and an atrial septal defect most commonly cause volume overload of the right ventricle with paradoxical septal motion during diastole. Pulmonic stenosis would cause pressure overload which is represented by paradoxical motion of the septum during systole.

10. **Answer: A**

    Rationale: Normally, the right ventricle is thin walled with RV free wall thickness (RVWT) < 5 mm at end-diastole. Right ventricular hypertrophy may be diagnosed when the RVWT is > 5 mm, while RVWT exceeding 10 mm (1 cm) is considered severe hypertrophy.

Chapter 11

1. **Answer: B**

   Rationale: The Eustachian valve is a sinus venosus remnant extending from the IVC, which directs blood from the IVC through the fossa ovalis during fetal circulation. It is located at the junction of the IVC and right atrium.

2. **Answer: C**

   Rationale: The ligament of Marshall, also called the coumadin ridge, is a remnant of the oblique vein of the left atrium and is located echocardiographically between the LAA and LUPV in a midesophageal two-chamber view.

3. **Answer: A**

   Rationale: All TTE/TEE atrial measurements should be performed at end-systole, prior to the mitral valve opening, when the atria are at their greatest size.

4. **Answer: D**

   Rationale: Linear dimension is obtained with TTE in the parasternal long-axis and apical four-chamber views. With TEE, linear measurement is performed in the midesophageal four-chamber (ME4C), aortic valve short-axis (ME AV SAX), and aortic valve long-axis views (ME AV LAX). Measurements made with TEE in the ME 4C view correlate with the TTE A4C view, whereas the ME AV SAX and LAX views correlate with the TTE PLAX view. Of note, it is often difficult to adequately visualize all sides of the LA with TEE due to the close proximity of the LA to the esophagus.

5. **Answer: D**

   Rationale: Left atrial volume has strong prognostic value in various cardiac diseases. Compared to linear dimensions, left atrial volume is a stronger predictor of outcomes.

6. **Answer: C**

   Rationale: The LA functions to regulate LV filling as a reservoir, conduit, and pump. As a reservoir, it typically contributes roughly 40% of LV systolic volume. During early ventricular diastole, the LA becomes a passive conduit for PV blood flow into the LV. This normally contributes approximately 35% of LV systolic volume. During late ventricular diastole, the LA acts as a pump to augment ventricular filling. Active contraction of the LA normally contributes about 25% of LV systolic volume. The sinoatrial (SA) node, which generates electrical current, is typically located in the right atrium, within the sulcus terminalis at the junction of the SVC.

7. **Answer: A**

   Rationale: The RA is formed from the division of the primitive atria into a right side that fuses with the sinus venosus and joins at a groove called the sulcus terminalis. The RA is positioned anteriorly relative to the LA. The anterior wall is comprised mainly of the right atrial appendage (RAA), which is triangular in shape and is demarcated laterally from the posterior wall by the sulcus terminalis. The posterior wall of the RA is largely comprised of the IAS. The sulcus terminalis internally corresponds to the crista terminalis, which is the origin of the pectinate muscles forming the anterior wall and RAA. The crista terminalis separates the pectinate anterior wall from the smooth posterior wall, formed by the sinus venosus and the IAS.

8. **Answer: D**

   Rationale: Pulsed-wave Doppler can aid the evaluation for LAA thrombus. The sample volume should be placed in the proximal 1/3 segment. Normal peak emptying velocities range from 50 ± 6 cm/s to 83 ± 25 cm/s. Velocities < 40 cm/s on PWD require a closer inspection, and velocities < 20 cm/s are associated with a high incidence of thromboembolism. Increased density of spontaneous echo contrast is correlated with increased risk of thromboembolism.

9. **Answer: C**

   Rationale: The presence of an interatrial septal aneurysm is present when the movement of the septum exceeds 1.5 cm distance from the midline. Patients with an interatrial septal aneurysm have a higher prevalence of patent foramen ovale, and elevated risk of cryptogenic stroke.

10. **Answer: D**

    Rationale: A total LA EF $\leq$ 49% has been shown to have increased risk of mortality and new-onset atrial fibrillation and atrial flutter. Up to 25% of patients may have a patent foramen ovale that may be detectable with echocardiography using color flow Doppler. A patent foramen ovale typically occurs at the superior rim of the fossa ovalis. The minimum LA volume (LA_{min}) occurs at end-diastole with MV closing, while the maximum atrial volume (LA_{max}) occurs at end-systole prior with MV opening.

Chapter 12

1. **Answer: D**

   Rationale: There are four main phases of diastole, in order: isovolumetric relaxation, early rapid filling, diastasis, and atrial contraction.

2. **Answer: C**

   Rationale: The two main properties that govern chamber filling are relaxation (the ability to decrease pressure to create a gradient, also called lusitropy) and compliance (the ability to create an increase volume to receive blood). Elastance ($\Delta P/\Delta V$) is the inverse of compliance and relates to elastic recoil (the ability to return to rebound after stretching). Strain rate is the rate at which the distances of adjacent particles change with respect to time.

3. **Answer: A**

   Rationale: The higher velocity S-wave is a result of active LA relaxation during early systole. As the mitral valve opens during early diastole, forward flow from the pulmonary veins travels down the pressure gradient into the LA and eventually into the LV, corresponding to the D-wave on the LA inflow profile. Atrial contraction during late diastole causes diastolic regurgitation into the pulmonary veins or an atrial reversal wave Doppler interrogation. The early diastolic (D-wave) VTI is typically not measured.

4. **Answer: B**

   Rationale: The peak E-wave velocity is primarily dependent on the LA-LV pressure gradient, which is a function of the large pressure drop in the LV during the IVRT phase, and *not* a result of a rise in LA pressure. Atrial contraction creates the A-wave. The deceleration time is the time it takes for atrial and ventricular pressures to equilibrate and is predicated upon the volume-pressure relationship or compliance ($\Delta V/\Delta P$) of the left ventricle. Diastasis, the third interval of diastole, marking the period in which the atrium and ventricle are in equilibrium with little flow moving into either chamber.

5. **Answer: B**

   Rationale: Pseudonormalization (moderate or intermediate diastolic dysfunction) is characterized by the combined presence of impaired relaxation and a compensatory elevation in LA pressure. The increase in LA pressure generates a reduction or blunting of the S-wave velocity. The additional increase in LA pressure (larger LA-LV gradient) produces an increase in the E-wave velocity, resulting in an apparent normalization of the *E* and *A* transmitral velocities. The *restrictive* form is manifested by the presence of impaired relaxation, elevated LA pressures, and elevated LV pressures (from poor compliance). As a result, ventricular filling typically occurs quickly, with less atrial contribution. The *E*/*e*’ ratio increases with impaired relaxation (larger *e*’).

6. **Answer: D**

   Rationale: A restrictive filling pattern is characterized by a predominate early filling of the ventricle (E-wave much larger than A-wave). The increased early velocity depends on a large pressure gradient between the left atrium and left ventricle, created by high elastance (low compliance) of the ventricle. The increased early ventricular filling results in less late-diastolic filling, and a smaller A-wave. While LV end-diastolic volume may increase, it does not explain the change in the diastolic filling pattern.

7. **Answer: B**

   Rationale: A normal diastolic filling pattern results in more early diastolic filling of the ventricle (the E-wave is larger than the A-wave). A pseudonormal filling pattern has a similar *E*/*A* ratio), but is the consequence of increased left atrial pressure in the setting of impaired ventricular relaxation. Myocardial tissue velocity or pulmonary venous flow pattern may help make this distinction. Normal filling will have normal myocardial velocity during relaxation ($e' > 10$ cm/s), and an S-wave predominant pulmonary venous inflow, while impaired relaxation (and a pseudonormal filling pattern) will have decreased myocardial tissue velocity and a blunted S-wave or D-wave predominant pulmonary inflow pattern. E-wave deceleration time would be expected to increase following nitroglycerin administration, as the relaxation would improve. A fluid bolus would be expected to shift impaired relaxation “to the right,” i.e., to a pseudonormal pattern, not the reverse.

8. **Answer: C**

   Rationale: Blunting of the S-wave following intravascular volume administration suggests that either left atrial relaxation is impaired, or there is a higher atrial pressure decreasing the pressure gradient coming from the pulmonary veins. Increased cardiac output alone would be expected to increase the S-wave, as would a decrease in systemic vascular resistance. Blunting of the S-wave is describing the transition from normal to impaired relaxation ("right shift"), while a shift from pseudonormal to impaired relaxation would not be expected to decrease S-wave velocity.

9. **Answer: B**

   Rationale: A restrictive filling pattern result in rapid filling of the ventricle and a shortened deceleration time. As a consequence, atrial contraction is less likely to flow into the ventricle, which is "already full," and instead creates regurgitant pressure into the pulmonary veins, which may contribute to pulmonary edema.

10. **Answer: B**

    Rationale: Impaired relaxation is characterized by a poor ventricular relaxation leading to an inability of the left ventricle to lower its pressure adequately. Pool LV compliance and elevations in LA pressure are characteristics of more advanced levels of diastolic dysfunction.

Chapter 13

1. **Answer: B**

   Rationale: The ability to differentiate true from false lumens serves to confirm the presence of an aortic dissection, rule out imaging artifacts, and allow confirmation of surgical repair. The true lumen is often the smaller and round-shaped lumen, while the false lumen tends to be the larger, irregularly shaped structure. Systolic motion involves the expansion of the true lumen with systolic ejection, while the false lumen will compress during systole. With color flow Doppler, the true lumen has early-systolic laminar flow, while the false lumen has late-systolic turbulent flow. Spontaneous echo contrast or thrombus may be identified in the false lumen.

2. **Answer: C**

   Rationale: The false lumen tends to be crescent-shaped and concave toward the true lumen, which is typically smaller. The true lumen generally has early laminar systolic flow, during which the intimal flap will expand toward the false lumen. The false lumen tends to have late-systolic turbulent flow.

3. **Answer: A**

   Rationale: Aortic dissection may allow transudative fluid to leak through the adventitial layer, leading to pleural or pericardial effusion. Dissection into a coronary ostium may lead to myocardial ischemia or infarction. Prolapse of the dissection flap into the aortic valve or dilation of the aortic annulus may cause malcoaptation, leading to aortic insufficiency. Aortic stenosis is not commonly a consequence of an aortic dissection.

4. **Answer: B**

   Rationale: While TEE has several advantages over TTE for assessment of the thoracic aorta, TTE provides the advantage of being less invasive and easily accessible and allows the visualization of the TEE "blind spot" from the interposition of the trachea between the aorta and esophagus. The aortic root and ascending aorta can be visualized through the parasternal windows. The suprasternal long-axis view of the aorta provides a complete view of the aortic arch as it wraps around the right pulmonary artery. TTE is less helpful for evaluation of the descending aorta; however, it may be visualized in cross section in the far field of the imaging sector in the parasternal long-axis view. TEE allows better visualization of the descending aorta, with improved specificity and sensitivity for aortic dissection. Both modalities together can complement each other for a more complete evaluation of the thoracic aorta.

5. **Answer: D**

   Rationale: Atheromatous disease of the aorta may be graded echocardiographically. Grade 1 describes a normal aorta with minimal intimal thickening. Grade 2 is an aorta with extensive intimal thickening. A calcified aortic plaque less than 5 mm qualifies as grade 3, while a calcified plaque > 5 mm is grade 4. Any mobile or ulcerated plaque is grade 5, regardless of its size.

6. **Answer: B**

   Rationale: The arrow indicates the sinotubular junction, between the sinuses of Valsalva and the tubular ascending aorta. The aortic root is the portion of the aorta proximal to this junction (to the left of the image).

7. **Answer: C**

   Rationale: Aortic aneurysm is defined by a dilation of all three layers of the vessel greater than 150% of the normal size of the aortic diameter. Vessels greater than 100% but less than 150% of the normal diameter are referred to as ectatic. Normal adult thoracic aortic diameters are approximately 3.5–4.0 cm for the aortic root and less than 3.0 cm for the ascending and descending thoracic aorta.

8. **Answer: D**

   Rationale: The Stanford system separates any involvement of the ascending aorta into Stanford type A, which is a surgical emergency, while Stanford type B involves only the descending thoracic aorta below the left subclavian artery take-off, which are often treated medically. The DeBakey system divides aortic dissections into three types: type 1 involves the ascending and descending aorta, and type 2 involves the ascending aorta only, while type 3 involves only the descending aorta below the left subclavian artery take-off.

9. **Answer: D**

   Rationale: The suprasternal long-axis view of the aorta provides a complete view of the aortic arch as it wraps around the right pulmonary artery, which is not visible via TEE due to the interposition of the air-filled trachea and left main stem bronchus. Unique to TTE, the suprasternal view allows assessment of the distal ascending aorta, aortic arch with each of its three great vessels, and proximal descending aorta.

10. **Answer: C**

    Rationale: Reverberation artifact from a calcified aortic wall is often confused with an intimal dissection flap. Changing the orientation of the probe so that the incident angle is not perpendicular can help minimize this artifact. Findings should be viewed from multiple angles to assure that they are not artifactual, but an orthogonal view with the same incident angle may show the same artifact. An intimal flap should have motion independent of the aortic wall, while an artifact is more likely to move as surrounding structures move. Adjusting the imaging depth will not change the positioning of most artifacts.

Chapter 14

1. **Answer: C**

   Rationale: The transverse sinus is the potential space at the base of the heart anterior to the superior vena cava, superior to the atria, and posterior to the great vessels. In the midesophageal two-chamber view, it may be visible surrounding the left atrial appendage. In the midesophageal right ventricular inflow-outflow view, it may be visible between the aortic valve and main pulmonary artery. In the midesophageal long-axis and ascending aorta short-axis views, the sinus may be seen between the ascending aorta and left atrium or right pulmonary artery, respectively. It is generally not visible from the midesophageal bicaval view.

2. **Answer: A**

   Rationale: It is important to distinguish epicardial fat from a pericardial effusion. Epicardial fat is less echogenic than myocardium, but more echogenic than a simple pericardial effusion and moves with the myocardium, while an effusion does not. Epicardial fat generally has a subtle speckled appearance, and is not associated with cardiac chamber collapse. Epicardial fat is located between the myocardium and visceral pericardium, while pericardial fat is adherent and external to the parietal pericardium.

3. **Answer: B**

   Rationale: During normal respirophasic conditions, negative intrathoracic pressure during spontaneous inspiration results in increased venous return to the right heart, and decreased filling of the left heart, as venous pooling is increased. Positive pressure ventilation results in decreased filling of the right heart, and increased filling of the left heart, as blood is "squeezed" out of the pulmonary vasculature.

4. **Answer: A**

   Rationale: During normal respirophasic conditions, spontaneous expiration results in less negative intrathoracic pressure, reduced right heart filling and output, and increased left heart filling and output. Left heart afterload is decreased as the relative increase in intrathoracic pressure helps "push" blood out of the left ventricle. Spontaneous inspiration has the opposite effect, increasing right heart filling and output, and decreasing left heart filling and output. Positive pressure inspiration decreases right heart filling and increases afterload, while it has the opposite effect on the left heart, increasing filling and decreasing afterload. Positive pressure exhalation increases right heart filling and output, while decreasing left heart filling and output.

5. **Answer: A**

   Rationale: Constrictive pericarditis causes an exaggerated response to the loading conditions during both positive and negative pressure ventilation.

6. **Answer: D**

   Rationale: The physiologic effects of a pericardial effusion depend on both the size of the effusion and rate of fluid accumulation. A small but rapidly accumulating effusion may have more hemodynamic consequence than a larger slower-developing effusion. Brief collapse of the right atrium may occur during diastole in the setting of low right atrial pressure, without tamponade. A localized pericardial lesion (e.g., loculated effusion) may cause preferential compression of isolated portions of the heart, so the left heart may be compressed without causing collapse of the right heart. Because the ventricles share the interventricular septum, differential pressures between the chambers may affect the filling volumes (e.g., elevated RV pressure may shift the septum to the left and decrease LV filling), known as ventricular interdependence.

7. **Answer: B**

   Rationale: With cardiac tamponade, respirophasic changes in loading conditions are exaggerated. As a result, during spontaneous inspiration, increased filling of the right heart and an increased transtricuspid inflow velocity are expected. Conversely, a reduction in left heart filling and a decreased transmitral inflow velocity are expected. An exaggerated reduction of > 30% of the peak mitral E-wave velocity is suggestive of tamponade.

8. **Answer: C**

   Rationale: A linear measurement perpendicular to the myocardial wall at end-diastole may help provide a semiquantitative estimate of the effusion volume. Effusions measuring less than 5 mm have an estimated volume 50–100 mL, 5–10 mm suggests a volume of 100–250 mL, 10–20 mm suggests 250–500 mL, and a transverse measurement > 20 mm suggests an effusion > 500 mL.

9. **Answer: D**

   Rationale: Constrictive pericarditis is often associated with a thickened pericardium, with or without calcification or pericardial adhesion, enlarged atria, with normal size and function of the left ventricle. A restrictive mitral inflow pattern is common. Paradoxical septal motion is also common because of exaggerated ventricular interdependence, giving the appearance of a septal "bounce." A decreased septal tissue velocity suggests restrictive cardiomyopathy, as septal tissue velocity is typically preserved with constrictive pericarditis.

10. **Answer: B**

    Rationale: In contrast to cardiac tamponade, in which there is primarily an exaggeration of respirophasic variation during spontaneous ventilation, with CP there is an exaggeration of respirophasic variation during both spontaneous ventilation and positive pressure ventilation. Positive pressure variation leads to overall reduced velocities in cardiac tamponade. Ventricular interdependence leading to septal "bounce" and differential ventricular loading with respiration causing pulsus paradoxus are expected in both conditions.

Chapter 15

1. **Answer: A**

   Rationale: The patient in this scenario has multiple potential sources of hypotension, including cardiogenic (e.g., systolic dysfunction), hypovolemic (e.g., acute blood loss), distributive (e.g., anesthetic effect), obstructive processes (e.g., IVC compression), or a combination of multiple causes. Without any additional information, the most appropriate choice from the options provided would be to elicit more information with point-of-care echocardiography.
2. **Answer: D**

   Rationale: The images show a normal end-diastolic diameter, and a small end-systolic diameter, suggesting hyperdynamic LV function, which excludes systolic heart failure as a cause of the hypotension. There is no evidence of a dilated right ventricle, which may suggest hypotension from a pulmonary embolism or other pulmonary process. The large end-diastolic diameter suggests that hypovolemia is a less likely cause of hypotension than a distributive shock process, and the normal right upper quadrant view from the FAST exam makes a large volume of intraperitoneal hemorrhage unlikely.
3. **Answer: D**

   Rationale: Significant mitral regurgitation is identified in the image provided. With the hemodynamic instability the patient is developing, this can be addressed while other causes of hypotension are evaluated. The quantification of the exact degree of mitral regurgitation is unnecessary to initiate management, and from the options provided, epinephrine would be an appropriate intervention to increase heart rate and contractility to promote forward flow. Phenylephrine would increase LV afterload, which may exacerbate the regurgitant lesion.
4. **Answer: D**

   Rationale: The image, taken during systole, reveals significant aortic stenosis, as evidenced by the restricted valve opening. Severe aortic stenosis is present with a valve opening less than 8 mm, as in this case. Epinephrine is unlikely to improve cardiac output against a fixed flow rate from aortic stenosis. Similarly, increased intravascular volume is unlikely to improve perfusion and may result in increased pulmonary edema. Norepinephrine infusion may be a reasonable method to increase coronary perfusion, but his diastolic pressure appears to be adequate. Lowering the heart rate to allow increased time for flow through the aortic valve is likely to have more of a positive effect on increasing cardiac output.
5. **Answer: B**

   Rationale: The images provided show a parasternal long-axis view during systole and diastole, reflecting a very low ejection fraction. While starting a vasopressor with some inotropy (norepinephrine) may be appropriate, and agent with increased inotropic activity (epinephrine) would be more appropriate in the setting of the severely depressed systolic function. Additional intravascular volume is unlikely to improve cardiac output and may have deleterious effects. While the imaging field is deeper than desired for the structure of interest (left ventricle), the diagnosis is apparent from the images provided, and a clinical decision can be made.
6. **Answer: B**

   Rationale: The image demonstrates a dilated right ventricle, which may be contributing to his hypotension. While pulmonary embolism is a cause of right ventricular failure, any cause of increased pulmonary vascular resistance can cause a similar appearance, including significant lung pathology (e.g., COPD) and elevated ventilator pressures. In this case, the patient's increased respiratory rate and limited expiratory flow have led to air trapping and increased intrathoracic pressure, and managing his airway pressures would be the appropriate intervention.

7. **Answer: C**

   Rationale: The image shows B-lines originating from the pleural line and extending to the edge of the image. This suggests that at this point, there are 2 contiguous layers of pleura. The B-lines suggest that the pleura or interlobular septae are thickened, which may be a consequence of pulmonary edema or interstitial lung disease and would require additional information to make a distinction regarding the cause. It can be said that no pneumothorax is present at the area where this image was obtained; however, a significant pneumothorax may still be present in other areas, including on the other side of the chest.

8. **Answer: A**

   Rationale: The images provided demonstrate a hyperdynamic ventricle with a low end-diastolic area, suggesting hypovolemia. In the setting of traumatic injuries, the most likely cause for his hypovolemia is bleeding, and the source of bleeding should be identified. A focused assessment with sonography in trauma (FAST) exam is appropriate in this setting to rapidly evaluate for sources of bleeding. While CT may be appropriate for evaluation, it should not be the next step in evaluation for a hypotensive patient. Similarly, surgery or vasopressors may be a part of his management, but without additional information, they would not be the next step.

9. **Answer: C**

   Rationale: The image reveals a large pericardial effusion from an apical four-chamber view. Ascites can be appreciated in the near field, and bilateral pleural effusions are apparent in the far field. Her hypotension is likely a consequence of decreased vascular resistance from anesthesia and decreased preload from positive pressure ventilation. Mitral inflow velocity may help confirm the diagnosis of tamponade, but perfusion should be supported immediately. Pericardiocentesis or surgical drainage of the pericardium may be appropriate, but as a temporizing measure, intravascular pressure can be increased to improve chamber filling by giving an intravascular volume bolus. Vasopressor infusion may also help hemodynamics, but with the degree of extravascular volume present, intravenous volume repletion would be the more appropriate initial step.

10. **Answer: C**

    Rationale: The patient has developed an unstable rhythm and immediate cardioversion/defibrillation is the appropriate intervention. Echocardiography is incredibly useful in helping differentiate different causes of hypotension, but in the case, the cause is already apparent and further evaluation with echocardiography would only delay intervention.

Chapter 16

1. **Answer: D**

   Rationale: The ultrasound beam bouncing back and forth between strong reflectors creates reverberation artifacts. Strong reflectors are present in different areas of the body (e.g., calcified aorta, aerated lung tissue), but the ultrasound probe itself is an important component of the reverberation artifact in many places. As ultrasound is reflected from a close structure, the energy is subsequently reflected off the transducer and reflected again from the close structure. This leads to twice the amount of transit time and an artifact that is twice as deep as the actual structure.

2. **Answer: B**

   Rationale: The velocity of an ultrasound wave in soft tissue is 1540 m/s (1.54 km/s).

3. **Answer: A**

   Rationale: Mirror artifact is a result of misinterpretation of received ultrasound waves reflected from two strong reflectors that lead to increased transit time. Sidelobe artifacts are a result of waves reflected from side lobes of the ultrasound beam. Acoustic shadowing refers to the "dropout" behind a strong reflector (e.g., bone), a consequence of most of the waves already having been reflected from the strong reflector. Acoustic enhancement is the apparent increase in signal deep to a hypoechoic region (e.g., fluid-filled bladder).

4. **Answer: C**

   Rationale: Papillary fibroelastomas are benign tumors that are typically attached to the aortic side of the AV. Because they are prone to embolization, they often require surgical resection. Lambl's excrescences are typically identified on the endocardial surface of the AV, at the site of valve closure. They are less likely to embolize, but may considered for anticoagulation or resection for patients who suffer from multiple cerebrovascular accidents. Nodules of Arantius are thickened central areas on the AV cusps. Aortic regurgitation has been attributed to the fibrosis and hypertrophy of the nodules of Arantius in some patients, but they are not known to embolize. A Chiari network is an inferiorly located, mobile, and heavily fenestrated structure in the RA. It is associated with patent foramen ovale and atrial septal aneurysms, and is not known to embolize.

5. **Answer: D**

   Rationale: The crista terminalis is a smooth fibromuscular ridge located in the RA, which separates the smooth RA from the right atrial appendage. A Chiari network is an inferiorly located, mobile, and heavily fenestrated structure, also in the RA. The Eustachian valve is an embryologic remnant between the IVC and RA, whose purpose was to shunt oxygenated blood from the RA to the LA through the foramen ovale during fetal development. The coumadin ridge describes the normal muscular ridge in the left atrium between the left upper pulmonary vein and left atrial appendage.

6. **Answer: A**

   Rationale: The arrow indicates a prominent moderator band in a patient with dilated right ventricle. A Chiari network is a mobile and heavily fenestrated structure located in the RA. The crista terminalis is a smooth fibromuscular ridge separating the smooth RA from the right atrial appendage, also located in the RA. The coumadin ridge is the normal muscular ridge between the left upper pulmonary vein and left atrial appendage, in the LA.

7. **Answer: B**

   Rationale: Aliasing is the result of measuring a velocity above the Nyquist limit, which is one-half the pulse repetition frequency (PRF). Changing the angle of insonation will affect the Doppler shift measured (Doppler shift is proportional to the cosine of the angle of incidence), but will also make velocity measurement less accurate. Decreasing the velocity scale decreases the PRF, which will lower the Nyquist limit and increase aliasing. Using a lower frequency transducer or decreasing the sector depth increase PRF and the Nyquist limit.

8. **Answer: C**

   Rationale: The crista terminalis is a smooth fibromuscular ridge located in the RA, which separates the smooth RA from the right atrial appendage. The interatrial septum separates the right and left atria. The coumadin ridge separates the left upper pulmonary vein from the left atrial appendage. The sinotubular junction is between the sinuses of Valsalva and the cusps of the aortic valve in the proximal aortic root.

9. **Answer: D**

   Rationale: Lipomatous hypertrophy of the interatrial septum is a benign fatty infiltration of the septum that spares the fossa ovalis, creating a cross-sectional appearance similar to a "barbell." The coumadin ridge is a muscular ridge in the left atrium between the left upper pulmonary vein and left atrial appendage, which usually has an appearance more like a "Q-tip." Ebstein's anomaly is a rare heart defect in which the tricuspid valve does not form properly. The Thebesian valve is an embryonic remnant of the sinoatrial valve at the junction of the coronary sinus and right atrium.

10. **Answer: B**

Rationale: Beam width artifact is a consequence of inadequate lateral resolution, where side-by-side reflectors close together may appear as a single reflector. Mirror artifact is a result of misinterpretation of received ultrasound waves reflected from a strong reflector. Reverberation artifact is a result of the ultrasound beam bouncing back and forth between strong reflectors (e.g., calcified aorta, aerated lung tissue, or the ultrasound transducer itself), resulting in a "step ladder" appearance at equally spaced distances along a scan line. Aliasing (with pulsed-wave or color flow Doppler) occurs when the velocity being measure is greater than the Nyquist limit, which is half of the pulse repetition frequency. This results in velocities being displayed on the opposite side of the zero baseline.

Chapter 17

1. **Answer: D**

Rationale: Cardiac thrombi account for 15–40% of ischemic strokes. The left atrial appendage is the most common site for left-sided thrombus formation. Right-sided thrombi are more commonly a result of peripheral thrombosis embolization (e.g., deep venous thrombosis). Right-sided (paradoxical) emboli passing to the left side through a shunt (e.g., patent foramen ovale) are a less-common cause of CVA.

2. **Answer: B**

Rationale: Valvular vegetations resulting from infective endocarditis typically attach to the low-pressure side of the valve: the atrial side of the tricuspid and mitral valves and the ventricular side of the aortic and pulmonic valves.

3. **Answer: B**

Rationale: Infective endocarditis can lead to destruction of the valve or distortion of the valvular or subvalvular apparatus, resulting in valvular prolapse, regurgitation, flail leaflets, or perforation. Vegetations rarely result in stenosis of the valve.

4. **Answer: C**

Rationale: Primary cardiac tumors are rare, and only 25% of them are malignant. While sarcomas are the most common malignant primary cardiac tumor (~95% of primary cardiac malignancies), hematologic metastasis from an extracardiac malignancy is a more common etiology for an intracardiac malignancy.

5. **Answer: B**

Rationale: Atrial myxomas are the most common primary intracardiac tumor in adults (rhabdomyomas are more common in children under the age of 15). The most common location is the left atrium (75%), with 20% in the right atrium, and 5% in the ventricles. Papillary fibroelastomas account for ~8% of cardiac tumors, most commonly on the aortic side of the aortic valve.

6. **Answer: A**

Rationale: Carcinoid tumors are neuroendocrine tumors that can metastasize to the heart. They typically originate in the gastrointestinal tract and secreted vasoactive substances travel via the portal venous circulation, where they are metabolized prior to reaching the heart. However, once the carcinoid tumor metastasizes into the liver, the vasoactive products can enter the caval circulation without being metabolized, leading to cardiac manifestations, preferentially on the right side of the heart. This is often a combination of regurgitation and stenosis from a relatively fixed valvular position.

7. **Answer: D**

Rationale: Placement of PACs under TEE visualization is a useful technique and allows for visualization of the catheter tip as it enters into the main pulmonary artery. PACs will be most easily visualized in the midesophageal four-chamber, RV inflow-outflow, and ascending aorta short-axis views (TEE), or with the parasternal RV inflow or parasternal short-axis views (TTE). The midesophageal ascending aorta short-axis view provides the best view of the pulmonary artery from the options provided.

8. **Answer: B**

 Rationale: IABP inflation during diastole augments diastolic perfusion, while deflation during systole decreases afterload and promotes forward flow. Therefore, the optimal timing for inflation is immediately after closure of the aortic valve. Earlier inflation may increase left ventricular afterload, and later timing may provide suboptimal augmentation of diastolic pressure.

9. **Answer: D**

 Rationale: Renal cell cancer is comprised of several subtypes, including clear cell carcinoma (75–85%), papillary renal cell carcinoma (10–15%), chromophobe renal cell carcinoma (5–10%), and oncocytomas (3–5%). Variants of clear cell carcinoma are highly vascular and have a high propensity for metastasis to the right atrium and ventricle through direct invasion of the inferior vena cava, in approximately 4–10% of cases.

10. **Answer: D**

 Rationale: The Impella CP® device uses a microaxial blood pump to provide up to 4 L/min of cardiac output and is typically placed via a percutaneous technique retrograde across the aortic valve. With echocardiography, assessment may be performed with midesophageal long-axis and five-chamber views (TEE) or apical four- or five-chamber and parasternal long-axis views (TTE). This should include evaluating the position of the device, any evidence of acute right heart failure, assessment of the intraventricular septum, new valvular lesions, and evidence of direct myocardial injury during device placement.

Chapter 18

1. **Answer: C**

 Rationale: The interatrial septum is best visualized from a midesophageal bicaval view. While a transthoracic apical four-chamber view may visualize the interatrial septum, it is in the far field and generally has inferior resolution to the midesophageal view.

2. **Answer: A**

 Rationale: The most common of the four subtypes of ventricular septal defects (VSDs) is the perimembranous VSD, occurring in 75–80% of all VSDs. The other types of VSD include inlet, outlet, and muscular defects.

3. **Answer: B**

 Rationale: A patent ductus arterosus is amenable to closure surgically or with a percutaneous device. Sinus venosus ASD and complete AV cushion defects are generally not amenable to percutaneous closure. Situs inversus is transposition of the organs, thus cannot be reversed with a closure device.

4. **Answer: B**

 Rationale: Upon release of a Valsalva maneuver, venous return to the right heart transiently increases, which may induce a right-to-left shunt through a patent foramen ovale and allow visualization of Doppler flow or agitated saline (bubbles) with echocardiography.

5. **Answer: A**

 Rationale: A pressure gradient between two chambers can be calculated from the modified Bernoulli equation: $\mathbf{\Delta P = 4}\boldsymbol{v}^{\mathbf{2}}$. If ΔP = LVSP – RVSP, and in the absence of valvular stenosis, the left ventricular pressure during systole (LVSP) is equal to the systolic arterial blood pressure (110 mmHg). Then RVSP = 110 mmHg - $4(4\ \text{m/s})^2$ = 46 mmHg.

6. **Answer: C**

 Rationale: High velocity, turbulent flow through the defect is indicative of a restrictive shunt, whereas low velocity, non-turbulent flow denotes a nonrestrictive defect. Generally, a nonrestrictive defect indicates a more severe lesion, which is easier to detect with 2D imaging. Because of the high velocity of flow through a restrictive VSD, decreasing the Nyquist limit is likely to cause more aliasing, which may make identification more difficult.

7. **Answer: A**

   Rationale: Release of a Valsalva maneuver transiently increases venous return to the right atrium and right atrial pressure. If the right atrial pressure exceeds the left atrial pressure, flow will occur across a patent foramen ovale, toward the probe and the right side of the screen. When left atrial pressure exceeds right atrial pressure, there is no flow through the "one-way valve" created by the overlap of the septum primum and the septum secundum. Lowering the color scale may improve the ability to detect lower-velocity flow using color Doppler, even without the aid of bubble contrast.
8. **Answer: D**

   Rationale: Coronary sinus dilation may be the result of an anatomical variation (e.g., unroofed coronary sinus) or a condition which results in increased right atrial pressure. A persistent left SVC drains into the coronary sinus in 90% of cases, which also results in its dilation. The presence of a Eustachian valve is a normal anatomic variant and does not typically result in dilation of the coronary sinus.
9. **Answer: B**

   Rationale: Transthoracic views are well-oriented with and closer to the interventricular septum, making them very useful for the evaluation of VSDs. A low Qp/Qs ratio suggests that there is a significant right-to-left shunt, while a high Qp/Qs ratio suggests a left-to-right shunt. Bubble studies are commonly used for evaluation of a shunt, and flow is typically from the higher-pressure left side toward the lower-pressure right side.
10. **Answer: C**

    Rationale: An ostium primum ASD is the result of incomplete development of the septum primum, resulting in a lack of fusion with the endocardial cushion. It is the second most common type of ASD, after ostium secundum ASD, which is a result of failure of fusion between the septum primum and the septum secundum. An ostium primum ASD is a communication between the foramen ovale and the ostium primum, while an ostium secundum ASD is a communication between the foramen ovale and the ostium secundum.

Chapter 19

1. **Answer: C**

   Rationale: The image of the patient's left upper quadrant shows a moderate amount of free fluid and with multiple septations. This suggests the presence of some type of intra-abdominal infection and the decrease in the patient's blood pressure is concerning for severe sepsis or shock. Thus, the next best step would be to administer antibiotics and perform a more definitive diagnostic test. A CT scan of the abdomen is not unreasonable, particularly if there is concern for primary bacterial peritonitis; however, this should be done after appropriate resuscitation and treatment of presumed sepsis. Because hemoperitoneum from trauma is not the likely cause of the hypotension, further diagnostic studies should be completed prior to transfer to the operating room.
2. **Answer: C**

   Rationale: The Focused Assessment with Sonography in Trauma (FAST) examination has excellent specificity (94–100%) and moderate sensitivity (69–98%), which depends on the quantity of free fluid present, patient positioning, and operator experience. This highlights the importance of serial exams if ongoing bleeding is suspected, as a small volume of hemorrhage may be missed initially. Fortunately, small volumes of hemorrhage are not generally responsible for hemodynamic instability.
3. **Answer: D**

   Rationale: This patient has evidence of hemodynamic instability following blunt trauma. The ultrasound image shows evidence of free fluid surrounding the tip of the liver. A positive FAST examination in a hypotensive patient following trauma should be assumed to be hemorrhage until proven otherwise, and this patient has a clear indication to go to the operating room for definitive diagnosis and control of bleeding. A repeated FAST examination or a CT of the patient's abdomen would be appropriate if the patient was hemodynamically stable, depending on the clinical scenario.

4. **Answer: D**

   Rationale: The sonographic appearance of solid organ, diaphragmatic, and hollow organ injury can be very subtle and easily missed, even by experienced sonographers. The FAST examination relies on the presence of free fluid to detect traumatic organ injury. Solid organ injury, typically the liver and spleen, results in accumulation of blood in potential spaces as a proxy for injury. Hollow organ injury is less common in blunt trauma and less likely to generate adequate levels of free fluid for detection. The abdominal aorta is a retroperitoneal structure and thus not assessed by the FAST examination unless catastrophic rupture occurs. A CT scan of the abdomen is the more appropriate study to identify diaphragmatic, hollow organ and aortic injury.

5. **Answer: C**

   Rationale: Although categorized as a deep vein, the soleal vein is a below-the-knee (distal) muscular vein. Deep vein thrombosis in this location bears a lower risk of propagation and may resolve spontaneously. In an asymptomatic patient, this isolated DVT can be managed conservatively with attention to serial surveillance imaging over 2 weeks per the 2016 ACCP guideline for antithrombotic therapy for VTE disease (Grade 2C). The femoral vein and popliteal vein are both proximal deep veins, and DVT in these locations should be treated with therapeutic anticoagulation. Although the great saphenous vein is a superficial vein, an SVT located within 3–5 cm to the saphenofemoral junction carries a high risk of propagation into proximal DVT. The ACCP guideline suggests prophylactic anticoagulation for 45 days in this scenario (Grade 2B).

6. **Answer: C**

   Rationale: Manually squeezing the muscle bulk distal to the ultrasound probe will augment the venous return flow signal. When the lumen of the proximal vein is interrogated with Doppler, the augmented blood flow should produce a Doppler signal coming to the probe if there is no blockage between the sites (i.e., thrombus). Placing the patient in Trendelenburg position will improve central venous return; however, it is not likely to produce an easily detectable Doppler signal. Additionally, Trendelenburg position (head down) may decrease the size of the lower extremity veins and make the DVT exam more difficult. Applying compression with the ultrasound probe is the maneuver to perform compression ultrasonography. Decreasing the Nyquist limit (i.e., scale) is reasonable and sometimes necessary to optimize the Doppler signal amplitude. However, this will not augment the blood flow.

7. **Answer: A**

   Rationale: It is important to interrogate the saphenofemoral junction (SFJ) as superficial thromboses in the great saphenous vein frequently propagate into DVT at this location. Studies have shown significantly increased sensitivity when the femoral vein is included in the DVT exam. The popliteal vein is another proximal deep vein where DVTs are frequently identified. The deep femoral vein is harder to interrogate, as it quickly moves outside of the ultrasound field when it travels distally, making it less practical for a point-of-care DVT exam.

8. **Answer: A**

   Rationale: The presence of an undulating flap is 99–100% specific for the presence of abdominal aortic dissection. However, the absence of a flap does not effectively exclude an aortic dissection. If there is concern for an aortic dissection and there is no dissection flap noted in the abdominal aorta, then a more definitive imaging modality (e.g., computed tomography with contrast) should be pursued.

9. **Answer: B**

   Rationale: Saccular aneurysms are asymmetric outpouchings of an aortic segment. Failure to properly evaluate the entire abdominal aorta in transverse and longitudinal views may result in a missed aneurysm. Fusiform aneurysms are more symmetric and thus less likely to be missed when performing point-of-care ultrasound. Obtuse is not a term used to describe abdominal aortic aneurysms.

10. **Answer: A**

    Rationale: This image shows a large abdominal aortic aneurysm with a significant amount of thrombus, most suggestive of a ruptured abdominal aortic aneurysm. Although there is no evidence of free fluid in this image, this should be presumed to be the etiology of the patient's hypotension. Although computed tomography may help better characterize the aortic aneurysm, it should not preclude immediate discussion with the vascular surgeon.

Chapter 20

1. **Answer: D**

   Rationale: The goal of intravascular volume resuscitation goal is to increase stroke volume and cardiac output, thereby increasing oxygen delivery to the tissues and improving organ function. However, depending on how sensitive the ventricles are to additional preload, the stroke volume response is variable. Increasing intravascular volume will increase venous pressure, and if there is not a commensurate increase in stroke volume and cardiac output, the increased venous pressure will decrease the organ perfusion gradient (arterial minus venous pressure), in addition to increasing interstitial tissue edema, both of which may decrease oxygen delivery and organ function.

2. **Answer: D**

   Rationale: Dynamic measures of preload reflect changes in circulation induced by changes in the loading conditions of the heart, for example, with respiratory variation. Static measures of preload less reliably predict volume responsiveness, although they can indicate preload, as related to end-diastolic wall tension. Static markers include central venous pressure, pulmonary capillary wedge pressure, and ventricular volumes, while pulse pressure variation and peak systolic velocity variation are dynamic markers. Velocity time integral (VTI) itself reflects stroke volume, and a single value does not provide useful information to predict preload response, but VTI *variation* throughout the respiratory cycle may a useful dynamic measure of preload responsiveness.

3. **Answer: C**

   Rationale: Calculation of cardiac output with echocardiography is most commonly achieved via measurement of flow through the left ventricular outflow tract. Assuming the LVOT is a circle, its area can be calculated as $\pi \times (\text{LVOT radius})^2$. Multiplying the LVOT area by the LVOT VTI provides the stroke volume. Lastly heart rate multiplied by stroke volume provides cardiac output.

4. **Answer: B**

   Rationale: Dynamic measures of preload are gained from provoking the circulation by inducing changes in the loading conditions of the heart. Some examples of dynamic markers are stroke volume variation, pulse pressure variation, and peak velocity variation throughout the respiratory cycle. Arrhythmias may be a confounding cause of beat-to-beat stroke volume variation. Low tidal volumes or an open chest may underestimate changes in stroke volume, and high intraabdominal pressures may overestimate the effects of changes in intrathoracic pressure.

5. **Answer: A**

   Rationale: In hypovolemic patients with dynamic LV outflow tract (LVOT) obstruction, hypovolemia accentuates the obstruction as the anterior leaflet of the mitral valve may be pushed into the LVOT during systole. There are several physiologic reasons for this, including narrowing of the outflow tract and high systolic outflow velocity, resulting in anterior movement of the anterior leaflet, causing further obstruction. Aortic insufficiency depends largely on afterload, which is less affected by hypovolemia, although significant hypovolemia may decrease systemic arterial pressure, decreasing the degree of aortic regurgitation. Mitral stenosis is unlikely to worsen from hypovolemia, though a decrease in atrial pressure may cause lower velocities across the stenotic valve (appearing as less severe). Diastolic dysfunction is unlikely to worsen with hypovolemia, but patients with significant diastolic dysfunction are prone to more exacerbated response to low or high filling conditions.

6. **Answer: C**

   Rationale: Stroke volume variation caused by changes in LV preload throughout the respiratory cycle is reflected in changes in the LVOT VTI, assuming that LVOT diameter stays constant. Less than 10% variation suggests that changes in preload do not have a significant effect on stroke volume (not volume responsive), while VTI variation greater than 14% suggests a volume-responsive state. Values in between 11% and 13% are considered "indeterminate" and have a lower predictive value.

7. **Answer: A**

   Rationale: Right ventricular failure can result in exacerbated stroke volume and VTI variation, falsely indicating a volume-responsive state. Distributive shock may result in significant stroke volume variation, but is also likely to be volume-responsive. Aortic stenosis is likely to underestimate stroke volume variation, due to a limited stroke volume from the stenotic lesion. Aortic regurgitation may result in increased pulse pressure and may decrease the percent change in stroke volume or pulse pressure variation, underestimating the likelihood for volume responsiveness.

8. **Answer: C**

   Rationale: The IVC diameter is > 2.1 cm, with < 50% collapse, suggesting a CVP 10–20 mmHg. An IVC diameter ≤ 2.1 cm with > 50% collapse suggests a CVP < 5 mmHg, while an IVC diameter > 2.1 cm with > 50% collapse suggests a CVP 5–10 mmHg. Dilated hepatic veins would suggest CVP > 20 mmHg.

9. **Answer: A**

   Rationale: Respirophasic IVC variation can be exacerbated by large tidal volumes (> 10 mL/kg ideal body weight) or increased respiratory effort, abdominal hypertension or IVC compression, pericardial effusion/tamponade, or restrictive pericarditis, which may underestimate CVP or falsely suggest a volume-responsive state. IVC variation may be decreased by low tidal volume ventilation or decreased respiratory effort, RV dysfunction or tricuspid regurgitation, or increased intrathoracic pressure (e.g., high PEEP), which may overestimate CVP or falsely suggest a nonresponsive state.

10. **Answer: C**

    Rationale: The image displays measurement of a LVOT VTI. The known LVOT diameter of 2 cm (radius 1 cm) suggests that this represents a stroke volume of 54 mL ($17.2 \times 3.14 \times 1^2$). With a heart rate of 100 bpm, this equates to a cardiac output of 5.4 liters per minute, which is unchanged from prior to the fluid bolus. Since there was no improvement in stroke volume with the additional preload, it is unlikely that additional intravascular volume will improve cardiac output (neither by 30 mL/kg fluid bolus nor passive leg raise maneuver). Although there may be a role for inotropy with dobutamine, this is not obvious from the information provided. Because the mean arterial pressure is still low, norepinephrine infusion would be the most appropriate next step.

Chapter 21

1. **Answer: C**

   Rationale: This patient has a left-sided pneumothorax, as evidenced by the lack of lung sliding and positive lung point. A lack of lung sliding is suggestive of pneumothorax, but the diagnosis should be confirmed by identifying a lung point prior to insertion of a chest tube.

If lung sliding is absent but a lung point cannot be identified (as in D), then additional radiographic imaging should be obtained. Absent lung sliding can also be caused by other disease such as bronchial obstruction, hypoventilation, and pleural inflammation/adhesions. A chest tube may be counterproductive in such cases.

B-lines can be a sign of pneumonia (if unilateral or heterogeneous) or pulmonary edema (if bilateral). However, 2 or less B-lines per rib space can be a normal finding due to interlobular septa. If the patient had more than 3 B-lines bilaterally, then treatment for pulmonary edema (answer A) would be appropriate.

A COPD exacerbation (answer B) would usually demonstrate a normal bilateral lung profile with lung sliding and A-lines, although the lung sliding may be decreased secondary to air trapping. The patient will likely have wheezing on examination and prolonged expiration.

2. **Answer: A**

   Rationale: This patient is having flash pulmonary edema from congestive heart failure. Cardiogenic pulmonary edema will usually be homogenous and therefore generate bilateral B-lines. Treatment is with preload reduction (nitroglycerin), afterload reduction (positive pressure ventilation), and diuresis if volume overloaded.

   A COPD exacerbation (answer B) would usually demonstrate a normal bilateral lung profile with lung sliding and A-lines, although the lung sliding may be decreased secondary to air trapping. The patient will likely have wheezing on examination and prolonged expiration.

   The patient has bilateral lung sliding, so a pneumothorax (answer C) is unlikely.

   Pneumonia (answer D) would not usually have bilateral homogenous B-lines. Pneumonia can have a number of heterogeneous profiles, including unilateral B-lines, consolidation (C-profile), or pleural effusion.

3. **Answer: B**

   Rationale: A-lines are a normal finding and represent a reverberation artifact between the pleural line and skin. They are present even in the case of pneumothorax, but will be absent and replaced by B-lines in the case of pulmonary edema.

   B-lines (answer A) are comet-tail artifacts created by reverberation between the pleural line and fluid-filled alveoli. Because the pleural and alveoli are in such close proximity, the individual reverberations are not easily visible. Instead the B-lines appears a solid beam deep to the pleural line.

   Shadowing (answer C) is a dark or blind area behind a solid object. For example, bones are solid and will reflect almost all ultrasound waves, not allowing any to pass deeper. Because of this, ultrasound is unable to visualize structures beyond solid bone.

   T-lines (answer D) are signs of subtle or intermittent lung sliding on M-Mode. The lung pulse could also be considered a type of T-line. Remember, any change in the pleural/artifact space that starts at the pleura must be from the lung. Motion artifact will also include the subcutaneous tissue.

4. **Answer: C**

   Rationale: If the anterior lungs are clear to ultrasound, as in this case, the next step is to look for DVT as a sign of likely PE. If the veins are clear, then the posterolateral lungs are evaluated. Effusion or consolidation in the posterolateral areas would likely indicate pneumonia, while clear lungs there as well would suggest COPD or asthma exacerbation.

   A COPD exacerbation (answer B) is possible in this case and would also show normal lungs on ultrasound, but the next step is to evaluate the veins for DVT.

   Pulmonary edema (answer A) would show bilateral B-lines.

   Pneumonia may be possible in this case if located in the posterolateral areas; however, the next step is to evaluate for DVT.

5. **Answer: C**

   Rationale: A-lines (lack of B-lines) are 90% specific for PAOP < 18 and 93% specific for PAOP < 13. The patient can likely tolerate additional fluid resuscitation. However, B-lines are not specific for elevated POAP, as B-lines may be caused by non-cardiogenic processes such as pneumonia and ARDS. Answers B and D are incorrect as the lung profile does not correlate with CVP, which is better evaluated with vena cava diameter and motion.

6. **Answer: D**

   Rationale: This patient has a right-sided pneumonia as evidenced by the unilateral B-lines and B-lines without lung sliding. Unilateral B-lines suggest a focal rather than homogenous edema process, which is more likely pneumonia. B-lines without lung sliding suggest an inflammatory process that has caused adhesion of the lung to the pleura. Remember, B-lines rule out pneumothorax even if there is no lung sliding.

   Cardiogenic pulmonary edema (answer A) will usually be homogeneous and therefore generate bilateral B-lines. Treatment is with preload reduction (nitroglycerin), afterload reduction (CPAP), and diuresis if volume overloaded.

   A pulmonary embolism (answer B) will generally have a normal lung appearance bilaterally. The pulmonary embolism is diagnosed by locating residual DVT in the veins after finding the normal anterior lungs. Rarely a PE can also have small pleural effusions or a C-profile.

   The patient has lung sliding on one side and B-lines on the other, so a pneumothorax (answer C) is unlikely.

7. **Answer: C**

   Rationale: While there are several different estimation equations that have been published, most will approximate a 2 cm interpleural distance to have roughly 400 mL of effusion. 1.5 cm is a commonly-used cutoff for safe thoracentesis, which may be both diagnostic and therapeutic. Traditional CXR has been shown to miss pleural effusions even up to 525 mL in volume, while ultrasound is 92% sensitive compared to CT.

8. **Answer: C**

   Rationale: This patient has obstructive atelectasis. Lung that is either consolidated or collapsed will have the appearance of liver or tissue. Air bronchograms are generated from the bronchioles within the collapsed lung. Normally, the bronchioles should grow and shrink with ventilation (dynamic air bronchograms). However, if the lobar bronchus is blocked (e.g., mucus plug), then there will be no air movement to the bronchioles past the obstruction. Bronchoscopy will likely be needed to remove the obstruction.

   While the patient may have pneumonia (answer A) as a cause of lobar collapse, the static air bronchograms suggest obstruction as the most acute cause of hypoxia.

   Increasing PEEP (answer B) has been shown to improve the ultrasound appearance of collapsed or edematous lung. However, it is unlikely to help with a mechanical obstruction.

   Pneumothorax (answer D) is wrong because the lung is able to be visualized directly, indicating effusion or consolidation rather than air.

9. **Answer: D**

   Rationale: Because lung ultrasound relies on certain artifacts, no special modes or filters should be used. Multiple probes have been used including linear, phased array, curvilinear, and microconvex.

10. **Answer: C**

    Rationale: Any signal originating from the lung must start at the pleura and deeper. Motion artifact from the patient or ultrasound probe will cover the entire height of the image, including both above and below the pleura.

Chapter 22

1. **Answer: D**

   Rationale: This patient has clinical findings of tamponade, including hypotension, tachycardia and elevated jugular venous pressure, with a pericardial effusion demonstrated on ultrasound. Point-of-care echocardiogram has been shown to be reliable in emergency situations with high degree of accuracy. One should be able to determine the difference between pericardial and pleural effusions with echo. Pericardial fluid will traverse the aorta anteriorly (along the posterior border of the ventricle), whereas a pleural effusion will not. Epinephrine may increase inotropy and contractility but would not address the tamponade. Phenylephrine may increase diastolic filling pressure, but also does not address the underlying pericardial effusion. There is no evidence of pleural effusion/hemothorax in the images provided.

2. **Answer: B**

   Rationale: This patient has a pneumothorax with tension physiology, as suggested by the developing hypotension and jugular venous distention. Pneumothorax would be expected to produce a lack of lung sliding in the area where the pleural layers are separated. A lung point may be visible at the transition between the pneumothorax and normal pleural apposition, but in the case of a large pneumothorax (as in this case), there will not be a visible transition point, thus no lung point. The tension physiology would also be expected to demonstrate a dysfunctional right ventricle.

3. **Answer: A**

   Rationale: This patient has a presentation consistent with severe sepsis. After initial volume resuscitation of 30 mL/kg, she shows little hemodynamic improvement, and worsening respiratory function. The ultrasound evaluation of her IVC shows a large IVC without significant respiratory variation, suggesting that hypovolemia is likely not the predominant derangement, and further volume resuscitation is unlikely to improve her cardiac output. Comparing a VTI measurement before and after a volume bolus may provide more precise evaluation of the change in stroke volume elicited from a volume bolus, but because there is no "before" measurement, an isolated VTI measurement is difficult to interpret. Radiographic evaluation of the chest may be appropriate as a part of her evaluation, but is not the appropriate next step while she remains hypotensive with evidence of hypoperfusion, and there is enough information to suggest a distributive component of her shock. Norepinephrine to increase her mean arterial pressure is the preferred intervention from the options listed.

4. **Answer: C**

   Rationale: The ultrasound image demonstrates a dilated right ventricle (left side of the image), which is larger than the left ventricle in this case. In the apical four-chamber view, a normal RV to LV ratio is < 0.6. A ratio of 0.6–1 is moderate dilation, and a ratio ≥ 1 is severe RV dilation. Although pneumonia and sepsis may be consistent with his initial presentation, RV dilation would not be an expected finding. Similarly, hypovolemia would be expected to show underfilled ventricles, and his blood pressure would not be likely to decrease after volume repletion. RV dysfunction in the setting of recent orthopedic surgery raises the suspicion for massive pulmonary embolism as the cause for his shock.

5. **Answer: D**

   Rationale: The patient presents in cardiac arrest with a wide-complex (shockable) rhythm. Resuscitation efforts should be focused on supporting circulation (chest compressions) and optimizing defibrillation attempts. If an alternative reversible cause for arrest is suspected (e.g., tension pneumothorax), it is reasonable to perform evaluation without compromising concurrent with resuscitation attempts. Most commonly, sources of arrest apparent with ultrasound would not result in a wide-complex tachycardia and would more likely result in PEA.

6. **Answer: C**

   Rationale: This patient has acute pulmonary edema and cardiogenic shock as the result of mitral regurgitation (MR). Acute MR may occur as the result of myocardial ischemia (functional) or a structural defect (e.g., papillary muscle rupture following MI). In this case, the posterior leaflet has prolapsed, causing an anteriorly directed mitral regurgitant jet. Clinical instability in the setting of acute MR should be considered a surgical emergency, although some medical interventions may help temporize the situation. Positive pressure ventilation, afterload reduction (e.g., nitroglycerin infusion), and inotropy/chronotropy (e.g., dobutamine) may all improve the regurgitant flow, but may be challenging in the setting of hypotension. Diuresis may also benefit the pulmonary edema but will not have an immediate benefit. Surgical repair should be obtained as soon as possible.

7. **Answer: A**

   Rationale: This patient has a presentation concerning for infective endocarditis. Blood cultures should be drawn, and antibiotics started as soon as possible. Evaluation of the IVC may facilitate preload assessment, but in this image, the aorta is the hypoechoic structure visualized, and the IVC is not visible. The IVC may be difficult to visualize in a patient with significant hypovolemia, so it is important to ensure that it is not confused with the aorta, which may be larger and lack collapsibility. Visualization of the IVC should be confirmed by following its entry into the right atrium and observing the confluence of the hepatic veins. Empirical fluid administration may be reasonable, but an accurate ultrasound assessment would be preferred to help guide management, since it is immediately available.

8. **Answer: A**

   Rationale: The patient has cardiogenic shock with acute pulmonary edema, demonstrated by point-of-care assessment. She has a dilated cardiomyopathy, with a large end-diastolic diameter, which can be identified by the EKG tracing on the lower left part of the image. In addition, the ventricular walls are very thin, suggesting some chronic development, which would be consistent with a peripartum cardiomyopathy. Acute septic physiology would be expected to have low ventricular filling volumes. Acute pulmonary embolism (including amniotic fluid embolism) would be expected to have dilated right ventricle and underfilled left ventricle. Hypocalcemia is an important cause of hypotension after blood product transfusion but would not be expected to cause a dilated cardiomyopathy. While mechanical circulatory support may be necessary for cardiogenic shock, inotropic support and expert consultation would be the next step.

9. **Answer: B**

   Rationale: A FAST exam is not sensitive for a small volume of intraperitoneal blood. While, initially, his hypotension was not attributable to a large volume of peritoneal blood, ongoing bleeding may cause this to develop. For this reason, repeated exams are necessary to evaluate for ongoing bleeding, especially in the setting of changing clinical status. CT to evaluate for additional causes of bleeding (e.g., retroperitoneal hemorrhage) may be appropriate, if the patient is stable, but would not be the next step. Exploratory laparotomy would not be indicated if the repeat FAST exam was negative, as the source of hypotension would not be attributed to hemoperitoneum, and alternative causes should be addressed. Serial hemoglobin evaluation may be an appropriate part of his evaluation but would not be the next step.

10. **Answer: B**

    Rationale: Extensive abdominal surgical procedures are associated with a large volume of insensible losses, which can lead to hypovolemia. The low BP, tachycardia, and low urine output may be a consequence of low intravascular volume. Giving a small intravascular bolus and assessing its effect is a reasonable strategy in this situation. This can be done with clinical signs of perfusion (e.g., mental status, urine output), or more directly as measures of hemodynamics, like changes in stroke volume (as measured by change in VTI). Because of her history of significant heart failure, a large volume bolus may cause excess intravascular volume, leading to deleterious effects (e.g., pulmonary edema). Her pain should certainly be addressed, but analgesia would not address the hypotension or hypoperfusion suggested by her low urine output. Inotropic support (e.g., dobutamine) may be indicated if her systolic dysfunction is significant enough, but that is not evident by the information provided.

Chapter 23

1. **Answer: C**

   Rationale: The image shows color Doppler evaluation of the radial artery. However, no Doppler flow is detected. This can be a consequence of an occluded artery; however, in this case, there is also no flow seen in the nearby veins, suggesting that the lack of flow may be a consequence of flow perpendicular to the angle of insonation. The Doppler shift observed is relative to the cosine of the angle of incidence; thus, there is no Doppler shift if the wave is perpendicular to the direction of flow (cos 90° = 0), as in this case. By angling the probe to be more aligned with the direction of flow, a more proper assessment can be made.

2. **Answer: C**

   Rationale: The cross-sectional appearance of a portion of the needle within the vessel does not provide information about the location of the tip of the needle, as any cross section will appear similar. Continuous (dynamic) tracking of the needle tip entering the plane, then advancing the imaging plane, and then watching the needle tip enter the plane in a step-wise fashion can facilitate visualization. Alternatively, a long-axis view may help identify the needle trajectory. Advancing the needle without localizing the needle tip risks injuring surrounding structures, and it is possible that the needle has already passed through the backwall of the vessel. While it may be reasonable to withdraw the needle and advance again, it would be preferred to localize the needle tip without first manipulating it further, to minimize risk and discomfort to the patient from multiple attempts. Agitating the needle is not an effective means to localize the needle tip, as, again, any cross section of the needle will move adjacent tissues in the same fashion, and the movement risks injuring adjacent structures.

3. **Answer: D**

   Rationale: In general, larger central venous catheters, and those with more lumens have a higher risk for infections. Subclavian central venous catheters have the lowest risk for infection (1.5–4%) and thrombosis (1.2–1.9%). Internal jugular catheters have an infection rate of 4–8% and a thrombosis rate of 7.6%. The femoral site has the highest incidence of both infection and thrombosis at 19.8% and 21.5%, respectively.

4. **Answer: A**

   Rationale: The pulmonary artery catheter tip can be positioned in the main pulmonary artery or proximal right pulmonary artery in the ascending aorta SAX view. A midesophageal modified bicaval tricuspid valve view or a midesophageal RV inflow-out view may be useful for manipulations of the catheter during placement, but do not provide visualize the final position of the catheter tip. Ultrasound guidance has not been shown to improve time to placement, although it may be useful in many situations.

5. **Answer: D**

   Rationale: A represents the superficial femoral artery, lateral to the venous structures. B represents the deep femoral artery. Both arteries have thicker-appearing vascular walls. The remaining structures represent the confluence of the common femoral vein (C) and the saphenous vein (D), which is suspicious for some thrombosis. Likely, more proximally, the common femoral vein will be adjacent to the arterial structures, and more easily accessed without risking arterial puncture. In addition, the vein should be investigated with compression and/or Doppler to evaluate for thrombosis prior to cannulation.

Index

T. M. Maus, C. R. Tainter (eds.), *Essential Echocardiography*,
https://doi.org/10.1007/978-3-030-84349-6

MIX
Papier aus verantwortungsvollen Quellen
Paper from responsible sources
FSC® C105338

If you have any concerns about our products,
you can contact us on
ProductSafety@springernature.com

In case Publisher is established outside the EU,
the EU authorized representative is:
Springer Nature Customer Service Center GmbH
Europaplatz 3, 69115 Heidelberg, Germany

Printed by Libri Plureos GmbH
in Hamburg, Germany